Practical Clinical Oncology

Second Edition

Practical Clinical Oncology

Second Edition

Edited by

Louise Hanna
Consultant Clinical Oncologist, Department of Oncology, Velindre Cancer Centre, Cardiff, UK

Tom Crosby
Consultant Clinical Oncologist, Department of Oncology, Velindre Cancer Centre, Cardiff, UK

Fergus Macbeth
Associate Director of the Wales Cancer Trials Unit, Cardiff University, Cardiff, UK

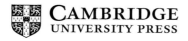

CAMBRIDGE
UNIVERSITY PRESS

CAMBRIDGE
UNIVERSITY PRESS

University Printing House, Cambridge CB2 8BS, United Kingdom

Cambridge University Press is part of the University of Cambridge.

It furthers the University's mission by disseminating knowledge in the pursuit of education, learning and research at the highest international levels of excellence.

www.cambridge.org
Information on this title: www.cambridge.org/9781107683624

© Cambridge University Press (2008) 2015

First published 2008
Second edition 2015
3rd printing 2016

Printed in the United Kingdom by TJ International Ltd. Padstow Cornwall

A catalogue record for this publication is available from the British Library

Library of Congress Cataloguing in Publication data
Practical clinical oncology / edited by Louise Hanna, Tom Crosby, Fergus
Macbeth. – Second edition.
    p. ; cm.
Includes bibliographical references and index.
ISBN 978-1-107-68362-4 (paperback)
I. Hanna, Louise, editor.   II. Crosby, Tom, editor.   III. Macbeth, Fergus, editor.
[DNLM: 1. Neoplasms–therapy.   2. Neoplasms–diagnosis. QZ 266]
RC261
616.99'4–dc23   2015022581

ISBN 978-1-107-68362-4 Paperback

Every effort has been made in preparing this book to provide accurate and up-to-date information which is in accord with accepted standards and practice at the time of publication. Although case histories are drawn from actual cases, every effort has been made to disguise the identities of the individuals involved. Nevertheless, the authors, editors and publishers can make no warranties that the information contained herein is totally free from error, not least because clinical standards are constantly changing through research and regulation. The authors, editors and publishers therefore disclaim all liability for direct or consequential damages resulting from the use of material contained in this book. Readers are strongly advised to pay careful attention to information provided by the manufacturer of any drugs or equipment that they plan to use.

Table of contents

List of contributors

Jacinta Abraham
Consultant Clinical Oncologist, Velindre Cancer Centre, Velindre Hospital, Cardiff, UK

Richard Adams
Reader and Honorary Consultant in Clinical Oncology, Cardiff University and Consultant Clinical Oncologist, Velindre Cancer Centre, Velindre Hospital, Cardiff, UK

Seema Safia Arif
Consultant Clinical Oncologist, Velindre Cancer Centre, Velindre Hospital, Cardiff, UK

Jim Barber
Consultant Clinical Oncologist, Velindre Cancer Centre, Velindre Hospital, Cardiff, UK

Alison Brewster
Consultant Clinical Oncologist, Velindre Cancer Centre, Velindre Hospital, Cardiff, UK

Mick Button
Consultant Clinical Oncologist, Velindre Cancer Centre, Velindre Hospital, Cardiff, UK

Samantha Cox
Specialty Registrar in Clinical Oncology, Velindre Cancer Centre, Velindre Hospital, Cardiff, UK

Tom Crosby
Consultant Clinical Oncologist, Velindre Cancer Centre, Velindre Hospital, Cardiff, UK

Rhian Sian Davies
Specialty Registrar in Clinical Oncology, Velindre Cancer Centre, Velindre Hospital, Cardiff, UK

Sean Elyan
Consultant Clinical Oncologist, Cheltenham General Hospital, Cheltenham, UK

Mererid Evans
Consultant Clinical Oncologist, Velindre Cancer Centre, Velindre Hospital, Cardiff, UK

Eve Gallop-Evans
Consultant Clinical Oncologist, Velindre Cancer Centre, Velindre Hospital, Cardiff, UK

Sarah Gwynne
Consultant Clinical Oncologist, South West Wales Cancer Centre, Singleton Hospital, Swansea, UK

Louise Hanna
Consultant Clinical Oncologist, Velindre Cancer Centre, Velindre Hospital, Cardiff, UK

Emma Harrett
Specialty Registrar in Clinical Oncology, Velindre Cancer Centre, Velindre Hospital, Cardiff, UK

Robert Hills
Reader in Translational Statistics, Department of Haematology, Cardiff University, Cardiff, UK

Emma Hudson
Consultant Clinical Oncologist, Velindre Cancer Centre, Velindre Hospital, Cardiff, UK

Najmus Sahar Iqbal
Specialty Registrar in Clinical Oncology, Velindre Cancer Centre, Velindre Hospital, Cardiff, UK

Nayyer Iqbal
Associate Professor of Medicine, Saskatoon Cancer Centre, University Of Saskatchewan, Canada

Rashmi Jadon
Advanced Radiotherapy Research Fellow, Velindre Cancer Centre, Velindre Hospital, Cardiff, UK

Rachel Jones
Consultant Medical Oncologist, Velindre Cancer Centre, Velindre Hospital, Cardiff, UK

Satish Kumar
Consultant Medical Oncologist, Velindre Cancer Centre, Velindre Hospital, Cardiff, UK

Andrew Lansdown
Clinical Research Fellow, Institute of Molecular and Experimental Medicine, Cardiff University School of Medicine, Cardiff, UK

Jason Lester
Consultant Clinical Oncologist, Velindre Cancer Centre, Velindre Hospital, Cardiff, UK

Fergus Macbeth
Associate Director, Wales Cancer Trials Unit, Cardiff University, Cardiff, UK

Usman Malik
Principal Pharmacist, Clinical Services, Velindre Cancer Centre, Velindre Hospital, Cardiff, UK

Julie Martin
Consultant Dermatologist, Royal Glamorgan Hospital, Mid Glamorgan, UK

Anthony Millin
Medical Physicist, Velindre Cancer Centre, Velindre Hospital, Cardiff, UK

Sankha Suvra Mitra
Consultant Clinical Oncologist, The Sussex Cancer Centre, Royal Sussex County Hospital, Brighton and Sussex University Hospitals NHS Trust, Brighton, UK

Carys Morgan
Consultant Clinical Oncologist, Velindre Cancer Centre, Velindre Hospital, Cardiff, UK

Laura Moss
Consultant Clinical Oncologist, Velindre Cancer Centre, Velindre Hospital, Cardiff, UK

Somnath Mukherjee
Senior Clinical Researcher, Consultant Clinical Oncologist, CRUK/MRC Oxford Institute For Radiation Oncology, University of Oxford, Churchill Hospital, Oxford Cancer Centre, Oxford, UK

Simon Noble
Reader and Honorary Consultant in Palliative Care, Royal Gwent Hospital, Newport, UK

Waheeda Owadally
Consultant Clinical Oncologist, Bristol Haematology and Oncology Centre, University Hospitals Bristol, Bristol, UK

Nachi Palaniappan
Consultant Clinical Oncologist, Velindre Cancer Centre, Velindre Hospital, Cardiff, UK

Kate Parker
Consultant Clinical Oncologist, South West Wales Cancer Centre, Singleton Hospital, Swansea, UK

Catherine Pembroke
Specialty Registrar in Clinical Oncology, Velindre Cancer Centre, Velindre Hospital, Cardiff, UK

James Powell
Consultant Clinical Oncologist, Velindre Cancer Centre, Velindre Hospital, Cardiff, UK

Delia Pudney
Consultant Clinical Oncologist, South West Wales Cancer Centre, Singleton Hospital, Swansea, UK

Amy Quinton
Specialty Registrar in Medical Oncology, South West Wales Cancer Centre, Singleton Hospital, Swansea, UK

Aled Rees
Reader and Consultant Endocrinologist, Centre For Endocrine and Diabetes Sciences, School of Medicine, Cardiff University, Cardiff, UK

Philip Savage
Consultant Medical Oncologist, BC Cancer Agency, Victoria, BC, Canada

Siwan Seaman
Consultant in Palliative Medicine, Marie Curie Hospice Cardiff and the Vale, Penarth, UK

Paul Shaw
Consultant Clinical Oncologist and Honorary Senior Lecturer, School of Biosciences, Cardiff University, Cardiff, UK

John Staffurth
Reader in Oncology, Cardiff University, Consultant Clinical Oncologist, Velindre Cancer Centre, Velindre Hospital, Cardiff, UK

Loretta Sweeney
Specialty Registrar in Clinical Oncology, Velindre
Cancer Centre, Velindre Hospital, Cardiff, UK

Jacob Tanguay
Consultant Clinical Oncologist, Velindre Cancer
Centre, Velindre Hospital, Cardiff, UK

Betsan Mai Thomas
Specialty Registrar in Clinical Oncology, Velindre
Cancer Centre, Velindre Hospital, Cardiff, UK

Hywel Thomas
Consultant Histopathologist, University Hospital of
Wales, Cardiff, UK

Owen Tilsley
Consultant Clinical Oncologist, Velindre Cancer
Centre, Velindre Hospital, Cardiff, UK

Andrew Tyler
Medical Physicist, Velindre Cancer Centre, Velindre
Hospital, Cardiff, UK

John Wagstaff
Professor, Swansea University, Consultant Medical
Oncologist, Singleton Hospital, Swansea, UK

Preface to the first edition

This book is intended primarily for trainees in clinical oncology, but members of other professions such as medical oncology, surgery, palliative care, nursing and radiography will also find it useful. The book started life as a set of lecture notes from the Cardiff Annual FRCR Part II course, but has since grown to include more topics than could possibly be covered during the three days of that course. Our approach in producing this volume has been to focus on practical suggestions appropriate to day-to-day decision making during the treatment of oncology patients. We are very grateful to our colleagues from Velindre and elsewhere, who are listed on page xi, for reviewing specific chapters and ensuring that the advice contained within is as widely applicable as possible.

The first seven chapters cover 'generic' topics which provide background information on cancer treatments. These are chemotherapy, biological and hormonal treatments, radiotherapy planning, research, emergencies and palliative care. The chapters which follow each focus on a tumour site or tumour type. In this latter group, the chapter layout is fairly consistent to help the reader navigate through the book. Thus, each chapter begins with background information on tumour types, anatomy, incidence, epidemiology, risk factors and aetiology. Next there are sections on pathology, routes of spread and, where appropriate, screening. These are followed by clinical sections on presentation, investigations, treatment and prognosis. Most of the chapters also discuss areas of current interest and clinical trials, reflecting the rapidly changing nature of clinical oncology where many areas of practice are open to debate. Where references are given, we have tried as much as possible to include those key publications which have influenced clinical practice. Towards the end of the book there is a series of 'single best answer' multiple choice questions, which will give the reader the opportunity to test their knowledge.

In a book of this length, it is not possible to provide as much of the subject as would be found, for example, in the larger multivolume oncology textbooks. Nevertheless, an attempt has been made to give an overview of clinical oncology practice at the present time, which we hope will be of interest and benefit to trainees.

The idea for writing this book came about several years ago when two of the editors (TC and LH) were studying for their FRCR part II examination. They have since become consultants in Velindre Hospital with FM and all three now teach on the Cardiff Annual FRCR part II course.

Preface to the second edition

It is now seven years since the first edition of this book was published and during that time there have been major changes in the non-surgical management of patients with cancer with new systemic treatments and new radiation technology becoming more widely available. We have reflected these changes by thoroughly updating all the topics. The aim of the book remains the same – to provide all health professionals training in cancer-related specialties with succinct, up-to-date summaries of current practice.

As before, the book starts with introductory chapters covering generic topics such as chemotherapy, biological and hormone treatments, radiotherapy planning, research and palliative care. We have added new generic chapters on pathology and advanced external beam radiotherapy to reflect recent developments in these areas. The chapters on oncological emergencies and cancer of unknown primary have been placed together to recognise the developing concept of acute oncology. After the generic topics, the chapters each address the management of specific tumour types. The topics on the use of radiotherapy in benign diseases have been incorporated within these chapters. As with all textbooks of this type, there is a limit to the amount of detailed information that can be included and, in particular, topics in which there is rapid change or active research may become dated quite quickly. We have asked the authors to flag up important current clinical trials and potential new developments. There is a series of multiple choice questions at the end of the book. For readers who wish to test their knowledge, further multiple choice questions set at the level of the Final FRCR examination can be found in Oncopaedia (www.oncopaedia.com/ accessed February 2015).*

Although the book is still firmly rooted in the revision course run at Velindre Hospital in Cardiff for trainees taking the Final FRCR examination and reflecting contemporary clinical practice in the UK, we hope that it will still be informative for those from other specialties and from other countries. We hope you will enjoy reading and learning from this new edition.

* Please note that this website is recommended by the Editors but is not formally endorsed by Cambridge University Press.

Acknowledgements

We are very grateful to the staff of Cambridge University Press, particularly Jane Seakins, Nisha Doshi and Sarah Payne, together with Jenny Slater of Out of House Publishing. James Williams helped prepare some of the figures, together with Owain Woodley of the Medical Physics Department, Velindre Cancer Centre, who also prepared the cover illustration. Alison Brewster provided the paragraphs on the treatment of benign conditions. Finally, we thank our families for their unending support during the preparation of this book.

Abbreviations

General

1D	1-dimensional
2D	2-dimensional
3D	3-dimensional
34βE12	mouse monoclonal antibody to high molecular weight cytokeratin
4D	4-dimensional
5AC	MUC subtypes A and C
5-ALA	5-aminolevulinic acid
5-FU	5-fluorouracil
5-HIAA	5-hydroxy-indoleacetic acid
5-HT3	5-hydroxy-tryptamine 3
5YS	five-year survival
αFP	alpha feto-protein
βhCG	beta human chorionic gonadotrophin
AAPM	American Association of Physicists in Medicine
ABC	activated B-cell-like; advanced bladder cancer
ABCSG	Austrian Breast and Colorectal Cancer Study Group
ABL	ABL proto-oncogene, non-receptor tyrosine kinase
ABPI	accelerated partial-breast irradiation
ACA	adenocarcinoma
ACE	anticholinesterase
ACh	acetylcholine
ACP	advanced care planning
ACTH	Adrenocorticotrophic hormone
ADC	apparent diffusion coefficient
ADH	antidiuretic hormone
ADI-PEG20	arginine deiminase formulated with polyethylene glycol
ADT	androgen deprivation therapy
AF	activating function
AFIP	American Forces Institute of Pathology
AFP	alpha feto-protein
AFX	atypical fibroxanthoma
AGES	age, grade, extent, size
AGITG	Australasian GastroIntestinal Tumour Group
AHT	adjuvant hormone therapy
AI	aromatase inhibitor
AIDS	aquired immune deficiency syndrome
AIN	anal intraepithelial neoplasia
AJCC	American Joint Committee on Cancer
AKT	thymoma viral proto-oncogene
ALK	anaplastic lymphoma kinase
ALL	acute lymphoblastic leukaemia
ALM	acral lentiginous melanoma
ALND	axillary lymph node dissection
AMES	age, metastases, extent, size
AML	acute myeloid leukaemia

AMP	adenosine monophosphate		BCIRG	Breast Cancer International Research Group
ANC	absolute neutrophil count		BCL	B-cell CLL/lymphoma
ANO1	anoctamin 1, calcium-activated chloride channel		BCNU	bis-chloroethylnitrosurea; carmustine
APBI	accelerated partial breast irradiation		BCR	breakpoint cluster region
A-P	anterior–posterior		BCS	breast-conserving surgery
AP-1	activator protein-1		BCSH	British Committee for Standards in Haematology
ApC	antigen-presenting cell		BCT	breast conservation therapy
APC	*adenomatosis polyposis coli*		b.d.	bis in die (twice a day)
AP/PA	anterior–posterior/posterior–anterior 'parallel-opposed'		BED	biologically effective dose
APR	abdominoperineal resection		Ber-EP4	antibody against EpCAM; epithelial cell adhesion molecule
APUD	amine precursor uptake and decarboxylation		BEV	beam's eye view
AR	androgen receptor		BGND	bilateral groin node dissection
ARE	androgen response element		BIG	Breast International Group
ARSAC	Administration of Radioactive Substances Advisory Committee		BIR	British Institute of Radiology
			BMD	bone mineral density
ASC	active symptom control		bNED	biochemical disease-free survival
ASCO	American Society of Clinical Oncology		BNLI	British National Lymphoma Investigation
ASH	American Society of Hematology			
ATAC	Arimidex, Tamoxifen, Alone or in Combination		BOADICA	Breast and Ovarian Analysis of Disease Incidence and Carrier Estimation Algorithm
ATD	amino-terminal domain			
ATLAS	Adjuvant Tamoxifen: Longer Against Shorter		BP	blood pressure
			bpm	beats per minute
ATP	adenosine triphosphate		BR	borderline resectable
AUC	area under curve		BRAF	B-Raf proto-oncogene, serine/threonine kinase
AVM	arteriovenous malformation			
B12	vitamin B12		BRCA	breast cancer gene
BAP1	BRCA-associated protein		BSA	body surface area
BC	British Columbia		BSC	best supportive care
BCC	basal cell carcinoma		BSCC	British Society for Clinical Cytology
BCG	bacillus Calmette–Guérin		BSO	bilateral salpingo-oophorectomy
			BTA	British Thyroid Association

BTK	Bruton's tyrosine kinase	CML	chronic myelocytic leukaemia
BTOG	British Thoracic Oncology Group	CNS	central nervous system; Clinical Nurse Specialist
BTS	British Thoracic Society	COG	Children's Oncology Group of North America
CA	cancer antigen		
CAIX	carbonic anhydrase IX	COMS	Collaborative Melanoma Study
CALGB	Cancer and Leukaemia Group B	CONSORT	Consolidated Standards of Reporting Trials
CBCT	cone beam CT		
CD	cluster of differentiation	COPD	chronic obstructive pulmonary disease
CD117	KIT; v-kit Hardy–Zuckerman 4 feline sarcoma viral oncogene homolog	CR	complete response
CDCA1	cell division cycle associated 1	CRAF	C-Raf proto-oncogene, serine/threonine kinase: approved gene symbol = RAF1; approved gene name = Raf-1 proto-oncogene, serine/threonine kinase
CDH1	cadherin 1		
CDK	cyclin-dependent kinase		
CDKN2A	cyclin-dependent kinase inhibitor 2A		
CDX	caudal-type homeobox	CRH	corticotropin-releasing hormone
CE	conversion electron	CRC	colorectal cancer
CEA	carcino-embryonic antigen	CRM	circumferential resection margin
CG	Clinical Guideline	CRMPC	castration-resistant metastatic prostate cancer
CgA	chromogranin A		
CFS	colostomy-free survival	CRP	c-reactive protein
CHART	continuous hyperfractionated accelerated radiotherapy	CRPC	castrate-refractory prostate cancer
		CRT	chemoradiotherapy
CI	confidence interval	CRT-S	chemoradiation followed by surgery
CIN	cervical intraepithelial neoplasia	CRUK	Cancer Research UK
CIS	carcinoma *in situ*	CSF	cerebrospinal fluid
CK	cytokeratin	CSS	cause-specific survival
C-Kit	KIT; v-kit Hardy–Zuckerman 4 feline sarcoma viral oncogene homolog	cT	clinical tumour stage
		ct	calcitonin
CLA	common leukocyte antigen	CT	computed tomography
CLIPi	Cutaneous Lymphoma International Prognostic Index	CTAG	cancer/testis antigen
		CTCAE	common toxicity criteria
CLL	chronic lymphocytic leukaemia	CTCL	cutaneous T-cell lymphoma
CM	complete mole	Ct DT	calcitonin doubling time
c-Met	MET; MET proto-oncogene, receptor tyrosine kinase		

CTLA4	cytotoxic T lymphocyte-associated protein 4	DOPA	dihydroxyphenylalanine
CTNNB1	catenin (cadherin-associated protein), beta 1, 88 kDa	DOTA	1,4,7,10-tetraazacyclododecane-1,4,7,10-tetraacetic acid
CTV	clinical target volume	DOTANOC	DOTA-1-NaI-octreotide
CTZ	chemoreceptor trigger zone	DOTATATE	DOTA-octreotate
CUP	carcinoma of unknown primary	DOTATOC	DOTA-octreotide
CVP	central venous pressure	DPC4	SMAD4; SMAD family member 4
CX	characteristic X-ray photon	DRE	digital rectal examination
CXR	chest X-ray	DRR	digitally reconstructed radiograph
CYP	cytochrome P450	DSM	disease-specific mortality
D2	dopamine D2	DT	doubling time
DAB	3,3-di-aminobenzidine tetra hydrochloride	DTC	differentiated thyroid cancer
DAHANCA	Danish Head and Neck Cancer	DVH	dose–volume histogram
DCC	deleted in colon cancer	DW	diffusion-weighted
DCE	dynamic contrast enhancement	EBCTCG	Early Breast Cancer Trialists Collaborative Group
DCIS	ductal carcinoma *in situ*	EBRT	external beam radiotherapy
dCRT	definitive chemoradiation	EBUS	endobronchial ultrasound
DDT	dichloro-diphenyl-trichloroethane	EBV	Epstein–Barr virus
DES	diethylstilboestrol	ECG	electrocardiogram
DEPDC1	DEP domain containing 1	ECOG	Eastern Cooperative Oncology Group
DFS	disease-free survival	ECS	extracapsular spread
DHA	dihydroxyandrostenedione	EDTA	ethylenediaminetetraacetic acid
DHT	5α dihydrotestosterone	eGFR	estimated glomerulofiltration rate
DLBCL	diffuse large B-cell lymphoma	EGFR	epidermal growth factor receptor
DM	diabetes mellitus	EIC	extensive intraductal component
d_{max}	depth of maximum dose	ELND	elective lymph node dissection
DMC	Data Monitoring Committee	EM	electron microscopy
DMSA	dimercapto succinic acid	EMA	epithelial membrane antigen
DMSO	dimethyl sulfoxide	eMC	electronic Medicines Compendium
DNA	deoxyribonucleic acid	EMR	endoscopic mucosal resection
DOG1	ANO1; anoctamin 1, calcium-activated chloride channel	EMP	extramedullary plasmacytoma

ENETS	European Neuroendocrine Tumor Society
ENT	ear nose and throat
EORTC	European Organisation for Research and Treatment of Cancer
EPI	electronic portal imaging
EPIC	European Prospective Investigation into Cancer and Nutrition
EPID	electronic portal imaging device
EPO	erythropoietin
EPP	extrapleural pneumonectomy
EPSE	extrapyramidal side effects
EQD2	equivalent dose at 2 Gy
ER	oestrogen receptor
ERBB1	erb-b2 receptor tyrosine kinase 1: EGFR; epidermal growth factor receptor
ERBB2	erb-b2 receptor tyrosine kinase 2
ERBB3	erb-b2 receptor tyrosine kinase 3
ERBB4	erb-b2 receptor tyrosine kinase 4
ERCP	endoscopic retrograde cholangiopancreatogram
ERE	oestrogen response element
ERG	v-ets avian erythroblastosis virus E26 oncogene homolog
ESA	Employment and Support Allowance
ESMO	European Society for Medical Oncology
ESPAC	European Study Group for Pancreatic Cancer
ESR	erythocyte sedimentation rate
ESTRO	European Society for Therapeutic Radiology and Oncology
EU	European Union
EUA	examination under anaesthetic
EURAMOS	European and American Osteosarcoma Study Group
EUS	endoscopic ultrasound
EWS	EWSR1; Ewing sarcoma breakpoint region 1
FA	folinic acid
FAK	focal adhesion kinase
FAP	familial adenomatous polyposis
FBC	full blood count
Fc	constant region
FDA	Food and Drug Administration
FDG	fluorodeoxyglucose
FEV-1	forced expiratory volume in 1 second
FGF	fibroblast growth factor
FGFR	fibroblast growth factor receptor
FIGO	Fédération Internationale de Gynécologie et d'Obstétrique
FISH	fluorescent *in situ* hybridisation
FL	follicular lymphoma
FLI1	Friend leukaemia virus integration 1
FLIPI	Follicular Lymphoma International Prognostic Index
FLT3	fms-related tyrosine kinase 3
fms	peptide deformylase
FNA	fine-needle aspiration
FNAC	fine-needle aspiration cytology
FOB	faecal occult blood
FRCR	Fellow of the Royal College of Radiologists
FSH	follicle-stimulating hormone
FT4	free T4
FTC	follicular thyroid carcinoma
FU	follow-up
GBq	giga-Becquerel

GCB	germinal centre B cell-like	H2	histamine H2
G-CSF	granulocyte colony-stimulating factor	H_2O_2	hydrogen peroxide
		HAART	highly active anti-retroviral therapy
GCP	good clinical practice	HAL	hexyl ester hexaminolevulinate
GCS	Glasgow coma score	HBF	heterotopic bone formation
GCT	germ cell tumour	HBV	hepatitis B virus
GD2	ganglioside G2	HCC	hepatocellular carcinoma
GEC-ESTRO	Groupe Européen de Curiethérapie and European Society for Radiotherapy and Oncology	hCG	human chorionic gonadotrophin
		HCV	hepatitis C virus
GELA	Groupe d'Etude des Lymphomes de l'Adulte	HDC	high dose chemotherapy
		HDC/ASCT	high dose chemotherapy with autologous stem cell transplant
GFR	glomerular filtration rate	HDCT	high dose chemotherapy
GHSG	German Hodgkin Study Group	HDR	high dose rate
GI	gastrointestinal	HDU	high dependency unit
GINET	GI-related neuroendocrine tumours	H+E	haematoxylin and eosin
GIST	gastrointestinal stromal tumour	HER	human epidermal growth factor receptor
GLI	GLI family zinc finger 1	HER1	human epidermal growth factor receptor 1: EGFR; epidermal growth factor receptor
GM-CSF	granulocyte–macrophage colony-stimulating factor		
GnRH	gonadotrophin-releasing hormone	HER2	human epidermal growth factor receptor 2: ERBB2; erb-b2 receptor tyrosine kinase 2
GO	gastro-oesophageal		
GOG	Gynaecologic Oncology Group	HER3	human epidermal growth factor receptor 3: ERBB3; erb-b2 receptor tyrosine kinase 3
GOJ	gastro-oesophageal junction		
GORD	gastro-oesophageal reflux disease		
GP	general practitioner	HER4	human epidermal growth factor receptor 4: ERBB4; erb-b2 receptor tyrosine kinase 4
GPA	granulomatosis with polyangiitis (Wegener's granulomatosis)		
GSTM1	glutathione *S*-transferase mu 1	HES	hospital episode statistics
GTT	gestational trophoblast tumour	HGF	hepatocyte growth factor
GTV	gross tumour volume	HGFR	hepatocyte growth factor receptor
GU	genitourinary	HGG	high grade glioma
Gy	Gray	HH	hedgehog
GYN	gynaecological	HHV	human herpesvirus

HIFU	high intensity focussed ultrasound		ICORG	Irish Clinical Oncology Research Group
HIR	high intermediate risk		ICP	intracranial pressure
HIV	human immunodeficiency virus		ICRU	International Commission on Radiation Units and Measurements
HL	Hodgkin lymphoma		IELSG	International Extranodal Lymphoma Study Group
HMB	human melanoma black			
HNPCC	hereditary non-polyposis colorectal cancer		IFN	interferon
HNSCC	head and neck squamous cell carcinoma		IFNAR	interferon (alpha and beta) receptor
hpf	high-powered field		IFNGR	interferon gamma receptor
HPOA	hypertrophic pulmonary osteo-arthropathy		IFRT	involved-field radiotherapy
			Ig	immunoglobulin
HPV	human papilloma virus		IGBT	image-guided brachytherapy
HR	hazard ratio		IGCCCG	International Germ Cell Consensus Collaborative Group
HR-CTV	high-risk CTV			
HRT	hormone replacement therapy		IGCN	intratubular germ cell neoplasia
HSP	heat shock protein		IGF	insulin-like growth factor
HT	hormone therapy		IGRT	image-guided radiotherapy
HTP	hydroxytryptophan		IHC	immunohistochemistry
hTERT	human telomerase reverse transcriptase		IHD	ischaemic heart disease
HTLV-1	human T-cell lymphotropic virus-1		IL	interleukin
IASLC	International Association for the Study of Lung Cancer		ILT	intraluminal brachytherapy
			i.m.	intramuscular
IBCSG	International Breast Cancer Study Group		IM	internal margin
			IMN	internal mammary node
IBIS	International Breast Cancer Intervention Study		IMP	investigational medicinal product
ICAM1	intercellular adhesion molecule 1		IMRT	intensity-modulated radiation therapy
ICC	interstitial cells of Cajal		INPC	International Neuroblastoma Pathology Classification
ICD-10	International Statistical Classification of Diseases 10th revision			
ICD-O-3	International Classification of Diseases for Oncology, 3rd Edition		INRT	involved node radiotherapy
			IPI	International Prognostic Index
ICRI	International Rare Cancers Initiative		I-PSS	International Prostate Symptom Score
ICON	International Collaborative Ovarian Neoplasm study		IQ	intelligence quotient
			IR-CTV	intermediate-risk CTV

IRAS	integrated research application system	LDL	low density lipoprotein
IRS	Intergroup Rhabdomyosarcoma Studies	LDR	low dose rate
ISO	International Organisation for Standardisation	LEEP	loop electro-excision procedure
		LFT	liver function tests
ISH	*in situ* hybridisation	LGG	low-grade glioma
ISRT	involved-site radiotherapy	LH	luteinising hormone
ITT	intention to treat	LHRH	luteinising hormone releasing hormone
ITU	intensive therapy unit		
ITV	internal target volume	LHRHa	luteinising hormone releasing hormone agonist
IU	international units		
i.v.	intravenous	LLETZ	large loop excision of the transformation zone
IVC	inferior vena cava		
IVU	intravenous urogram	LMM	lentigo maligna melanoma
IWG	International Working Group	LN	lymph node
JVP	jugulo-venous pressure	LOH	loss of heterozygosity
Ki-67	MKI67; marker of proliferation Ki-67	LR	local recurrence
KIF20A	kinesin-like protein	LUCADA	National Lung Cancer Audit Database
KIT	v-kit Hardy–Zuckerman 4 feline sarcoma viral oncogene homolog	MAb	monoclonal antibody
		MAB	maximal androgen blockade
KOC1	IGF II mRNA binding protein 3	MACH-NC	Meta-Analysis of Chemotherapy on Head and Neck Cancer
KPS	Karnofsky performance status		
KRAS	Kirsten rat sarcoma viral oncogene homolog	MACIS	metastases, age, completeness of surgery, invasion of extrathyroidal tissues, size
LACE	Lung Adjuvant Cisplatin Evaluation		
LAK	lymphokine-activated killer	MAG 3	mercaptoacetyltriglycerine
LAPC	locally advanced pancreatic cancer	MAGE	melanoma antigen expression family
LAR	long-acting release		
LCIS	lobular carcinoma *in situ*	MAGIC	Medical Research Council Adjuvant Gastric Infusional Chemotherapy
LCNEC	large cell neuroendocrine carcinoma		
LCNED	large cell neuroendocrine differentiation	MALT	mucosa-associated lymphoid tissue
		MAMS	multi-arm multi-stage
LD	latissimus dorsi	MAOI	monoamine oxidase inhibitor
LDFS	local disease-free survival	MAPK	mitogen-activated protein kinase
LDH	lactate dehydrogenase	MART	melanoma antigen recognised by T cells

MASCC	Multinational Association for Supportive Care in Cancer		MRI	magnetic resonance imaging
MBC	metastatic breast cancer		mRNA	messenger ribonucleic acid
MBq	mega-Becquerel		MRS	magnetic spectroscopy
MCF-7	Michigan Cancer Foundation-7		MRSA	methicillin-resistant *Staphylococcus aureus*
MCL	mantle cell lymphoma		MS	median survival
mCRC	metastatic colorectal cancer		MSCC	malignant spinal cord compression
MDFS	metastatic disease-free survival		MSH	DNA mismatch repair gene
MDR	medium dose rate		MSI	microsatellite instability
MDT	multidisciplinary team		MSKCC	Memorial Sloan-Kettering Cancer Center
MEN	multiple endocrine neoplasia			
MET	MET proto-oncogene, receptor tyrosine kinase (synonym = hepatocyte growth factor receptor)		MSTR1	macrophage-stimulating 1 receptor (c-met-related tyrosine kinase)
			MSU	mid-stream urine
MF	mycosis fungoides		MTC	medullary thyroid carcinoma
M:F	male to female		MTD	maximally tolerated dose
MGMT	O^6 methylguanine-DNA methyltransferase		MTOR	mechanistic target of rapamycin (serine/threonine kinase)
MGUS	monoclonal gammopathy of undetermined significance		MUC	mucin
			MUGA scan	multigated acquisition scan
MIB-1	antibody to Ki-67		MUM1	melanoma-associated antigen (mutated) 1
MIBC	muscle-invasive bladder cancer			
MIBG	meta-iodobenzylguanidine		MUO	metastatic malignancy of unknown origin
MLC	multileaf collimator			
MM	malignant melanoma		MV	megavoltage
MMC	mitomycin C		MW	molecular weight
MMAE	monomethyl auristan E		MYC	v-myc myelocytomatosis viral oncogene homolog
MMR	mismatch repair			
MMS	multimodal screening		MYCN	v-myc avian myelocytomatosis viral oncogene neuroblastoma derived homolog
mp	multiparametric			
MPHOSPH1	M phase phosphoprotein 1			
MRC	Medical Research Council		MYOD1	myogenic differentiation 1
MRCP	magnetic resonance cholangiopancreatogram		MZL	marginal zone lymphoma
			NAC	nipple areola complex
			NAHT	neoadjuvant hormone therapy

NALP7	NLRP7; NLR family, pyrin domain containing 7	NS	not significant
NAT	*n*-acetyltransferase	NSAA	non-steroidal anti-androgen
NCCN	National Comprehensive Cancer Network	NSABP	National Surgical Adjuvant Breast and Bowel Project
NCCTG	North Central Cancer Treatment Group	NSAID	non-steroidal anti-inflammatory drug
NCI	National Cancer Institute	NSCLC	non-small-cell lung cancer
NCRI	National Cancer Research Institute	NSGCT	non-seminomatous germ cell tumour
NCRN	National Cancer Research Network	NST	no specific type
Nd-YAG	neodynium-doped yttrium–aluminium–garnet	NTCP	normal tissue complication probability
NET	neuroendocrine tumour	NY-ESO-1	cancer/testis antigen
NEU	neuro/glioblastoma-derived oncogene homolog: HER2; erb-b2 receptor tyrosine kinase 2	OAR	organs at risk
		OC	oesophageal cancer; oral contraceptive
NF	neurofibromatosis	OCT3/4	POU5F1; POU class 5 homeobox 1
NHL	non-Hodgkin lymphoma	OFA	oncofetal antigen
NHS	National Health Service	OFS	ovarian function suppression
NI	Nottingham prognostic index	OPC	oropharyngeal carcinoma
NICE	National Institute for Health and Care Excellence	OPT	orthopantogram
		OR	odds ratio
NIH	National Institute of Health	OS	overall survival
NIHR	National Institute for Health Research	p16	CDKN2A; cyclin-dependent kinase inhibitor 2A
NK	natural killer		
NLPHL	nodular lymphocyte predominant Hodgkin lymphoma	p16INK4a	p16: CDKN2A; cyclin-dependent kinase inhibitor 2A
NM	nodular melanoma	p450	cytochrome p450
NMIBC	non-invasive bladder cancer	PanIN	pancreatic intraepithelial neoplasia
n-myc	MYCN; v-myc avian myelocytomatosis viral oncogene neuroblastoma-derived homolog	PAP	prostatic acid phosphatase
		PATCH	Prostate Adenocarcinoma: TransCutaneous Hormones
NNT	number needed to treat		
nocte	at night	PAX8	paired box 8
NOS	not otherwise specified	PCI	prophylactic cranial irradiation
NPC	nasopharyngeal carcinoma	PCNSL	primary central nervous system lymphoma
NRIG	National Radiotherapy Implementation Group		
		PCP	*pneumocystis carinae* pneumonia

pCR	pathological complete response		PNET	primitive neuroectodermal tumour
PD-1	PDCD1; programmed cell death 1		p.o.	*per os* (by mouth)
PDA	poorly differentiated adenocarcinoma		PORT	postoperative radiotherapy
PDC	poorly differentiated carcinoma		PORTEC	PostOperative Radiation Therapy in Endometrial Cancer
PDD	percentage depth dose		PP	pancreatic polypeptide
PDE5	phosphodiesterase type 5 inhibitor		PPPD	pylorus-preserving pancreatico-duodenectomy
PDGF	platelet-derived growth factor			
PDGFR	platelet-derived growth factor receptor		PPE	palmar–plantar erythrodysaesthesia
PD-L1	programmed death-ligand 1		PPI	proton pump inhibitor
PDN	poorly differentiated neoplasm		PPRT	prostate and pelvic radiotherapy
PDR	pulsed dose rate		PR	partial response
PDT	photodynamic therapy		PR-A	progesterone receptor A
PDVR	pancreaticoduodenectomy with vein resection		PR-B	progesterone receptor B
			p.r.n.	*pro re nata* (as required)
PEI	percutaneous ethanol injection		PrRT	prostate radiotherapy
PET	positron emission tomography		PRRT	peptide-receptor radionuclide therapy
PFS	progression-free survival		PRV	planning organ at risk volume
PGF	placental growth factor		PS	WHO performance status
PGP	protein gene product		PSA	prostate-specific antigen
PgR	progesterone receptor		PSTT	placental site trophoblast tumour
PhRMA	Pharmaceutical Research and Manufacturers of America		PTC	in thyroid cancer = papillary thyroid carcinoma; in hepatobiliary cancer = percutaneous transhepatic cholangiograph
PI3K	phosphatidyl inositol 3 kinase			
PICC	peripherally inserted central catheter			
PIK3CA	phosphatidylinositol-4,5-bisphosphate 3-kinase, catalytic subunit alpha		PTCH	patched gene
			PTEN	phosphatase and tensin homolog
PIP	Personal Independent Payment		PTH	parathyroid hormone
PLAP	placental alkaline phosphatase		PTH-RP	parathyroid hormone-related peptide
PLDH	pegylated liposomal doxorubicin hydrochloride		PTV	planning target volume
PM	partial mole		PUVA	psoralen plus ultraviolet A
PMS	PMS1 postmeiotic segregation increased 1		PV	*per vagina* (through the vagina)
			PVC	poly (vinyl-choride)
PMS2	PMS2 postmeiotic segregation increased 2 (*S. cerevisiae*)		PVI	protracted venous infusion
			QA	quality assurance

q.d.s.	*quater die sumendum* (four times a day)
QART	Quality Assurance in Radiation Therapy
QLQ	quality of life questionnaire
qmax	maximum flow
QOL	quality of life
QT	QT interval
R0	complete resection
R1	microscopic involved margins
R2	macroscopic involved margins
RA	rheumatoid arthritis
RAF	rapidly accelerated fibrosarcoma
RAF1	Raf-1 proto-oncogene, serine/threonine kinase
RAGE	renal antigen expression family
RANK	approved gene symbol = TNFRSR11A; name = tumour necrosis factor receptor superfamily, member 11a, NFKB activator
RANKL	TNFSF11; tumour necrosis factor (ligand) superfamily, member 11
RAS	rat sarcoma viral oncogene homolog
Rb	retinoblastoma
RB1	retinoblastoma 1 (including osteosarcoma)
RBE	radiobiologically equivalent dose
RC	radical cystectomy
RCC	renal cell carcinoma
RCCM	renal cell carcinoma marker
RCR	Royal College of Radiologists
RCT	randomised controlled trial
REAL	revised European–American lymphoma
RECIST	response evaluation criteria in solid tumours
RET	ret proto-oncogene
RFA	radiofrequency ablation
RFS	recurrence-free survival
rhTSH	recombinant human thyroid-stimulating hormone
RIC	reduced intensity conditioning
RMI	relative malignance index
RON	Recepteur d'Origine Nantais: MSTR1; macrophage-stimulating 1 receptor (c-met-related tyrosine) kinase
RPLND	retroperitoneal lymph node dissection
RR	response rate; relative risk
RRA	radioiodine remnant ablation
RS	recurrence score
rT	recurrent tumour
RT	radiotherapy
RTOG	Radiation Therapy Oncology Group
S100	S100 calcium-binding protein
SAB	same as before
SABR	stereotactic ablative body radiation therapy
SACT	systemic anti-cancer therapy
SAE	serious adverse event
SBP	solitary bone plasmacytoma
SBRT	stereotactic body radiotherapy
s.c.	subcutaneous
SCC	squamous cell carcinoma
SCF	supraclavicular fossa
SCFR	mast/stem cell growth factor receptor
SCGB2A2	secretoglobin family 2A member 2 (Mammaglobin-A)
SCLC	small cell lung cancer
SCT	stem cell transplant
SDH	succinate dehydrogenase complex
SEER	Surveillance Epidemiology and End Results

SEP	solitary extramedullary plasmacytoma		STAT3	signal transducer and activator of transcription 3
SERM	selective oestrogen receptor modulator		SV 40	simian virus 40
SH	SRC homology		SVC	superior vena cava
SI	sacro-iliac		SVCO	superior vena cava obstruction
S-I	superior–inferior		SWENOTECA	Swedish and Norwegian Testicular Cancer Group
SIADH	syndrome of inappropriate antidiuretic hormone		SWOG	Southwest Oncology Group
SIGN	Scottish Intercollegiate Guidelines Network		SXR	superficial X-ray
SIOP	Société Internationale d'Oncologie Pédiatrique		T3	liothyronine
			T4	thyroxine
SIRT	selective internal radiation microsphere therapy		TA	technology appraisal
SLE	systemic lupus erythematosus		TACE	transarterial chemo-embolisation
SLL	small lymphocytic lymphoma		TAH	total abdominal hysterectomy
SLN	sentinel lymph node		TB	tuberculosis
SLNB	sentinel lymph node biopsy		TBI	total body irradiation
SM	set-up margin		TCC	transitional cell carcinoma
SMA	smooth muscle actin		TCP	tumour control probability
SMAD4	SMAD family member 4		t.d.s.	*ter die sumendum* (three times a day)
SMAS	superficial musculo-aponeurotic system		TEK	TEK tyrosine kinase, endothelial
SMC	Scottish Medicines Consortium		TEM	trans-anal endoscopic microscopy
SMO	smoothened receptor		TFE3	transcription factor binding to IGHM enhancer 3
SMV	superior mesenteric vein			
SNB	sentinel node biopsy		Tg	thyroglobulin
SPECT	single photon emission computed tomography		TGF-β	transforming growth factor beta
SRC	SRC proto-oncogene, non-receptor tyrosine kinase		THW	thyroid hormone withdrawal
			TIE2	tunica interna endothelial cell kinase: TEK; TEK tyrosine kinase, endothelial
SRH	stigmata of recent haemorrhage			
SS	Sézary syndrome		TKI	tyrosine kinase inhibitor
SSD	source–skin distance		TLD	thermoluminescence dosimetry
SSM	superficial spreading melanoma		TLM	transoral laser microsurgery
SSP	statutory sick pay		TLS	tumour lysis syndrome
SSRS	somatostatin receptor scintigraphy			

TME	total mesorectal excision
TMR	tissue maximum ratio
TNF	tumour necrosis factor
TNFSF11	tumour necrosis factor (ligand) superfamily, member 11
TNM	tumour nodes metastases
TORS	transoral robotic surgery
TP53	tumour protein p53
TPR	tissue phantom ratio
TRAIL	tumour necrosis factor apoptosis-inducing ligand: TNFSF10; tumour necrosis factor (ligand) superfamily, member 10
TROG	Trans Tasman Radiation Oncology Group
TRUS	transrectal ultrasound
TSC	trial steering committee
TSEBT	total skin electron beam therapy
TSH	thyroid-stimulating hormone
TTF-1	thyroid transcription factor 1
TTK	TTK protein kinase
TURBT	transurethral resection of bladder tumour
TURP	transurethral resection of the prostate
TVS	transvaginal ultrasound
U+E	urea and electrolytes
UFT	tegafur–uracil
UC	ulcerative colitits
UICC	International Union Against Cancer
UK	United Kingdom
UKINETS	UK and Ireland Neuroendocrine Tumour Society
URLC10	upregulated in lung cancer 10
US	ultrasound scan
USA	United States of America

UTI	urinary tract infection
UV	ultraviolet
VAIN	vaginal intraepithelial neoplasia
VATS	video-assisted thoroscopic surgery
VC	vomiting centre
VEGF	vascular endothelial growth factor
VEGFR	vascular endothelial growth factor receptor
VHL	Von Hippel Lindau
VIN	vulval intraepithelial neoplasia
VIP	vasoactive intestinal peptide
VMAT	volumetric modulated arc therapy
VSIM	virtual simulation software
VTE	venous thromboembolism
WA	wedge angle
WAF1	cyclin-dependent kinase inhibitor
WBC	white blood cell
WBrRT	whole breast radiotherapy
WBRT	whole brain radiotherapy
WCB	Wales Cancer Bank
WCC	white cell count
WHO	World Health Organisation
WLE	wide local excision
WNT	wingless-type MMTV integration site family
wt	wild-type
WT1	Wilms tumour 1
XRT	X-ray treatment

Chemotherapy regimens

ABVD	doxorubicin, bleomycin, vinblastine, dacarbazine
AC	doxorubicin, cyclophosphamide

BEACOPP	bleomycin, etoposide, doxorubicin, cyclophosphamide, vincristine, procarbazine, prednisolone		EOX	epirubicin, oxaliplatin, capecitabine
			EP	etoposide, cisplatin
BEAM	carmustine, etoposide, cytarabine, melphalan		EP-EMA	etoposide, cisplatin–etoposide, methotrexate, actinomycin-D
BEC	bleomycin, etoposide, carboplatin		Epi-CMF	epirubicin, cyclophosphamide, methotrexate, 5-FU
BEP	bleomycin, etoposide, cisplatin		ESHAP	etoposide, methylprednisolone, cytarabine, cisplatin
BOP	bleomycin, vincristine, cisplatin			
BuCy	busulphan, cyclophosphamide		FAC	5-FU, doxorubicin, cyclophosphamide
CAF	cyclophosphamide, doxorubicin, 5-FU			
CAP	cyclophosphamide, doxorubicin, cisplatin		FEC	5-FU, epirubicin, cyclophosphamide
CAPOX	capecitabine, oxaliplatin		FEC-T	5-FU, epirubicin, cyclophosphamide then docetaxel
CAV	cyclophosphamide, doxorubicin, vincristine		FF	folinic acid, 5-FU
CHOP	cyclophosphamide, doxorubicin, vincristine, prednisolone		FOLFIRI	5-FU, folic acid, irinotecan
			FOLFIRINOX	5-FU, folic acid, irinotecan, oxaliplatin
CMF	cyclophosphamide, methotrexate, 5-FU			
COPDAC	cyclophosphamide, vincristine, dacarbazine, predniolone		FOLFOX	5-FU, folic acid, oxaliplatin
			GDP	gemcitabine, dexamethasone, cisplatin
CTD	cyclophosphamide, thalidomide, dexamethasone			
CVAD	cyclophosphamide, vincristine, doxorubicin, dexamethasone		GEMCAP	gemcitabine, capecitabine
			Gem-cis	gemcitabine, cisplatin
CVP	cyclophosphamide, vincristine, prednisolone		HD-MTX	high-dose methotrexate
			HD-AC	high-dose cytarabine
Cy	cyclophosphamide		ICE	ifosfamide, carboplatin, etoposide
CYVADIC	cyclophosphamide, vincristine, doxorubicin, dacarbazine		IE	ifosfamide, etoposide
			IGEV	ifosfamide, gemcitabine, prednisolone, vinblastine
DAT	daunorubicin, ara-C (cytarabine), thioguanine			
			IVA	ifosfamide, vincristine, dactinomycin
DHAP	dexamethasone, cytarabine, cisplatin			
EC	epirubicin, cyclophosphamide		IVADo	ifosfamide, vincristine, dactinomycin, doxorubicin
ECF	epirubicin, cisplatin, 5-FU			
ECX	epirubicin, cisplatin, capecitabine		JEB	carboplatin, etoposide, bleomycin
EMA-CO	etoposide, methotrexate, dactinomycin, cyclophosphamide, vincristine		MAP	methotrexate, doxorubicin, cisplatin
			M-CAVI	methotrexate, carboplatin, vinblastine

MTX	methotrexate
MVAC	methotrexate, vinblastine, doxorubicin, cisplatin
MVP	mitomycin, vinblastine, cisplatin
OEPA	vincristine, etoposide, prednisolone, doxorubicin
OFF	oxaliplatin, folinic acid, 5FU
PEI	cisplatin, etoposide, ifosfamide
PF	cisplatin, 5-FU
PLaDo	cisplatin, doxorubicin
R-CHOP	rituximab, cyclophosphamide, doxorubicin, vincristine, prednisolone
R-CVP	rituximab, cyclophosphamide, vincristine, prednisolone
R-FC	rituximab, fludarabine, cyclophosphamide
R-GCVP	rituximab, gemcitabine, cyclophosphamide, vincristine, prednisolone
R-CODOX-M/R-IVAC	rituximab, cyclophosphamide, vincristine, doxorubicin, cytarabine, methotrexate, etoposide, ifosfamide
TAC	docetaxel, doxorubicin, cyclophosphamide
TC	docetaxel, cyclophosphamide
TE-TP	paclitaxel, cisplatin; paclitaxel etoposide
TIP	paclitaxel, ifosfamide, cisplatin
TPF	docetaxel, cisplatin and 5-FU

VAC	vincristine, dactinomycin, cyclophosphamide
VACA	vincristine, dactinomycin, cyclophosphamide, doxorubicin
VAI	vincristine, dactinomycin, ifosfamide
VAIA	vincristine, dactinomycin, ifosfamide, doxorubicin
VACD	vincristine, dactinomycin, cyclophosphamide, doxorubicin
VC	vincristine, cyclophosphamide
VDC	vincristine, doxorubicin, cyclophosphamide
VEC-CDDP	vincristine, etoposide, cyclophosphamide, cisplatin
VIDE	vincristine, ifosfamide, etoposide
VIP	etoposide, ifosfamide, cisplatin
XELOX	capecitabine, oxaliplatin

Radioisotopes

^{11}C	carbon-11
^{60}Co	cobalt-60
^{51}Cr	chromium-51
^{137}Cs	caesium-137
^{18}F	fluorine-18
^{68}Ga	gallium-68
^{123}I	iodine-123
^{125}I	iodine-125
^{131}I	iodine-131
^{111}In	indium-111
^{192}Ir	iridium-192
^{177}Lu	lutetium-177
^{103}Pd	palladium-103
^{106}Ru	ruthenium-106
^{99m}Tc	technetium-99m
^{90}Y	yttrium-90

Chapter

1

Practical issues in the use of systemic anti-cancer therapy drugs

Usman Malik and Philip Savage

Introduction

The role of systemic anti-cancer therapy (SACT) in the management of cancer is evolving rapidly with widening indications for treatment and, in many diagnoses, additional therapies and lines of treatment now available. In 2015, there are now over 140 drugs licensed to be used for cancer treatment and it is not practical within this chapter to give a comprehensive description of each drug or treatment regimen. More detailed information can be found in chemotherapy textbooks, at the manufacturers' websites, the electronic Medicines Compendium (eMC) or from oncology pharmacy websites (e.g. http://www.medicines.org.uk/emc and www.bccancer.bc.ca, accessed January 2015). However, we hope this chapter, which focuses mainly on classic cytotoxic chemotherapy drugs, will provide SACT prescribers, pharmacists and administrators with sufficient information to discuss treatment with patients, to prescribe and deliver drugs safely and to recognise common treatment-related side effects.

Over the last decade there has been a major increase in activity and workloads within chemotherapy treatment units. The 2009 National Cancer Advisory Group report described an increase in overall activity of 60% in just a four year period (NCAG, 2009). This rise in activity is in part a result of increased numbers of patients but there has also been a major expansion in the indications for which there is effective treatment, the upper age range of patients treated and, in many malignancies, the number of lines of therapy available for use. Whilst the newer drugs are predominantly oral agents, the recent development of maintenance monoclonal antibody therapies for breast cancer and non-Hodgkin lymphoma and the more modern prolonged and complex regimens in gastrointestinal malignancies

have added considerable pressure to the workload of pharmacy and chemotherapy treatment units.

A summary of the rapid increase in both the number of new cancer treatment drugs and the change in identity of new SACT agents can be see in Table 1.1 that shows both the historical and modern trends in new cancer drugs. This demonstrates the change from the initial cancer treatment drugs of the 1970s/80s/90s that were predominantly classic cytotoxic chemotherapy agents to a new, varied range of agents including monoclonal antibodies, TKI and MTOR inhibitors and other new agents (Savage and Mahmoud, 2013).

This increase in the number and variety of anti-cancer drugs seems set to continue as there are nearly 1000 new cancer drug trials in the USA alone at present (PhRMA, 2012). One of the consequences of the increased numbers of new drugs is the financial challenge in providing the facilities and manpower to deliver care, and to pay for the drugs themselves. This is a problem for all healthcare systems, whether paid by insurance or state-funded, and it is likely that the increasing numbers and cost of cancer drug treatment will continue to influence clinical, economic and political decision making (Sullivan *et al.*, 2011).

Aims of systemic anti-cancer therapy

There are three main indications for the use of SACT drugs.

- Curative: the management of patients with chemotherapy-curable advanced malignancies including gestational choriocarcinoma, testicular cancer, ovarian germ cell tumours, acute leukaemia, Hodgkin lymphoma, high-grade non-Hodgkin lymphoma (NHL) and some rare childhood malignancies.

Practical Clinical Oncology, Second Edition, ed. Louise Hanna, Tom Crosby and Fergus Macbeth. Published by Cambridge University Press. © Cambridge University Press 2015.

Table 1.1 Historical and modern trends in new cancer drugs

Drug class	Pre 1975	1975–1999	2000–2009	2010–13	Total
Cytotoxic	15	30	5	5	55
Hormonal	0	13	3	2	18
Cytokine	0	2	0	0	2
Peptide	0	2	0	1	3
MAb	0	1	5	5	11
TKI	0	0	5	6	11
MTOR	0	0	1	1	2
Other	0	0	3	0	3

The table shows the number of new cancer treatment drugs licensed during each of the time periods and the total currently available in each therapeutic class. MAb = antibody; MTOR: mechanistic target of rapamycin (serine/threonine kinase); TKI: tyrosine kinase inhibitor.

- Adjuvant: the preoperative or postoperative treatment of clinically localised malignancies, primarily breast cancer and colorectal cancer.
- Palliative: the treatment of patients with advanced incurable malignancies, where the main aims of treatment include prolonging life and reducing disease-related symptoms.

Before starting a course of SACT, the prescriber and the patient should both be clear about the aims and realistic expectations of treatment and ideally use consent forms specific to individual regimens and indications giving detailed information on the risks and benefits of treatment.

For patients with curable malignancies or receiving adjuvant therapy, it is important to avoid treatment delays or dose reductions and to maintain the calculated dose and schedule of the standard treatment protocols. The importance of this has been shown in the cure rates for testicular cancer (Toner *et al.*, 2001) and lymphoma (Lepage *et al.*, 1993) and also in the adjuvant treatment of breast cancer, where the rate of relapse is higher when the dose intensity is reduced (Budman *et al.*, 1998).

Generally, the chemotherapy regimens used in the curable malignancies have significant side effects including neutropenia and the use of granulocyte colony stimulating factor (G-CSF) is frequently required to keep treatment on schedule. However because there is the clear intent of achieving either cure or, in adjuvant treatment, an increased chance of cure, these side effects and treatment-related risks and costs are seen as acceptable temporary issues. In contrast, for patients having non-curative chemotherapy the benefits of treatment need to be balanced against quality of life and dose reductions may be made to ensure that the patient tolerates the treatment safely.

Cytotoxic chemotherapy

Cytotoxic chemotherapy drugs aim to kill or slow the growth of tumour cells while being relatively sparing to normal non-malignant cells. The sensitivity of different tumour types to the actions of cytotoxic drugs varies widely among the cells of origin and across the range of drugs. This variation in part reflects native metabolism of the tumour cell and differing metabolic pathways, drug handling, abilities to repair DNA and sensitivity to the induction of apoptosis.

In general tumour cells are more sensitive to cytotoxic drugs than their parent cell types and also often more sensitive than the usually dose limiting cells of the bone marrow. Whilst chemotherapy treatment brings routine cures in the rare chemotherapy curable malignancies, for the common malignancies cure of metastatic disease with chemotherapy is not a realistic outcome. The ability of chemotherapy treatment to cure patients with these limited numbers of chemo curable malignancies, listed above, started in the 1950s and was firmly established by the end of the 1970s. Since then, despite many new classic cytotoxic drugs being subsequently introduced, this pattern of chemotherapy curable malignancies has not changed. Whilst there has been enormous endeavour looking at the mechanisms of chemotherapy resistance, other explanations based on the natural genetic processes occurring in the parent cells of the chemotherapy curable malignancies may offer an alternate perspective (Masters and Köberle 2003, Savage *et al.*, 2009).

The action of cytotoxic chemotherapy drugs has traditionally been classified as being either 'cell-cycle specific' or 'cell-cycle non-specific.' The cycle-specific drugs, (such as the anti-metabolites methotrexate, fluorouracil and gemcitabine) mainly interact with cells that are actively synthesising DNA in the synthesis (S) phase and so are most effective in tumours with high mitotic rates and kill more cells when given in prolonged exposures.

The cell-cycle non-specific drugs interact with cells in all parts of the cycle and can affect more slowly proliferating tumour cells. These include the alkylating agents (e.g. cyclophosphamide, bendamustine, ifosfamide) and the anti-tumour antibiotics (e.g. bleomycin, doxorubicin, epirubicin). These drugs are active in all phases of the cell cycle, and their effect is more closely related to the total dose rather than to the duration of administration.

More modern research suggests that this distinction is relatively crude and that most drugs affect both dividing and resting cells. However, it is still quite useful for predicting the side effects of chemotherapy, because the extended use of cell-cycle specific drugs can cause more neutropenia and mucosal damage, and for designing combination regimens.

Combination chemotherapy regimens

Most cytotoxic drugs were originally used as single agents and were then incorporated into clinical trials of combination chemotherapy schedules. The combination of drugs with different modes of action and patterns of toxicity led to major improvements in the treatment of testicular cancer and lymphoma and made these tumours routinely curable in the 1970s (Li et al., 1960, Freireich et al., 1964, DeVita et al., 1970). In the adjuvant and palliative setting, combination treatments often also give enhanced results with acceptable toxicity.

The key principles for selecting the chemotherapy drugs for use in combinations include the following.

- Each drug has activity against the tumour as a single agent.
- There are no clinically important drug interactions between the agents.
- Combinations should avoid drugs of the same class or those with similar modes of action.
- The drugs should have different dose-limiting toxicities.

For example, BEP (bleomycin, etoposide, cisplatin) is now the regimen of choice for advanced testicular cancer. The drugs all have significant activity as single agents, usually with a short duration of response, and have different dose-limiting toxicities. By combining them with their different toxicities, each can be used at nearly the full single-agent dose, resulting in increased effectiveness with little extra toxicity. This combination changed advanced testicular cancer from a diagnosis with a poor prognosis to one which was routinely curable (Williams et al., 1987).

The treatment of high-grade B-cell NHL is an example of the benefits of adding an additional modern drug with a completely different mode of action to an already effective regimen. After its introduction in the 1970s the combination of cyclophosphamide, doxorubicin, vincristine and prednisolone (CHOP) became standard treatment (McKelvey et al., 1976), and subsequent trials comparing CHOP with more complex and toxic regimens showed no greater effectiveness (Fisher et al., 1993). In contrast, addition of the anti-CD20 monoclonal antibody rituximab, with a different mode of action and minimal toxicity, to give the R-CHOP regimen has led to significant improvement in cure rates (Sehn et al., 2005).

Chemotherapy scheduling

In some regimens the cytotoxic drugs must be given in the correct order, for example the combination of paclitaxel and carboplatin for patients with ovarian cancer. Carboplatin is a cell-cycle non-specific drug and is best given as a single bolus dose, infused over 30 minutes, because of the risk of hypersensitivity. The usual administration cycle is 28 days when used as a single agent because the myelosuppression nadir is between 14 and 21 days. Paclitaxel is cell-cycle specific and so should be given in multiple fractions over a prolonged period and is now usually given as a 3-hour infusion (ICON Group, 2002). Its nadir of myelosuppression occurs after 10 days, implying a maximum cycle length of 21 days, and so combining the two drugs presents a problem deciding what interval there should be between doses. However, studies have shown that giving paclitaxel before carboplatin appears to give some bone marrow protection and 21-day cycles do not produce unacceptable myelosuppression. However, recent trials giving paclitaxel weekly in combination with 3-weekly carboplatin, a 'dose-dense' schedule, showed greater effectiveness but more toxicity (Katsumata et al., 2013).

SACT protocols and guidelines

The introduction of peer-reviewed treatment policies in the NHS has led to the development of local protocols for approved SACT regimens, which should be familiar to all the health professionals who prescribe, dispense and administer them. 'Off-protocol' regimens should generally not be prescribed unless there is good evidence in the research literature.

Electronic prescribing systems for SACT have reduced the risk of prescribing errors, improved administration scheduling and provided accurate data on prescribing patterns (Ammenwerth *et al.*, 2008).

Dose calculation

Body surface area

Ideally, calculating the appropriate dose of a cytotoxic drug would take into account its pharmacokinetic properties – how the body delivers the drug to its site of action and the patient's metabolism and excretion. The dose could then be adjusted according to the toxicity seen in each patient. Although this method of chemotherapy drug dosing has been advocated, routine cytotoxic chemotherapy doses continue to be calculated according to the patient's body surface area (BSA) (Veal *et al.*, 2003).

There are several formulae for calculating BSA. The most commonly used is that of DuBois and DuBois, which dates from 1916 and was based on data from only eight adults and one child (DuBois and DuBois, 1916). Other formulae using both electronic and manual methods (nomograms and slide rules) are available, and there is generally good correlation between them.

Dose capping

Whether to dose chemotherapy according to the patient's actual weight or their calculated ideal body weight is controversial (Hall *et al.*, 2013). Using the calculated BSA in large or obese patients may lead to relative overdosing and a risk of increased toxicity. Placing an upper limit on the dose has been suggested and some centres will use 2.2 m^2 as an upper limit of BSA for curative and adjuvant treatments and 2.0 m^2 for palliative treatments. However, when prescribing for tall but non-obese individuals there is a potential risk of underdosing if the BSA is capped at 2.2 m^2. The only commonly agreed exception is in the use of vincristine, for which the dose is usually capped at 2 mg. At present there is no consensus on this, and local policies should always be checked, especially when treating patients with chemotherapy-curable tumours.

Area under the curve dosing

Carboplatin is excreted unchanged by the kidneys and is the only commonly used agent for which the dose is calculated from the renal function. A formula (the Calvert equation) has been developed based on renal function (Calvert *et al.*, 1989) by which the desired AUC (area under the curve of serum levels against time) is chosen, and the dose is calculated by the following formula:

$$\text{Dose (mg)} = \text{desired AUC} \times (\text{GFR mL/min} + 25)$$

GFR is the glomerular filtration rate, which may be calculated by ^{51}Cr-EDTA clearance, using a 24-h urine collection, or from the Cockcroft–Gault equation which derives it from a measure of serum creatinine, weight, age and sex. It is important to know which value of BSA is used in routine reporting of GFR and whether the value relates to the actual body size or to a standardised 1.73 m^2 BSA.

Body weight dosing

Body weight alone is not sufficent for calculating doses of most cytotoxic drugs except for some of the newer drugs, such as trastuzumab.

Flat dosing

Bleomycin is the only commonly used cytotoxic drug for which a fixed dose is used routinely. In the BEP regimen a fixed dose of 30,000 units on days 1, 8 and 15 is used irrespective of the patient's size. Also, many of the new SACT agents, particularly the TKI and MTOR drugs (see Chapter 2) are generally used at a standard flat dose irrespective of the patient's size and age.

Dose reduction

It is important to avoid unnecessary routine dose reductions solely on the basis of transient toxicity, particularly in curative and adjuvant treatments. Most modern protocols and clinical trial publications give clear advice on how best to reduce doses either across the regimen or for individual drugs in response to excess toxicity and using these can help maintain optimal care.

Elderly patients

Appropriately used chemotherapy can bring similar benefits in the elderly as in younger patients. However, the elderly metabolise drugs more slowly and are less resistant to side effects or complications. Whilst it is important that elderly patients have access to SACT treatments, it is also prudent to consider organ dysfunction carefully when starting treatment, often with dose adjustments from standard doses when starting. The emerging subject of geriatric oncology is exploring this area and many revised protocols for the elderly are being published.

Pretreatment procedures and investigations

Informed consent

Printed information on individual drugs or regimens is usually available and should be used to supplement oral information. The NHS patient 'information prescription' system has large amounts of local and national information readily available. All patients should be given a clear explanation of the purpose of treatment, its possible benefits and risks, clear advice about watching out for possible neutropenic fever and other serious toxicities and what to do if they occur. The advice must include essential 24-hour contact telephone numbers at the hospital, which must also be sent to the patient's GP.

Cardiotoxic drugs

Patients treated with cardiotoxic drugs such as anthracyclines and trastuzumab should have a pretreatment cardiac assessment, such as a multi-gated acquisition (MUGA) scan. This is especially important if the patient is elderly or has a history of cardiac disease, previous anthracycline exposure or mediastinal radiotherapy. Repeat monitoring should be performed according to the specific regimen protocol. Care should be taken to avoid exceeding the recommended total lifetime doses of anthracyclines, particularly when different courses of chemotherapy are given over long periods of time or at different hospitals.

Renal function

A number of drugs including methotrexate and carboplatin are excreted by the kidney and an assessment of renal function by ^{51}Cr-EDTA clearance should be done before starting treatment. The renal function may change during treatment, particularly when using a nephrotoxic drug such as cisplatin, and repeat measurements of renal function by ^{51}Cr-EDTA or calculated values are important to avoid toxicity. If there is

significant decline in GFR below 50–60 mL/min, carboplatin at an AUC of 4–5 replaces cisplatin in many regimens. Information on the appropriate dose reduction in renal impairment will be found in most protocols or national guidelines.

Hepatic function

The majority of SACT drugs are wholly or partly metabolised in the liver. The capacity of the liver to handle the drugs is large and the need for dose reduction is relatively uncommon. However, some drugs, including doxorubicin, do need dose reductions in the presence of hepatic impairment, and liver function tests, bilirubin, transaminases and alkaline phosphatase should be reviewed before treatment. Increase in the alkaline phosphatase, alone or accompanied by slight increases in transaminases, does not usually require dose reduction. However, the dose of drugs metabolised in the liver should be reduced if bilirubin is raised, particularly if accompanied by increases in transaminases. The dose of irinotecan, which is excreted in the bile, has to be reduced if the serum bilirubin level is raised. The treatment protocols in most units include advice on appropriate dose reductions. Other sources of advice include the websites of the British Columbia Cancer Agency and the London Cancer Alliance (http://www.bccancer.bc.ca/ and http://www.londoncanceralliance.nhs.uk/, accessed January 2015).

Baseline assessments of tumour

A baseline and regular objective measurements of response are required to assess whether the patient is benefiting from SACT treatment, except for those having adjuvant treatment. This may be by direct physical measurement of visible or palpable tumour, radiological examination, biochemical tests or measurement of tumour markers. When the main aim is symptom control, the patient's symptoms should be monitored carefully and balanced against the treatment toxicity.

Central venous access

Patients who have chemotherapy through ambulatory infusion devices must have central venous access, using a Hickman® or PICC line. Patients with poor veins or those who are to receive multi-day infusions may also need central lines early in their treatment. Although many patients do not have any problems with these lines, up to 11% develop line-related thromboses and 19% line infections. Patients should therefore be monitored regularly for these problems (Minassian *et al.*, 2000) and the use of subcutaneous ports in place of external catheters should be considered (Estes *et al.*, 2003).

Height and weight

To calculate BSA, height and weight measurements are needed. The patient's body weight should be measured before each new course of chemotherapy, and again if there is reason to suspect that it has altered by more than 5%. If the dose is calculated on the body weight alone, small changes in weight will have a greater impact on the dose and the patient's weight should be checked regularly; for example, every three months, or if the body weight is thought to have changed by more than 5%.

Checks before each SACT cycle

Full blood count

The patient's full blood count should be taken on the day of treatment or the day before. A finding of significant neutropenia or thrombocytopenia will mean a treatment delay. Patients who are anaemic rarely require a delay in chemotherapy (see below). Patients who are admitted with neutropenic fever or who have had more than one delay in treatment during a course of chemotherapy will require a dose reduction if receiving palliative treatment or support with growth factors if they are receiving curative or adjuvant treatment.

Biochemical, renal, liver and bone profile

A full biochemical profile is required before treatment to ensure that there has been no significant change in renal or hepatic function. If there is deteriorating renal or hepatic function, some drugs may need dose reduction or to be changed to an alternative, according to the local protocols. Some patients who experience disease-related hepatic or renal impairment may no longer need a dose reduction if these improve with treatment.

Some drugs have individual specific toxic effects that require additional monitoring. For example, cisplatin treatment frequently increases the renal excretion of potassium and magnesium and in addition to supplements in the i.v. hydration regimen additional oral supplements may be needed. Some of the newer SACT agents have novel side effects including hypothyroidism that may need specific monitoring.

Tumour markers

In malignancies with circulating tumour markers, measuring them can be a rapid, simple way of monitoring the response to treatment. Tumour markers are most useful in gestational choriocarcinoma, in which human chorionic gonadotrophin (hCG) is produced by all tumours (Sita-Lumsden *et al.*, 2012). In advanced testicular cancers, approximately 60% of tumours make one or both of hCG and alpha feto-protein (AFP). These can be used to monitor response or to prompt a change to second-line therapy when the rate of fall is inappropriately slow (Toner *et al.*, 1990). Other tumour markers which can be used for monitoring include CA125 in ovarian cancer, CA15-3 in breast cancer, CA19-9 in pancreatic cancer, carcino-embryonic antigen (CEA) in lower GI malignancies and prostate-specific antigen (PSA) in metastatic prostate cancer.

Major toxicities and their management

This section looks at practical issues in managing SACT toxicities. The main toxicities of individual cytotoxic chemotherapy drugs are summarised in the Appendix (see p. 7).

Myelosuppression

Primary and secondary prophylaxis

If a patient receiving palliative chemotherapy is admitted with neutropenic fever or has persistently low neutrophil counts without fever the dose of the next course should be reduced. However, patients receiving curative (including adjuvant) treatment should receive granulocyte colony stimulating factor (G-CSF) as secondary prophylaxis. For patients on very myelosuppressive regimens the ASH/ASCO guidelines recommend the use of G-CSF from cycle 1 for regimens with a greater than 20% risk of neutropenic sepsis in the first cycle (Smith *et al.*, 2006), as primary prophylaxis, although this is not widely accepted UK practice.

There are some practical problems with the timing and administration of growth factors which can be

Appendix Cancer treatment drugs and their major toxicities

Drug/class	Myelosuppression (0/+/++/+++)	Emetogenic risk (0–5)	Other major toxicities	Notes
Alkylating agents				
Bendamustine	++	3	Hypersensitivity	
Cyclophosphamide	++	4–5	Haemorrhagic cystitis	May need mesna
Dacarbazine	+++	5	Hepatotoxic	Vesicant
Ifosfamide	++	3	Haemorrhagic cystitis Encephalopathy	Needs mesna routinely to prevent haemorrhagic cystitis
Lomustine	+++ Delayed myelosuppression	3	Pulmonary Renal	Capsules 40 mg
Anthracyclines				
Doxorubicin	+++	4	Cardiotoxic Alopecia	Vesicant, give by bolus injection or centrally
Epirubicin	+++	4	As above	As above
Liposomal doxorubicin	+++	2	PPE Cardiotoxic	Exfoliant
Mitomycin	+++ Delayed myelosuppression	2	Renal	Vesicant
Mitozantrone	+++	2	Cardiotoxic	Exfoliant
Anti-metabolites				
Capecitabine	+	2	PPE	Tablets 500 mg, 300 mg and 150 mg
Fludarabine	+++	1	Diarrhoea	Consider PCP prophylaxis
Fluorouracil	+	2	Diarrhoea	PPE with long infusion
Gemcitabine	+	2	Influenza-like reactions after infusion	
Methotrexate	+	3	Mucositis and renal toxicity in high dose	Note drug interactions. Avoid in patients with pleural effusions or ascites
Pemetrexed	+++	2	Mucositis and hepatic toxicity	Toxicity reduced with folate and B12 supplement
Vinca alkaloids and etoposide				
Vincristine	Minimal	1	Neurotoxic	Must be given by intravenous injection only. Vesicant. Max. dose 2 mg
Vinblastine	+	1	Neurotoxic	Must be given by intravenous injection only. Vesicant. Max. dose usually 10 mg

Appendix *(cont.)*

Drug/class	Myelosuppression (0/+/++/+++)	Emetogenic risk (0–5)	Other major toxicities	Notes
Vinorelbine	+	1	Neurotoxic	Oral form (capsules) or intravenous injection only. Vesicant. Max. i.v. dose 60 mg
Vinflunine	+++	3	Constipation	
Etoposide	++	2	Alopecia.	Oral form (large capsules) twice i.v. dose
Platinums				
Cisplatin	+	5	Nephrotoxic Neurotoxic	Exfoliant. Check renal function carefully; good pre- and post-hydration essential
Carboplatin	++ Especially platelets	4	Less nephrotoxic than cisplatin	Hypersensitivity reactions common
Oxaliplatin	++	3	Neurotoxic	Exfoliant. Hypersensitivity reactions
Taxanes				
Cabazitaxel	++	1	Hypersensitivity Diarrhoea	Premedicate prior to infusion
Paclitaxel	++	2	Alopecia Neurotoxic	Vesicant. Hypersensitivity reactions – needs premedication
Docetaxel	+++	2	Alopecia	Vesicant. Hypersensitivity reactions – needs premedication
Topoisomerase 1 inhibitors				
Irinotecan	++	3	Diarrhoea Cholinergic syndrome	May need atropine
Topotecan	+++	2	Alopecia	Exfoliant
Other cytotoxics				
Bleomycin	No	1	Pulmonary Skin	
Eribulin	++	1	Alopecia, fatigue, neuropathy	
Procarbazine	+	5		Weak MAOI; avoid alcohol
Trabectedin	+++	2	Hepatic toxicity	Pretreatment dexamethasone must be given

MAOI, monoamine oxidase inhibitor; PCP, pneumocystis pneumonia; PPE, palmar–plantar erythrodysaesthesia.

overcome with the use of pegylated G-CSF (Neulasta®), needing only a single administration, generally 24 hours after chemotherapy. Studies have shown Neulasta® to be more successful in preventing neutropenic sepsis and better tolerated than daily G-CSF. Although Neulasta® is currently more expensive than daily G-CSF, it may be more cost-effective overall.

Prophylactic antibiotics

The results of the significant trial showed that patients given a prophylactic quinolone antibiotic had fewer admissions for neutropenic fever (Cullen *et al.*, 2005) and so these are now often incorporated into some chemotherapy protocols. Regimens that cause prolonged myelosuppression, particularly lymphoma regimens with long-term steroid administration, also often include co-trimoxazole to reduce the risk of *Pneumocystis carinii* infection.

Anaemia

Many cytotoxic drugs, particularly cisplatin, cause a gradual reduction in haemoglobin levels over the course of treatment. This usually does not lead to dose reductions or delays in treatment, but can significantly affect the patient's quality of life, and an elective blood transfusion may be appropriate. In some patients, erythropoietin may be a reasonable option, but has side effects such as nausea, pyrexia, headache, arthralgia and an increased risk of thrombosis.

Nausea and vomiting

The problems of chemotherapy-associated nausea and vomiting are much less since the introduction of the 5-HT3 antagonist drugs such as ondansetron and granisetron. It is now very unusual for patients to require hospital admission for control of vomiting. So, although many new cancer patients will expect nausea and vomiting to be a major problem, they can be reassured that, with appropriate use of anti-emetics, this is now very unlikely.

Anticipatory nausea and vomiting

Anticipatory nausea and vomiting occur before and during administration of chemotherapy, and are mainly due to the psychological effects associated with previous treatment and poor control of emesis. The problem can be managed by offering lorazepam 0.5–1 mg sublingually or orally immediately before chemotherapy and/or on the previous evening.

Acute nausea and vomiting

Acute nausea and vomiting are defined as occurring up to 24 hours after chemotherapy administration. The drugs used in prevention depend on the emetogenic potential of the regimen, and they are used in a step-wise fashion (Herrstedt *et al.*, 2005). All chemotherapy units will have guidance on which anti-emetics to use with each chemotherapy drug or regimen. Oral metoclopramide or domperidone are usually recommended for drugs of low emetogenic potential, such as bleomycin, vindesine or gemcitabine. However, the majority of drugs and regimens require more powerful anti-emetics, generally a 5-HT3 antagonist such as ondansetron and granisetron, and dexamethasone, on the day of treatment and for one to two days afterwards.

Some new anti-emetic drugs have been developed and licensed recently, including aprepitant, a neurokinin-1 receptor antagonist, useful in patients with poorly controlled emesis, and palonosetron, a long-acting 5-HT3 antagonist and the dissolving film form of ondansetron, which is easier for patients to take.

Delayed nausea and vomiting

The incidence of delayed nausea and vomiting is higher when there is poor control during the acute phase. The 5-HT3 antagonists are generally ineffective in controlling delayed nausea and vomiting, and metoclopramide is usually added to anti-emetic regimens. Cyclizine may be used during prolonged oral regimens if metoclopramide is ineffective in controlling delayed nausea and vomiting.

Cardiotoxicity

Cumulative cardiac toxicity is a problem associated with anthracyclines, and treatment should remain within the standard guidelines for the total lifetime dose – 450 mg/m^2 for doxorubicin. Cardiac function should be monitored more closely in patients with pre-existing cardiac problems and in patients who have received previous treatment with anthracyclines or mediastinal radiotherapy. A number of other drugs can also occasionally cause cardiotoxicity: fluorouracil may cause cardiac ischaemia and arrhythmias and cisplatin can occasionally cause vasospasm and angina or, rarely, stroke.

Renal toxicity

Although renal function is monitored before each chemotherapy cycle in most regimens, particular attention is needed for drugs that are either renally toxic in themselves or are excreted by the kidneys. Renal toxicity is most often caused by cisplatin. Appropriate treatment modifications should be made if there is a significant rise in the serum creatinine while on therapy, pending a more accurate assessment of renal function such as a ^{51}Cr-EDTA clearance. High-dose methotrexate can also cause renal toxicity and both cyclophosphamide and ifosfamide can cause both renal toxicity and haemorrhagic cystitis.

Diarrhoea

Diarrhoea can be a dose-limiting toxicity with capecitabine and fluorouracil and may also occur as part of the cholinergic syndrome caused by irinotecan. It is important to recognise the symptoms early and to start treatment with fluids, rehydration salts and loperamide.

Palmar–plantar erythrodysaesthesia (hand-foot syndrome)

Palmar–plantar erythrodysaesthesia (PPE) consists of swelling, redness, pain and, occasionally, blistering on the palms of the hands and/or the soles of the feet. It is a common dose-limiting toxicity with capecitabine and liposomal doxorubicin. Patients should be encouraged to use emollients, but effective prevention is difficult. A dose delay is usually required for grade 2 or greater PPE.

Alopecia

Alopecia can be a very distressing side effect of chemotherapy treatment for some patients. The problem can be minimised to some extent by the use of scalp hypothermia in patients receiving bolus injections or short infusions of doxorubicin, epirubicin and docetaxel. However, many patients do develop significant alopecia and they need to be aware of this possibility. Arrangements should be offered for the provision of wigs and alternatives such as head scarves.

Post-chemotherapy fertility

Chemotherapy can affect the patient's fertility. The regimens used in the treatment of testicular cancer, Hodgkin lymphoma, and high-grade NHL tend to have a relatively modest impact on fertility, but it is good practice to offer sperm storage for men undergoing chemotherapy. The situation for women is less satisfactory because techniques for the preservation of oocytes or ovarian tissue are not yet reliable or widely used. Embryo storage is time-consuming and may cause an inappropriate delay in starting treatment.

Surprisingly, the incidence of foetal abnormalities born to patients who have previously completed chemotherapy appears to be similar to that in the normal population. Patients should be advised to defer pregnancy for 12 months after the completion of treatment, but there is little evidence to say whether or not this is too cautious. In addition to the potential risk of foetal abnormalities, the risk of relapse needs to be taken into account when giving patients advice about the timing of future pregnancies. More detailed information on cancer treatment, chemotherapy and fertility is readily available (Lee et al., 2006).

Phlebitis and extravasation

Phlebitis is a common problem with irritant drugs such as dacarbazine, the alkylating agents and vinca alkaloids. These drugs should always be given as bolus injections through a fast-flowing drip or central line. Some drugs, especially anthracyclines, are vesicant and, in the event of extravasation, can cause local tissue necrosis. The patient may report pain on injection, but there may not be any obvious local reaction. There are a number of general and individual drug-specific measures for the treatment of suspected extravasation and the problem should be dealt with as an emergency (see Chapter 8). If extravasation occurs, the drug infusion should be stopped immediately and the local policy on management followed, including referral to plastic surgery if needed. Fortunately, significant extravasations are rare in modern chemotherapy units, but an advance awareness of the local extravasation policy may help urgent care to be delivered more effectively in the event of an occurrence.

Safe administration of chemotherapy

In the UK, there are national standards for the safe prescribing, dispensing and administering of chemotherapy. The standards, and methods of auditing these, vary in detail, but every organisation that provides chemotherapy has the responsibility to maintain policies and procedures to ensure that these standards are met. Training, competency and adequate facilities are the keys to safely prescribing, dispensing and administering chemotherapy. All healthcare staff involved in chemotherapy must be aware of their local policies.

Intrathecal chemotherapy

Sadly there have been a number of fatalities from the inadvertent administration of vinca alkaloids intrathecally. There has been a major NHS initiative to minimise this risk by both training and regulation of who can be involved in intrathecal chemotherapy and also by delivering vinca alkaloids in mini-bags that cannot be physically linked to an intrathecal needle. As a result of these simple changes there have been no further episodes in the UK since 2001. To maintain this safety record, the prescription and administration of intrathecal chemotherapy can be performed only by specially trained medical staff, and only suitably trained pharmacists and nurses can take part in their key roles in this complex procedure. All staff involved with SACT therapy must be aware of the national rules and local arrangements for intrathecal chemotherapy and must refuse to undertake any procedure for which they have not been trained and appropriately documented.

Hypersensitivity and anaphylaxis

Some cytotoxic drugs, especially platins, taxanes and bleomycin and most monoclonal antibodies, can produce hypersensitivity reactions, ranging from a 'flu-like' syndrome to anaphylactic shock. Premedication with corticosteroids, antihistamines and paracetamol is usually recommended and is built into most electronic prescribing systems. Full resuscitation facilities must be available for patients receiving their first dose of these drugs, and this means treatment in a hospital setting at a time when staffing levels and skill mix are appropriate to deal with emergencies. Subsequent doses may be given outside hospital depending on the risk of future reactions. The treatment of anaphylaxis should follow local policies but will include epinephrine (adrenaline) and oxygen (see Chapter 8).

Cholinergic syndrome

Irinotecan may cause a cholinergic syndrome, characterised by flushing, sweating and diarrhoea. The treatment is with atropine, and premedication with this is recommended for subsequent cycles. Late-onset diarrhoea (more than 24 hours after infusion) may occur, best treated with loperamide, rehydration and possibly antibiotics. Patients must be taught to recognise these symptoms and to take appropriate action.

Oesophageal—pharyngeal syndrome

Oxaliplatin may cause a sensation of dysphagia or dyspnoea without any evidence of respiratory distress, laryngospasm or bronchospasm. Although it is uncommon, it can be very distressing for the patient, who may confuse this symptom with respiratory or cardiac arrest. Avoiding cold liquids and food and not exposing the body to sudden cold will usually prevent this and patients can be reassured if they are warned in advance that it is transient. Treatment is symptomatic (warm drinks often help) and prolonging infusion times may reduce the chance of recurrence.

Oral chemotherapy and overcompliance

One of the most frequent causes of serious chemotherapy toxicity is with oral capecitabine. Patients may not be aware of or ignore the potentially serious adverse effects, such as diarrhoea, and continue treatment and become significantly dehydrated. Careful patient education is essential and capecitabine treatment must not be started until the prescriber is sure that the patient fully understands how to take the medication, the use of supportive medication, the circumstances when treatment should be discontinued, and how to obtain help.

Acknowledgements

The authors would like to acknowledge the contribution of Sian Evans to this chapter.

References

Ammenwerth, E., Schnell-Inderst, P., Machan, C., *et al.* (2008). The effect of electronic prescribing on medication errors and adverse drug events: a systematic review. *J. Am. Med. Inform. Assoc.*, **15**, 585–600.

Budman, D., Berry, D., Cirrincione, C., *et al.* (1998). Dose and dose intensity as determinants of outcome in the adjuvant treatment of breast cancer. The Cancer and Leukemia Group B. *J. Natl Cancer. Inst.*, **90**, 1205–11.

Calvert, A. H., Newell, D. R., Gumbrell, L. A., *et al.* (1989). Carboplatin dosage: prospective evaluation of a simple formula based on renal function. *J. Clin. Oncol.*, **7**, 1748–56.

Cullen, M., Steven, N., Billingham, L., *et al.* (2005). Antibacterial prophylaxis after chemotherapy for solid tumors and lymphomas. *N. Engl. J. Med.*, **353**, 988–98.

DeVita, V. T. Jr., Serpick, A. A. and Carbone, P. P. (1970). Combination chemotherapy in the treatment of advanced Hodgkin's disease. *Ann. Intern. Med.*, **73**, 881–95.

DuBois, D. and DuBois, E. F. (1916). A formula to estimate the approximate surface area if height and weight be known. *Arch. Intern. Med.*, **17**, 863–71.

Estes, J. M., Rocconi, R., Straughn, J. M., *et al.* (2003) Complications of indwelling venous access devices in patients with gynecologic malignancies. *Gynecol. Oncol.*, **91**, 591–95.

Fisher, R. I., Gaynor, E. R., Dahlberg, S., *et al.* (1993). Comparison of a standard regimen (CHOP) with three intensive chemotherapy regimens for advanced non-Hodgkin's lymphoma. *N. Engl. J. Med.*, **328**, 1002–06.

Freireich, E. J., Karon, M. and Frei, E., III. (1964). Quadruple combination therapy (VAMP) for acute lymphocytic leukemia of childhood. *Proc. Am. Assoc. Cancer Res.*, **5**, 20.

Hall, R. G., Jean, G. W., Sigler, M., *et al.* (2013). Dosing considerations for obese patients receiving cancer chemotherapeutic agents. *Ann. Pharmacother.*, **47**, 1666–74.

Herrstedt, J., Aapro, M. S., Roila, F., *et al.* (2005). ESMO minimum clinical recommendations for prophylaxis of chemotherapy-induced nausea and vomiting (NV). *Ann. Oncol.*, **16** (Suppl. 1), i77–79.

ICON Group. (2002). Paclitaxel plus carboplatin versus standard chemotherapy with either single-agent carboplatin or cyclophosphamide, doxorubicin, and cisplatin in women with ovarian cancer: the ICON3 randomised trial. *Lancet*, **360**, 505–15.

Katsumata, N., Yasuda, M., Isonishi, S., *et al.* (2013). Long-term results of dose-dense paclitaxel and carboplatin versus conventional paclitaxel and carboplatin for treatment of advanced epithelial ovarian, fallopian tube, or primary peritoneal cancer (JGOG 3016): a randomised, controlled, open-label trial. *Lancet Oncol.*, **14**, 1020–26.

Lee, S. J., Schover, L. R., Partridge, A. H., *et al.* (2006). American Society of Clinical Oncology recommendations on fertility preservation in cancer patients. *J. Clin. Oncol.*, **24**, 2917–31.

Lepage, E., Gisselbrecht, C., Haioun, C., *et al.* (1993). Prognostic significance of received relative dose intensity in non-Hodgkin's lymphoma patients: application to LNH-87 protocol. The GELA (Groupe d'Etude des Lymphomes de l'Adulte). *Ann. Oncol.*, **4**, 651–56.

Li, M. C., Whitmore, W. F. Jr., Golbey, R., *et al.* (1960). Effects of combined drug therapy on metastatic cancer of the testis. *J. Am. Med. Assoc.*, **174**, 1291–99.

Masters, J. and Köberle, B. (2003). Curing metastatic cancer: lessons from testicular germ-cell tumours. *Nat. Rev. Cancer*, **3**, 517–25.

McKelvey, E. M., Gottlieb, J. A., Wilson, H. E., *et al.* (1976). Hydroxyldaunomycin (Adriamycin) combination chemotherapy in malignant lymphoma. *Cancer*, **38**, 1484–93.

Minassian, V. A., Sood, A. K., Lowe, P., *et al.* (2000). Longterm central venous access in gynecologic cancer patients. *J. Am. Coll. Surg.*, **191**, 403–09.

NCAG. (2009). *Chemotherapy Services in England: Ensuring Quality and Safety*. London: National Chemotherapy Advisory Group.

PhRMA. (2012). *Medicines in Development: Cancer*. Washington, DC: Pharmaceutical Research and Manufacturers of America, available online at www.pharma.org

Savage, P. and Mahmoud, S. (2013). Development and economic trends in cancer therapeutic drugs: an updated analysis of modern and historical treatment costs compared to the contemporary GDP per capita. *J. Clin. Oncol.* **31**, Suppl. 31, abstract 259.

Savage, P., Stebbing, J., Bower, M., *et al.* (2008). Why does cytotoxic chemotherapy cure only some cancers? *Nat. Clin. Pract. Oncol.*, **6**, 43–52.

Sehn, L. H., Donaldson, J., Chhanabhai, M., *et al.* (2005). Introduction of combined CHOP plus rituximab therapy dramatically improved outcome of diffuse large B-cell lymphoma in British Columbia. *J. Clin. Oncol.* **23**, 5027–33.

Sita-Lumsden, A., Short, D., Lindsay, I., *et al.* (2012). Treatment outcomes for 618 women with gestational trophoblastic tumours following a molar pregnancy at the Charing Cross Hospital, 2000–2009. *Br. J. Cancer*, **107**, 1810–14.

Smith, T. J., Khatcheressian, J., Lyman, G. H., *et al.* (2006). 2006 update of recommendations for the use of white blood cell growth factors: an evidence-based clinical practice guideline. *J. Clin. Oncol.*, **24**, 3187–205.

Sullivan, R., Peppercorn, J., Sikora, K., *et al.* (2011). Delivering affordable cancer care in high-income countries. *Lancet Oncol.*, **12**, 933–80.

Toner, G. C., Geller, N. L., Tan, C., *et al.* (1990). Serum tumor marker half-life during chemotherapy allows early prediction of complete response and survival in nonseminomatous germ cell tumors. *Cancer Res.*, **50**, 5904–10.

Toner, G. C., Stockler, M. R., Boyer, M. J., *et al.* (2001). Comparison of two standard chemotherapy regimens for good-prognosis germ-cell tumours: a randomised trial. Australian and New Zealand Germ Cell Trial Group. *Lancet*, **357**, 739–45.

Veal, G. J., Coulthard, S. A. and Boddy, A. V. (2003). Chemotherapy individualization. *Invest. New Drugs*, **21**, 149–56.

Williams, S. D., Birch, R., Einhorn, L. H., *et al.* (1987). Treatment of disseminated germ-cell tumors with cisplatin, bleomycin, and either vinblastine or etoposide. *N. Engl. J. Med.*, **316**, 1435–40.

Chapter

2

Biological treatments in cancer

Amy Quinton and Rachel Jones

Introduction

The management of many cancers has changed as more biological agents have become available. For some, such as renal cell cancer and melanoma, in which chemotherapy has only limited effectiveness, targeted agents are now the mainstay of treatment. For others, where developments in chemotherapy have improved survival rates but increased toxicity, biological agents provide additional benefit with manageable toxicity, when alone or in combination with chemotherapy.

The licensed indications for new drugs are changing rapidly. A useful resource for up-to-date information can be found in the electronic Medicines Compendium (www.medicines.org.uk/emc, accessed January 2015). However, although they are licensed, several of these biological agents are not available for routine use in the UK.

This chapter is an overview of the biological agents in current use in the UK, and covers their mode of action and side effects. Their specific clinical indications will be described in the individual tumour chapters. This chapter will concentrate on five areas:

- protein kinase inhibitors and small molecule drugs,
- monoclonal antibodies,
- cytokines,
- haemopoietic colony-stimulating factors, and
- vaccines

Protein kinase inhibitors

Protein kinase inhibitors are predominantly oral agents, often with different, non-overlapping toxicities from chemotherapy, which allow them to be safely combined with chemotherapy and radiotherapy or to be given alone.

The targets for these drugs are the tyrosine and serine/threonine kinases. These enzymes transfer phosphate groups from ATP to specific amino acid residues on a protein through phosphorylation. The protein kinase inhibitors act by binding to the intracellular kinase region, directly competing with ATP, and thus preventing autophosphorylation. This in turn blocks the intracellular signalling cascades involved with the promotion of tumour growth, invasion, angiogenesis and resistance to apoptosis. They can be subdivided into receptor and non-receptor kinases.

The receptor kinase is an integral part of the receptor molecule spanning the cell membrane. Ligand binding to the receptor activates signalling pathways, and affects the activity of transcription factors and DNA synthesis. These include the epidermal growth factor receptor (EGFR), and the vascular endothelial growth factor receptor (VEGFR).

Non-receptor kinases are intracellular enzymes, transmitting regulatory signals when their phosphorylated form is recognised by SH (SRC homology) domains on other binding proteins. Although usually cytoplasmic, they may be membrane-bound. Examples of non-receptor serine/threonine kinases include RAF and MTOR.

An overview of these drugs is given in Table 2.1.

Small molecule drugs

A limited number of 'small molecule' drugs have been developed with specific intracellular targets.

Vismodegib

Vismodegib is an inhibitor of the hedgehog signalling pathway, involved in angiogenesis, as well as cellular proliferation, survival and differentiation. It binds to the G-protein-coupled SMO (smoothened) receptor transmembrane protein, and is licensed for use in basal

Practical Clinical Oncology, Second Edition, ed. Louise Hanna, Tom Crosby and Fergus Macbeth. Published by Cambridge University Press. © Cambridge University Press 2015.

Table 2.1 An overview of the currently licensed protein kinase inhibitor drugs, detailing their cellular targets, clinical indications and major toxicities

Name	Target	Tumour type/indication	Toxicities
Tyrosine kinase inhibitors			
Imatinib	BCR-ABL KIT (CD117/SCFR) PDGFRα PDGRFβ	Philadelphia+ CML Philadelphia+ ALL Myelodysplastic/proliferative disease Unresectable/metastatic KIT mutation+ GIST Unresectable/metastatic dermatofibrosarcoma protuberans	Myelosuppression Rash Diarrhoea Arthralgia Myalgia Oedema Visual disturbance
Erlotinib	EGFR (HER1/ERBB1)	Locally advanced/metastatic EGFR mutation+ (exon 19 deletion/exon 21 (L858R) substitution) adenocarcinoma of lung Recurrent/progressive NSCLC Unresectable/advanced/metastatic pancreatic cancer	Acneiform rash Paronychia Hair changes Diarrhoea Stomatitis Interstitial lung disease
Gefitinib	EGFR (HER1/ERBB1)	Locally advanced/metastatic EGFR mutation+ (exon 19 deletion/exon 21 (L858R) substitution) adenocarcinoma of lung	As erlotinib Liver dysfunction
Afatinib	EGFR (HER1/ERBB1) HER2 (ERBB2) HER3 (ERBB3) HER4 (ERBB4)	Locally advanced/metastatic EGFR mutation+ (exon 19 deletion/exon 21 (L858R) substitution) NSCLC	Acneiform rash Paronychia Diarrhoea Stomatitis
Lapatinib	EGFR (HER1/ERBB1) HER2 (ERBB2)	HER2+ metastatic breast cancer	Rash Diarrhoea Stomatitis Liver dysfunction Congestive cardiac failure Interstitial lung disease
Sunitinib	VEGFR1 VEGFR2 VEGFR3 PDGFRα PDGRFβ KIT (CD117/SCFR) FLT3	Advanced/metastatic renal cell carcinoma Pancreatic neuroendocrine carcinoma	Myelosuppression Rash Skin/hair depigmentation PPE Diarrhoea Stomatitis Hypertension Haemorrhage Venous thromboembolism Hypothyroidism
Pazopanib	VEGFR1 VEGFR2 VEGFR3 PDGFRα PDGRFβ KIT (CD117/SCFR)	Advanced/metastatic renal cell carcinoma Soft tissue sarcoma	As sunitinib Liver dysfunction

Table 2.1 (*cont.*)

Name	Target	Tumour type/indication	Toxicities
Axitinib	VEGFR1 VEGFR2 VEGFR3	Advanced/metastatic renal cell carcinoma	PPE Diarrhoea Gastrointestinal perforation Hypertension Haemorrhage Arterial and venous thromboembolism Posterior reversible leukoencephalopathy syndrome Dysphonia
Vandetanib	VEGFR2 EGFR (HER1/ERBB1) RET	Aggressive, symptomatic unresectable/metastatic medullary thyroid cancer	Myelosuppression Rash Diarrhoea Hypertension Prolonged QT/torsades de Pointes Posterior reversible leukoencephalopathy syndrome
Crizotinib	ALK MET (HGFR) MSTR1 (RON)	ALK mutation+ advanced NSCLC	Visual disturbance Peripheral oedema Diarrhoea Stomatitis
Serine/threonine kinase inhibitors			
Vemurafenib	BRAF	BRAF mutation+ unresectable/metastatic melanoma	Rash PPE Photosensitivity Squamous cell carcinoma Alopecia Diarrhoea Arthralgia
Dabrafenib	BRAF	BRAF mutation+ unresectable/metastatic melanoma intolerant of vemurafenib	Rash PPE Hyperkeratosis Alopecia Diarrhoea Cough Arthralgia Myalgia
Everolimus	MTOR	Advanced/metastatic renal cell carcinoma ER/PgR+ HER2– advanced/metastatic breast cancer Progressive unresectable/metastatic well-/moderately differentiated neuroendocrine pancreatic cancer	Myelosuppression Rash Diarrhoea Stomatitis Hyperglycaemia Electrolyte disturbance Interstitial lung disease

Table 2.1 (cont.)

Name	Target	Tumour type/indication	Toxicities
Temsirolimus	MTOR VEGF synthesis	Advanced/metastatic renal cell carcinoma Relapsed/refractory mantle cell lymphoma	Myelosuppression Rash Diarrhoea Stomatitis Hyperglycaemia Electrolyte disturbance Interstitial lung disease
Multi-kinase inhibitors			
Sorafenib	VEGFR2 VEGFR3 PDGFRβ KIT (CD117/SCFR) FLT3 BRAF RAF1 (CRAF)	Advanced/metastatic renal cell carcinoma Unresectable/advanced /metastatc hepatocellular carcinoma	Palmar/plantar erythrodysaesthesia syndrome Impaired wound healing Diarrhoea Stomatitis Liver dysfunction Hypertension Haemorrhage Cardiac ischaemia Dysphonia Arthralgia
Regorafenib	VEGFR2 VEGFR3 PDGFRβ FGFR KIT (CD117/SCFR) FLT3 BRAF RAF1RETTEK (TIE2)	Unresectable GISTs Metastatic colorectal cancer	Rash Palmar/plantar erythrodysaesthesia syndrome Impaired wound healing Diarrhoea Gastrointestinal perforation Liver dysfunction Hypertension Haemorrhage Cardiac ischaemia Dysphonia Posterior reversible leukoencephalopathy syndrome

ABL, ABL proto-oncogene, non-receptor tyrosine kinase; ALK, anaplastic lymphoma receptor tyrosine kinase; ALL, acute lymphoblastic leukaemia; BCR, breakpoint cluster region; BRAF, B-Raf proto-oncogene, serine/threonine kinase; CD, cluster of differentiation; CML, chronic myelogenous leukaemia; CRAF, C-Raf proto-oncogene, serine/threonine kinase; EGFR, epidermal growth factor receptor; ER, oestrogen receptor; ERBB1, epidermal growth factor receptor; FGFR, fibroblast growth factor receptor; FLT3, fms-related tyrosine kinase 3; GIST, gastrointestinal stromal tumour; HER, human epidermal growth factor receptor; HGFR, hepatocyte growth factor receptor; KIT, 'kitten': derived from v-kit Hardy–Zuckerman 4 feline sarcoma viral oncogene homolog; MET, MET proto-oncogene, receptor tyrosine kinase; MSTR1, macrophage stimulating 1 receptor (c-met-related tyrosine kinase); MTOR, mechanistic target of rapamycin (serine/threonine kinase); NSCLC, non-small-cell lung cancer; PDGFR, platelet-derived growth factor receptor; PgR, progesterone receptor; PPE, palmar–plantar erythrodysaesthesia; QT, QT interval; RAF1, Raf-1 proto-oncogene, serine/threonine kinase; RET, ret proto-oncogene; RON, Recepteur d'Origine Nantais; SCFR, mast/stem cell growth factor receptor; TEK, TEK tyrosine kinase, endothelial; TIE2, tunica interna endothelial cell kinase; VEGF(R), vascular endothelial growth factor (receptor).

Table 2.2 Nomenclature of monoclonal antibodies

Type	Origin	Nomenclature
Murine	Mouse	'-omab'
Chimeric	65–90% human murine variable regions	'-ximab'
Humanised	95% human 5% murine hypervariable region	'-zumab'
Human	Human	'-umab'

Adapted from Wick (2004).

cell carcinoma which is otherwise untreatable or has metastasised.

Aflibercept

Aflibercept is a recombinant fusion protein, made up of the VEGF-binding portions found on the extracellular domains of human VEGF receptors 1 and 2, fused to the Fc portion of IgG1. It acts as a soluble decoy receptor, binding VEGF with higher affinity than the native receptors, blocking receptor-mediated intracellular signalling. It is licensed for use in metastatic colorectal cancer that has progressed following an oxaliplatin-based chemotherapy regimen.

Monoclonal antibodies

Monoclonal antibodies (MAbs) are identical antibodies, produced in culture by cloning hybridised B cells ('hybridomas') that have been selected to target a specific antigenic epitope. All therapeutic MAbs are derived from B cells, and are immunoglobulins of isotype IgG. Hybridomas are typically splenic cells from inoculated mice fused with myeloma cells. Early attempts at using MAbs were limited by the strong immune responses evoked by the resulting murine antibodies. Advances in genetic engineering have provided increasingly humanised antibodies and better-tolerated preparations.

Nomenclature and classification

The MAbs are named according to the origin of their components (see Table 2.2).

Structurally, all antibodies consist of four polypeptides: two heavy chains and two light chains, which are joined together by disulphide bonds to form a 'Y' shape. Each chain has a variable amino acid sequence at its tip, which is the antigen binding site. The constant region (Fc) determines the mechanism that destroys the antigen, and is used to classify antibodies as IgA, IgD, IgE, IgM or IgG. As the therapeutic MAbs are derived from B cells, they are of the immunoglobulin isotype IgG.

The following are tumour antigen characteristics that are ideal for targeting by antibodies (Harris, 2004).

- The antigen should be expressed stably and homogeneously by tumour cells.
- There should be limited expression of the antigen in normal tissues.
- There should be minimal or no soluble form of the antigen (to avoid rapid clearance or extracellular binding of the antibody).
- The antigen should be present on the cell surface to allow clear access for the antibody.

MAbs act through a direct effect on tumour cells by activating either complement-mediated or antibody-dependent cell-mediated cytotoxicity, as well as through inhibition of signalling cascades involved in cellular proliferation and angiogenesis.

There are several antibodies routinely used as systemic therapy in the management of malignancy as single agents or in combination with chemotherapy (Table 2.3).

Monoclonal antibodies are also being used as vectors for radioactive isotopes. Ibritumomab is a CD20-specific recombinant murine IgG1 monoclonal antibody, which is radiolabelled with yttrium-90 and is licensed for the treatment of follicular lymphoma.

Cytokines

Cytokines are proteins which bind to specific effector-cell surface receptors and initiate intracellular signalling cascades that change the functioning of the effector cell. The cytokines are a complex group of molecules, and their number is expanding with further research. Several classification systems are in use, based on their presumed function, cell of secretion, target of action or molecular structure. There are five recognised major cytokine families:

- Type I cytokines (interleukins),
- Type II cytokines (interferons),
- the tumour necrosis factor family,

Table 2.3 An overview of the monoclonal antibodies in current clinical use in the UK

Name	Origin/subclass	Target	Tumour type/ indications	Toxicities
Bevacizumab	Humanised IgG1	VEGF	Advanced/metastatic breast cancer Metastatic colorectal cancer Metastatic/ recurrent NSCLC Advanced/metastatic renal cell cancer Advanced epithelial ovarian, fallopian tube and primary peritoneal cancer	Leucopenia Impaired wound healing Diarrhoea Gastrointestinal perforation Hypertension Haemorrhage Congestive cardiac failure Arterial and venous thromboembolism Proteinuria
Cetuximab	Chimeric IgG1	EGFR (HER1/ERBB1)	RAS wild-type metastatic colorectal cancers Squamous cell head and neck cancers	Rash Diarrhoea Mucositis Liver dysfunction Venous thromboembolism Interstitial pneumonitis Electrolyte disturbance
Trastuzumab	Humanised IgG1	HER2 (ERBB2)	HER2+ breast cancer Metastatic HER2+ gastric/ gastro-oesophageal junction adenocarcinoma	Myelosuppression Rash Diarrhoea Hypertension Congestive cardiac failure Arrhythmia Interstitial lung disease
Rituximab	Chimeric IgG1	CD20	Follicular lymphoma CD20-positive diffuse large B cell lymphoma CLL, RA, GPA and microscopic angiitis	Myelosuppression Rash Alopecia Bronchitis
Brentuximab	Chimeric IgG1 Conjugated with anti-microtubule drug MMAE	CD30	CD30+ Hodgkin lymphoma Relapsed/refractory systemic anaplastic large cell lymphoma	Myelosuppression Stevens Johnson syndrome Diarrhoea Hyperglycaemia Tumour lysis syndrome Peripheral sensory-motor and demyelinating polyneuropathy
Pertuzumab	Humanised IgG1	HER2 (ERBB2)	HER2+ locally recurrent/metastatic breast cancer	Neutropenia Rash Diarrhoea Left ventricular dysfunction

Table 2.3 (cont.)

Name	Origin/subclass	Target	Tumour type/ indications	Toxicities
Panitumumab	Fully human IgG2	EGFR	RAS wild-type metastatic colorectal cancer	Rash Paronychia Diarrhoea Stomatitis
Ipilimumab	Fully human IgG1	CTLA4	Advanced/metastatic melanoma	Rash Toxic epidermal necrolysis Colitis Gastrointestinal perforation Hepatitis Neuritis Adrenal, thyroid and pituitary dysfunction Visual disturbance
Denosumab	Fully human IgG2	TNFSF11 (RANKL)	Prevention of skeletal-related events including pathological fractures, spinal cord compression and the requirement for radiotherapy or surgery to bones in adults with bone metastases from solid tumours	Rash Diarrhoea Dyspnoea Osteonecrosis of the jaw

CLL, chronic lymphocytic leukaemia; CTLA4, ytotoxic T-lymphocyte-associated protein 4; EGFR, epidermal growth factor receptor; ERBB1, erb-b2 receptor tyrosine kinase 1; GPA, granulomatosis with polyangiitis; HER, human epidermal growth factor receptor; Ig, immunoglobulin; MMAE, monomethyl auristatin E; NSCLC, non-small-cell lung cancer; RA, rheumatoid arthritis; RANKL, receptor activator of nuclear factor kappa-B ligand; RAS, rat sarcoma oncogene; VEGF, vascular endothelial growth factor.

- the immunoglobulin supergene family, and
- the chemokines.

Although over a hundred cytokines have been identified, only interleukin-2, interferon alpha and tumour necrosis factor alpha have established roles in the management of cancer. Their use in cancer therapy is decreasing because of significant toxicity and the development of better-tolerated and more effective protein kinase inhibitors.

Interleukin-2 (IL-2)

IL-2 was first identified as a T-cell growth factor in 1976. It is released by T-helper cells and induces activation of both T-helper cells and cytotoxic T-cells. *In vitro* incubation of lymphoid cells with recombinant IL-2 leads to the generation of lymphokine-activated killer (LAK) cells, which are able to lyse fresh tumour suspensions.

IL-2 is given by continuous i.v. infusion or subcutaneously. It has been used in metastatic renal cancer (Coppin *et al.*, 2004), but is contraindicated in patients with a poor WHO performance status (PS), multiple sites of metastatic disease, and more than 24 months between initial diagnosis and treatment (Palmer *et al.*, 1992). It has also been used in metastatic melanoma (Atkins *et al.*, 2000).

IL-2 is very toxic, causing capillary leak syndrome, hypotension, cardiac arrhythmias, pulmonary oedema, fever and death. Therefore, patients should be selected carefully and only treated in centres with experienced clinicians and the facility to provide haemodynamic support.

Interferon alpha (IFNα)

Interferons (IFNs) have anti-viral, anti-proliferative and immunomodulatory effects and are of three types: alpha (α), beta (β) and gamma (γ). Only IFNα is used as cancer therapy.

Naturally occurring IFNα is produced by many cells, including T- and B-lymphocytes, fibroblasts, endothelial cells and osteoblasts. It acts by stimulating macrophages, natural killer cells and cytotoxic T-lymphocytes.

IFNα has been used in metastatic renal cancer, in melanoma both as adjuvant treatment and for metastatic disease and in the following haematological malignancies: hairy cell leukaemia, Philadelphia-positive CML, cutaneous T-cell lymphoma and follicular non-Hodgkin lymphoma, as well as asymptomatic AIDS-related Kaposi's sarcoma.

Its main toxicities are flu-like symptoms, fatigue, depression, neutropenia and reversible hepatotoxicity. Long-term treatment (12–18 months) may be difficult to tolerate, and is associated with hypothyroidism.

Tumour necrosis factor alpha (TNFα)

TNFα is a cytokine involved in cell signalling of the acute inflammatory response and is produced by macrophages and a variety of other haemopoietic cells. It has been used in isolated limb perfusion in combination with melphalan for unresectable melanoma of the extremities.

Haemopoietic colony-stimulating factors

Granulocyte colony-stimulating factor (G-CSF)

Recombinant G-CSF is available for clinical use in short- and long-acting (pegylated) forms. It can reduce the morbidity and mortality of neutropenia, and prevent treatment delays in patients receiving chemotherapy. Indications are:

- Primary prophylaxis with the first cycle of chemotherapy (see Chapter 1).
- Secondary prophylaxis in subsequent cycles following the first episode of febrile neutropenia (see Chapter 1).
- Therapeutically, to reduce duration of neutropenia during acute infective episode (see Chapter 6).

- To allow the delivery of dose-dense chemotherapy regimens (chemotherapy regimens in which the cycle length has been reduced).

The aim of dose-dense chemotherapy is to deliver multiple, reduced-interval treatment cycles, using G-CSF to support the recovery from myelosuppression. There is evidence of a survival benefit with this approach in NHL (Pfreundschuh *et al.*, 2004) and breast cancer (Citron *et al.*, 2003). However the administration schedule is not yet standardised, and different regimens are the subject of clinical trials.

Granulocyte–macrophage colony-stimulating factor (GM-CSF)

GM-CSF is a growth factor which stimulates the proliferation and differentiation of haemapoietic progenitor cells to form neutrophils, monocytes/macrophages and myeloid-derived dendritic cells, as well as activating mature granulocytes and macrophages. It is licensed in the US, although not currently in Europe or the UK, for use in acute myeloid leukaemia, to mobilise autologous peripheral stem cells before harvesting for bone marrow transplantation and for myeloid repopulation following stem cell transplant.

Erythropoietin

Recombinant human erythropoietin, analogous to the native glycoprotein hormone produced predominantly by the kidneys which regulates erythrocyte production, is an alternative to blood transfusion in cancer patients. It reduces the risks associated with transfusion including alloimmunisation, severe complications if mismatched blood is given and the transfer of blood-borne viral infections. Multiple recombinant erythropoietins are licensed for use in patients receiving chemotherapy who have symptomatic anaemia with a haemoglobin level less than 100 g/L, including epoetin alfa, beta, theta and zeta, and the longer-acting hyperglycosylated darbepoetin alfa. There remain concerns about the effects of erythropoietin analogues on tumour progression, and increased cardiovascular risks, especially thromboembolism.

The National Institute for Health and Care Excellence (NICE) recommends the use of these drugs in combination with intravenous iron for chemotherapy-induced anaemia (NICE, 2014).

Table 2.4 Examples of tumour-associated antigens that are potential targets for cancer vaccines

Tumour-associated antigen	Tumour
Alpha feto-protein (*a*FP)	Hepatocellular
B catenin	Melanoma
Cancer/testis antigen (CTAG; also called NY-ESO-1)	Testis, ovary, glioma, melanoma, ovarian, sarcoma, breast or non-small-cell lung cancer
Carcino-embryonic antigen (CEA)	Colon, bladder, breast
Caspase 8	Head and neck tumours (squamous cell carcinoma)
Cell division cycle associated 1 (CDCA1)	Brain, gastrointestinal, lung, breast, head and neck
DEP domain containing 1 (DEPDC1)	Lung
Epidermal growth factor receptor variant III (EGFRvIII)	Glioblastoma
Epstein Barr Virus (EBV) antigen	Nasopharyngeal cancers
Gangliosides	Melanoma
Human epidermal growth factor receptor 2 (HER2/ERBB2)	Breast, ovarian, colon, prostate, pancreas, lung
Human telomerase reverse transcriptase (hTERT)	Breast, pancreas, lung
IGF II mRNA binding protein 3 (KOC1)	Lung
Kinesin-like protein (KIF20A)	Lung
Mammaglobin-A (secretoglobin family 2A member 2, SCGB2A2)	Breast
Melanoma antigen expression family (MAGE)	Melanoma, breast, bladder (normal testicular proteins)
Melanoma antigen recognised by T-cells 1/Melan A (MART)	Melanoma
M phase phosphoprotein 1 (MPHOSPH1)	Lung
Mucin 1 (MUC1)	Breast, pancreatic, lung, renal cell, colorectal, bladder
Oncofetal antigen (OFA)	Breast
p16INK4a/human papilloma virus (HPV) antigen	HPV-associated cervical, vulvar, vaginal, penile, anal and head and neck squamous cell carcinomas
Prostate-specific antigen (PSA)	Prostate
Prostatic acid phosphatase (PAP)	Prostate
Renal antigen expression family (RAGE)	Melanoma, kidney
Survivin	Melanoma, pancreas, colon, cervix
TTK	Lung
Transforming growth factor β (TGF-β) receptor II	Colorectal
Upregulated gene in lung cancer 10 (URLC10)	Lung
Vascular endothelial growth factor receptor (VEGFR)	Lung, pancreas

Data collated from Espinoza-Delgado (2002), Janeway *et al.* (2001) and Rosenberg *et al.* (2004) and from the National Cancer Institute and the UK Clinical Research Network (www.cancer.gov/clinicaltrials/ and http://public.ukcrn.org.uk/search/, accessed January 2015).

Vaccines

Vaccination has been investigated as a treatment option in the prevention and management of cancer. In cancers where there is a known infectious cause, vaccination provides a prevention strategy. A major advance has been the development of two vaccines against human papilloma virus (HPV), the main cause of cervical cancer. In the US, vaccination against hepatitis B is recommended as prophylaxis against hepatocellular cancer.

The aim of vaccination as treatment for an established tumour is to stimulate a cellular immune response against specific tumour-associated antigens that will lead to the death of the tumour cell. To achieve this:

- the tumour antigen needs to be recognised on an antigen-presenting cell (ApC) by interaction with a cytotoxic T-cell receptor;
- the ApCs need to be co-stimulated through members of the B7 family and various adhesion molecules (e.g. ICAM1);
- effector mechanisms need to be generated (e.g. secretion of cytokines causing tumour cell destruction);
- immune-suppressive factors produced by the tumour (e.g. TGF-β) need to be avoided.

Tumour-associated antigens are usually proteins, but they can also be carbohydrates (e.g. gangliosides) or glycoproteins. Their expression by cancer cells may differ from normal cells only in a quantitative manner (i.e. they are present in significantly greater amounts than in normal cells). There are a number of tumour-associated antigens currently being investigated as targets for vaccination, as shown in Table 2.4.

Antigen vaccines

Viral proteins from cancer-causing viruses may be used as antigens to prevent infection by the virus. HPV virus types 16 and 18 are responsible for about 70% of cervical cancers. Two vaccines have been developed which use non-infectious virus-like particles of the major capsid protein L1. Cervarix® prevents infection by HPV types 16 and 18 and shows some cross-protection against other oncogenic HPV viruses, such as HPV 31 and 45 (Harper *et al.*, 2006). Gardasil® prevents infection by HPV 16 and 18, and by the HPV types 6 and 11, which are responsible for genital warts (Ault, 2007). In the UK, Gardasil® is offered to girls aged 12 and 13, as a regimen of 3 intramuscular injections over a maximum of 12 months, with the optimal scheduling being at 0, 1 and 4–6 months. It is hoped that HPV vaccines will have a major impact on the incidence of cervical cancer in the future.

Currently, research is focussing on peptides derived from tumour-associated antigens or gangliosides (which are sialated glycolipid antigens) as potential vaccines. However, at present, only sipuleucel-T, which combines a peptide-based vaccine with cellular immunotherapy, is commercially available (see next paragraph).

Cellular vaccines

Cellular vaccines can be based on whole cells, tumour lysates or antigens that have been shed from the surface of tumour cells grown *in vitro*. Sipuleucel-T is an intravenously administered vaccine targeted against the glycoprotein prostatic acid phosphatase (PAP) antigen which is expressed by most prostate cancers. It is licensed for the treatment of asymptomatic or minimally symptomatic castrate-resistant metastatic (non-visceral) prostate cancer, when chemotherapy is not clinically indicated. Dendritic cells are potent antigen-presenting cells, which can be manipulated to present a tumour-associated antigen, and thus increase the chances of an immune response. Their use, and that of a number of other potential vaccines, is currently restricted to clinical trials.

Vaccines as immune stimulants

Live attenuated *Mycobacterium bovis* bacillus Calmette–Guerlin (BCG) vaccine has been used since the 1980s as intravesical treatment for superficial transitional cell cancers of the bladder, either alone or as an adjuvant after transurethral resection. It is not specifically targeted at tumour antigens, and its exact mechanism of action is unclear. It is thought to evoke strongly cytotoxic immune responses, involving T-cell and macrophage induction, and increased expression within the bladder and in the urine of multiple cytokines including IFNγ, IL-1, IL-2, IL-6, IL-8, IL-12, TNFα and tumour necrosis factor apoptosis-inducing ligand (TRAIL), as well as being a direct suppressor of tumour growth (Lockyer, 2001; Schenk-Braat, 2005; Rosevear *et al.*, 2009).

Clinical results

A review of cancer vaccines by the National Cancer Institute (USA) showed that the objective response rate in 440 patients with established tumours was only 2.6% (Rosenberg *et al.*, 2004). However, since this publication, the field of cancer vaccine research has grown significantly. The expectation is that with increasing understanding of the mechanisms of immune responses to tumours, targeted therapies (including vaccines) are likely to play an ever more important role in cancer prevention and treatment.

References

Atkins, M. B., Kunkel, L., Sznol, M., *et al.* (2000). High-dose recombinant interleukin-2 therapy in patients with metastatic melanoma: long-term survival update. *Cancer J. Sci. Am.*, **6**(Suppl. 1), S11–14.

Ault, K. A. (2007). Effect of prophylactic human papillomavirus L1 virus-like-particle vaccine on risk of cervical intraepithelial neoplasia grade 2, grade 3, and adenocarcinoma in situ: a combined analysis of four randomised clinical trials. *Lancet*, **369**, 1861–68.

Citron, M. L., Berry, D. A., Cirrincione, C., *et al.* (2003). Randomized trial of dose-dense versus conventionally scheduled and sequential versus concurrent combination chemotherapy as postoperative adjuvant treatment of node-positive primary breast cancer: first report of Intergroup Trial C9741/Cancer and Leukemia Group B Trial 9741. *J. Clin. Oncol.*, **21**, 1431–39.

Coppin, C., Porzsolt, F., Autenrieth, M., *et al.* (2004). Immunotherapy for advanced renal cell cancer. *Cochrane Database of Systematic Reviews*, Issue 3. Art. No.: CD001425.

Espinoza-Delgado, I. (2002). Cancer vaccines. *Oncologist*, 7(Suppl. 3), 20–33.

Harper, D. M., Franco, E. L., Wheeler, C. M., *et al.* (2006). Sustained efficacy of up to 4.5 years of a bivalent L1 virus-like particle vaccine against human papillomavirus types 16 and 18: follow-up from a randomised control trial. *Lancet*, **367**, 1247–55.

Harris, M. (2004). Monoclonal antibodies as therapeutic agents for cancer. *Lancet Oncol.*, **5**, 292–302.

Janeway, C. A., Travers, P., Walport, M., *et al.* (2001). *Immunobiology: The Immune System in Health and Disease*, 5th edn. New York: Garland.

Lockyer, C. R. W. and Gillat, D. A. (2001). BCG immunotherapy for superficial bladder cancer *J. R. Soc. Med.* **94**, 119–23.

NICE. (2014). *Erythropoiesis-stimulating agents (epoetin and darbepoetin) for treating anaemia in people with cancer having chemotherapy (including review of TA142) (TA323)*. London: National Institute for Health and Care Excellence.

Palmer, P. A., Vinke, J., Philip, T., *et al.* (1992). Prognostic factors for survival in patients with advanced renal cell carcinoma treated with recombinant interleukin-2. *Ann. Oncol.*, **3**, 475–80.

Pfreundschuh, M., Trumper, L., Kloess, M., *et al.* (2004). Two-weekly or 3-weekly CHOP chemotherapy with or without etoposide for the treatment of young patients with good-prognosis (normal LDH) aggressive lymphomas: results of the NHL-B1 trial of the DSHNHL. *Blood*, **104**, 626–33.

Rosenberg, S. A., Yang, J. C. and Restifo, N. P. (2004). Cancer immunotherapy: moving beyond current vaccines. *Nat. Med.*, **10**, 909–15.

Rosevear, H. M., Lightfoot, A. J., O'Donnell, M. A., *et al.* (2009). The role of neutrophils and TNF-related apoptosis-inducing ligand (TRAIL) in bacillus Calmette–Guérin (BCG) immunotherapy for urothelial carcinoma of the bladder *Cancer Metast. Rev.*, **28**, 345–53.

Schenk-Braat, E. A. M. and Bangma, C. H. (2005). Immunotherapy for superficial bladder cancer. *Cancer Immunol. Immun.*, **54**, 414–23.

Wick, J. (2004). What's in a drug name? *J. Am. Pharm. Assoc.*, **44**, 12–14.

Hormones in cancer

Jacinta Abraham and John Staffurth

Introduction

Hormonal therapies are some of the oldest active systemic anti-cancer therapies in use today. In 1896, Beatson demonstrated that surgical oophorectomy resulted in tumour regression in some premenopausal women with metastatic breast cancer, and, by doing so, he was the first to identify a link between ovarian function and breast cancer (Beatson, 1896).

Substantial evidence now exists that hormones play a key role in both the cause and the outcome of several cancers. Although this is most clearly seen in breast and prostate cancer, other cancers that may exhibit hormone dependence include endometrial, ovarian and testicular cancers.

Hormones are classified into two groups:

- non-steroidal hormones including peptides, polypeptides or derivatives of amino acids, generally acting via cell-membrane-localised receptors which trigger second messengers within the cytoplasm; and
- steroidal hormones, such as oestrogens, androgens and progestins, bind to intracellular receptors to mediate their action.

This chapter will focus primarily on steroidal hormones that are of particular importance in breast and prostate cancer: oestrogens, progestins and androgens. It should be read in conjunction with the relevant site-specific chapters (Chapters 19 and 22). This chapter provides some background knowledge of the production and functioning of hormones and their receptors, which will help in the understanding of commonly used therapies. The aetiology of hormone-related cancers is discussed in the relevant site-specific chapters.

Steroidal hormones have the potential to activate oncogenes or inactivate tumour-suppressor genes, producing a sequence of changes within the cell that ultimately lead to cancer. The continued growth of the cancer often depends on continuing hormone stimulation and so removing the hormonal stimulus causes the cancer to regress. Anti-cancer hormone therapies work in a number of different ways – by affecting hormone synthesis, metabolism or action, or by altering hormone receptor expression within the cell.

A summary of the major historical landmarks in anti-cancer hormonal therapy since Beatson's observation in 1896 is listed here.

- Large doses of oestrogenic steroids inhibit gonadotropin secretion in women (Zondek, 1940).
- Surgical orchidectomy results in the regression of advanced prostate cancer (Huggins and Hodges, 1941).
- Adrenalectomy results in regression of advanced breast and prostate cancers (Huggins and Bergenstal, 1952).
- Prolonged exposure to oestrogens or androgens, alone or in combination, leads to breast and prostate cancers in rats (Noble, 1980).

Hormone synthesis

Oestrogen synthesis

In premenopausal women, oestrogens are synthesised from cholesterol. Oestrogen synthesis takes place mainly in the granulosa cells of the ovaries; production is cyclical and is controlled by positive and negative feedback via the hypothalamic–pituitary–gonadal axis (see Figure 3.1). Inhibin is a polypeptide which is also produced by ovarian granulosa cells, and it inhibits follicle-stimulating hormone (FSH) release by pituitary gonadotrophs.

Practical Clinical Oncology, Second Edition, ed. Louise Hanna, Tom Crosby and Fergus Macbeth. Published by Cambridge University Press. © Cambridge University Press 2015.

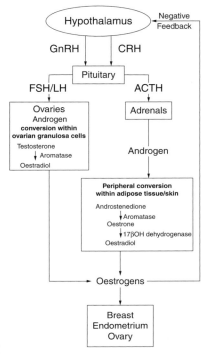

Figure 3.1 The hypothalamic–pituitary–gonadal axis in the female. ACTH, adrenocorticotrophic hormone; CRH, corticotropin-releasing hormone; FSH, follicle-stimulating hormone; GnRH, gonadotropin-releasing hormone; LH, luteinising hormone.

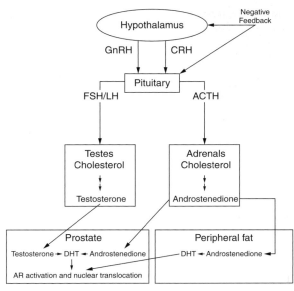

Figure 3.2 The hypothalamic–pituitary–gonadal axis in the male. ACTH, adrenocorticotrophic hormone; AR, androgen receptor; CRH, corticotropin-releasing hormone; DHT, 5α-dihydrotestosterone; FSH, follicle-stimulating hormone; GnRH, gonadotropin-releasing hormone; LH, luteinising hormone. Testosterone, DHT, androstenedione and circulating oestrogens contribute to negative feedback.

In postmenopausal women, the main site of oestrogen synthesis is the adipose tissue, via the enzyme aromatase, and production may vary depending on environmental and genetic factors such as obesity.

In men, 30% of plasma oestrogens originate from the testis and 70% arise from peripheral aromatisation of androstenedione and testosterone; testosterone is converted to oestradiol by the enzyme aromatase. Although only 0.5% of the total daily production of testosterone is converted, oestradiol is a much more potent gonadotropin inhibitor than testosterone.

Androgen synthesis

In men, the main circulating androgen is testosterone, 95% of which is produced by the Leydig cells of the testis (see Figure 3.2). The remaining circulating androgens, including dihydroxyandrostenedione (DHA), androstenedione, and DHA sulphate, are produced in the adrenal cortex from cholesterol. These androgens diffuse passively into the prostate and are metabolised to the more biologically active 5α-dihydrotestosterone (DHT), which binds to the androgen receptor (AR) with a three- to five-times greater affinity than testosterone.

Hormone receptors

Oestrogen receptor

There are two oestrogen receptors (ERs) which are encoded by separate genes:

- oestrogen receptor alpha (ERα) is encoded by a gene on chromosome 6;
- oestrogen receptor beta (ERβ) is encoded on chromosome 14.

The two receptors have a similar structure, but they share only 47% amino acid homology.

Not all ER-positive breast cancers respond to hormonal treatments, and there is some evidence that different expression of the two ERs in breast cancer cells affects hormone responsiveness and hormone resistance. For example, ERα is often markedly upregulated in breast cancer and it is the marker that can best predict responsiveness to hormonal treatments. However, ERβ may modulate the ability of cells to respond to oestrogen, and its expression has been implicated in tamoxifen resistance (Miller *et al.*, 2006).

Oestrogen receptor functioning

To understand how anti-oestrogen treatments work, it is necessary to be aware of three important domains on the ER: activating functions 1 and 2 (AF1 and AF2), which carry out the effector functions of the receptor, and the ligand-binding domain. First, oestradiol binds to the ER in the nucleus via the ligand binding domain on AF2, and this causes dimerisation, phosphorylation and a conformational shape change. This allows the ER to bind to DNA oestrogen response elements (EREs), which are upstream of oestrogen-responsive genes. Second, the transcriptional activity of the genes that contain EREs is modulated by AF1 and/or AF2. Third, co-regulator proteins can also influence ER-mediated transcription; depending on the ligand, the ER interacts with either co-repressors or co-activators to inhibit or enhance its transcriptional activity on target genes (Milano *et al.*, 2006).

Tamoxifen blocks AF2 when it competes with oestradiol for ER binding, but AF1 remains functional, which accounts for the oestrogenic activity seen in some tissues. Aromatase inhibitors block the production of oestrogens, and in doing so they effectively prevent the action of both AF1 and AF2.

Oestrogenic effects

The following is a list of the effects of oestrogen.

- Development of female secondary sexual characteristics.
- Endometrial growth.
- Bone formation in both women and men.
- Procoagulant.
- Reduced low-density lipoprotein (LDL).

Progesterone receptor

There is one gene for the progesterone receptor (PgR), but it exists as two isoforms, A (PR-A) and B (PR-B), which have different physiological functions. PgR is important in mammary gland development, and an excess production of PR-B is associated with breast cancer risk. However, PR-A can repress PR-B and ER and its expression is related to tamoxifen resistance (Hopp *et al.*, 2004).

Main actions of progesterone

Progesterone performs the following actions.

- Causes endometrial secretory phase.
- Increases the viscosity of cervical mucus.
- Facilitates mammary gland development.

Receptor status in breast cancer and response to hormone therapy

At present, it is standard practice to measure ER and PgR status in breast cancer, but it is not usual to distinguish between the subtypes. Approximately 75% of postmenopausal and 50% of premenopausal women with breast cancer will have hormone-receptor-positive tumours. Whether the cancer is sensitive to hormone treatment is related to the degree of ER and PgR positivity, but receptor status alone is not the only determinant of hormone responsiveness.

- ER+/PgR+ disease confers the highest response rates of up to 70%. The response is less for ER+/PgR– cancers.
- In contrast, ER–/PgR– cancers, with current testing, have a response rate to hormone therapy of less than 5% and patients with these tumours are likely to derive a greater benefit from chemotherapy.
- ER–/PgR+ cancers account for 5% of all breast cancers and they should be regarded as being hormone-responsive because they will have response rates of up to 30%.
- An ER-negative status may be detected in metastatic or recurrent disease even when the primary tumour is ER-positive. It is not clear if this represents a change in ER expression or a heterogeneous primary tumour in which the ER-negative component has a survival advantage, allowing it to metastasise.

Androgen receptor

The AR gene is on the long arm of the X chromosome, q11-13, and has eight exons. In contrast to breast cancer, the measurement of AR in patients with prostate cancer is not performed routinely because both hormone-dependent and hormone-independent prostate cancers possess functioning AR; AR status provides no prognostic or diagnostic value. There is, however, evidence for the prognostic value of androgen receptor expression in subtypes of breast cancer such as ER-negative or triple negative disease, where loss of expression of the androgen receptor may predict a worse prognosis.

Androgen receptor functioning

DHT binds to the AR via the ligand-binding domain, and this binding results in separation from heat shock protein 90 (HSP-90; a protein that maintains the AR in an inactive state), dimerisation to form a DHT–AR complex, phosphorylation and a conformational shape change. The complex is translocated to the nucleus of prostate cells, allowing DNA binding of the AR to androgen response elements (AREs) upstream of androgen-regulated genes. The activity of genes containing AREs can be modulated by transcription factors via the highly variable amino-terminal domain (ATD).

Androgenic effects

The effects of androgen include the following.

- Virilisation and development of secondary sexual characteristics.
- Development of prostate and seminal vesicles.
- Increased muscle mass.
- Increased bone density.
- Increased libido and frequency of erection.

Breast cancer treatment: ovarian function suppression (OFS)

In premenopausal women, the most obvious and direct way to reduce oestrogen production is to suppress ovarian function, by chemical, radiotherapeutic or surgical treatments. Chemical ablation uses gonadotropin-releasing hormone (GnRH/LHRH) agonists such as goserelin, which is currently the treatment of choice, particularly in early breast cancer, because its effects are reversible. The hormonal effects of goserelin may be observed by measuring plasma levels of luteinising hormone (LH), FSH, and oestradiol.

In advanced disease, all three techniques are essentially equivalent and they produce response rates of 25–30%, with a median response duration of 9–12 months. In early breast cancer, OFS has been shown to produce a survival benefit equivalent to that achieved by chemotherapy (EBCTG, 2005). The various roles of OFS, endocrine therapy and chemotherapy in early breast cancer are now the subject of clinical

trials coordinated by the International Breast Cancer Study Group (IBCSG).

Breast cancer treatment: other hormone therapies

Table 3.1 summarises some hormonal therapies used in breast cancer.

Anti-oestrogens

Tamoxifen

Tamoxifen is the most studied and widely used anti-oestrogen in breast cancer; it has been the mainstay of endocrine therapy for breast cancer for many years. Tamoxifen is a selective oestrogen receptor modulator (SERM) because of its agonist and antagonist activities, which cause a varied effect on genes, cells, and tissues.

Mode of action of tamoxifen

- SERMs modulate oestrogen activity by binding to the ER, resulting in a conformational shape change. This alters the balance of co-activator and co-repressor complexes and affects the regulation of activation domain AF2. AF1 remains active, accounting for the oestrogenic effects of tamoxifen.
  - Impaired transcription of oestrogen-dependent genes occurs in the breast.
  - Tamoxifen also reduces plasma levels of the potent cancer mitogen IGF1.

Clinical studies of adjuvant tamoxifen

Five years of postsurgical adjuvant tamoxifen reduces the annual recurrence rate by 41% and annual mortality rate by 34% in ER-positive early breast cancer (EBCTCG, 2005). A meta-analysis showed that 5 years of tamoxifen therapy (EBCTCG, 2011) reduced the 15-year risk of breast cancer recurrence and death.

There is evidence for a reduction in breast cancer recurrence and mortality by continuing tamoxifen in ER-positive disease for 10 years rather 5. In the ATLAS (Adjuvant Tamoxifen: Longer Against Shorter) trial, continuing rather than stopping tamoxifen reduced breast cancer recurrences (617 versus 711 recurrences; $p = 0.002$), breast cancer mortality (331 versus 397 deaths; $p = 0.01$) and overall mortality (639 versus 722 deaths; $p = 0.01$; Davis et al., 2013).

Table 3.1 Selected hormonal therapies in breast cancer

Drug	Type	Dose/route	Mode of action
Tamoxifen	Antioestrogen	20 mg daily p.o.	Competes with oestradiol for ER binding
Anastrazole	Non-steroidal aromatase inhibitor	1 mg daily p.o.	Competitive aromatase inhibition
Letrozole	Non-steroidal aromatase inhibitor	2.5 mg daily p.o.	Competitive aromatase inhibition
Exemestane	Steroidal aromatase inhibitor	25 mg daily p.o.	Irreversible aromatase inhibition
Fulvestrant	ER antagonist	Loading dose 250 mg 2-weekly followed by 250 mg (5 mL) monthly i.m.	Downregulation of the ER protein
Megestrol acetate	Progestin	80–160 mg daily p.o.	Cellular action not fully understood; downregulation of ovarian steroidogenesis
Aminoglutethimide	First generation aromatase inhibitor	250 mg twice daily p.o.	Inhibits the aromatase enzyme; is given with hydrocortisone to prevent adrenal insufficiency; rarely used because of side effects including rash, dizziness, nausea and drowsiness

ER, oestrogen receptor.

In the aTTom trial, 10 years of tamoxifen was associated with a significant 15% reduction in the risk of recurrence (relative risk [RR] 0.85, 95% CI [0.76, 0.95]; $p = 0.003$) and a significant 25% reduction in the risk of breast cancer mortality starting at year 10 (RR 0.75, 95% CI [0.63, 0.90]; $p = 0.007$) compared with 5 years of tamoxifen, in the 6953 women enrolled in the trial (Gray *et al.*, 2013).

Tamoxifen is beneficial in both pre- and postmenopausal women.

Adverse effects and beneficial effects of tamoxifen

- Increased adverse effects compared to placebo: hot flushes (64% versus 48%), vaginal discharge (30% versus 15%), irregular menses (25% versus 19%), and thrombotic events (1.7% versus 0.4%) (Fisher *et al.*, 1989).
- Thrombotic events; deep vein thrombosis and pulmonary embolism. The risk is increased further when tamoxifen is co-administered with chemotherapy. Tamoxifen should be avoided in individuals at increased risk of thrombosis.
- An increased risk of endometrial changes, including hyperplasia and polyps, caused by oestrogen agonist effects, and a small but statistically significant increase in endometrial cancer. Women on tamoxifen with abnormal vaginal bleeding should be investigated promptly.
- Beneficial effects of the weak agonist effect of tamoxifen are a reduction in cholesterol levels, decreased cardiac morbidity and increased bone mineral density in postmenopausal women.

Fulvestrant

Fulvestrant is an ER antagonist that competitively binds and downregulates the ER protein; no oestrogen agonist effect has been demonstrated. It is licensed for use in postmenopausal hormone-positive advanced breast cancer that has progressed following anti-oestrogen therapy. Side effects include gastrointestinal symptoms, headache, back pain, hot flushes and pharyngitis.

Table 3.2 Summary of main studies of early breast cancer that compare AIs with tamoxifen; updated results

Trial	Study design	Patients (n)	Median FU	DFS	Other
ATAC	Upfront anastrazole vs tamoxifen for 5 years or in combination (included ER unknown and negative)	9366	120 months	Improved for anastrazole (HR 0.91, 95% CI 0.83–0.99, $p = 0.04$)	No benefit for combination arm; benefit greater in receptor-positive patients
BIG-98	Letrozole (L) vs tamoxifen (T); 5 years T or 5 years L or 2 years T, 3 years L or 2 years L, 3 years T	8010	76 months	Improved for letrozole (HR 0.88, 95% CI 0.78–0.99, $p = 0.03$)	Results account for 25% of patients crossing over from tamoxifen to letrozole after unblinding
IES	Tamoxifen for 5 years vs 2–3 years tamoxifen and switch to 2–3 years exemestane	4742	91 months	Improved for exemestane (HR 0.81, 95% CI 0.71–0.92, $p = 0.001$)	Overall survival benefit in the ER+ group for switching to exemestane: HR 0.86, 95% CI 0.75–0.99, $p = 0.04$
MA.17	Tamoxifen for 5 years followed by letrozole for 5 years or placebo for 5 years	5187	64 months	Improved for letrozole (HR 0.52, 95% CI 0.45–0.61, $p < 0.001$)	Overall survival benefit with letrozole compared to placebo adjusting for crossover effect: HR 0.61, 95% CI 0.45–0.61, $p < 0.001$

CI, confidence interval; DFS, disease-free survival; ER, oestrogen receptor; FU, follow-up; HR, hazard ratio. Adapted from Bliss *et al.*, 2012; Cuzick *et al.*, 2010; Jin *et al.*, 2012; Joerger *et al.*, 2009.

Aromatase inhibitors (AIs)

Types

The first-generation AIs include aminoglutethimide. It has significant side effects and has been largely superseded by third-generation AIs which are better tolerated.

AIs are either type 1 steroidal inhibitors, which irreversibly inactivate aromatase (e.g. exemestane and formestane), or type 2 non-steroidal competitive inhibitors such as anastrozole and letrozole.

Mode of action

AIs inhibit or inactivate the p450 enzyme aromatase, and significantly reduce serum oestradiol. They are contraindicated in premenopausal women because ovarian suppression would lead to feedback on the hypothalamic–pituitary–gonadal axis, resulting in gonadal stimulation. When AIs are indicated in these patients, the AIs should be given only after suppression of ovarian function.

Use in early postmenopausal breast cancer

Several studies of early breast cancer have shown that AIs are safe and effective and increase disease-free survival when compared with tamoxifen. These studies have helped redefine the optimal hormonal strategy for breast cancer patients as shown in Table 3.2. A greater understanding of primary resistance to tamoxifen (in particular, being able to predict who is going to have tamoxifen-resistant disease) and longer-term follow-up data may help identify the subgroups that might benefit most from initial or subsequent AIs.

Use in premenopausal breast cancer

AIs are contraindicated in premenopausal women unless they are undergoing OFS. In early premenopausal breast cancer, the role of concurrent use of OFS and AI is the subject of ongoing clinical trials coordinated by Breast International Group (BIG)/IBCSG. In advanced disease, there is clearly a role for OFS and AI use in women who have advanced disease and receptor-positive tumours and who have progressed on tamoxifen.

AIs alone should be used with caution in premenopausal women who have become amenorrhoeic after chemotherapy. AIs may promote recovery of ovarian function in some of these women, even up to the age of 50 and after many months of amenorrhoea (Smith *et al.*, 2006). It is suggested that serial measurements of oestradiol, LH and FSH levels should be performed, but these measurements require validated, sensitive immunoassays which are not available in all centres.

Adverse effects of aromatase inhibitors

The comparative studies of AIs and tamoxifen have provided excellent toxicity data. Tamoxifen is associated more with thromboembolic events, vaginal discharge and endometrial hyperplasia or cancers, whereas the AIs are linked more with osteoporosis, fractures and arthralgia.

AIs are associated with an increased risk of musculoskeletal events, including arthralgia, fractures and reduced bone mineral density (BMD). The clinical relevance of this reduction in BMD and how it should be monitored while the patient receives an AI are unclear. The ATAC bone substudy showed that women who had normal BMD at the outset and were treated with an AI did not become osteopenic or osteoporotic after 5 years (Howell *et al.*, 2005). Those with a reduced BMD at the start were more at risk of developing a further reduction. Individuals who are at a high risk of osteoporosis (see list that follows) should be monitored and given strong advice on diet and lifestyle (i.e. high-calcium diet and smoking cessation). The role of bisphosphonates in early breast cancer patients at risk of osteoporosis is a subject of current clinical trials.

Risk factors for osteoporosis include the following:

- Radiographic evidence of osteopenia and/or vertebral deformity.
- Loss of height, thoracic kyphosis.
- Previous fragility fracture.
- Prolonged corticosteroid use.
- Premature menopause (< 45 years).
- Prolonged secondary amenorrhoea (> 1 year).
- Primary hypogonadism.
- Maternal history of osteoporosis.
- Low body mass index (< 19 kg/m^2).

The rate of thrombotic events is reduced when using AIs rather than tamoxifen. The rates of hot flushes are similar.

Progestins

The two most widely used progestins are megestrol acetate and medroxyprogesterone acetate. These compounds are thought to act directly via the PgR, but they also have an indirect action on the ER. Their biochemical effects are complex and not well understood. Progestins decrease the circulating levels of gonadotropins, interfere with steroid synthesis, and exhibit glucocorticoid activity, which can lead to corticosteroidal side effects and adrenocorticotrophic hormone suppression.

The optimal progestin dose is controversial. High doses have been used in premenopausal women, but this is also associated with increased side effects. The several side effects seen with their use include weight gain, fluid retention, breast tenderness, nausea and hypertension.

Breast cancer treatment: mechanisms of resistance

Hormone-positive tumours may show resistance to endocrine therapy, either at first exposure (*de novo*) or after a period of time (acquired). Understanding the mechanisms of resistance will help to predict the likely response to specific treatments and will help in the development of new agents targeted at endocrine-resistant pathways at the molecular level.

Nearly all patients with advanced breast cancer who initially respond to hormone therapy will ultimately become hormone-refractory. The development of resistance to tamoxifen does not necessarily predict resistance to an AI; patients initially responding to tamoxifen have a 50% response rate to AIs.

De novo resistance

A strongly ER-positive tumour is likely to respond better to tamoxifen than one with a weakly positive ER status. However, ER status alone does not accurately predict for intrinsic resistance.

Possible mechanisms of resistance include the following.

- Some of the actions of oestrogens appear to be mediated through transcription factors such as activator protein 1 (AP-1). Enhanced activation of AP-1 transcription factors has been associated with tamoxifen resistance in both human breast cancers and xenografts.
- Expression of ERβ has been seen to activate AP-1-regulated genes when bound to tamoxifen. Increased expression of ERβ is implicated in tamoxifen resistance.
- ERs located in the membrane can activate growth-factor-signalling pathways; this bidirectional crosstalk between signalling pathways may be active in endocrine resistance, for example, binding of oestrogen, and even tamoxifen in membrane ER can activate the epidermal growth factor family receptors (Milano et al., 2006).

Acquired resistance

Peptide growth factor receptor pathways such as epidermal growth factor receptor (EGFR) and human epidermal growth factor receptor 2 (HER2) become selectively upregulated in breast cancer cells that acquire resistance to tamoxifen during prolonged exposure, and they are an alternative mechanism stimulating cell growth. Enhanced expression of EGFR and subsequent downstream mitogen-activated protein kinase (MAPK) activation have been found in MCF-7 breast cancer cells that become resistant to tamoxifen over time. In addition, the effect of low levels of oestrogen stimulation induced by tamoxifen and AIs may result in sensitisation of the ER.

The agonist activity of tamoxifen is also an important mechanism of resistance; that is, tamoxifen may become an ER agonist in breast cancer cells. This concept is supported by the fact that withdrawal responses may occur, albeit rarely.

Role of the progesterone receptor in hormone resistance

In ER-positive disease, a PgR-negative status is associated with a reduced chance of response to tamoxifen, but not necessarily with AI resistance. Tamoxifen resistance may be linked to growth factor receptor pathways such as HER2. Excessive growth factor signalling or overexpression of HER2 downregulates expression of the PgR gene. Crosstalk may also occur between the ER and growth factor receptor pathways such as HER2, and so oestrogen or tamoxifen might stimulate these alternative pathways.

Support for this hypothesis comes from the ATAC study in which the benefit of time to recurrence seen with anastrozole compared with tamoxifen was greater in the ER-positive/PgR-negative subgroup compared to the ER-positive/PgR-positive subgroup (Dowsett et al., 2005). This effect was not seen in a subgroup analysis in the BIG 1–98 trial, and it remains a continuing area of research.

Non-hormonal approaches to overcoming resistance: signal transduction inhibitors

EGFR expression in cells studied during research is associated with increased proliferation and resistance to apoptosis. There is interest in whether EGFR inhibitors may overcome hormone resistance. There are several ongoing trials combining signal transduction inhibitors with hormonal therapies, e.g. aromatase inhibitors, and the results of these studies are eagerly awaited.

Breast cancer: prevention

Breast cancer chemoprevention is an area of current interest with drugs such as tamoxifen, raloxifene, exemestane and anastrazole showing activity in preventing breast cancer in unaffected women at high risk of developing the disease.

Raloxifene is a nearly pure oestrogen antagonist with no stimulatory effects on the endometrium. The STAR study of tamoxifen and raloxifene in breast cancer prevention showed that raloxifene is as effective as tamoxifen in reducing the incidence of invasive breast cancer in postmenopausal women and is associated with fewer thromboembolic events and endometrial cancers (Vogel, 2009).

For aromatase inhibitors, the IBIS-II study randomised 3864 postmenopausal women at high risk of breast cancer to anastrozole or placebo every day for 5 years. After a median follow-up of 5 years, 40 (2%) of 1920 women in the anastrozole group and 85 (4%) of 1944 in the placebo group had developed breast cancer (HR 0·47, 95% CI 0.32–0.68, $p < 0.0001$). There was no difference in breast cancer-specific or all-cause mortality (Cuzick et al., 2014).

Table 3.3 Selected hormonal therapies in prostate cancer

Drug	Type	Dose/route	Mode of action
Goserelin	LHRH agonist	3.6 mg every 28 days or 10.8 mg every 3 months s.c.	Reduces pituitary production of LH and FSH
Leuprorelin	LHRH agonist	3.75 mg every 28 days or 11.25 mg every 3 months s.c./i.m.	Reduces pituitary production of LH and FSH
Degarelix	LHRH antagonist	Loading dose 240 mg then 80 mg every 28 days s.c.	Reduces pituitary production of LH and FSH
Bicalutamide	Non-steroidal anti-androgen	50–150 mg daily p.o.	Competitive AR inhibition
Flutamide	Non-steroidal anti-androgen	250 mg t.d.s. p.o.	Competitive AR inhibition
Enzalutamide	Non-steroidal anti-androgen	160 mg daily p.o.	Inhibits AR and prevents translocation to nucleus
Abiraterone	CYP17 inhibitor	1g daily p.o. taken with prednisolone 10 mg daily p.o.	Reduces adrenal and intraprostatic production of androgens
Dexamethasone	Corticosteroid	0.5–1.5 mg daily p.o.	Reduces adrenal production of androgens
Diethylstilboestrol	Oestrogen	1–5 mg daily p.o.	Reduces pituitary production of LH and FSH

AR, androgen receptor; CYP17, cytochrome P45, 17a-hydroxylase/C17,20-lyase; FSH, follicle-stimulating hormone; LH, luteinising hormone; LHRH, luteinising hormone-releasing hormone.

Prostate cancer: hormonal therapies

The hormonal therapies most commonly used in prostate cancer are summarised in Table 3.3.

Androgen deprivation therapy

Androgen deprivation therapy (ADT) can be achieved by either castration or single agent bicalutamide (150 mg daily). Castration can be surgical (subcapsular orchidectomy) or medical (with LHRH agonists or antagonists), and it produces serum testosterone levels of less than 50 ng/mL. LHRH antagonists have the advantage of avoiding a testosterone surge and not requiring anti-androgen therapy; they can be used in emergency situations, such as impending spinal cord compression, as can diethylstilboestrol (3–5 mg daily p.o.), cyproterone acetate (100 mg t.d.s. p.o) or ketoconazole.

In advanced or recurrent prostate cancer, ADT produces responses in at least 85% of patients, often with dramatic reversal of the clinical picture.

The median duration of response is approximately 18 months, with evidence that the prostate-specific antigen (PSA) doubling time before and the PSA nadir following ADT are of prognostic significance (D'Amico et al., 2006; Rodrigues et al., 2006). Eventually, and inevitably, patients will relapse. Trials investigating adjuvant therapies that might prolong the time to relapse have generally shown no effect or only minimal benefit. However, the ongoing MRC STAMPEDE study is investigating the benefits of zoledronic acid, docetaxel, abiraterone and local radiotherapy in addition to ADT.

Mode of action

LHRH agonists, such as goserelin, leuprorelin acetate and triptorelin, are synthetic analogues of the decapeptide LHRH which have increased affinity for the LHRH receptor and reduced susceptibility to protease degradation, resulting in increased binding to the receptor. After an initial surge in LH and FSH and a rise in testosterone (unless temporary anti-androgens are used), downregulation of LHRH receptors and desensitisation of the gonadotroph to the normal pulses of LHRH occur. LH and FSH fall and castrate testosterone levels are reached in 10–20 days.

Reduced serum testosterone leads to reduced expression of androgen-regulated gene products. Some cells undergo apoptosis (androgen-dependent), some cell-cycle arrest (androgen-sensitive) and some are unaffected (androgen-insensitive). Oral administration is ineffective because LHRH agonists are rapidly cleared by the liver, but subcutaneous or intramuscular delivery gives 94% bioavailability. LHRH agonists can be given as monthly or three-monthly depot injections. The temporary rise in testosterone (flare) should be prevented by giving 3 weeks of anti-androgens (bicalutamide 50–150 mg daily, flutamide 250 mg t.d.s. or cyproterone acetate 100 mg t.d.s.), starting at least 1 week before the first LHRH agonist injection.

The LHRH antagonist, degarelix, achieves castrate levels of testosterone (≤ 0.5 ng/mL) without an initial surge in 96% of patients after 3 days and 100% after 1 month with a starting dose of 240 mg s.c. Injections are then continued at 80 mg every 4 weeks.

Clinical use

Advanced disease

LHRH agonists have been used for more than 15 years for the management of metastatic prostate cancer, as a medical alternative to orchidectomy. Trials show equivalent response rates and survival, although they have been too small to show true equivalence. However, medical castration is reversible, and it has become the preferred management approach.

Deferred therapy in locally advanced or asymptomatic metastatic disease

Patients with locally advanced or asymptomatic metastatic disease are incurable, and the balance between quality and quantity of life is very important. They may not need immediate hormonal therapy. ADT has well-documented acute and late side effects that may be avoidable for a considerable time in certain clinical situations. Deferred therapy is an option for patients with locally advanced disease who are not having radical therapy or for those with asymptomatic early metastatic disease (e.g. painless rib metastases only; Anonymous, 1997). Patients should be closely supervised and made aware of the symptoms of progressive disease. Single-agent bicalutamide may also be considered as an alternative to castration in certain situations, although it is not licensed for single-agent use in metastatic disease.

Intermittent therapy in advanced disease

Intermittent therapy may allow androgen-dependent cells to repopulate the tumour, thereby delaying the development of androgen-resistant clones, and

may reduce the side effects of long-term castration. Intermittent androgen suppression is not inferior to continuous androgen suppression for overall survival in patients with a rising PSA (at least 3 ng/mL) at least one year after radical radiotherapy for localized prostate cancer (Crook et al., 2012). In patients with newly diagnosed, metastatic, hormone-sensitive prostate cancer, a study comparing intermittent with continuous androgen was inconclusive because the event rate was low (Hussain et al., 2013). The median overall survival was 5.8 years in the continuous arm and 5.1 years in the intermittent arm (HR for death 1.10; 90% confidence interval (CI) 0.99 to 1.23).

Hormone therapy as an adjunct to radical radiotherapy

The major randomised trials investigating the combination of hormone therapy and radical radiotherapy are summarised in Table 3.4. Hormone therapy can be used either neoadjuvantly and concurrently with radiotherapy (neoadjuvant hormone therapy, NAHT) and/or as an adjuvant following radiotherapy (adjuvant hormone therapy, AHT). Early trials included predominantly patients with locally advanced or node-positive disease, but more recent trials have included those with intermediate- or high-risk localised disease. Interpretation of these trials is complicated by changes in radiotherapy technique, such as dose escalation.

Neoadjuvant hormone therapy

NAHT causes cytoreduction, maximal at around 3 months, and may radiosensitise cells. In patients with bulky tumours, NAHT reduces the volume of rectum irradiated (Zelefsky and Harrison, 1997). Radiosensitisation would be expected to improve *local* control, which is also improved with dose escalation. Multiple trials have shown convincing improvement in outcomes for patients with locally advanced disease. TROG 96.01 showed longer metastasis-free survival, cause-specific survival and overall survival with 6 months of NAHT compared to no androgen suppression. This was not seen with just 3 months of NAHT (Denham et al., 2011). Four months of NAHT has been shown to improve overall survival in intermediate-risk localised prostate cancer patients in RTOG 9408 (Jones et al., 2011). The ability of longer-duration hormonal therapy to eradicate micrometastatic disease has been studied in various trials. Three years of AHT improved 5-year overall survival in patients with locally advanced disease who were treated with prostate and pelvic radiotherapy (Bolla

Table 3.4 Studies of neoadjuvant and/or adjuvant hormonal therapies in prostate cancer; updated results

Trial	Patient group	Study design	n	Median FU (yrs)	Disease-free survival	Other results/ issues
Neoadjuvant studies						
RTOG 8610	Bulky or locally advanced	PPRT ± 4 months of MAB starting 2 months pre-RT	456	12	10-yr DFS better with NAHT (11% vs 3%, $p < 0.0001$)	Reduced 10-yr CSS and bNED with AHT
TROG 96.01	Locally advanced	Prostate and seminal vesicle RT + 0, 3, or 6 months of MAB starting 2 or 5 months pre-RT	818	10.6	Improved event-free survival with NAHT (HR 0.63, $p < 0.0001$ for 3 months; HR 0.51, $p < 0.0001$ for 6 months)	6 months NAHT only improved MDFS, CSS and OS
L101	T2–3	PrRT ± 3 months MAB starting 3 months pre-RT	161	5	Improved bNED for NAHT (HR 0.59, $p = 0.009$)	See section on combined studies, below
Crook *et al.*	T1c–T4	PrRT with 3 or 8 months MAB NAHT	378	6.6	No difference in overall trial	Improved 5-yr DFS with 8 months in high-risk group (71% vs 42%, $p = 0.01$)
RTOG 9408	T1b–T2b PSA < 20	PrRT ± 4 months of MAB starting 2 months pre-RT	1979	9.1	Improved with NAHT	Improved 10-yr OS (HR 1.17, $p = 0.03$) and DSM (HR 1.87, $p = 0.001$) with NAHT
ICORG 97-01	Intermediate or high-risk localised disease	PrRT with 4 or 8 months of NAHT	276	8.5	No difference at 5 yrs	No difference in 5-yr OS or CSS
Adjuvant studies						
MRC PR02	T2–4	Orchiectomy vs PrRT vs orchiectomy + PrRT	277			Delayed time to metastatic disease with orchiectomy
RTOG 8531	T3–4 or N1 (some pT3)	PPRT + immediate (in last week of RT) or delayed (at relapse) LHRHa	945	7.3	AHT improved 10 yrs bNED (HR 0.77, $p < 0.0001$)	Improved LDFS, MDFS, CSS, and OS with AHT; 10-yr OS 53 vs 38% (HR 0.76, $p < 0.004$)
EORTC 22863	T1–4	PPRT + concurrent and 3 yrs of AHT or LHRHa at relapse	401	5.5	AHT better (HR 0.43, $p = 0.0001$)	AHT improved CSS and OS; 5-yr OS 78 vs 62% (HR 0.59, $p = 0.0002$)

Table 3.4 (*cont.*)

Trial	Patient group	Study design	n	Median FU (yrs)	Disease-free survival	Other results/ issues
Early Prostate Cancer Trial	T1–4, N0–1, M0	PrRT ± adjuvant bicalutamide 150 mg daily for 2–5 yrs	1370	5.3	AHT better (HR 0.72, $p = 0.002$)	Improved outcome significant on subgroup analysis for locally advanced disease (T3–4) (HR 0.58, $p = 0.003$); no difference in OS
Combined studies						
L101	T2–3	PrRT + 0, 3 or 10 months of MAB starting 3 months pre-RT	161	5	No difference NAHT and NAHT/AHT	Both improved bNED compared to no HT (HR 0.59 and 0.53, $p = 0.009$)
L200	T2–3	PrRT + 5 or 10 months of MAB starting 3 months pre-RT	325	3.7	No difference NAHT and NAHT/AHT	
RTOG 9202	T2c–4	PPRT + 4 months of MAB starting 2 months pre-RT ± 2 yrs of AHT	1554	11.3	10-yr DFS improved with AHT (13% vs 23%, $p < 0.0001$)	AHT improved CSS, MDFS, and LDFS; unplanned subgroup analysis showed OS advantage for high-grade tumours ($p = 0.006$)
EORTC 22961	T1–4, N0–1	PPRT + 6m MAB ± 2.5 yrs adjuvant LHRHa	970	6.4		Additional HT improved CSS and OS; 5-yr OS 19% vs 15% (HR 1.42)
D'Amico	Intermediate or high-risk localised disease	PrRT ± 6 months MAB	206	7.6		Improved overall survival 44 vs 30 deaths with AHT (HR 1.8; $p = 0.01$)

AHT, adjuvant hormone therapy; bNED, biochemical disease-free survival; CSS, cause-specific survival; DSM, disease-specific mortality; FU, follow-up; HR, hazard ratio; HT, hormone therapy; LDFS, local disease-free survival; LHRHa, luteinising hormone-releasing hormone agonist; MAB, maximal androgen blockade; MDFS, metastatic disease-free survival; n, number of patients; NAHT, neoadjuvant hormone therapy; OS, overall survival; PPRT, prostate and pelvic radiotherapy; PrRT, prostate radiotherapy; RT, radiotherapy.
Adapted from Armstrong *et al.*, 2011, Bolla *et al.*, 1997, 2009; Crook *et al.*, 2009; D'Amico *et al.*, 2008; Denham *et al.*, 2011; Fellows *et al.*, 1992; Horwitz *et al.*, 2008; Jones *et al.*, 2011; Laverdiere *et al.*, 2004; Pilepich *et al.*, 2005; Roach *et al.*, 2008; Tyrrell *et al.*, 2005.

et al., 2002). EORTC 22961 and RTOG 92-02 both compared short-course and long-course ADT in high risk, locally advanced and/or node-positive patients. RTOG 92-02 showed improved overall survival only in high-grade tumours (Horwitz *et al.*, 2008). EORTC 22961 showed improved 5-year cause-specific and overall survival in patients of whom 73% had T3 tumours (Bolla *et al.*, 2009).

Adjuvant hormonal therapy following surgery

Two trials have investigated the role of AHT following radical prostatectomy. One showed no benefit in terms of overall survival from the addition of flutamide in patients with locally advanced, node-negative disease. At a median of 11.9 years, the second trial showed improved overall survival with immediate ADT in patients with involved pelvic lymph nodes (HR 1.84; p = 0.04). Progression-free and cause-specific survival were also improved (Messing *et al.*, 2006).

Adverse events

ADT causes hot flushes, sweats, weight gain and mood changes, especially emotional lability and depression. The depression can be profound, and depressive psychoses have been reported. Patients become impotent and have decreased libido. They may notice tiredness, weakness and reduced energy levels.

Men with advanced prostate cancer have been shown to have reduced BMD at presentation compared with controls (40% versus 27%; Hussain *et al.*, 2003). ADT also causes a 4–10% loss of BMD within the first year of therapy. There is an increased rate of all-site and hip fractures (13% versus 20% and 2% versus 4%, respectively) in prostate cancer patients treated with ADT compared to those treated without (Shahinian *et al.*, 2005). Bisphosphonates can prevent BMD loss in men who are starting ADT (Smith *et al.*, 2003), although their effect on fracture rate has not been reported.

There are reports of an increased risk of cardiovascular death (D'Amico *et al.*, 2007), but this is not confirmed in larger cohorts (Bolla *et al.*, 2009).

Non-steroidal anti-androgens: bicalutamide, flutamide and enzalutamide

Mode of action

The modes of action of non-steroidal anti-androgens include the following.

- Competitive inhibition of the AR prevents the binding of DHT in the prostate; binding results in a conformational shape change, altering the balance of co-activator and co-repressor complexes and reducing the effects of DHT.
- Stimulation of the hypothalamus results in LH secretion, which leads to the production of testosterone, thus reducing many of the side effects associated with LHRHa, including impotence.
- Bicalutamide can be used in combination with LHRHa (dose = 50 mg daily) for maximal androgen blockade (MAB) or as a single agent at 150 mg daily.
- Enzalutamide has greatly increased affinity for the AR and cause a greater degree of inhibition.

In addition, it prevents nuclear translocation of activated AR and inhibits the association of activated AR with DNA. It is used in castrate-refractory metastatic disease in addition to LHRHa (dose = 160 mg daily).

Clinical uses

Single-agent bicalutamide 150 mg daily is less effective than surgical castration in patients with metastatic disease in terms of time to progression and overall survival; the outcome for patients with non-metastatic locally advanced disease was not statistically different (Iversen *et al.*, 2000).

MAB has been compared with medical and surgical castration alone in several trials and meta-analyses. There seems to be a small overall survival advantage of approximately 7 months (2–5% improvement in 5-year overall survival) when MAB is used (with bicalutamide as the preferred anti-androgen). The largest benefit may be for patients with minimal disease. However, advisory groups on both sides of the Atlantic have questioned the cost-effectiveness of MAB, and standard therapy remains LHRHa alone (Schmitt *et al.*, 2000).

The Early Prostate Cancer Trials assessed the role of bicalutamide alone, or as an adjunct, in 3 studies including 8113 patients with localised or locally advanced prostate cancer (McLeod *et al.*, 2006). At 7.4 years' median follow-up, there was no benefit from early or adjuvant bicalutamide in men with localised disease, and there was a trend towards decreased survival (HR 1.16 [95% CI 0.99 to 1.37]; p = 0.07). In patients with locally advanced disease who received radiotherapy (n = 305), bicalutamide significantly reduced the risk of disease progression by 44% (HR 0.56 [95% CI 0.40 to 0.78]; p < 0.001) and death by 35% (HR 0.65 [95% CI 0.44 to 0.93]; p = 0.03; See and Tyrrell, 2006).

Enzalutamide has been shown to prolong survival in men with castrate refractory metastatic prostate cancer in the post-docetaxel setting (Scher *et al.*, 2012) and results of trials in other disease states are awaited.

Adverse events

Approximately 70% of men suffer breast pain and gynaecomastia; 10% report hot flushes, asthenia, rash and impotence; 6% report alopecia and weight gain (Wirth *et al.*, 2004).

The breast-related side effects can be most effectively managed by using adjuvant tamoxifen 10–20 mg daily, although the long-term effects on the cancer and the patient are not yet known. Breast bud irradiation and anastrazole are less effective alternatives. Tamoxifen may also have a role in patients who have already developed gynaecomastia (Boccardo et al., 2005; Perdona et al., 2005).

There are well-documented beneficial effects of bicalutamide on BMD (presumably due to increased testosterone and oestradiol levels), but unfortunately bicalutamide cannot be used to reverse the loss of BMD seen with the previous use of LHRHa.

Enzalutamide is well tolerated and the only additional notable toxicity is a 0.8% risk of seizure.

Anti-androgen withdrawal

Withdrawing anti-androgen therapy has been reported to give response rates of up to 30% *in patients who have been responding to antiandrogen therapy*. This response is thought to be due to mutation in the AR, which results in stimulation by the anti-androgen rather than inhibition. Re-challenging with an alternative anti-androgen may result in further responses (e.g. bicalutamide following flutamide or nilutamide following bicalutamide).

CYP17 inhibitors: abiraterone acetate

Abiraterone acetate is licensed for use in castration-resistant metastatic prostate cancer (CRMPC) in both the pre- and post-docetaxel setting.

Mode of action

Abiraterone acetate inhibits both the 17α-hydroxylase and C17-20-lyase components of CYP17. This leads to suppression of the production of adrenal androgens and mineralocorticoids. It is now understood that intraprostatic production of androgens occurs following the same pathway and this is also suppressed.

Clinical uses

Abiraterone acetate prolongs survival in men with CRMPC in the post-docetaxel setting (Fizazi et al., 2012). Prior to chemotherapy, abiraterone increased time to radiological progression, but the improvement in overall survival was non-significant (Ryan et al., 2013). Abiraterone acetate is licensed for both indications, however. Results of trials in other disease states are awaited.

Adverse events

The side effects are all related to its mechanism of action and include fluid retention, hypertension and hypokalaemia. This is reduced by co-administration with prednisone or prednisolone (typically at 10 mg daily) or eplerenone. Asymptomatic transaminitis can also occur and requires monitoring. Reversal usually occurs after withdrawal of abiraterone and most patients can tolerate reintroduction with a lower dose.

Steroidal anti-androgens: cyproterone acetate, megestrol acetate and medroxyprogesterone acetate

Cyproterone acetate is licensed for use in advanced prostate cancer and for suppression of tumour flare with initial LHRHa.

Mode of action

The biochemical effects of steroidal anti-androgens are multiple, complex and not well defined:

- anti-androgenic;
- reduced LHRH and LH release;
- reduced steroid synthesis leading directly to reduced testosterone levels;
- interference with the intracellular binding of DHT to the androgen receptor; and
- progestational and glucocorticoid activities. The main clinical use of steroidal anti-androgens is to prevent LHRHa-induced tumour flare.

Adverse events

Fluid retention can precipitate congestive cardiac failure and cause ankle oedema. Steroidal anti-androgens are associated with thromboembolic disease. Their hepatotoxicity includes jaundice, hepatitis and abnormal liver function tests. Reduced libido and erectile dysfunction also occur.

Exogenous oestrogens: diethylstilboestrol and ethinyloestradiol

Diethylstilboestrol (DES) is the only oestrogen used in standard clinical practice.

Mode of action

The exact mode of action is not understood, but it is likely that DES functions in multiple ways to reduce androgenic activity:

- suppression of adrenal androgen production;
- reduced LH/FSH production from the pituitary;
- reduced testicular production of testosterone.

Pharmacokinetics

DES can be given orally and undergoes first-pass metabolism within the liver to form its active metabolites.

Clinical use

DES (3–5 mg daily) can be used as a single agent to achieve rapid castrate testosterone levels. It can also be used in combination with LHRHa at 1 mg for hormone-refractory disease. Transcutaneous application may bypass the first-pass metabolism and thus reduce the liver, cardiac and thromboembolic side effects (which is being assessed in the ongoing MRC PATCH study).

Adverse events

DES causes sodium retention with oedema and can precipitate congestive cardiac failure. It can cause thromboembolic disease. Hepatotoxicity can occur with jaundice, hepatitis and abnormal liver function tests. It should be given with aspirin 75 mg daily or full anticoagulation to prevent the thromboembolic disease. Gynaecomastia occurs, which is prevented with the use of pre-DES radiotherapy (7–10 Gy). Nausea and impotence also occur.

Glucocorticoids: prednisolone or dexamethasone

Mode of action

The mode of action of glucocorticoids involves suppression of adrenal androgen production.

- Response rates to prednisolone/prednisone (5–20 mg daily) and hydrocortisone (30 mg daily) are in the order of 30% (PSA decrease of at least 50%), with a median duration of response of about 2 months.
- Dexamethasone (0.5–2 mg daily) is highly active, with response rates of up to 80%, and up to 30% of patients may get an 80% reduction in PSA. The median time to progression is approximately 7 months. PSA responders have a median survival of approximately 15 months.

Adverse effects

Typical glucocorticoid toxicities include proximal myopathy, cushingoid facies, thin skin with easy bruising, hypertension, mental changes including hyperactivity and confusion and increased risk of osteoporosis. The lowest effective dose should be prescribed.

Prostate: mechanisms of resistance

The underlying mechanism for hormone resistance is still largely unknown. Because the adrenal glands produce 5–10% of circulating androgens, the majority of successful hormonal manoeuvres used in LHRHa-refractory disease reduce adrenal androgen production. However, even with MAB, patients relapse. It is now understood that intraprostatic androgen production occurs.

After ADT, some cells undergo apoptosis (androgen-dependent) and some undergo cell-cycle arrest (androgen-sensitive) while others are unaffected (androgen-insensitive). It is thought that before treatment with ADT there is a predominance of androgen-sensitive cells, but after ADT the less-dependent cells grow more and become the dominant clones.

It has been suggested that the malignant cells are prostate cancer stem cells, whose progeny are primarily androgen-sensitive in the presence of androgens. However, in the absence of androgens or with low circulating levels of androgens, the progeny become increasingly androgen-resistant.

An alternative hypothesis is that androgen-sensitive cells initially enter cell-cycle arrest, but over time they develop molecular pathways that overcome the low/absent circulating androgens. These include the following.

- Upregulated levels of AR mRNA and protein – this occurs because androgen levels are low and AR is not internalised.
- AR mutation – increased activation by low levels of androgens or low-potency androgens. This may lead to auto-activation, with AR activation even in the absence of androgens.
- Upregulation of the ARE in the absence of activated AR (e.g. via upregulated transcription factors such as those in the EGFR pathway).
- Upregulated survival pathways (i.e. reduced apoptosis, e.g. via BCL2 or survivin).

Prostate cancer: areas of current interest

Additional novel hormonal therapies

Orterenol is an even more selective CYP17 inhibitor that may allow suppression of the C17-20 lyase enzyme activity without affecting the

17α-hydroxylase activity. This could avoid the need for concurrent prednisolone therapy. Galeterone is earlier still in the developmental pathway, but has the additional advantage of having some direct AR antagonistic function. ODM-201 is a novel anti-androgen that potentially has even higher affinity for the AR than enzalutamide, with the same blockade of AR nuclear translocation.

Resistance to novel hormones

One area of intense research is the mechanism behind *de novo* or acquired resistance to abiraterone and/or enzalutamide and therapeutic approaches to overcome these. Current approaches include combinations with each other and with non-hormonal agents, predominantly inhibitors of pathways relevant to hormonal functionality – such as AKT inhibitors.

Timing of novel hormones

The high efficacy and low toxicity of the two main classes of novel hormonal agents has led to many trials looking at the various agents in different disease states, from use in hormone-sensitive disease, e.g. abiraterone acetate in the MRC STAMPEDE trial, at first relapse on LHRH agonists and in the pre-chemotherapy setting. Much is still to be learnt.

References

Anonymous. (1997). Immediate versus deferred treatment for advanced prostatic cancer: initial results of the Medical Research Council Trial. The Medical Research Council Prostate Cancer Working Party Investigators Group. *Br. J. Urol.*, **79**, 235–246.

Armstrong, J. G., Gillham, C. M. and Dunne, M. T. (2011). A randomized trial (Irish Clinical Oncology Research Group 97-01) comparing short versus protracted neoadjuvant hormonal therapy before radiotherapy for localized prostate cancer. *Int. J. Radiat. Oncol. Biol. Phys.*, **81**, 35–45.

Beatson, G. T. (1896). On the treatment of inoperable cases of carcinoma of the mamma. Suggestions for a new method of treatment with illustrative cases. *Lancet*, **ii**, 104–107.

Bliss, J., Kilburn, L. S., Coleman, R. E., *et al.* (2012). Disease-related outcomes with long-term follow-up: an updated analysis of the Intergroup Exemestane Study. *J. Clin. Oncol.*, **30**, 709–717.

Boccardo, F., Rubagotti, A., Battaglia, M., *et al.* (2005). Evaluation of tamoxifen and anastrozole in the prevention of gynecomastia and breast pain induced by bicalutamide monotherapy of prostate cancer. *J. Clin. Oncol.*, **23**, 808–815.

Bolla, M., Gonzalez, D., Warde, P., *et al.* (1997). Improved survival in patients with locally advanced prostate cancer treated with radiotherapy and goserelin. *N. Engl. J. Med.*, **337**, 295–300.

Bolla, M., Collette, L., Blank, L., *et al.* (2002). Long-term results with immediate androgen suppression and external irradiation in patients with locally advanced prostate cancer (an EORTC study): a phase III randomised trial. *Lancet*, **360**, 103–106.

Bolla, M., de Reijke, T. M., Van Tienhoven, G., *et al.* (2009). Duration of androgen suppression in the treatment of prostate cancer *N. Engl. J. Med.*, **360**, 2516–2527.

Crook, J. M., Ludgate, C., Malone, S., *et al.* (2009). Final report of multicenter Canadian Phase III randomized trial of 3 versus 8 months of neoadjuvant androgen deprivation therapy before conventional-dose radiotherapy for clinically localized prostate cancer. *Int. J. Radiat. Oncol. Biol. Phys.*, **73**, 327–333.

Crook, J. M., O'Callaghan, C. J., Duncan, G, *et al.* (2012). Intermittent androgen suppression for rising PSA level after radiotherapy. *N. Engl. J. Med.*, **367**, 895–903.

Cuzick, J., Sestak, I, Baum, M., *et al.* (2010). Effect of anastrozole and tamoxifen as adjuvant treatment for early-stage breast cancer: 10 year analysis of the ATAC trial. *Lancet Oncol.*, **11**, 1135–1141.

Cuzick, J., Sestak, I. and Forbes, J. F. (2014). Anastrozole for prevention of breast cancer in high-risk postmenopausal women (IBIS-II): an international, double-blind, randomised placebo-controlled trial. *Lancet*, **383**, 1041–1048.

D'Amico, A. V., Kantoff, P., Loffredo, M., *et al.* (2006). Predictors of mortality after prostate-specific antigen failure. *Int. J. Radiat. Oncol. Biol. Phys.*, **65**, 656–660.

D'Amico, A. V., Denham, J. W., Crook, J. M., *et al.* (2007). Influence of androgen suppression therapy for prostate cancer on the frequency and timing of fatal myocardial infarctions. *J. Clin. Oncol.*, **25**, 2420–2425.

D'Amico, A. V., Chen, M-H., Renshaw, A. A., *et al.* (2008). Androgen suppression and radiation vs radiation alone for prostate cancer. *J. Am. Med. Ass.*, **299**, 289–295.

Davis, C., Pan, H., Godwin, J., *et al.* (2013). Long-term effects of continuing adjuvant tamoxifen to 10 years versus stopping at 5 years after diagnosis of oestrogen receptor-positive breast cancer: ATLAS, a randomised trial. *The Lancet*, **381**, 805–816.

Denham, J. W., Steigler, A. and Lamb, D. S. (2011). Short-term neoadjuvant androgen deprivation and radiotherapy for locally advanced prostate cancer: 10-year data from the Trans-Tasman Radiation Oncology Group 96.01 randomised controlled trial. *Lancet Oncol.*, **12**, 451–459.

Dowsett, M., Cuzick, J., Wale, C., *et al.* (2005). Retrospective analysis of time to recurrence in the ATAC trial according to hormone receptor status: an hypothesis-generating study. *J. Clin. Oncol.*, **23**, 7512–7517.

EBCTCG. (2005). Effects of chemotherapy and hormonal therapy for early breast cancer on recurrence and 15-year survival: an overview of the randomised trials. *Lancet*, **365**, 1687–1717.

EBCTCG. (2011). Relevance of breast cancer hormone receptors and other factors to the efficacy of adjuvant tamoxifen: patient-level meta-analysis of randomised trials. *Lancet*, **378**, 771–784.

Fellows, G. J., Clark, P. B., Beynon, L. L., *et al.* (1992). Treatment of advanced localised prostatic cancer by orchiectomy, radiotherapy, or combined treatment. A Medical Research Council Study. Urological Cancer Working Party – Subgroup on Prostatic Cancer. *Br. J. Urol.*, **70**, 304–309.

Fisher, B., Costantino, J., Redmond, C., *et al.* (1989). A randomized clinical trial evaluating tamoxifen in the treatment of patients with node-negative breast cancer who have oestrogen-receptor-positive tumors. *N. Engl. J. Med.*, **320**, 479–484.

Fizazi, K., Scher, H., Molina, A., *et al.* (2012). Abiraterone acetate for the treatment of metastatic castrate-resistant prostate cancer: final overall survival analysis of the COU-AA-301 randomised, double-blind, placebo-controlled phase 3 trial. *Lancet Oncol.*, **13**, 983–992.

Gray, R. G., Rea, D., Handley, K., *et al.* (2013). aTTom: long-term effects of continuing adjuvant tamoxifen to 10 years versus stopping at 5 years in 6953 women with early breast cancer. *J Clin Oncol.*, **31** (Suppl.), abstr. 5.

Horwitz, E. M., Bae, K., Hanks, G. E., *et al.* (2008). Ten-year follow-up of radiation therapy oncology group protocol 92-02: a phase III trial of the duration of elective androgen deprivation in locally advanced prostate cancer. *J. Clin. Oncol.*, **26**, 2497–2504.

Hopp, T. A., Weiss, H. L., Hilsenbeck, S. G., *et al.* (2004). Breast cancer patients with progesterone receptor PR-A-rich tumors have poorer disease-free survival states. *Clin. Cancer Res.*, **10**, 2751–2760.

Howell, A., Cuzick, J., Baum, M., *et al.* (2005). Results of the ATAC (Arimidex, Tamoxifen, Alone or in Combination) trial after completion of 5 years' adjuvant treatment for breast cancer. *Lancet*, **365**, 60–62.

Huggins, C. and Bergenstal, D. M. (1952). Inhibition of human mammary and prostatic cancers by adrenalectomy. *Cancer Res.*, **12**, 134–141.

Huggins, C. and Hodges, C. V. (1941). Studies on prostate cancer. The effects of castration, of oestrogen and of androgen injection on serum phosphatases in carcinoma of the prostate. *Cancer Res.*, **1**, 293–297.

Hussain, S. A., Weston, R., Stephenson, R. N., *et al.* (2003). Immediate dual energy X-ray absorptiometry reveals a high incidence of osteoporosis in patients with advanced prostate cancer before hormonal manipulation. *BJU Int.*, **92**, 690–694.

Hussain, S. A., Tangen, C. M., Berry, D. L., *et al.* (2013). Intermittent versus continuous androgen deprivation therapy in prostate cancer. *N. Engl. J. Med.*, **368**, 1314–1325.

Iversen, P., Tyrrell, C. J., Kaisary, A. V., *et al.* (2000). Bicalutamide monotherapy compared with castration in patients with nonmetastatic locally advanced prostate cancer: 6.3 years of followup. *J. Urol.*, **164**, 1579–1582.

Jin, H., Tu, D., Zhao, N.,*et al.* (2012). Longer-term outcomes of letrozole versus placebo after 5 years of tamoxifen in the NCIC CTG MA.17 Trial: Analyses Adjusting for Treatment Crossover. *J. Clin. Oncol.*, **30**, 718–721.

Joerger, M. and Thurlimann, B. (2009). Update of the BIG 1–98 trial: where do we stand? *Breast*, **18**, 78–82.

Jones, C. U., Hunt, D., McGowan, D. G., *et al.* (2011). Radiotherapy and short-term androgen deprivation for localized prostate cancer. *N. Engl. J. Med.*, **365**, 107–118.

Laverdiere, J., Nabid, A., De Bedoya, L. D., *et al.* (2004). The efficacy and sequencing of a short course of androgen suppression on freedom from biochemical failure when administered with radiation therapy for T2–T3 prostate cancer. *J. Urol.*, **171**, 1137–1140.

McLeod, D. G., Iversen, P., See, W. A., *et al.* (2006). Bicalutamide 150 mg plus standard care vs standard care alone for early prostate cancer. *BJU Int.*, **97**, 247–254.

Messing, E. M., Manola, J., Yao, J., *et al.* (2006). Immediate versus deferred androgen deprivation treatment in patients with node-positive prostate cancer after radical prostatectomy and pelvic lymphadenectomy. *Lancet Oncol.*, **7**, 472–479.

Milano, A., Dal Lago, L., Sotiriou, C., *et al.* (2006). What clinicians need to know about antioestrogen resistance in breast cancer therapy. *Eur. J. Cancer*, **42**, 2692–2705.

Miller, W. R., Anderson, T. J., Dixon, J. M., *et al.* (2006). Oestrogen receptor beta and neoadjuvant therapy with tamoxifen: prediction of response and effects of treatment. *Br. J. Cancer*, **94**, 1333–1338.

Noble, R. L. (1980). Production of Nb rat carcinoma of the dorsal prostate and response of estrogen-dependent transplants to sex hormones and tamoxifen. *Cancer Res.*, **40**, 3547–3550.

Perdona, S., Autorino, R., De Placido, S., *et al.* (2005). Efficacy of tamoxifen and radiotherapy for prevention and treatment of gynaecomastia and breast pain caused by bicalutamide in prostate cancer: a randomised controlled trial. *Lancet Oncol.*, **6**, 295–300.

Pilepich, M. V., Winter, K., Lawton, C. A., *et al.* (2005). Androgen suppression adjuvant to definitive radiotherapy in prostate carcinoma – long-term results of phase III RTOG 85–31. *Int. J. Radiat. Oncol. Biol. Phys.*, **61**, 1285–1290.

Roach, M. 3rd, Bae, K. and Speight, J. (2008). Short-term neoadjuvant androgen deprivation therapy and external beam radiotherapy for locally advanced prostate cancer: long-term results of RTOG 8610. *J. Clin. Oncol. Biol. Phys.*, **26**, 585–591.

Rodrigues, N. A., Chen, M. H., Catalona, W. J., *et al.* (2006). Predictors of mortality after androgen-deprivation therapy in patients with rapidly rising prostate-specific antigen levels after local therapy for prostate cancer. *Cancer*, **107**, 514–520.

Ryan, C. J., Smith, M., de Bono, J. S., *et al.* (2013). Abiraterone in metastatic prostate cancer without previous chemotherapy. *N. Engl. J. Med.*, **368**, 138–148.

Scher, H., Fizazi, K., Saad, F., *et al.* (2012). Increased survival with enzalutamide in prostate cancer after chemotherapy. *N. Engl. J. Med.*, **367**, 1–11.

Schmitt, B., Bennett, C., Seidenfeld, J., *et al.* (2000). Maximal androgen blockade for advanced prostate cancer. *Cochrane Database Syst. Rev.*, **2**, CD001526.

See, W. A. and Tyrrell, C. J. (2006). The addition of bicalutamide 150 mg to radiotherapy significantly improves overall survival in men with locally advanced prostate cancer. *J. Cancer Res. Clin. Oncol.*, **132** (Suppl. 13), 7–16.

Shahinian, V. B., Kuo, Y. F., Freeman, J. L., *et al.* (2005). Risk of fracture after androgen deprivation for prostate cancer. *N. Engl. J. Med.*, **352**, 154–164.

Smith, I. E., Dowsett, M., Yap, Y. S., *et al.* (2006). Adjuvant aromatase inhibitors for early breast cancer after chemotherapy-induced amenorrhoea: caution and suggested guidelines. *J. Clin. Oncol.*, **24**, 2444–2447.

Smith, M. R., Eastham, J., Gleason, D. M., *et al.* (2003). Randomized controlled trial of zoledronic acid to prevent bone loss in men receiving androgen deprivation therapy for nonmetastatic prostate cancer. *J. Urol.*, **169**, 2008–2012.

Tyrrell, C. J., Payne, H., See, W. A., *et al.* (2005). Bicalutamide ('Casodex') 150 mg as adjuvant to radiotherapy in patients with localised or locally advanced prostate cancer: results from the randomised Early Prostate Cancer Programme. *Radiother. Oncol.*, **76**, 4–10.

Vogel, V. G. (2009). The NSABP Study of Tamoxifen and Raloxifene (STAR) trial. *Expert. Rev. Anticancer Ther.*, **9**, 51–60. Erratum in *Expert. Rev. Anticancer Ther.*, **9**, 388.

Wirth, M. P., See, W. A., McLeod, D. G., *et al.* (2004). Bicalutamide 150 mg in addition to standard care in patients with localized or locally advanced prostate cancer: results of the second analysis of the early prostate cancer program at median followup of 5.4 years. *J. Urol.*, **172**(5 Pt. 1), 1865–1870.

Zelefsky, M. J. and Harrison, A. (1997). Neoadjuvant androgen ablation prior to radiotherapy for prostate cancer: reducing the potential morbidity of therapy. *Urology*, **49** (Suppl. 3A), 38–45.

Zondek, B. (1940). Effect of prolonged administration of oestrogen on uterus and anterior pituitary of human beings. *J. Am. Med. Ass.*, **114**, 1850–1854.

Chapter

4

Pathology in cancer

Hywel Thomas and Mick Button

Introduction

Histopathology plays an essential role in oncology, both in the initial tissue diagnosis of the tumour and later in the detailed examination of the surgical specimen. The information gained from the macroscopic and microscopic examination of the specimen will guide further treatment and establish prognostic and predictive markers for the patient. Pathologists will often demonstrate the morphology of tumours to the members of the multidisciplinary team (MDT). This is an excellent opportunity to question the pathologist on morphological descriptions and it provides a teaching experience for medical students through to senior consultants. Mutual understanding of working practices and interpretation of results among all members of the MDT improves team working and patient care.

Immunohistochemistry has revolutionised histopathology over the last 20–30 years and a number of tumours now require immunohistochemistry for their accurate diagnosis or subclassification. It has also, along with cytogenetics, significantly changed the analysis of lymphoreticular tumours with the REAL classification, which was adopted by the WHO and published in 2001 and updated in 2008 (Jaffe *et al.*, 2001 and Swerdlow *et al.*, 2008).

Molecular genetic analysis is also an important and rapidly developing area of histopathology with tissue used for diagnostic and prognostic purposes. It is beyond the scope of this chapter to list all the molecular investigations available, as these are covered in specific chapters.

It is not essential for an oncologist to have a detailed knowledge of histopathology, but a general understanding of pathological terms, tumour morphology, laboratory techniques and limitations is helpful. This chapter describes:

- specimen types,
- important microscopic descriptions of tumours,
- essential and practical immunohistochemical results and
- important aspects of working with pathologists within busy MDTs.

Practical MDT information relating to pathology

Before obtaining a biopsy, the risks and benefits for the individual patient should be considered, especially when deciding which site is likely to most easily give a complete and accurate diagnosis, balancing the risk of failing to get a tissue diagnosis with the possible morbidity of the procedure. The patient will almost certainly be very anxious and any delays from repeated negative biopsies will not only make this worse but also delay treatment decisions. Sometimes a biopsy may not be necessary if treatment options are very limited. Biopsy procedures often have an associated risk of morbidity; for instance, up to 5% of patients may require a therapeutic chest drain after a lung biopsy (Hiraki *et al.*, 2010) and liver biopsy may have a mortality rate of up to 1% (West and Card, 2010).

When requesting a pathology report, it is important for the requesting clinician to put all relevant clinical details on the request form including radiological information, symptoms, tumour markers, suspected diagnosis and previous cancer diagnosis (if relevant) to allow the pathologist to perform the most helpful tests as rapidly as possible.

Advances in both pathology and oncology have changed working practices significantly. There are now more tools available to pathologists to guide treatment decisions (e.g. ER/PgR and HER2 testing in breast cancer and differentiating adenocarcinoma from squamous cell carcinoma in non-small-cell lung cancer (NSCLC)) and in elucidating a primary tumour when none may be apparent clinically (e.g. by immunohistochemistry). Additional genetic tests (e.g. epidermal growth factor mutation testing in NSCLC) have also changed working practices and a tissue diagnosis may now be needed when none was needed previously, with more tissue required for all the necessary tests. This means good teamwork to ensure that the most appropriate tissue is available to make an accurate, complete and timely diagnosis.

Specimen type

The pathologist will receive a variety of different types of specimen, each of which has advantages and limitations for making a diagnosis.

Fine-needle aspirate cytology (FNAC)

This is a simple, cost-effective and relatively painless procedure often undertaken by a radiologist. The sample can be made into direct smears and reported quickly by a pathologist, as happens in 'one stop' breast clinics. In skilled hands, FNAC has a high sensitivity and specificity. It is also possible to perform immunohistochemistry on an FNAC sample either by decolourising the smear or by making a cell block from any remaining sample (Fowler and Lachar, 2008). The cell block method is preferred because decolourising the smear can lead to unpredictable results.

A disadvantage of FNAC is that the cellularity of the specimen depends on the skill and experience of the operator. A smear with too few cells can prevent an accurate diagnosis and accurate definition of the histological subtype because of loss of the architecture. It may also be difficult to distinguish invasive from *in situ* lesions with an FNAC sample of a breast mass and so, many pathologists prefer tissue core biopsies, as they can assess the overall architecture of the tumour and perform more immunohistochemical tests.

Exfoliative cytology (non-gynaecology)

Exfoliative cytology specimens include pleural and peritoneal fluids, urine, cerebro-spinal fluid (CSF), sputum, bronchial washings and brushings. These samples are relatively rapid to process, although not as rapid as FNAC, and the cellularity depends on the disease process involved. In skilled hands, high sensitivity and specificity can be obtained and immunohistochemistry

can be performed using the cell block method, which may, however, be more difficult to interpret than a core biopsy. Samples can also be sent for flow cytometry if required.

The disadvantages are also similar to those of FNAC specimens. It may be difficult to accurately sub-type tumours on cytological grounds alone and poor cellularity of the sample may be a problem.

Frozen section

A frozen section is useful for a rapid answer to an issue that arises during an operation. There may, for instance, be a suspicious peritoneal nodule during an anterior resection of a colonic carcinoma, or a need to examine margins to establish complete surgical excision.

Frozen sections can provide a rapid result, but the morphology of cells in frozen section specimens differs from that in conventional paraffin-embedded, haematoxylin and eosin-stained slides. False positive and negative results are possible and in a difficult case the pathologist would issue a cautious report while awaiting more definitive paraffin sections.

Tissue core, endoscopic and excision biopsies

This is the commonest type of specimen. Depending on the size of the tissue, the sample tends to be fixed in formaldehyde for a period ranging from a few hours to overnight. The morphology from a good-quality long core of tissue is often excellent, enabling the pathologist to assess the overall architecture and cytonuclear features. It is possible to perform histochemical stains (for example, to look for mucin) and also immunohistochemical stains. Tissue can also be prepared for flow cytometry and sent for molecular analysis if required.

The drawback of most core biopsies is that the fixation and processing of the tissue can delay the reporting of the specimen, although it can usually be diagnosed and reported on the day after reaching the laboratory. There are now microwave processors that enable a much more rapid assessment of the tissue and a 'same-day' diagnosis, but their cost prohibits their use in many pathology laboratories. Another problem may be the quality of the sample, and a tumour in a difficult anatomical location may produce fragmented, small-volume cores leading to a cautious or unhelpful pathology report.

Large cancer resections

Following fixation in formaldehyde for at least 24 hours, the pathologist will examine the gross morphology carefully and decide on the appropriate tissue blocks of tumour, background, margins and lymph nodes. These will be processed overnight and cut and stained into slides the following day. The advantage of this specimen is that there will usually be abundant tissue to examine. Gross photographs of the specimen are taken and, with appropriate consent, tissue can easily be collected for research or for the local cancer bank. One very successful example is the Wales Cancer Bank (WCB), launched in June 2004. Located across several hospitals in north and south Wales, the WCB consents patients with a variety of cancer types and collects normal and tumour tissue to be used by a wide variety of research organisations. Approximately 10,000 patients have already been consented for the WCB, including pre-consent for using their tissue/tumour for future research questions (WCB Annual report, 2014; www.walescancerbank.com, accessed August 2014).

Microscopic features of common malignant tumours

The following section is a brief overview of the histological appearances of some of the common tumour subtypes.

Squamous cell carcinoma

Squamous epithelium may be simple or stratified; the latter covers many parts of the body, including skin, oral cavity, oesophagus, cervix, vagina and anal canal. The epithelium is typically robust and can withstand mechanical stresses placed on it.

Dysplasia of the squamous epithelium may progress to invasive squamous cell carcinoma that invades through the basement membrane into the underlying supporting connective tissue. The usual appearance of the tumour depends on the degree of differentiation. There are different grading systems, but typically high-grade squamous tumours will exhibit reduced keratinisation and intercellular bridging and increased cytonuclear pleomorphism and mitotic activity. There are several variants of squamous cell carcinoma, including basaloid and spindle cell types.

Adenocarcinoma

Adenocarcinomas arise from glandular epithelium, of which there are many different types and functions in the body. Some glandular epithelia have a secretory or absorptive role, while others, such as ciliated columnar epithelium, have a propulsion role.

The sheer number and diversity of adenocarcinoma cannot be covered in this chapter. They are found in a wide variety of sites including breast, lung, colon, stomach, pancreas, prostate, kidney, liver, ovary, uterus and thyroid, among many others. When a lung biopsy of a mass shows an adenocarcinoma, the pathologist must use a combination of histological appearance, immunohistochemistry and clues from the clinical history and radiology to determine whether it is a primary lung adenocarcinoma or a metastasis. Many adenocarcinomas show similar morphology to each other, but some show subtle clues as to their primary site:

1. a cord-like pattern of lobular carcinoma of breast or the trabecular appearance of hepatocellular carcinoma;
2. comedonecrosis (central necrosis in a rounded epithelial island) as seen in some breast and salivary duct carcinomas;
3. central necrosis ('dirty necrosis') seen in the enteric-type epithelium of colonic adenocarcinoma;
4. signet ring adenocarcinomas are a feature of diffuse gastric adenocarcinoma, but can also occur in tumours from other locations;
5. prominent perineural invasion is often seen in adenoid cystic carcinoma of the salivary glands and in prostate adenocarcinoma;
6. a papillary growth pattern is seen in several types of adenocarcinoma, such as kidney, ovary and thyroid; and
7. cribriform ('sieve-like') architecture is seen in prostate, breast and some endometrial adenocarcinomas.

Other adenocarcinomas show distinctive cytonuclear features that can point to a primary site.

1. The cytoplasm of clear cell renal cell carcinoma is distinctive, but clear cell adenocarcinoma variants are also present in the ovary and endometrium and several other sites.
2. The optically clear nuclei of thyroid papillary carcinoma, so-called 'Orphan Annie' nuclei.

Malignant melanoma

The diagnosis of malignant melanoma can be tricky for the pathologist. In the primary cutaneous form, the diagnosis is relatively straightforward when there are nests of atypical melanocytes displaying epidermal pagetoid spread and an infiltrative pattern in the dermis. Melanin pigment may be abundant and the cells can show pleomorphism. The problem is that there are a significant number of histological variants of melanoma, with some displaying small bland nuclei and others a prominent spindle cell component. The latter would fall into a wide differential diagnosis including spindle cell squamous carcinoma, cutaneous sarcomas or an atypical fibroxanthoma.

Metastatic deposits of malignant melanoma can occur in various clinical situations and anatomical sites, can show a wide variety of cellular appearances and often require immunohistochemistry for diagnosis. Pathologists always have melanoma in their differential for a tumour of unknown origin.

Small cell carcinoma

This is a poorly differentiated neuroendocrine carcinoma which can be found in many different parts of the body, with the lung being the commonest primary site. The tumour is often found centrally in the lung, and morphology shows a solid distribution of cells, although other patterns can be seen, including rosettes, ribbons and tubules. The cells have a distinctive small size with very dark (hyperchromatic) nuclei. The chromatin pattern is granular and there is minimal cytoplasm present. Nuclei may show moulding and in small endoscopic biopsies the nuclei may become elongated and distorted, causing diagnostic problems. In necrotic areas nuclear debris may be smeared into blood vessel walls – a phenomenon known as the Azzopardi effect. In a limited and partly crushed endoscopic biopsy, immunohistochemistry for neuroendocrine markers would be essential to confirm the diagnosis because lymphoma would be in the differential.

Lymphoreticular tumours

There is great morphological diversity in the histopathology of lymphomas. From a broad division into non-Hodgkin and Hodgkin lymphoma, the pathologist has a low to high power approach when assessing the microscopy. On low power the lymphoid infiltrate is divided into nodular/follicular or diffuse, and on high power the individual cell morphology is assessed. For example, a nodular/follicular architecture composed of small cleaved centrocytes would suggest grade 1 follicular lymphoma, while a diffuse population of large atypical blasts would suggest a diffuse large B cell lymphoma.

Pathologists very rarely report lymphomas based on morphology alone. Since the REAL classification of 2001 was adopted by the WHO, pathologists use a combination of morphology, immunohistochemistry and cytogenetics to arrive at a diagnosis. The differential diagnosis of a lymph node replaced with a nodular/follicular proliferation of small to medium-sized lymphoid cells would include follicular lymphoma, small cell lymphoma, mantle cell lymphoma and marginal zone lymphoma. Immunohistochemistry would be relatively straightforward to distinguish these tumours. Many lymphomas are now reported by pathologists with a dedicated interest in haematopathology.

Germ cell tumours

There are a wide variety of tissue types within the spectrum of germ cell tumours. Completely differentiated somatic-type tissues can be seen in both male and female tumours. Germ cell tumours in men are broadly divided into two types.

1. Seminoma: sheets of cells separated by fibrous septae. The cells are well-defined and show enlarged nuclei with usually clear cytoplasm and varying degrees of lymphocyte infiltration.
2. Non-seminomatous germ cell tumour (NSGCT) consists of a number of different tumours including:
   - embryonal carcinoma: pleomorphic cells with a wide variety of architectural growth patterns;
   - yolk sac tumour: several growth patterns exist with a microcystic pattern being one of the commonest showing mild to moderately pleomorphic cells;
   - choriocarcinoma: a markedly haemorrhagic tumour with both syncytiotrophoblast and cytotrophoblast elements; and
   - mature teratoma: somatic tissue present.

The tumours present either as pure forms or as a mixture of tumour types.

Soft tissue and bone tumours

Malignant soft tissue and bone tumours are uncommon and the average pathologist will see only a small number of cases per year. Their appearance will depend on the anatomical site, the cell of origin and the degree of differentiation. For example, a differentiated leiomyosarcoma should show some morphological similarities to normal smooth muscle. Poorly differentiated sarcomas are often a diagnostic challenge and may require immunohistochemistry to identify the original cell type. Sarcomas are usually diagnosed and treated by a dedicated MDT and so if sarcoma is suspected, it is better to refer to the sarcoma MDT who will arrange for the biopsy to be performed in a way that will not affect subsequent management.

Immunohistochemical features in pathology

Immunohistochemistry was first described in the 1940s (Coons *et al.*, 1941). During the last 20–30 years, it has developed into an essential tool for pathologists in the diagnosis, classification and prognosis of tumours. However, it should not be a substitute for good morphological evaluation using a haematoxylin and eosin (H+E) slide.

Principles of immunohistochemistry

Antigens found at intracellular and extracellular sites may be identified by commercially produced antibodies. This binding reaction is not visible and a labelling method must be used to make the reaction visible on light microscopy.

After sections are cut for immunohistochemistry, the tissue must first undergo a process of antigen retrieval. This unmasks epitopes that have been hidden because of cross-linkage during formaldehyde fixation. The primary antibody is introduced to the tissue with a secondary biotin-labelled antibody. To amplify the signal and increase the sensitivity of the reaction, a streptavidin–biotin complex will attach to the secondary antibody. The final step involves adding a chromogen to produce a visible reaction. The chromogen (3,3-di-aminobenzidine tetra hydrochloride; DAB) will react with the combination of horseradish peroxidase enzyme combined with hydrogen peroxide H_2O_2 to form a coloured reaction that is insoluble in alcohol (Hsu *et al.*, 1981).

Immunohistochemistry in routine clinical practice

Tables 4.1 and 4.2 list some of the most useful markers. These tables are not exhaustive and histopathology textbooks contain comprehensive accounts. All results have to be interpreted in the light of clinical information and, like all tests, immunohistochemistry (IHC) results do not have 100% sensitivity or specificity. For example, results on poorly differentiated tumours or from FNAC samples may be less reliable.

Cytokeratins (keratins)

Cytokeratins (CKs) are a family of intermediate filaments that form the cytoskeleton of epithelial cells. There are 20 CKs in routine use and they are numbered 1–20 based on their molecular weight – the higher the number, the lower the molecular weight. Carcinomas arise from different types of epithelium and the majority will be cytokeratin-positive, but the grade of the tumour plays an important role in determining the strength of the reaction. A poorly differentiated carcinoma may show only weak or focal cytokeratin staining. Most pathologists use a cytokeratin 'cocktail' (such as AE1/AE3) that contains multiple cytokeratins in one antibody to increase the sensitivity of the reaction.

Two particular cytokeratins deserve a special mention. CK7 and CK20 can be used to help the pathologist narrow down the search for an unknown primary. Table 4.2 is a summary of the main reactions (for adenocarcinoma, unless otherwise stated).

Immunohistochemical results should not be viewed as definitive. Exceptions do occur, for example, a small percentage of colorectal adenocarcinomas may be CK7+ve. Cytokeratins can also show positive staining reactions with some non-epithelial tumours, for example, embryonal carcinoma of the testis, mesothelioma and some sarcomas.

Malignant melanoma

S100 is a low molecular weight protein found in many cells, especially melanocytes, glial cells, Schwann cells, neurons, Langerhans cells, cartilage and adipose tissue.

Other melanoma markers include HMB45 and Melan A, which are often used as part of a panel with S100.

Table 4.1 Common immunohistochemical markers

Marker	Reactivity
ALK	Anaplastic large cell lymphoma, inflammatory myofibroblastic tumour
CA125	Not specific (cervix, endometrium, GI tract, thyroid, breast)
Calretinin	Mesothelioma (+ve) versus adenocarcinoma (-ve)
CD3	T lymphocytes
CD5	T lymphocytes, B-CLL/SLL and mantle cell lymphoma
CD10	Endometrial stromal tumours, follicular lymphoma, RCC + many others
CD15	Reed Sternberg cells, AML
CD20	B lymphocytes
CD23	B-CLL/SLL
CD30	Reed Sternberg cells, embryonal carcinoma
CD31 and CD34	Vascular tumours
CD45	Stains all leucocytes
CD117 (C-Kit)	GISTs, seminoma, AML
CEA	Many carcinoma +ve (GI tract, pancreas, lung, medullary thyroid cancer)
Chromogranin	Neuroendocrine tumours
Cyclin D1	Mantle cell lymphoma
Cytokeratins:	
AE1/AE3 (cocktail)	Most normal epithelia and carcinomas
CK7 and CK20	Can be used to differentiate certain tumours (e.g. colorectal carcinoma are CK7– CK20+ and ovarian serous carcinomas are CK7+ CK20–
Desmin	Smooth and striated muscle
EMA	Many carcinomas, mesothelioma, plasma cell tumours, meningioma
ER	Breast, ovary, endometrial + some vulval stromal tumours
HER2	Detects overexpression of EGFR
HMB45	Malignant melanoma
Calcitonin	Medullary carcinoma of thyroid
PLAP and OCT3/4	Seminoma, embryonal carcinoma
PSA	Prostate carcinoma
S100	Neurons, Schwann cells, naevi/melanoma, fat and cartilage
SMA	Smooth muscle, myoepithelial cells
Thyroglobulin	Thyroid tumours
TTF-1	Primary lung adenocarcinoma and small cell carcinoma, thyroid tumours
Vimentin	Several mesenchymal tissue types, some epithelia
Tumour type	**Main immunohistochemical markers used**
Carcinomas	AE1/AE3 (among others)
Melanoma	HMB45. S100 and Melan A
Sarcomas	Depends on histological subtype
Mesothelioma	As part of panel: calretinin, thrombomodulin, CK5/6
Germ cell tumours	PLAP, OCT-3/4
Lymphoma	CD45 to confirm haematological origin. Many others for subtyping

ALK, anaplastic lymphoma kinase; AML, acute myeloid leukaemia; CA, cancer antigen; CD, cluster of differentiation; CEA, carcino-embryonic antigen; CK, cytokeratin; C-Kit, = KIT (kitten: v-kit Hardy–Zuckerman 4 feline sarcoma viral oncogene homolog); CLL, chronic lymphocytic leukaemia; EMA, epithelial membrane antigen; ER, oestrogen receptor; GI, gastrointestinal; GIST, gastrointestinal stromal tumour; HER2, human epidermal growth factor receptor 2; HMB, human melanoma black; OCT-3/4, octamer-binding transcription factor 3/4; PLAP, placental alkaline phosphatase; PSA, prostate-specific antigen; RCC, renal cell carcinoma; SLL, small lymphocytic lymphoma; S100, S100 calcium binding protein; SMA, smooth muscle actin; TTF-1, thyroid transcription factor 1.

Table 4.2 Cytokeratin 7 and 20 profile for common tumours

	CK20+	CK20-
CK7+	Stomach Pancreas Ovarian mucinous Urothelial carcinoma	Breast Lung Ovarian serous Endometrial + endocervical Mesothelioma
CK7-	Colorectal Merkel cell	Kidney clear cell Prostate Liver Lung squamous cell carcinoma Adrenal

The adenocarcinomas in the CK7+CK20+ box (especially stomach, pancreas and ovarian mucinous) often show unpredictable CK20 staining. They should perhaps be regarded as CK7+CK20+/−.
Adapted from Tot, 2002 and Dennis et al., 2005.

Lymphoreticular tumours

There are over 200 'cluster of differentiation' (termed 'CD' for short) markers available for testing. A working knowledge of a subset of these is essential, as highlighted in Table 4.1. Common lymphomas and a brief summary of their immunohistochemical profile include the following:

Diffuse large B-cell lymphoma (DLBCL)

- CD45+ve, CD20+ve, BCL2+ve, CD10+ve (in germinal centre type).
- BCL 6, CD10 and MUM1 can be used to determine germinal centre type or non-germinal centre type.
- CD5 may be occasionally positive.

Follicular lymphoma (FL)

- CD45+ve, CD20+ve, CD10+ve, BCL2+ve (may be negative in some grade 3 tumours and cutaneous FL).
- CD5−ve, CD23−ve, Cyclin D1−ve.

Chronic lymphocytic leukaemia/small lymphocytic lymphoma (CLL/SLL)

- CD45+ve, CD20+ve, CD5+ve, CD23+ve.
- CD10−ve, Cyclin D1−ve.

Mantle cell lymphoma

- CD45+ve, CD20+ve, CD5+ve, Cyclin D1+ve.
- CD10−ve, CD23−ve.

Marginal zone lymphoma

- CD45+ve, CD20+ve.
- CD5−ve, CD10−ve, CD23−ve, Cyclin D1−ve.

Classical Hodgkin lymphoma

- Classical Reed Sternberg cells and mononuclear Hodgkin cells are CD45−ve, CD20−ve, CD15+ve, CD30+ve.

Germ cell tumours

Both placental alkaline phosphatase (PLAP) and Oct-3/4 are robust markers of germ cell tumours, although the latter is negative in yolk sac tumour and mature/immature teratoma. PLAP also shows positive staining of smooth and skeletal muscle tumours (which rarely cause diagnostic confusion). Overall they show good sensitivity and specificity.

Soft tissue tumours

A large number of antigens are available and their use will depend on the subtype of the tumour. Commonly used markers include the following:

- Vimentin: a type of intermediate filament found in the majority of mesenchymal cells. Unfortunately its use is somewhat restricted because of lack of specificity.
- Desmin: similar to cytokeratin, this is another type of intermediate filament found in muscle cells and is positive in leiomyosarcoma and rhabdomyosarcoma.
- MYOD1: this is a transcription factor and is positive in rhabdomyosarcoma.
- S100: positive in liposarcoma and chondrosarcoma (see melanoma section).
- CD31, CD34: these are endothelial markers and are positive in angiosarcoma.

Practical use of immunohistochemistry

Pathologists have a structured approach to the use of IHC in routine clinical practice based on a combination of the tissue morphology, clinical and radiological information. The humble H+E stain remains the most useful stain in determining which panel of markers to use. Indiscriminate use of IHC without considering the H+E appearance is costly and may lead to an incorrect diagnosis.

The commonest situations in which IHC is used are as follows.

1. To confirm a diagnosis on H+E.

    Example: a high molecular weight cytokeratin antibody (e.g. 34βE12 or CK5/6) will stain the basal cells of normal prostate glands. Prostate adenocarcinoma lacks a basal layer and therefore it is the absence of staining that is notable.

2. To ascertain if a tumour is primary to that organ.

    Example: a lung biopsy in a patient showing a moderately differentiated non-enteric type adenocarcinoma with clinical and radiological evidence of a lung primary would have a limited panel:

    - AE1/AE3: broad spectrum cytokeratin to confirm epithelial origin;
    - CK7: usually +ve in primary lung adenocarcinoma;
    - CK20: usually –ve in primary lung adenocarcinoma;
    - TTF-1: positive in > 75% of primary lung adenocarcinoma.

    If the CK7, CK20 and TTF-1 results were inconsistent, other markers would be used in a second panel to ascertain if the tumour was a metastasis (markers such as PSA, CDX2, thyroglobulin or CEA would be considered). This stepwise approach is commonly used with adenocarcinoma of uncertain origin (Dennis et al., 2005).

3. The problem of the tumour of unknown origin.

    Example: a neck biopsy in a patient showing a pleomorphic tumour would need a wide differential diagnosis. Clinical and radiological information would be considered. There may be subtle clues on morphology such as vague glandular formation in adenocarcinomas or some possible brown melanin pigment suggesting melanoma. The broad differential includes carcinoma, melanoma, lymphoma (such as anaplastic large cell lymphoma), sarcoma and (possibly less likely depending on the clinical scenario) germ cell tumours or mesothelioma.

The first immunohistochemical panel would include:

- AE1/AE3: broad spectrum cytokeratin to look for epithelial differentiation;
- S100, HMB45: markers to exclude metastatic malignant melanoma;
- CD45: (leucocyte common antigen) to exclude lymphoma.

Immunohistochemical markers for sarcomas, germ cell tumour and mesothelioma are often used in the second-line panel if the initial markers as listed above are negative.

If the pleomorphic tumour showed epithelial differentiation (AE1/AE3+ve) further markers would then be used to try to establish the site of origin. These markers would include: CK7, CK20, TTF-1, CEA, CDX2, PSA and thyroglobulin. (ER and CA125 may be used in females.) Neuroendocrine markers may also be used. Positive staining for S100 and HMB45 would indicate a diagnosis of malignant melanoma. If the CD45 was initially positive, additional lymphoma markers would then be used for definitive subclassification.

This stepwise approach of using immunohistochemical markers is essential, as every histopathology department faces time and financial pressures. Using every possible immunohistochemical marker from the outset on a pleomorphic tumour would not be cost-effective and would dramatically increase the time taken to report the case. It could also cause non-specific staining from uncommon IHC antigens leading to erroneous diagnoses.

The pathology report

A histopathology report should convey a combination of the stated clinical history, macroscopic description of the tissue, microscopic assessment and diagnosis. If the diagnosis is straightforward, the report should be concise, with a list of all prognostic information. If the tumour is difficult to classify, the report should reflect this with a list of differential diagnoses including a favoured diagnosis (depending on immunohistochemical and molecular investigations). A second expert opinion may be required.

The Royal College of Pathologists have published 'Tumour Datasets' (previously referred to as

Box 4.1 Example dialogue from a lung MDT

Consultant respiratory physician

The next case is an 87-year-old man, a lifelong smoker with a history of severe COPD, DM, IHD (angina on moderate exertion) and atrial fibrillation. He takes metformin, ramipril, statin, warfarin. He lives at home where his family help to care for him. His current PS is 3 and he is an inpatient under our care. He presented with weight loss and chest discomfort. Oxygen saturation is 89% on air.

Radiologist

A CT scan reveals emphysematous lungs with a 6 cm central, necrotic left-sided pulmonary mass in the upper lobe, invading the superior mediastinum with ipsilateral and contralateral mediastinal lymph nodes and also multiple liver metastases.

Respiratory physician

A CT lung biopsy would give a tissue diagnosis – a bronchoscopy wouldn't be tolerated that well.

Radiologist

This could be very risky – a pneumothorax would be devastating for him given his emphysema.

Respiratory physician

What about a liver biopsy, then?

Radiologist

Also risky: he is anti-coagulated and his liver function could be deranged.

Lung cancer CNS (patient's key worker)

This is a frail, elderly man who is unwell and who understands that he probably has advanced cancer. He and his family are keen for him to get home as soon as possible to spend what time he has left with his family.

Oncologist

Why are we getting a biopsy in this patient? Clinically and radiologically, he has advanced cancer. Treatment options are very limited: a short course of palliative radiotherapy could help his chest symptoms, but he may be better with supportive care only. A biopsy would not change treatment decisions. He is not a candidate for systemic therapy. So could we say that he has metastatic lung cancer based on clinical/radiological grounds and avoid the risks of a biopsy? We can then have an open conversation with him and plan discharge at an earlier date.

Palliative care consultant

He's known to our team – he is not well and just wants to be home. His symptoms have improved with low-dose opiates and prednisolone. If we agree that the plan is supportive care, we can start planning his discharge – organising a biopsy would delay this.

MDT decision

No need for biopsy in this case: we do not need it to merely confirm that he has cancer – it may cause complications and delay his discharge. Discharge is to be planned with involvement from the Community Palliative Care team. The lung clinical nurse specialist will be his key worker.

Box 4.2 Example dialogue from a lung MDT

Respiratory physician

The next case is a 48-year-old lady, a non-smoker with multiple bone metastases, liver metastases and a 5 cm peripheral lung mass. Her performance status is 2 and she has lost > 10% of her body weight.

Radiologist

Radiologically this may be a primary lung cancer – the upper lobe lung mass isn't typical of a metastasis, but it is hard to be certain. There are also mildly enlarged cervical and axillary lymph nodes, more prominent on the right.

Oncologist

I agree – this could be a primary lung cancer, or it could be metastatic disease from another site. She is a non-smoker and should be worked up for systemic therapy. We need a tissue diagnosis to help guide treatment decisions. Has she had a breast examination?

Respiratory physician

She has – it was normal. She has no systemic symptoms apart from weight loss, so no clue from history regarding what her primary cancer is. A bronchoscopy may not give a result: the lung mass is quite peripheral and in the upper lobe.

Lung cancer CNS (patient's key worker)

She is desperate to find out her diagnosis as soon as possible and start treatment if possible.

Radiologist

I can do an ultrasound-guided FNA of a lymph node tomorrow – that would get an answer very quickly.

Oncologist

A good plan, but are we certain that the lymph nodes are malignant, or what if the FNA isn't that cellular? We may not get a tissue diagnosis and would need to repeat a biopsy which would delay things for her. We also need to think about tissue for IHC/molecular studies – we may not get this from an FNA.

Lung cancer CNS

We need a diagnosis on our first investigation to minimise delays and anxiety for her. What is the best way to get a pathological diagnosis on our first attempt?

Pathologist

IHC may be essential to try and identify her primary, especially if this is an adenocarcinoma. This can be done on a cell block from a cellular FNA, but is less reliable than a core biopsy. I'd prefer a good tumour sample for us to work with, so a core biopsy would be best. It will help us to give you more information, if that is important for you clinically.

Oncologist

So – we need a core biopsy. We are not just doing this to confirm that she has cancer, but also to guide treatment decisions. Molecular testing may also be essential, e.g. for EGFR or ALK/MET mutation testing, if this is metastatic lung cancer. The question is what to biopsy?

Box 4.2 (*cont.*)

Radiologist

The options are bone, lymph node, lung or liver. Of these, I think lung is probably the best: lowest morbidity and most likely to get a result.

Oncologist

If it is a lung adenocarcinoma on pathology/IHC, could it be sent straight away for genetic testing for specific activating mutations, please?

MDT decision

For core biopsy of lung mass, then re-discuss. Although this is probably metastatic lung cancer, it may not be. The patient should stay in our MDT with the lung CNS as her key worker, until we have clear evidence that she should be under the care of another MDT. Investigations will happen more rapidly and she will benefit from having a key worker to support her.

'Minimum Datasets') since 1998. These are comprehensive and informative documents covering almost all cancer sites with an emphasis on practical handling of the pathological specimen, dissection of different specimen types and essential macroscopic and microscopic features to list in the pathology report. They also provide information on diagnostic coding, accurate staging, audit and quality indicators. An example of a recently updated data set is the second edition of the Royal College of Pathologists data set for tumours of the urinary collecting system (Shanks *et al.*, 2013). A cystoprostatectomy specimen report should have the following items listed.

Macroscopic

- Location, size and extent of tumours.
- Extent of invasion into bladder wall (macroscopic involvement of extravesical tissue by tumour is automatically pT3b).
- Margin status.
- Location and number of lymph nodes and measurement of tumour deposit in a lymph node if applicable.

Microscopic

- Type of tumour and grade (both WHO 1973 and 2004 grading schemes should be used). Histological variants of urothelial carcinoma should be noted, such as the micropapillary variant, as it has a worse prognosis.

- Microscopic extent of invasion into the wall (as in the TNM 7th edition).
- Presence or absence of lymphovascular invasion.
- Margin status (urethra, ureteric and circumferential soft tissue).
- Lymph node status (total number examined, number involved, size of largest deposit, presence or absence of extracapsular spread).
- Background – carcinoma *in situ*, examination of the prostate is performed – incidental finding of prostate adenocarcinoma may be found (if present this should be graded and allocated a tumour stage).

The above information is written as a 'proforma style' report with important prognostic information available and easy to read.

Boxes 4.1 and 4.2 show examples of dialogue from a lung MDT which illustrate how pathological information can guide the diagnosis and treatment of patients.

Summary

It is essential for all members of the MDT to work closely together and to understand the practices, language and limitations of each other's work. A sound understanding of the principles of pathological assessment of tumours is critical to this teamwork and to high-quality patient care. Advances in pathological/molecular testing alongside new, targeted therapies in oncology have revolutionised practice, but have created challenges in that additional processes and more complex diagnostic pathways have to be performed within tight time frames. It is incumbent on all MDT members to manage these challenges and to work well as a team to the best advantage of our patients.

References

Coons, A. H., Creech, H. J. and Jones, R. H. (1941). Immunological properties of an antibody containing a fluorescence group. *Proc. Soc. Exp. Biol. Med.*, **47**, 200–202.

Dennis, J. L., Hvidsten, T. R., Wit, E. C., *et al.* (2005). Markers of adenocarcinoma characteristic of the site of origin. Development of a diagnostic algorithm. *Clin. Cancer. Res.*, **11**, 3766–3772.

Fowler, L. J. and Lachar, W. A. (2008). Application of Immunohistochemistry to cytology. *Arch. Pathol. Lab. Med.*, **132**, 373–383.

Hiraki, T., Mimura, H., Gobara, H., *et al.* (2010). Incidence of and risk factors for pneumothorax and chest tube placement after CT fluoroscopy–guided percutaneous lung biopsy: retrospective analysis of the procedures conducted over a 9-year period. *Am. J. Roentgenol.*, **194**, 809–814.

Hsu, S-M., Raine, L. and Fanger, H. (1981). Use of avidin–biotin–peroxidase complex (ABC) in immunoperoxidase technique: a comparison between ABC and unlabeled antibody (PAP) procedures. *J. Histochem. Cytochem.*, **29**, 577–580.

Jaffe, E. S., Harris, N. L., Stein, H. *et al.* (2001). *World Health Organisation Classification of Tumours. Pathology and Genetics. Tumours of Haematopoietic and Lymphoid Tissues.* Lyon: IARC Press.

Shanks, J. H., Chandra, A., McWilliam, L., *et al.* (2013). *Standards and Datasets for Reporting Cancers. Dataset for Tumours of the Urinary Collecting System (Renal Pelvis, Ureter, Urinary Bladder and Urethra.* 2nd ed. London: The Royal College of Pathologists. Available at https://www.rcpath.org/Resources/RCPath/Migrated%20Resources/Documents/G/G044_Urologydataset_Apr13.pdf (accessed October 2014).

Swerdlow, S. H., Campo, E., Harris, N. L., *et al.* (2008). *World Health Organisation Classification of Tumours. Pathology and Genetics. Tumours of Haematopoietic and Lymphoid Tissues.* 4th ed. Lyon: IARC Press.

Tot, T. (2002). Cytokeratins 20 and 7 as biomarkers: usefulness in discriminating primary from metastatic adenocarcinoma. *Eur. J. Cancer*, **38**, 758–763.

West, J., and Card, T. R. (2010). Reduced mortality rates following elective percutaneous liver biopsies. *Gastroenterology*, **139**, 1230–1237.

Radiotherapy planning 1: fundamentals of external beam and brachytherapy

Andrew Tyler and Louise Hanna

Introduction

It is important to understand the basic techniques of radiotherapy planning because these will help when developing complex plans. These techniques, which are taught at the First FRCR level (Royal College of Radiologists), are used by the treatment centre's Physics Department for checking the validity of calculations before they are applied to patients, and anyone interpreting plans will need to be familiar with them to know whether it is worth adjusting treatment plans during review. Advanced radiotherapy techniques will be discussed in Chapter 6.

There are several useful reviews of radiotherapy physics in the literature. One by Shiu and Mellenberg (2001) includes sections on isodose planning. Another, by Purdy (2000), provides a perspective on future directions in 3D treatment planning. Radiotherapy is a rapidly developing field and it is important to ensure that new methods satisfy safety and effectiveness requirements before being adopted as routine treatments.

This chapter will deal with the general principles of developing isodose plans that are suitable for treatment and will use specific examples to highlight particular points. It will focus mainly on external beam radiotherapy with megavoltage photons; there will be shorter sections on the use of electrons and brachytherapy. Some aspects of radiotherapy planning using lower energy (kilovoltage) photons will be discussed in Chapter 36. The use of unsealed radiation sources for prostate, thyroid and childhood cancers are discussed in Chapters 22, 38 and 40, respectively.

Treatment planning overview

Radiotherapy planning can be divided into stages as follows.

- Patient preparation, position and immobilisation.

- Localisation method (e.g. orthogonal films, CT scanning, and image co-registration).
- Definition of target volumes and organs at risk.
- Radiotherapy technique, including beam arrangements, beam energy, size and shape, weighting, wedges and production of isodose plan.
- Prescription, including number of phases, dose, energy and fractionation.
- Verification (i.e. checking the geometrical set-up of the treatment). This can take place before treatment in the simulator or CT simulator, and/or during treatment using portal imaging.

Quality assurance (QA) is essential and it is of paramount importance for each member of the planning team to be familiar with the overall process.

Patient position and immobilisation

For radiotherapy to be effective it must be delivered accurately, and it is important to understand the methods of immobilisation and the inevitable uncertainties in the delivery of treatment. Patients must be positioned to allow the optimum delivery of the radiotherapy while maintaining comfort. Variables include whether the patient is prone or supine, and the position of the limbs or the neck. Radiotherapy treatments that require unusual treatment positions include total-body irradiation, when the patient may lie in the lateral position with the arms in front of the chest to provide lung compensation, and total skin electron treatment, when the patient may stand up, adopting the stance of a cross-country skier (one arm and the opposite leg forward, the other arm and leg back).

A wide variety of different immobilisation devices exists. The most appropriate one (or combination) depends on the position of the tumour, the need to

Practical Clinical Oncology, Second Edition, ed. Louise Hanna, Tom Crosby and Fergus Macbeth. Published by Cambridge University Press. © Cambridge University Press 2015.

protect adjacent structures, and the treatment intent. The following are some commonly used devices.

- Simple head, knee or ankle supports which help to stabilise the patient. For patients who do not have very mobile superficial tissues, treatments can be delivered to within ± 5 mm, providing that a careful set-up, suitable reference points, and calibrated couch movements are all used.
- Chest board with cross bar to fix the arms above the head (e.g. for breast treatments).
- Vacuum bags offer customised support (e.g. for limbs when it is necessary to support the limb in a position that allows access for beams).
- Vacuum-formed shells, moulded thermoplastic shells (heated in warm water) or Perspex® shells formed from individualised plaster moulds. By using well-fitted vacuum-formed shells for head and neck treatments, inaccuracies in set-up can be reduced to within 3 mm. However, vacuum-formed shells for other anatomical sites do not usually give this reliability.
- Complete fixation devices such as stereotactic frames with mouth bites give set-up accuracy to within about 1 mm. These also require high-level QA on treatment machines.

It is important to be certain that the immobilisation device is effective. For example, one study looked at the use of a customised immobilisation system (Vacfix® cushion) for the treatment of the prostate, and the authors concluded that the treatment accuracy was not improved when compared with the conventional technique (using standard ankle stocks) (Nutting et al., 2000).

Imaging the patient

Imaging the patient is essential to delineate gross tumour volume (GTV), to design the clinical target volume (CTV) and planning target volume (PTV), and to outline critical structures in accordance with ICRU reports 50 and 62 (ICRU, 1993, 1999).

CT simulation

A CT simulator is one of the mainstays of 3D conformal planning. It is typically a wide-bore CT scanner with virtual simulation software (VSIM) and radiotherapy accessories (e.g. flat couch, mounts for immobilisation devices, laser positioning, etc.). It provides precise imaging and positioning information for the treatment planning process.

Automatic electronic data transfer to a treatment planning system is required to enable the treatment calculation to be performed.

The wide bore, although theoretically providing a slight reduction in image quality, allows patients to be scanned in the treatment position and for reference marks, from which treatments can be set up, to be identified securely.

CT scans are taken over a few seconds, whereas a treatment fraction can take longer to deliver. Therefore, normal patient motion, such as breathing, may be 'frozen' at any point in the cycle on the CT scan and the expansion of the CTV to PTV must take this into account.

The planning CT scan is usually taken using a slice interval of 1.5–5 mm. The narrower the slice width, the better will be the resolution in the digital reconstructed radiograph (DRR). It is important to include the proposed target volume and the organs at risk in the scan to allow dose volume histograms (DVHs) to be calculated.

Administration of intravenous contrast helps to distinguish tumour from normal tissues. One example of this is during planning for lung cancer. There has been debate whether the use of contrast alters the dosimetry, but Lees et al. (2005) have found that it makes little difference in dose computation. 4D CT where a number of CT scans are taken at each phase of the breathing cycle is also in common use (see Chapter 31).

For some tumour sites, such as the brain, MRI scans are better than CT scans for delineating the GTV (see Chapter 35).

Nuclear medicine

Although radiopharmaceutical imaging tends to be used for diagnostic purposes, it is increasingly being used to inform the treatment planning process, especially with the advent of positron emission tomography (PET)/computed tomography (CT), where the automatic co-registration of the images can be used as a direct input into the planning process. Applications which have been studied include brain, head and neck, lung, lymphoma, GI, genitourinary (GU) and gynaecological cancers.

'Conventional' radiotherapy planning

Conventional radiotherapy planning has been largely superseded by CT planning. The target volumes are delineated on orthogonal X-ray images and then transferred onto an outline of the patient taken at one or more levels. Alternatively, for some treatments using simple beam arrangements such as a parallel opposed pair of fields, the field borders themselves are defined on a radiograph or simulator image. These borders represent the PTV with a small margin to take into account the beam penumbra. Tissue definition, particularly for soft tissues, is not clear when using orthogonal films.

Defining the target volumes

Standards

The publications ICRU 50 and ICRU 62 (ICRU, 1993, 1999) will be referred to throughout in this text. Anyone taking part in the planning process should be familiar with the terms defined within. As a brief recap, the following terms are used to ensure that accurate treatment records are kept (ICRU, 1993, 1999).

- Gross tumour volume (GTV) – the demonstrable tumour.
- Clinical target volume (CTV) – the GTV and/or suspected subclinical tumour.
- Planning target volume (PTV) – the CTV and a margin for uncertainties, which may be systematic or random, and are taken into account by:
  - the internal margin (IM), which is added to account for involuntary changes in the organs that surround the CTV;
  - the set-up margin (SM), which accounts for the uncertainties and lack of reproducibility in setting up the patient day by day.
- Treated volume – the volume enclosed by an isodose surface, selected and specified by the radiation oncologist as being appropriate to achieve the purpose of treatment (e.g. tumour eradication, palliation).
- Irradiated volume – the tissue volume that receives a dose that is considered significant in relation to normal tissue tolerance.
- Organs at risk (OARs) – critical normal structures the radiation sensitivity of which may significantly affect treatment planning and/or prescribed dose.
- Planning organ at risk volume (PRV) – the organs at risk with a suitable margin to account for movements and uncertainties in set-up.

Figure 5.1 shows tumour and target volumes as defined in ICRU 50 (ICRU, 1993).

The target volume is delineated with all the relevant clinical information available including medical

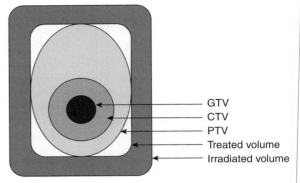

Figure 5.1 International Commission on Radiation Units volume definitions. CTV, clinical target volume; GTV, gross tumour volume; PTV, planning target volume. Redrawn with permission of the ICRU, 1993: ICRU Report 50. *Prescribing, Recording, and Reporting Photon Beam Therapy.* Bethesda, Maryland: International Commission on Radiation Units and Measurements; http:ICRU.org, accessed January 2015.

history, pretreatment diagnostic and staging investigation results, scan images, operation notes and pathology reports. The three volumes, GTV, CTV and PTV, can be defined, together with the OAR and PRV. There can be more than one OAR.

Any reduction in the treatment margins spares more normal tissues and introduces an opportunity for considering dose escalation for the tumour. When margins are smaller, it becomes more difficult to be sure that the tumour is being treated. Although the treatment machine delivers radiation with an accuracy supported by elaborate QA, there are many other uncertainties in the planning process, including our inability to define microscopic disease.

Delineating the GTV

Delineating the GTV involves outlining the demonstrable tumour. However, considerable variation between GTVs has been observed among different radiation oncologists (Logue *et al.*, 1998; Weiss and Hess, 2003). Discussion with the multidisciplinary team, dedicated radiotherapy planning meetings and involvement of a radiology specialist can facilitate this process. For example, in the head and neck, the tumour volumes may shrink during radiotherapy.

Growth from GTV to CTV

By definition, it is not possible to identify subclinical disease by imaging or clinical examination. Individual patient variation will add to the uncertainty (e.g. the internal mammary chain lymph nodes lie between 1 and 6 cm deep and up to 4 cm from the midline). Some organs are more difficult to delineate than others, but other imaging techniques such as magnetic resonance imaging (MRI) may be helpful. Guidelines have been produced for CTV definition in high-grade gliomas, head and neck, and lung tumours (Gregoire *et al.*, 2000; Jansen *et al.*, 2000; Senan *et al.*, 2004; Apisarthanarax *et al.*, 2006).

Forming the PTV

The dose delivered to the CTV or OARs will not be the same as that shown on the plan if they are not in exactly the same place during all the treatments. Internal movements are significant in the thorax, abdomen and pelvis. For example, the prostate and seminal vesicles can move with changes in the volume of the bladder or rectum, up to a centimetre each way anterior–posterior (A-P), and the CTV of tumours in the lung, particularly those nearest to the diaphragm, will move during breathing.

- Changes in the position or size of the CTV (both during and between fractions) must be taken into account. These natural variations are inevitable, but the size of the variation can to some extent be estimated and accounted for. These form the IM.
- Uncertainties of patient set-up, alignment of beams and so forth also need to be taken into account; these make up the SM.
- The combination of these two margins around the CTV forms the PTV (ICRU, 1999).
- The uncertainties associated with these margins have been estimated (BIR, 2003) and methods of calculation have been introduced that ensure that 95% of the prescribed dose covers the CTV in 90% of cases. The BIR (2003) document uses the concepts of systematic and random errors, and, as part of the document, some key examples by clinical site provide excellent guidance.
- Options such as image-guided radiation therapy (IGRT) and respiratory gating can be employed to reduce the required margins. Techniques to reduce tumour movement have been used in thorax treatments such as breath hold, active breathing control, or depressing the chest to reduce the movement. Lung tumour motion can be in the order of 2 cm during a normal breathing cycle, depending on the lobe of the lung affected (Seppenwoolde *et al.*, 2002).
- Automatic growth tools on the planning computer may help, but the mechanism should be understood before using them and they should always be used with care.

Delineating organs at risk

OARs are normal structures with a high sensitivity to radiation and it is important that they are delineated on the plan. Some, such as the spinal cord, may be described as being 'serial' with a high 'relative seriality'.

Others such as the lung may be described as 'parallel' and have a low 'relative seriality' (ICRU, 1999). Within some organs (e.g. the heart), there may be a combination of serial and parallel structures.

The function of serial organs may be seriously affected if even a small portion is irradiated above a tolerance dose. The effect of radiation on the function of parallel organs is more dependent on the volume irradiated. For a serial organ, the accuracy of treatment planning and delivery are important to ensure that tolerance is not exceeded. In a manner similar to the construction of the PTV, a margin must be added to make the planning organ at risk volume (PRV). In practice, this applies most commonly to the spinal cord.

Principles of the isodose plan: photons

Basic beam data

It is important that the concepts of basic beam data are understood. These are described briefly here, but in detail in other texts (e.g. Williams and Thwaites, 2000; Khan, 2003). These topics are all covered in the First FRCR course (RCR) and are discussed in ICRU 24 (ICRU, 1976).

Beam divergence. The width of the radiation beam increases linearly with distance from the treatment head.

Beam penumbra. At the edge of the radiation beam, the dose reduces over the distance of some millimetres. The penumbra is the distance between the 80% and 20% isodoses. In general it will be necessary to use a beam that is wider than the PTV to allow the 95% isodose to encompass the PTV.

Percentage depth dose. The dose is expressed as a percentage of the maximum dose deposited by the beam. This maximum dose occurs at a depth d_{max}. With mega-voltage beams the dose is deposited by secondary electrons, which travel primarily in a forward direction. As a result there is build-up of dose below the skin surface before d_{max} is reached.

Build-up changes also occur at interfaces between tissues of differing densities. In some centres the tissue phantom ratio (TPR) or tissue maximum ratio (TMR) is used instead of the percentage depth dose because each is easier to use with isocentric calculations.

Radial profile. The radial profile of a megavoltage beam changes with depth due to the differential hardening across the beam. This means that, if an asymmetric beam is created, the shape of the profile may also be noticeably asymmetric.

Changes with distance. As the distance from the treatment machine to the patient increases, the cross-sectional area of the beam increases because of divergence. The inverse-square law causes the intensity of the radiation beam to decrease but the percentage depth doses below d_{max} to increase.

Changes with field size. As the field size increases, the central axis receives more radiation per monitor unit because of increased scatter from the machine head and within the patient.

Beam arrangements

Typical beam arrangements are as follows.

- A single beam is used for superficial tumours such as skin cancers, or for tumours that are not at or near the midplane (e.g. spinal tumours having palliative treatment).
- For two beams, opposing beams are used for palliative treatments or for treatments in sites that have a relatively small separation, such as head and neck, breast and limbs;
  - non-opposing beams, for example, are set at right angles to the floor of the mouth and the maxillary antrum. Wedges are needed to reduce the inhomogeneities that arise in this situation. If the external contour of the patient is irregular in all directions around the central axis of the beam, then external tissue compensators or 'field-in-field' techniques using multi-leaf collimators (MLCs) will probably be required.
- Combinations of beams are usually used for radical treatments in sites such as the chest, pelvis and brain, where the use of multiple beams spares adjacent normal tissues.

It is also important to understand beam weighting so that the relative proportion of dose delivered to the tumour from each beam can be adjusted (Williams and Thwaites, 2000).

Choosing beam directions

For conventional planning the choice of beam directions will depend on the treatment intent and the locations of the PTV and OARs. For example, with radical oesophagus treatments, delivering the dose entirely by anterior and posterior parallel-opposed fields would exceed spinal cord tolerance. Similarly, using oblique laterals instead of the posterior beam would cause an excessive dose to the lungs. A two-phase technique that combines both of these approaches can prevent tolerance doses from being exceeded. In prostate planning, an anterior beam is combined with two wedged lateral fields. Use of lateral fields, rather than posterior obliques, allows beam shaping to be more effective in reducing the dose to the rectum. In head and neck treatments, the exit beams should avoid such critical structures as the contralateral eye and spinal cord. When performing IMRT/VMAT planning, different rules apply.

Treatment plans can frequently be improved with the use of non-coplanar beams, which can improve the dose distribution in the PTV and reduce the dose to organs at risk. Non-coplanar beam arrangements can be achieved easily by linear accelerators, by rotating the table and the gantry, but it is important to ensure that the beam direction can be achieved (e.g. there is no collision between the treatment head and the couch or the patient). Non-coplanar beams are particularly useful in central nervous system and head and neck treatments.

Isodose shapes for combinations of beams

The directions of the beams will influence the shape of the treated volume. By tracing the edges of the beams, it is possible to identify the general shape of the high-dose volume, provided that the beams are well balanced and that there is a homogeneous dose distribution across the PTV. In Figure 5.2, the treated volume in the plane shown will be approximately the hexagon enclosed by the beam edges.

It is important to identify potential regions of hot and cold dose. The global hot spot in a balanced multi-beam treatment is likely to lie close to the centre of the treated volume.

There are occasions when it may be difficult to prevent the dose to the PTV from dipping low. Examples include the following:

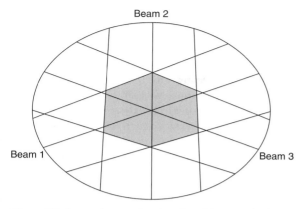

Figure 5.2 Beam edges creating the edge of the treated volume. In the scenario presented here, there are three beams (beams 1, 2 and 3). The shaded area represents the volume which received the highest radiation dose, and it is formed by the edges of the beams.

- The superior and inferior (S-I) ends of a coplanar plan because of the lack of dose scattering into the volume from outside the beams.
- When a wedged pair is used (e.g. with an anterior and a lateral field), it is common for the postero-medial aspect to be underdosed. It is possible to top up the beam with a small amount of dose from the contralateral side, but this obviously has implications for the dose to normal tissue on that side. Outside of the treated volume, the greatest doses for this type of plan will lie underneath the thin ends of the wedges.

Use of a field-in-field technique, where regions of underdose are topped up with small beamlets, can help to reduce inhomogeneities of dose.

Beam modifications: shape, wedges and tissue compensators

Beam shaping

Shaping the beam around the PTV spares more normal tissue. For example, randomised trials of prostate treatments have shown that the use of conformal radiotherapy reduces rectal toxicity compared with non-conformal treatments, and this has led to studies of dose escalation for improving local control (Dearnaley et al., 1999).

Traditionally, low-melting-point alloy blocks have been shaped individually for each field for megavoltage treatments, but in many cases field shaping can be achieved with MLCs. Making low-melting-point alloy

blocks requires time and handling of heavy and hazardous substances. The conformity achieved by MLCs is limited by the width of the leaves and their direction of movement. A potential problem is leakage between the abutted leaf ends; this can be reduced if the main collimator jaws are positioned as far as possible over the leaf abutments (Klein et al., 1995).

Wedges

Wedges are used in two situations where there is an unwanted dose gradient that is relatively uniform in one direction:

- To act as a tissue compensator for a sloping external surface (see discussion of surface obliquity that follows).
- To even out the dose when two or more beams intersect, in order to avoid hot and cold spots within the treated volume.

Surface obliquity

Surface obliquity will cause isodoses to tilt in the same directions as the surface. If the obliquity occurs only in one direction, it can be corrected for by placing a wedge in the beam. If it occurs in both the S-I and A-P directions, then it may be necessary to consider using a custom-built tissue compensator. Tissue compensators are used most frequently in head and neck treatments. They can also be used in other situations, such as 3D radiotherapy of the breast, although they will be needed less often in the future as advanced radiotherapy techniques such as IMRT develop.

Calculation cycle

Everybody involved in a patient calculation should know the whole calculation process and where each factor is applied in their own department, even if many of the factors are applied by the planning computer programs. The method of calculation varies from centre to centre, depending on how the factors are defined, and it is not possible to go through each variation in this chapter. Because of this, it is important to be familiar with the local method before starting any calculations involving patients. Factors (and their relative values) that need to be understood follow (Williams and Thwaites, 2000).

- Percentage depth dose (PDD) or tissue maximum ratio (TMR).
- Inverse-square law.

- Wedge factor.
- Field size (output) factor.
- Accessory factors (e.g. trays).

Using a 3D planning system

Production of the isodose plan

With a 3D planning system, the target volumes and PRVs can be delineated individually on each slice of a cross-sectional imaging study such as a CT scan. Software can allow co-registration of images from other modalities such as MRI or PET. After identifying the relevant volumes, it is then possible to simulate the positions of treatment beams and shielding and to use algorithms to calculate and display the resulting isodose curves.

The respective doses to the PTV and PRVs can be displayed in the form of a DVH, which is a line graph showing the proportion of the volume that receives at least a specified dose of radiation. DVHs are a convenient way of comparing different planning solutions for the same tumour in order to select the best dose distribution.

Data from the planning process can be used to create a 'beam's eye view' (BEV) image of the treatment fields, which can be superimposed on the digital reconstructed radiograph and used for verification purposes.

Selection of the ICRU reference point

The recommendation for reporting doses is based on the ICRU reference point. According to ICRU 50 (ICRU, 1993), the reference point is selected according to the following criteria.

- The point should be clinically relevant and representative of the dose throughout the PTV.
- It should be easy to define in a clear and unambiguous way.
- It should be selected where the dose can be accurately determined.
- It should be selected in a region where there is no steep dose gradient.

In practice, the ICRU reference point is often at the isocentre or at the intersection of beams, but sometimes this is not possible, in which case it should be selected to be in a place where dose specification is considered meaningful.

Inhomogeneities of density

When organs are of different densities, there will be changes in the penetration of the beam. For example, the dose in a central organ, such as the oesophagus, from a beam passing through an aerated lung can increase by as much as 15% when a correction is applied. This is because in a well-aerated lung, the extra penetration of the beam is usually slightly greater than 2% per centimetre of the lung traversed. In contrast, bones tend to have little effect on the dose; dense bone tends to lie in thin layers, and the core of long bones is almost unit density. Artificial hips are very high density and they can create particular problems during planning. In addition to the artefacts seen on CT imaging, the planning algorithm may not be able to correct properly for the very-high-density material. It is best to avoid passing beams through metal objects if possible.

Treatment planning systems will make corrections for changes of density pixel by pixel, by using the CT values. Nearly all planning systems will estimate these effects, but some of the so-called 3D planning systems still use 1D corrections, which means that only the primary beam is corrected. This can lead to uncertainties in dose when adjacent structures have different densities, because changes from scatter contributions will be significant. Many systems use a 2D correction which does reduce some of this uncertainty, but routine clinical use of a full 3D correction as given by Monte Carlo simulation is still some way off because of the very large computing power required.

Doses to organs at risk

Outside the PTV, significant volumes of normal tissue are irradiated to a high dose, and they would benefit from receiving a smaller dose. The OAR dose often limits the highest dose that can be delivered to the tumour. In general, it is best to try to avoid letting any part of the beam pass through an OAR, and skilful use of the beam edge and beam direction can often ensure that the beam passes through the PTV but avoids an OAR. However, it is not always necessary to avoid an OAR completely. For example, in the thorax it may be appropriate to pass a posterior beam through the spinal cord to reduce lung dose and meet the appropriate DVH constraint. If one or more beams exit through an OAR, it is important to check the tolerance doses carefully.

In addition to choosing appropriate beam directions, it is also possible to use wedges to reduce the doses in sensitive structures. For example, in Figure 5.3, a

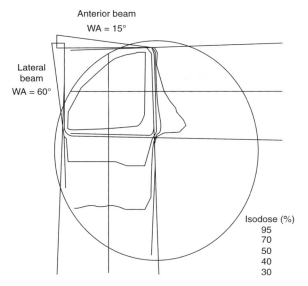

Anterior beam
WA = 15°

Lateral beam
WA = 60°

Isodose (%)
95
70
50
40
30

Figure 5.3 Drawing dose away from sensitive structures using wedges. A steep wedge angle on the lateral beam allows an extra dose to be given from the anterior beam, and can be used to spare a structure such as the contralateral eye or brain, but obviously at a cost of dose to the deeper structures posterior to the target volume, which could include the brain stem. WA, wedge angle.

steep wedge angle on the lateral beam allows extra dose to be given from the anterior beam, and this can be used to spare a structure such as the contralateral eye or brain, but obviously at a cost of dose to the deeper posterior structures which could include the brain stem.

Matching adjacent beams in complex treatments

Sometimes beams need to be adjacent to each other, for example, in combined breast and supraclavicular fossa radiotherapy, or craniospinal axis treatments. When two diverging beams are adjacent to each other, there will be an overlap and a potential gap, depending on the depth at which the beams meet. Various methods have been used to minimise any variations in dose that occur when beams are matched together. However, care must be taken because, although it is possible to produce what looks like a perfect plan with perfect junctions between the beams, patients can move between treatments even when they are in an immobilisation shell.

For craniospinal treatments, the junction can be moved twice during treatment to spread the effect of any uncertainty in positioning.

Other ways of minimising dose variations at junctions include half-beam blocking or couch rotations, both of which can compensate for the effect of beam

divergence, but the possibility of patient movement during treatment must still be considered.

When treating neck nodes with conventional radiotherapy, it is sometimes necessary to have an electron field next to a photon field, which can pose even more difficulties because the shapes of the isodoses are completely different. One solution has been to increase the number of photon fields with the intention of trying to avoid using the electron fields. This type of treatment is a prime case for advanced radiotherapy planning with intensity-modulated radiation therapy (IMRT).

Verification

Verification of the planned treatment

The treatment actually delivered will differ from that which has been planned because of set-up errors and internal movements during and between fractions. If possible, it is best to minimise these effects by careful immobilisation and the use of accurate and stable marks for beam set-up.

Otherwise, movements may require online megavoltage portal imaging or use of a kilovoltage CT imager attached to the linac gantry. Ultrasound-based guidance can also been used for prostate treatments.

Validity of the set-up

Indexed positioning, using identical simulation and treatment couches, has been developed to aid in quick and repeatable set-ups. Although portal imaging helps to verify the set-up in relation to bony landmarks, the organ of interest may not show up on the image, and internal organs may move during the course of treatment. A prostate gland can move more than 5 mm in 7 minutes; therefore, the position of the prostate can be significantly different from the time of scan to the time of treatment (Padhani *et al.*, 1999). Implanted markers, such as gold grains (e.g. in the prostate) which can be monitored on the portal image, have been shown to improve the accuracy of treatment set-up (Shimizu *et al.*, 2000).

The treatment position can be verified before treatment by using a simulator or CT simulator, and/or during treatment by using megavoltage portal imaging or kilovoltage CT imaging. By taking serial images it is possible to judge whether a set-up error is systematic or random. Correction of set-up errors by moving treatment fields should only be carried out for systematic errors, unless the movement is done on a daily basis as required and as part of an online IGRT strategy. See Chapter 6 for a further discussion of IGRT.

Verification of treatment dose

If the CTV receives less than the intended dose then the risk of recurrence is likely to increase. For example, as beam conformity increases, there may be a greater risk of a recurrence at the edge of the treatment field. It will become increasingly important to identify the position of recurrence within the PTV in conformal radiotherapy. At present, thermoluminescence dosimetry (TLD) is the only practical method of *in vivo* dosimetry, but it is usually used only at the skin surface. There is interest in evaluating electronic portal imaging devices to measure exit doses, which may provide some verification of the dose received from each portal.

Quality assurance of treatment planning systems

Reducing treatment errors

To treat patients safely, technical quality is essential but not enough: QA of the clinical process is also required. Systems such as 'Quality Assurance in Radiation Therapy' (QART) should be put in place to ensure overall control of the activities in the radiotherapy department (Kehoe and Rugg, 1999). In the UK it is a requirement for radiotherapy services to have a Quality Management System (e.g. ISO9000: 2008) and for all staff to be engaged with this. Towards Safer Radiotherapy provides a comprehensive overview of how to develop a risk aware culture and is now used as the basis of radiotherapy incident reporting (The Royal College of Radiologists *et al.*, 2008).

Increasing the complexity of treatments does not necessarily result in more treatment errors; automated data transfer and automated set-ups have considerably decreased errors without increasing treatment times. However, increasing the complexity of manual treatments does lead to more errors.

Modern 3D treatment planning systems provide a wealth of information which was previously not available, such as the density of internal body organs and DVHs, but using this information also needs careful QA to ensure that the data are valid (Purdy and Harms, 1998). New tests and phantoms have been designed to investigate the non-dosimetric functions of these systems.

Commissioning 3D treatment planning systems involves a large number of quality checks, including testing the reliability of the transfer of body outlines, of the values for tissue density and of the projection of reconstructions. 'TG53' is an important document produced by a topic group of the AAPM Radiation Therapy Committee which describes all the tests to be considered when commissioning a treatment planning system (Fraass *et al.*, 1998). Care needs to be taken when introducing what seem to be simpler treatments such as replacing physical wedges with dynamic ones. Implementation into the planning systems is complicated and entails significant QA before use in a clinical setting.

Other tools such as the DVH used in 3D planning can cause errors if they are not used correctly. For example, if the number of dose points used to form the DVH is low, this will give a false volume, or if there is a high dose gradient within a volume, the computer may be unable to evaluate the dose within that volume. Also, it may not be appropriate to define some organs (e.g. hollow structures like the rectum) simply by delineating their outer surface.

It is expected that the dose under MLCs will increase because of leaf penetration and interleaf leakage, but if the back-up collimators can be used, then the jaws will provide extra shielding and reduce the peripheral dose at these points.

Verification systems have helped the treatment process but, to reduce the risk of errors, further automation of data transfer is essential.

Critical analysis of treatment plans

Using the basic principles discussed earlier, the quality of a treatment plan can be reviewed and decisions can be made about whether to improve the distribution or whether a compromise must be made between delivery of the dose to the PTV and that to the adjacent OARs.

Three principles, backed up by ICRU 50, provide the basics for this analysis.

Homogenous dose to the PTV. When the dose is prescribed at the ICRU reference point (typically the crosspoint of the beams), the highest dose in the PTV is usually considerably less than the +7% maximum described in ICRU 50. However, it may be more difficult to ensure that the PTV is covered by the 95% isodose while not irradiating too much normal tissue.

Organs at risk. The plan should be designed to avoid overtreating any dose-limiting organ, but sometimes a compromise may have to be made, which will limit the overall delivery of dose to the PTV.

Other normal tissues. The high dose volume in the PTV should fall off rapidly in normal tissue. When the correct choice of energy and beams is used, the doses in normal tissue are not usually a problem, but there will always be higher doses at the entry points of the beams. The exit sites of all beams should be checked carefully to ensure that the dose to sensitive tissues is at a safe level.

Examples of plans that require improvement

Figure 5.4 shows two different plans for a two-field treatment for radical radiotherapy treatment for carcinoma of the larynx. In example (a), two lateral beams are used and the PTV dose homogeneity is not ideal, because of the oblique skin surface. The solution, shown in example (b), is to use fairly small-angled wedged beams (~15°) to act as tissue compensators. However, care must be taken here because any changes in the patient's contour in the S-I direction will not be accounted for, and a full compensator may be needed.

Figure 5.5 shows two different plans for a 3D conformal treatment with radical radiotherapy to the prostate. In plan (a), the 95% isodose lies considerably outside the lateral margins of the PTV. The solution to this problem is to make the anterior beam narrower, as shown in plan (b). Note that the DVHs for the PTV and rectum in both plans are identical. This shows that it is important to look at both the plan and the DVHs. This three-field plan requires 60° wedges on the lateral beams to compensate for the dose gradient caused by the anterior beam. The plan also illustrates the importance of using the correct beam direction. Using lateral beams rather than posterior obliques allows for greater sparing of the rectum, because the beam edge is used to try to provide the maximum dose gradient between the prostate and the rectum.

Figure 5.6 shows two plans for a 3D conformal treatment with radical radiotherapy for carcinoma of the bronchus delivering 55 Gy in 20 fractions. In example (a), all three beams pass through the spinal cord, and cord tolerance is exceeded. A solution is shown in example (b), where the posterior beam has been moved to a posterior oblique direction and the anterior oblique beam has been moved more laterally. As a result, only the exit beam from

(a)

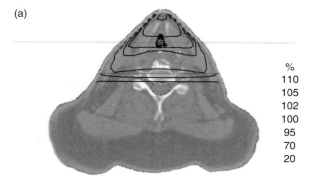

	%
	110
	105
	102
	100
	95
	70
	20

(b)

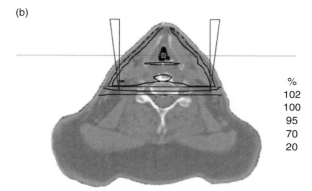

	%
	102
	100
	95
	70
	20

Figure 5.4 Two different plans for a radical radiotherapy treatment for carcinoma of the larynx treated with lateral opposed fields. In example (a), two lateral beams are used and the PTV dose homogeneity is not ideal, because of the oblique skin surface. The solution, shown in example (b), is to use fairly small-angled wedged beams (~15°) to act as tissue compensators (see text for further explanation).

the anterior direction passes through the spinal cord and the dose is now within tolerance. Note also that, by exiting through the cord, the anterior beam avoids the lung. Part (c) shows that the DVH for spinal cord is significantly better for plan (b), and although the lung DVH is worse for plan (b) it is still well within acceptable limits (V20 of less than 35%).

Electrons

Electron beam isodoses have a shape that is significantly different from that of photon beams. The fairly homogeneous dose distribution close to the surface and rapid fall-off at depth make electron doses ideal for treating superficial tumours. The reporting of electron doses should follow ICRU 71 (ICRU, 2004) in a way similar to that for photons. Figure 5.7 shows an electron isodose for an 18-MeV electron beam.

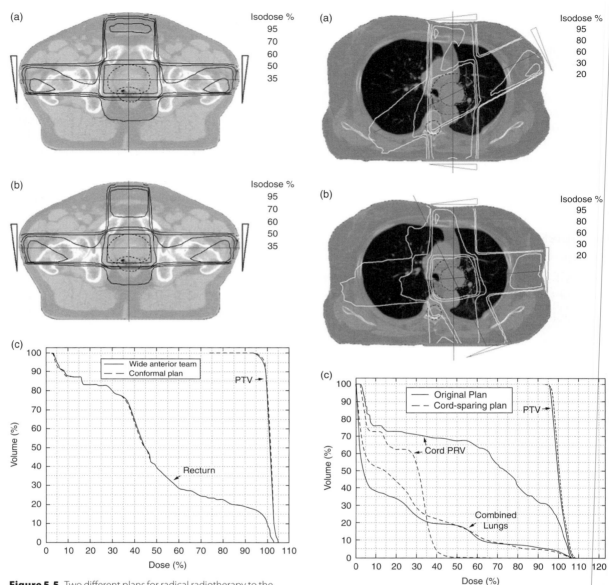

Figure 5.5 Two different plans for radical radiotherapy to the prostate treated with an anterior and two lateral fields. In example (a) for treating the prostate, the 95% isodose lies considerably outside the lateral margins of the PTV. The solution to this is to make the anterior beam narrower as shown in example (b). The DVHs for both plans are shown in (c). See text for further explanation.

Figure 5.6 Two plans for radical radiotherapy for carcinoma of the bronchus. In example (a), all three beams pass through the spinal cord and because of this, cord tolerance is exceeded. A solution is shown in example (b), where the posterior beam has been moved to a post-oblique direction and the ant-oblique beam has been moved more laterally. PRV, planning organ at risk volume; PTV, planning target volume. See text for further explanation.

Care is required when using electrons:

- high-dose treatment isodoses tend to pinch in, especially with small fields;
- low-dose isodoses tend to spread out and can impinge on local OARs; and
- a bolus is often required to increase the dose at the skin surface. The thickness of the bolus will need

to be taken into account when deciding on the electron energy.

The uncertainties are much greater than in photon beam treatments:

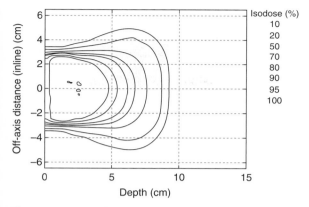

Figure 5.7 Isodoses for a 6 × 6 cm 18 MeV electron beam. Note how the higher isodoses become narrower with depth, while the lower isodoses become wider.

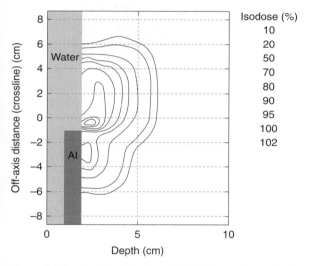

Figure 5.8 Isodoses for a 10 × 10 cm 12 MeV electron beam which has an aluminium (Al) insert. Note the hot spot. The isodoses have been normalised to the d_{max} of a beam with no insert.

- skin apposition rather than point placement of beams is used for set-up (*cf.* isocentric setups for photons);
- non-standard air gaps between the applicator and patient will affect the scattered dose;
- oblique surfaces will significantly alter the isodoses; and
- inhomogeneities within the patient such as air gaps or high-density structures may cause unexpected hot and cold spots as demonstrated in Figure 5.8, where an aluminium sheet has been placed in the phantom.

Brachytherapy

Introduction

Brachytherapy is radiation treatment given by placing a radioactive source near or in the target (usually a malignant tumour). It is possible to deliver a high dose of radiation to the target while sparing adjacent normal tissues; therefore, brachytherapy is a highly conformal type of therapy. It is also often accelerated radiotherapy. Tumours suitable for brachytherapy must be accessible, of moderate size, and able to be delineated.

Brachytherapy treatments are described according to the position of the radioactive source in relation to the body.

- Interstitial – in the target (may be permanent, as in iodine seeds, or temporary, as in iridium wires).
- Intracavitary – in a body cavity.
- Intraluminal – into a lumen.
- Intravascular – into an artery.
- Surface applications.

For radiation protection purposes, non-radioactive guides are placed first whenever possible, followed by 'afterloading' of the radioactive source. Afterloading may be either manual or remote, but there is an increasing trend towards the use of remote after-loading.

This section will describe the broad principles of brachytherapy. For more detail, the reader is referred to more comprehensive texts (see Further Reading).

Isotopes

The properties of some radionuclides used in brachytherapy are shown in Table 5.1.

Dose rates

The International Commission on Radiation Units and Measurements report 38 (ICRU, 1985) classified radiation dose rates at the point or surface where the dose is prescribed into low, medium and high, which have important differences in their radiobiological effects.

- Low dose rate (LDR): 0.4–2 Gy/h. N.B. dose may need to be modified if it exceeds 1 Gy/h.
- Medium dose rate (MDR): 2–12 Gy/h.
- High dose rate (HDR): > 12 Gy/h.

As the dose rate increases, it is necessary to reduce the total dose and fractionate the radiotherapy to avoid unacceptable late tissue damage.

Table 5.1 Properties of some radionuclides used in brachytherapy

Isotope	Approximate half-life	Disintegration	Average photon energy (keV)	Types of source
Caesium-137 (^{137}Cs)	30.2 years	β, γ	662	Needles, tubes, afterloading
Iridium-192 (^{192}Ir)	74 days	β, γ	380	Wires, pins, plaque, afterloading
Cobalt-60 (^{60}Co)	5.3 years	β, γ	1250	Needles, tubes, afterloading
Iodine-125 (^{125}I)	60 days	CE, CX, γ	28	Seeds
Palladium-103 (^{103}Pd)	16.9 days	CX	20–23 (mean 21)	Seeds
Ruthenium-106 (^{106}Ru)	374 days	β	3541	Plaque

CE, conversion electron; CX, characteristic X-ray photon.

Pulsed dose rate (PDR) is a hyperfractionated form of brachytherapy that uses remote afterloading and a single high-activity source that is stepped through dwell positions within the catheters to provide a multiple-fraction high-dose-rate treatment. It may act as an alternative to low-dose-rate brachytherapy, although differences in relative biological effectiveness must be taken into account.

Dosimetry

The radiation dose delivered to the tissues is primarily determined by the activity of the source, the length of time that the sources are in place, and the inverse-square law (dose is proportional to the inverse square of the distance from the source). Traditional methods of dosimetry use rules to govern the configuration of radiation sources and methods to calculate the dose received by the tissues.

Paris system

The Paris system was based on experience in the use of iridium-192 wires (Pierquin *et al.*, 1978). Rules for the Paris system are as follows.

- The linear activity of the sources must be uniform along the full length of the source and identical for each source.
- The radioactive sources must be linear, parallel and straight, and their centres must be in the same plane perpendicular to the direction of each source, which is called the central plane.
- In an implant all the sources must be separated equally from each other, but the source separation may vary from one implant to another.

- The separation between the sources may vary between implants, but the separation should be 0.8–2 cm.
- For volume implants the array of the source intersections in the central plane should be either in an equilateral triangle or a square configuration.
- The average length of the source should be 25–30% longer than the target volume, per uncrossed end. The dose is calculated as follows.
  - The basal dose rate is calculated in the central plane of the implant and is the arithmetic mean of the local minimum dose rates.
  - The reference dose rate is calculated as 85% of the basal dose rate and is the dose rate used for the tumour prescription and calculation time of the implant. The isodose surface that corresponds to the reference dose rate is called the reference isodose and this must encompass the PTV. For this to occur, the radiation sources must be longer than the PTV, unless the ends are crossed as in iridium hairpins. The volume enclosed in the reference isodose is known as the treated volume.

Manchester interstitial system

The Manchester interstitial system was based on experience in the use of radium sources and is also known as the Paterson–Parker system (Meredith, 1967). Its rules governed the distribution of radiation sources for different configurations including planar implants, volume implants and moulds. For further details, see Meredith (1967).

Gynaecological brachytherapy

For treating cervical cancer, in the Manchester system, the applicators are configured as a central uterine tube and two vaginal ovoids, with packing or a rectal retractor to push the rectum away from the high-dose volume. The resulting isodose distribution is a pear-shaped volume encompassing the uterus, cervix, paracervical tissues and upper vagina. The radiation dose is specified at point A, which is 2 cm lateral to the centre of the uterine canal and 2 cm above the lateral vaginal fornices (this latter level is sometimes described as the level of the cervical os or the level of the flange at the base of the intrauterine tube). Point B is 5 cm lateral to the midline at the level of point A. Other reference points are specified by ICRU 38 (ICRU, 1985), including the bladder and rectal points, which can be defined on the anterior and lateral radiographs. Reporting doses to these points allows comparison between centres.

New imaging techniques, computerised treatment planning and optimisation have opened new prospects for individualised treatment and reporting dose to OARs as described in the GEC ESTRO guidance (Pötter et al., 2006). The use of remote afterloading and CT and MRI planning with the treatment applicators in place has led to the development of image-guided brachytherapy, of which there are four defined levels (The Royal College of Radiologists, 2009).

1. Accurate verification of applicator position.
2. Accurate definition of normal tissue dosimetry.
3. Opportunity for conformal dose distributions to tumour volume and OAR.
4. Opportunity for dose escalation.

Isotopes used for gynaecological brachytherapy include caesium-137 for low and medium dose rate treatments or cobalt-60 and iridium-192 for high dose rate treatments. Remote afterloading is typically used. Brachytherapy for gynaecological cancer is discussed further in Chapters 26–28.

Brachytherapy procedures

Indications for brachytherapy include the following.

- Primary radical treatment (e.g. small tumours of tongue, floor of mouth, prostate).
- Treatment in combination with external beam radiotherapy.
- Treatment in combination with surgery (e.g. intraoperative sarcoma treatments).
- Re-irradiation within a previously treated volume (e.g. second primary tumours or locally recurrent tumours).
- Palliative treatments (e.g. bronchus, oesophagus).
- Benign conditions (e.g. keloids).

In the UK, the most widespread use of brachytherapy is for gynaecological cancer, head and neck cancer and, increasingly, prostate cancer. Brachytherapy for ocular melanoma is discussed in Chapter 37.

Practical steps in brachytherapy:

- the treatment is preplanned to determine the tumour volume, the target volume, the technique and the number/size of radiation sources required. An appropriate radionuclide is selected;
- the implant procedure itself takes place under general or local anaesthetic;
- with afterloading techniques, the guides for the active sources are placed first;
- the position of the sources is verified (e.g. using orthogonal X-rays, CT, MRI, ultrasound);
- the treatment time is calculated;
- the active sources are then placed;
- once the implant is complete, the radiation sources are removed, followed by the applicators.

ICRU 58 recommends that the brachytherapy treatment be reported in a standardised way, including information on target volume, description of sources and technique, dose prescribed and a description of the high- and low-dose volumes (ICRU, 1997).

Optimisation

Use of cross-sectional imaging, computer planning systems and treatment machines with moveable stepping sources allows the radiation oncologist to define the target volume, obtain dose volume histograms and achieve the best dose distribution. The dwell times for the source can be varied at different positions, enabling the dose to conform more accurately to the target volume. However, it is still important to take great care in positioning the brachytherapy sources, because optimisation cannot make a bad insertion good.

Quality assurance and radiation protection in brachytherapy

Local rules and systems of work must be drawn up that enable the centre to comply with current legislation. These rules include source storage and preparation, written systems of work for staff entering controlled radiation areas and contingency plans for emergency situations such as source sticking. On receipt of a radiation source, checks should be carried out that include independent measurements of the activity of the source and tests for leakage.

The quality of calculation methods needs to be properly ensured and a regular quality control programme should be in place. For computerised systems, this is especially important so that the transfer of patient image data and the validity of the data and calculations are verified. Any equipment used to measure the actual delivered dose needs to be calibrated against a recognised standard.

References

Apisarnthanarax, S., Elliott, D. D., El-Nagger, A. K., *et al.* (2006). Determining optimal clinical target volume margins in head-and-neck cancer based on microscopic extracapsular extension of metastatic neck nodes. *Int. J. Radiat. Oncol. Biol. Phys.*, **64**, 678–683.

BIR. (2003). *Geometric Uncertainties in Radiotherapy. Defining the Planning Target Volume. Prepared by a Working Party of the British Institute of Radiology.* London: British Institute of Radiology.

Dearnaley, D. P., Khoo, V. S., Norman, A. R., *et al.* (1999). Comparison of radiation side-effects of conformal and conventional radiotherapy in prostate cancer: a randomised trial. *Lancet*, **353**, 267–272.

Fraass, B., Doppke, K., Hunt, M., *et al.* (1998). American Association of Physicists in Medicine Radiation Therapy Committee Task Group 53: quality assurance for clinical radiotherapy treatment planning. *Med. Phys.*, **25**, 1773–1829.

Gregoire, V., Coche, E., Cosnard, G., *et al.* (2000). Selection and delineation of lymph node target volumes in head and neck conformal radiotherapy. Proposal for standardizing terminology and procedure based on the surgical experience. *Radiother. Oncol.*, **56**, 135–150.

ICRU. (1976). *ICRU Report 24. Determination of Absorbed Dose in a Patient Irradiated by Beams of X or Gamma rays in Radiotherapy Procedures.* Bethesda, MD: International Commission on Radiation Units and Measurements.

ICRU. (1985). *ICRU Report 38. Dose and Volume Specification for Reporting Intracavitary Therapy in Gynaecology.* Bethesda, MD: International Commission on Radiation Units and Measurements.

ICRU. (1993). *ICRU Report 50. Prescribing, Recording, and Reporting Photon Beam Therapy.* Bethesda, MD: International Commission on Radiation Units and Measurements.

ICRU. (1997). *ICRU Report 58. Dose and Volume Specification in Interstitial Brachytherapy.* Bethesda, MD: International Commission on Radiation Units and Measurements.

ICRU. (1999). *ICRU Report 62. Prescribing, Recording, and Reporting Photon Beam Therapy (Supplement to ICRU Report 50).* Bethesda, MD: International Commission on Radiation Units and Measurements.

ICRU. (2004). *ICRU Report 71. Prescribing, Recording, and Reporting Electron Beam Therapy. Journal of the ICRU*, 4 (No. 1). Oxford: Oxford University Press.

Jansen, E. P. M., Dewit, L. G. H., van Herk, M., *et al.* (2000). Target volumes in radiotherapy for high-grade malignant glioma of the brain. *Radiother. Oncol*, **56**, 151–156.

Kehoe, T. and Rugg, L. J. (1999). From technical quality assurance of radiotherapy to a comprehensive quality of service management system. *Radiother. Oncol.*, **51**, 281–290.

Khan, F. M. (2003). *The Physics of Radiation Therapy*, 3rd edn. Philadelphia, PA: Lippincott, Williams and Wilkins.

Klein, E. E., Harms, W. B., Low, D. A., *et al.* (1995). Clinical implementation of a commercial multileaf collimator: dosimetry, networking, simulation and quality assurance. *Int. J. Radiat. Oncol. Biol. Phys.*, **33**, 1195–1208.

Lees, J., Holloway, L., Fuller, M., *et al.* (2005). Effect of intravenous contrast on treatment planning system dose calculations in the lung. *Australas. Phys. Eng. Sci. Med.*, **28**, 190–195.

Logue, J. P., Sharrock, C. L., Cowan, R. A., *et al.* (1998). Clinical variability of target volume description in conformal radiotherapy planning. *Int. J. Radiat. Oncol. Biol. Phys.*, **41**, 929–931.

Meredith, W. J. (1967). *Radium Dosage: the Manchester System/Compiled from Articles, by Ralston Paterson (and Others).* Edinburgh: Livingstone.

Nutting, C. M., Khoo, V. S., Walker, V., *et al.* (2000). A randomized study of the use of a customized immobilization system in the treatment of prostate cancer with conformal radiotherapy. *Radiother. Oncol.*, **54**, 1–9.

Padhani, A. R., Khoo, V. S., Suckling, J., *et al.* (1999). Evaluating the effect of rectal distension and rectal movement on prostate gland position using cine MRI. *Int. J. Radiat. Oncol. Biol. Phys.*, **44**, 525–533.

Pierquin, B., Dutreix, A., Paine, C. H., *et al.* (1978). The Paris system in interstitial radiation therapy. *Acta Radiol. Oncol. Radiat. Phys. Biol.*, **17**, 33–48.

Pötter, R., Haie-Meder, C., Van Limbergen, E., *et al.* (2006). Recommendations from gynaecological (GYN) GEC ESTRO working group (II): concepts and terms in 3D image-based treatment planning in cervix cancer brachytherapy – 3D dose volume parameters and aspects of 3D image-based anatomy, radiation physics, radiobiology. *Radiother. Oncol.*, **78**, 67–77.

Purdy, J. A. (2000). Future directions in 3-D treatment planning and delivery: a physicist's perspective. *Int. J. Radiat. Oncol. Biol. Phys.*, **46**, 3–6.

Purdy, J. A. and Harms, W. B. (1998). Quality assurance for 3D conformal radiation therapy. *Strahlenther. Onkol.*, **174** (Suppl. 2), 2–7.

Senan, S., Chapet, O., Lagerwaard, F. J., *et al.* (2004). Defining target volumes for non-small cell lung carcinoma. *Semin. Radiat. Oncol.*, **14**, 308–314.

Seppenwoolde, Y., Shirato, H., Kitamura, K., *et al.* (2002). Precise and real-time measurement of 3D tumor motion in lung due to breathing and heartbeat, measured during radiotherapy. *Int. J. Radiat. Oncol. Biol. Phys.*, **53**, 822–834.

Shimizu, S., Shirato, H., Kitamura, K., *et al.* (2000). Use of an implanted marker and real-time tracking of the marker for the positioning of prostate and bladder cancers. *Int. J. Radiat. Oncol. Biol. Phys.*, **48**, 1591–1597.

Shiu, A. S. and Mellenberg, D. E. (2001). *General Practice of Radiation Oncology Physics in the 21st Century: AAPM Monograph no. 26*. Madison, Wisconsin: Medical Physics Publishing.

The Royal College of Radiologists. (2009). *Implementing Image-Guided Brachytherapy for Cervix Cancer in the UK*. London: The Royal College of Radiologists.

The Royal College of Radiologists, Society and College of Radiographers, Institute of Physics and Engineering in Medicine, National Patients Safety Agency,

British Institute of Radiology. (2008). *Towards Safer Radiotherapy*. London: The Royal College of Radiologists.

Weiss, E., and Hess, C. F. (2003). The impact of gross tumor volume (GTV) and clinical target volume (CTV) definition on the total accuracy in radiotherapy theoretical aspects and practical experiences. *Strahlenther. Onkol.*, **179**, 21–30.

Williams, J. R. and Thwaites, D. I. (2000). *Radiotherapy Physics in Practice*. Oxford: Oxford University Press.

Further reading

Bomford, C. K. and Kunkler, I. H. (2003). *Walter and Miller's Textbook of Radiotherapy. Radiation Physics, Therapy and Oncology*, 6th edn. Edinburgh: Churchill Livingstone.

Dobbs, J., Barrett, A. and Ash, D. (1999). *Practical Radiotherapy Planning*, 3rd edn. New York, NY: Arnold.

Gerbaulet, A., Pötter, R., Mazeron, J.-J., *et al.* (2002). *The GEC ESTRO Handbook of Brachytherapy*. Brussels: European Society for Therapeutic Radiology and Oncology.

Hoskin, P. (2006). *Radiotherapy in Practice. External Beam Therapy*. Oxford: Oxford University Press.

Hoskin, P. and Coyle, C. (2011). *Radiotherapy in Practice. Brachytherapy*, 2nd edn. Oxford: Oxford University Press.

Joslin, C. A. F., Flynn, A. and Hall, E. J. (2001). *Principles and Practice of Brachytherapy: Using Afterloading Systems*. London: Arnold.

Chapter 6

Radiotherapy planning 2: advanced external beam radiotherapy techniques

Anthony Millin

Introduction

Recent advances in technology have enabled more complex radiotherapy to be delivered routinely and the use of stereotactic or modulated techniques have become standard for many indications. These developments allow the radiation dose to conform more closely to the planning target volume (PTV) while more effectively avoiding normal tissue. This can allow the dose to be escalated without increasing the risks of normal tissue toxicity.

Some of these techniques require specialised machines, described later in the chapter, and recently there has also been interest in modifying conventional linear accelerators to achieve the same aim. For instance, the increased use of cranial stereotactic techniques for both malignant and non-malignant indications has led both to an increase in specific machines and to the development of linear accelerators which deliver advanced radiotherapy to both cranial and extracranial sites. Rotational therapy, a technique that was used by some centres in the 1960s, has been 'rediscovered' and, when combined with the modulated techniques of conventional intensity-modulated radiotherapy (IMRT), has led volumetric-modulated adaptive therapy (VMAT), delivering radiation in a way similar to tomotherapy.

Advances in imaging have also contributed to radiotherapy development. For example, use of pre-treatment MRI or PET scans can help to define planning target volumes, and cone beam CT scans during treatment can check on internal organ movement and set-up accuracy. The ability to 'fuse' these images with the CT planning scan has greatly assisted both radiotherapy planning and treatment delivery.

Intensity-modulated radiation therapy

Introduction

IMRT is a technique which uses beams that, unlike the flat or wedged beams of conventional RT, have changing dose intensity across them, as shown in Figure 6.1 (Webb, 2003; Bortfeld, 2006). Modulation was originally produced by using low melting point compensators, but is now usually generated by moving the multi-leaf collimators (MLCs) during 'beam on' time. The aim of this is to build up the desired dose distribution by producing appropriately modulated beams.

The basic principle of IMRT can be seen in Figure 6.2, which shows three modulated beams to cover a PTV with an isodose distribution that wraps around the organ at risk (OAR) and conforms well to the target volume. In practice more beams, usually between 5 and 9, are needed to give an acceptable distribution.

Modulated beams are generated by using beams composed of many different sized segments, each of which has the MLC leaves in a different position, building up an intensity profile as shown in Figure 6.3. This shows a very simple two-segment beam and the intensity profile created by adding the intensities of the two segments together. IMRT can be delivered in one of two ways. In 'step and shoot' IMRT, the beam is turned on for the first segment, turned off while the leaves move to the next position and turned on again when the leaves reach their planned positions. So the treatment is analogous to a multi-beam conventional technique and it is easier to commission and calculate doses during treatment planning. In 'sliding window' IMRT, the beam remains on while the MLCs move, enabling

Practical Clinical Oncology, Second Edition, ed. Louise Hanna, Tom Crosby and Fergus Macbeth. Published by Cambridge University Press. © Cambridge University Press 2015.

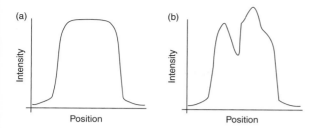

Figure 6.1 Intensity profiles of a standard beam (a) and an IMRT beam (b).

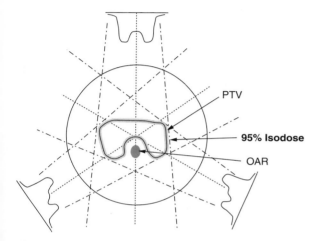

Figure 6.2 Schematic diagram of an IMRT plan showing how the intensity of the beams is modulated to produce an isodose distribution that covers the PTV and 'wraps' around an organ at risk. OAR, organ at risk; PTV, planning target volume.

a smoother intensity profile more closely matching the one planned. However, dose calculation and plan verification are more problematic.

Inverse treatment planning

In conventional treatment planning (*forward planning*) the planner selects beam angles, weights, wedges and other planning parameters and adjusts them until the dose distribution is appropriate. An experienced planner can optimise parameters and produce a deliverable plan quite quickly.

With intensity modulation, because the number of possible MLC positions and beam angles is so great, it is very difficult for the planner to determine prospectively what combination of beams and segment sizes will produce the optimal plan. Therefore, *inverse planning* techniques are used, starting with the planner describing the required dose distribution by defining points on a dose volume histogram (DVH) curve, and

then a module in the treatment planning system (called the optimiser) determines the modulations needed to produce the optimal treatment plan.

Figure 6.4 shows the DVHs of a plan produced using inverse optimisation. The planner has set PTV dose–volume constraints shown by the triangular marker pointing to the right, which shows the desired minimum dose, and the triangular marker pointing to the left, which shows the desired maximum dose. Ideally, the DVH curve for the PTV will lie between the minimum and maximum dose points. For OARs, maximum dose–volume constraints are used, shown by the triangles pointing to the left, with the expectation that the DVH curve for an OAR will lie to the left of these points. During optimisation the system tries to meet all the constraints by adjusting the size and relative weights of each of the beam segments. The system expresses the quality of the plan mathematically by describing how well the plan meets the set constraints in terms of both target volume coverage and OAR avoidance. If plans have very poor coverage of the target(s) and high doses to the OARs, the 'cost' or 'penalty' function will be at its highest. During optimisation, as the target coverage and OAR doses improve, the cost function decreases and when it falls below a certain level which has been specified by the planner, the computer considers the plan to be optimised and no further iterations are undertaken. The balance between covering the PTV and avoiding the OAR is achieved by adding relative weights to the required doses to define the relative importance of each planning aim. For most systems, this entails a lot of trial and error to achieve the optimal solution. Because the computer stops optimising when the required constraints are met, it is important that the constraints are not too easy for it to achieve. For this reason, the planner will sometimes set overly optimistic constraints in order to force the planning system to continue calculating to achieve the best possible plan. So even if the constraints are recorded as not having been met, the plan produced by the computer will be better than if the constraints had been set at an easier level. Ultimately, it is a clinical decision whether the plan is acceptable, regardless of whether it has 'passed' or 'failed' the constraints set for the computer.

Using this technique, complex dose distributions can be achieved covering different PTVs with different dose levels. Figure 6.5 shows a typical dose distribution for a head and neck IMRT plan in which a treatment

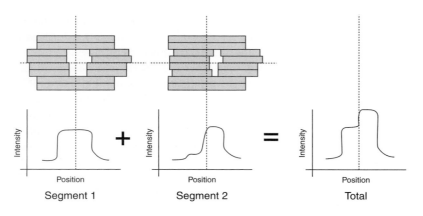

Figure 6.3 Illustration of the production of an intensity-modulated beam. The upper row shows two fields defined by MLCs that have intensity profiles shown by the second row and are added together to produce the intensity profile shown on the bottom right.

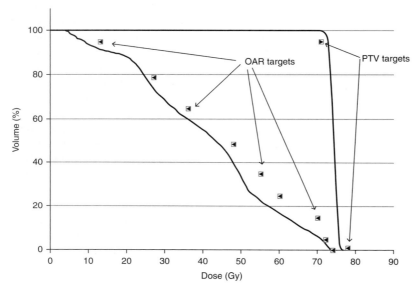

Figure 6.4 Typical DVH showing the dose volume targets and calculated DVHs of the optimised plan. OAR, organ at risk; PTV, planning target volume.

dose is delivered to the primary PTV and a prophylactic dose to bilateral targets. The parotid glands have been delineated and dose to the right parotid has been set to ensure that it receives a dose low enough to preserve its function. This would be very difficult to achieve using conformal radiotherapy.

Volumetric-modulated arc therapy

Volumetric-modulated arc therapy (VMAT) is an extension of the IMRT concept whereby the dose is delivered while both the gantry and the MLCs are moving. The treatment is usually given using one or two arcs, depending on the complexity of the plan, and may involve one or more full rotations or a partial arc or arcs. The exact technique will depend on the treatment site and the complexity of the volumes to be

treated and avoided. VMAT planning involves inverse planning techniques.

The advantage of VMAT is that gantry rotation allows more complex dose distributions to be planned (Alvarez-Moret et al., 2010; Rao et al., 2010) and faster treatment times than IMRT. Doses to the outlined OARs are usually lower than with IMRT, but this is achieved by distributing the dose outside the PTV to all tissues within the superior–inferior length of the beam. This effect can be seen in Figure 6.6, which shows typical isodoses of a VMAT plan applied to a prostate. The higher-dose regions are within or close to the target area and there is less of the higher dose spreading into the periphery of the patient than there would be with a static conformal or IMRT plan. This is accompanied by a 'low-dose bath' in the more

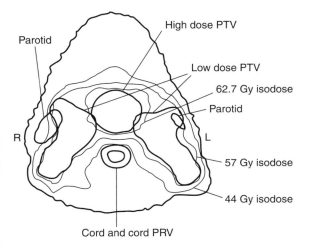

Figure 6.5 Typical doses planned with an IMRT technique to several dose volumes. This is an axial section of an oropharynx treatment with parotid sparing on the right side. In this case, a high-dose PTV has been drawn with a prescription dose of 66 Gy and two lower-dose volumes with 60 Gy prescriptions. The plan has been optimised aiming to limit the cord PRV to a dose of 44 Gy and to keep the parotid doses as low as possible. Note the parotid sparing on the right.

peripheral parts of the patient that may sometimes be clinically significant.

Technical issues

The complexity of modulated treatments may be challenging. The ability to confine the dose to more complex target volumes and to avoid OAR means that more precise, often irregular volumes have to be drawn. This takes more time and the roles of the different staff groups may be redefined so that tasks once only done by oncologists have now become the routine work of radiographers, dosimetrists and medical physicists.

The inverse planning algorithms employed by modern planning systems, although seemingly simple, are very different from traditional methods, and numerous options need to be explored in order to produce optimal plans quickly. This entails a lot of development work and training of users.

Handing over the optimisation of the plan to a mathematical algorithm can also be problematic, because during the forward planning process some issues are intuitively taken into account. For instance, the megavoltage build-up effect near the surface of the patient will reduce the dose and therefore the dose coverage of the PTV if it lies in this area. A human operator can instinctively either accept this lack of coverage

or account for it if this area of the irradiated volume is important. It is difficult to describe this mathematically and it is important to take this into account when producing a planning solution.

To produce the complex dose distributions using inverse planning is often time-consuming and to make the process more efficient, a site-specific class solution may be used. An optimal set of dose–volume constraints and plan optimisation volumes for each treatment site are developed to achieve optimal dose distributions. Using a single approach for each tumour site allows the process to be partly automated. A good class solution should produce an optimal plan for the majority, if not all, patients with a particular indication. If the plan is suboptimal, further work has to be done taking a few hours for simple indications but up to 10 hours for the most complex cases, meaning that more staff are needed for IMRT and VMAT planning.

Both IMRT and VMAT require more detailed dosimetry than conventional radiotherapy techniques to check the accuracy of the plan. Most centres have implemented this by measuring each individual plan using a dosimetric phantom before starting treatment, but as confidence in the technology has increased, an independent calculation algorithm as used for conventional planning techniques is more often used. Quality assurance to assess the performance of the machine now has to take account of these new techniques and many geometric and dosimetric tolerances have been tightened, leading to more staff time being devoted to quality assurance.

Image-guided radiation therapy

Image guided radiotherapy (IGRT) is used to ensure that the patient set-up is accurate. Traditionally, port films placed at the exit plane of the treatment beam, using the planned beam collimation or a wider field for a few monitor units, were used to verify the set-up. They confirm that the set-up was correct and beam delivery accurate and may prompt adjustments or replanning. Electronic portal imaging devices (EPIDs; Herman *et al.*, 2001) capture the image using detector arrays and produce an instant electronic image that can be viewed immediately. The image can be processed electronically to improve the contrast, making matching of the expected and acquired images easier. Imaging before each treatment can permit immediate corrections and increases the accuracy and consistency of treatment delivery.

(a)
Prescription isodose
25 Gy isodose
10 Gy isodose

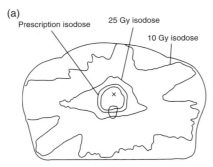

(b)
Prescription isodose
25 Gy isodose
10 Gy isodose

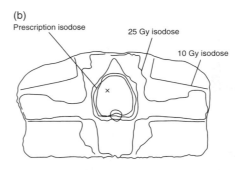

Figure 6.6 Typical doses delivered by VMAT (a) and IMRT (b) plans for a prostate and seminal vesicles treatment delivering 55 Gy in 20 fractions to the ICRU reference point to two different patients. The PTV coverage for both plans is quite similar, but while the 25 Gy isodose is closer to the PTV in the VMAT plan than the IMRT plan, the volume of patient irradiated to 10 Gy is more with VMAT than it is with IMRT.

The main disadvantage of EPIDs is that the poor contrast of the megavoltage image gives little information about soft tissues, and for most treatments, generally only allows matching against the bony anatomy. If the tumour is not fixed to bony anatomy the system is less useful. Newer techniques such as cone beam CT-based systems give better soft tissue contrast, but EPIDs can still give useful dosimetric and positional information (van Elmpt *et al.*, 2008) and are therefore likely to continue to have a role.

Kilovoltage X-rays, giving greater contrast, can be used to generate planar images from one or two X-ray sources or volumetric imaging such as in a cone beam CT (CBCT; Jaffray *et al.*, 2002). Most CBCT systems have a kilovoltage X-ray generator and image intensifier on the treatment machine at right angles to the therapy beam. Once the patient has been positioned the gantry is rotated around the patient before treatment and a full 3D volumetric image of the patient is acquired. The data can then be reconstructed into transverse slices and compared to the planning CT with volumes drawn on it to assess the spatial accuracy of the treatment. There is good soft tissue contrast and the images can be easily compared to the planning CT. However, it can take 2–3 minutes to acquire and process the image, lengthening the overall treatment time.

Clinical implementation of IGRT

The correct placement of radiation beams has been shown to be clinically important (Miralbell *et al.*, 1997) and IGRT can help to ensure that radiotherapy is delivered more accurately. Ideally, the patient would be imaged before every fraction, but:

- the cumulative additional dose from the imaging may be significant over a long course of treatment;
- the additional time may affect the patient's ability to maintain their position, leading to further adjustments and imaging, and decreasing the throughput on the machine; and
- clear, site-specific, local protocols are needed, describing the policies for both online and offline imaging.

With online imaging the patient is imaged before treatment and, after analysis of the image, may be moved to the correct treatment position for subsequent fractions. With offline imaging the patient is imaged before treatment on one or several fractions and an average displacement of the patient from the expected position calculated and this position used subsequently. Further periodic images may then be performed to check this position. Most offline techniques will include a move towards online imaging should discrepancies seen on imaging be particularly large or random.

A further advantage of IGRT, particularly CBCT-based systems where there is good soft tissue contrast, is that changes to the patient anatomy during treatment can be assessed and, if necessary, corrected for. If so, the data from a CBCT scan are not usually suitable for treatment planning dose calculation and the patient will need to have a repeat planning CT scan. Figure 6.7 illustrates the planning scan and CBCT image of a patient having radiotherapy to the head and neck. Following fusion of the data sets the volumes are shown on both images. The patient has lost a significant amount of weight since the planning scan, shown by air gaps between the CBCT-imaged skin surface and the skin surface drawn during the planning scan.

Finally, the correct training of treatment staff to ensure that the anatomy can be correctly identified

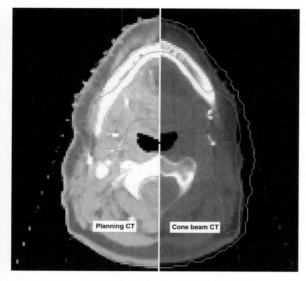

Figure 6.7 Illustration of the planning CT (left side) and cone beam CT (right side) of a patient undergoing radiotherapy for head and neck cancer. The volumes from the original planning CT are shown on both data sets following fusion of the two images. Note how the skin contour from the cone beam CT is slightly inside that of the planning CT; this is due to weight loss during radiotherapy. If patients lose significant amounts of weight, the treatment will need to be re-planned.

and the images analysed efficiently is an essential part of implementation. It is also important that audits of the accuracy of patient positioning are performed and used to determine the appropriate PTV margins applied during the planning process. The National Radiotherapy Implementation Group have produced guidance on the implementation and use of IGRT (NRIG, 2012).

Adaptive planning

An extension of IGRT is adaptive planning, adapting the plan during treatment because of changes in the position or size of the tumour or in the patient's shape. This may be based on either the CBCT or a repeat planning scan if gross changes in patient shape are seen. This can be very time-consuming, particularly if the patient is being treated with an advanced technique such as IMRT or VMAT. This can be prevented by prospectively developing plans based on expected changes in the patient's anatomy. For instance, a treatment in the pelvis may be affected by the degree of bladder filling at the time of treatment, and so several plans can be produced anticipating the different amounts of urine in the bladder. Each day the patient is imaged, the volume of the bladder assessed and the appropriate

plan chosen. Alternatively repeat planning scans can be done at defined points in the treatment process in anticipation of the tumour shrinking or the patient changing shape with a re-plan if necessary.

As with other advanced techniques, the implementation of adaptive radiotherapy requires the correct staff, correctly trained in the correct part of the treatment process and may involve staff having to change roles.

Gating

It is well known that tumours move during each treatment and for some tumour sites, such as the thorax, this movement may be several centimetres. Gated radiotherapy (Kubo and Hill, 1996) addresses this problem by switching the beam on only when the tumour is in a defined position. This requires monitoring tumour movement, either by monitoring the breathing cycle of the patient using belts or external markers and allowing the beam on only at defined parts of the breathing cycle, or by imaging the tumour itself, possibly using implanted fiducial markers. These are radio-opaque markers inserted into the tumour itself or into adjacent normal tissue which move in a similar way during respiration. Alternatively, patients can be coached in specific techniques such as a deep inspiration breath-holding. This can be used during left-sided breast radiotherapy and moves the heart outside the intended treatment area. In order to maintain reproducibility, sensors track the respiratory cycle, provide feedback to the patient and automatically switch the machine off if the patient is unable to maintain inspiration.

Advanced imaging tools and imaging modalities

Imaging modalities used in radiotherapy planning

For some years conformal radiotherapy has been based on CT scans, giving good geometric accuracy and reasonable soft tissue contrast. The Hounsfield units produced by a CT scanner are proportional to electron density and can be used for accurate dose calculation. However, other imaging modalities offer advantages such as higher image quality from small-bore diagnostic CT images and additional information provided by functional MRI and positron emission tomography

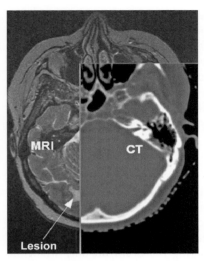

Figure 6.8 An example of an MRI and a CT scan of the brain of a patient undergoing radiotherapy. Note how the lesion can be seen on the MRI which is the main part of the figure but not on the CT.

(PET). Studies have shown differences between the target volumes drawn on CT and those using MRI (Kagawa *et al.*, 1997) even in sites such as the prostate with relatively well-defined anatomy. Figure 6.8 shows an MRI and CT scan of a patient being planned for intracranial radiotherapy. The lesion is clearly seen in the MRI but not on the CT.

Image fusion

When new imaging techniques are introduced into the radiotherapy planning process, there must be some way of merging the images into the planning system and so most modern treatment systems have image fusion functionality. This may involve either the user defining fixed anatomical markers or an automatic system, but both methods need to be checked once the operation has been performed.

Ideally, in patients for whom both imaging sets are needed for planning, the patient would be scanned in an identical position and coordinate system each time so that the images can be easily overlaid and the organs or tumour seen on one image series can be outlined on the other. This may be possible using PET-CT when the PET and CT scans are obtained at effectively the same time using the same coordinate system, but more often software-based fusion is required.

Figure 6.9 shows fusion using landmark points on each image. The user marks at least three identical points on each image series (not necessarily on the same transverse plane) and the software geometrically calculates the shift necessary to align the two images. In this case a clear rotation of the MRI image compared to the CT scan has been corrected to generate the fused image on the right of the figure. Tools such as a checkerboard pattern shown on the fused image are used to confirm the accuracy of the fusion.

Many modern systems are automatic and use software algorithms to arrive at a fused image. These may be rigid fusion in which only movements and rotations are used to transform the secondary image on to the primary image or elastic fusion in which as well as movements and rotation the secondary scan may be stretched or squashed until it matches the primary image. It is important that the user understands what process they are employing and to assess whether it is required. For instance, in fusing a planning CT with a diagnostic scan it may be appropriate to use an elastic fusion that will overlay the correct anatomy on the planning scan. It is also important to remember that while image fusion can help to define anatomy during radiotherapy planning, it does not give information on the changes in doses received by the PTV or OAR which might occur as a result of any internal movement or set-up inaccuracy during treatment.

Stereotactic radiotherapy

Stereotactic concept

The purpose of a stereotactic coordinate system is to eliminate the spatial uncertainties introduced by the scanning and treatment delivery devices. This means that the PTV margins can be reduced and more accurate radiotherapy given, enabling higher doses to be prescribed. A cranial stereotactic radiosurgical frame is used to immobilise the patient securely using steel rods fixed surgically to the skull. Bars on the side and top of the box define the coordinate systems on the planning scan.

Figure 6.10 shows a phantom scanned within a stereotactic frame. The computerised planning system has identified the bars and from knowledge of the precise position of the bars can generate a coordinate system independent of the scanner.

The plan is then produced conventionally, but all positional information is based on the stereotactic coordinate system and not that generated by the scanner as in a conventional plan. Once the plan is produced the positional information is transferred to a

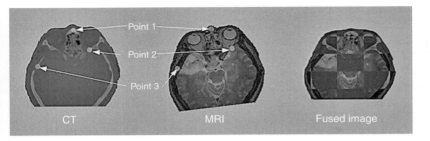

Figure 6.9 Illustration of fusion using a landmark matching technique. Placing three points on each scan at equivalent positions enables the computer to fuse the images and eliminate the effect of the rotation seen on the MRI scan. In the fused image the CT and MRI components can be seen in alternating squares of a chequer board pattern.

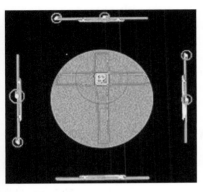

Figure 6.10 Transverse section through a phantom scanned in a stereotactic frame. The circles are the localiser rods automatically acquired by the stereotactic treatment planning system used to define the stereotactic coordinate system.

target positioner box, and the information used to set up the patient. In this way, all of the positional uncertainties associated with the scanner and accelerator are eliminated and accuracy depends only on how well the patient can be immobilised relative to the frame. For this reason for single fraction treatments (radiosurgery) invasive frames have been used to attach the patient firmly to the frame with positional uncertainties of a millimetre or less. For fractionated techniques (stereotactic radiotherapy), precise stereotactic masks, based on thermoplastic or vacuum-assisted mouth-bites, are usually used and they decrease the spatial uncertainty down to 2 mm or less.

Frameless techniques have been devised that use the patient's anatomical landmarks rather than a positioner box. Here the patient is positioned using images acquired on the treatment machine and adjustments made until the anatomy exactly matches that of the images generated by the planning system in stereotactic coordinates. In this way the stereotactic principle is maintained.

Because of greater accuracy, higher doses and shorter fractionation regimens have been introduced

with a clear clinical benefit both cranially and extracranially (Norihisa *et al.*, 2008; UK SBRT Consortium, 2011). As the difference between an image-guided and a stereotactic technique has become blurred, the term stereotactic has often become a synonym for a high-dose, low number of fractions regimen, but clearly there are dangers in losing the significance of the stereotactic concept.

Cranial stereotactic radiotherapy and radiosurgery

Cranial stereotactic radiosurgery has been used for over 50 years for both benign and malignant indications, using either invasive frames for radiosurgery in which the treatment is delivered in a single fraction or removable thermoplastic or similar masks that are used to immobilise the patient relative to the stereotactic frame. Framed systems as discussed above have been widely used for cranial stereotactic radiotherapy and radiosurgery, but the use of frameless systems has become increasingly widespread.

Extracranial stereotactic radiotherapy

Stereotactic ablative radiotherapy (SABR), also known as stereotactic body radiotherapy (SBRT), has been introduced in recent years, especially for the treatment of early-stage lung cancer. Linear accelerator-based systems use CBCT scans to guide the treatment using the patient's anatomy to define the coordinate system (UK SBRT Consortium, 2011). Target volumes are drawn using a 4D CT of the patient from which an internal target volume (ITV) is drawn, to which a PTV margin is added to account for set-up errors.

Margins can be reduced using immobilisation devices such as abdominal compression which splints the diaphragm and reduces respiratory movement, or by the application of gated radiotherapy (see above). In this case, the volume of the ITV (from which the PTV will be grown) will be reduced because the tumour moves less during 'beam on' time.

The dose for each fraction is much higher than in conventional radical radiotherapy. The UK SBRT Consortium (2011) suggests doses of 54 Gy in 3 fractions or 55 Gy in 5 fractions. The treatment times for each fraction will be longer, around 5 times that of a standard conformal therapy especially if gating techniques are used, and so it is important to ensure that the patient is able to maintain the treatment position. Several confirmation cone beam images may be required to ensure that the patient remains in the correct position, which may further prolong the time required.

Technical issues

Stereotactic radiotherapy and radiosurgery, as with IMRT and VMAT, require small field dosimetry which can cause problems in acquiring data for the planning system and validating its performance. However, it is a common practice to prescribe to the 80% or 50% isodoses to ensure that all the PTV receives at least the prescription dose. When prescribing to the 80% isodose the resultant plan delivers at least a 25% overdose to the conventional prescription point and so a dosimetric uncertainty of a few percent may be of far less significance than the geometric accuracy of the whole system.

Systems using a conventional linear accelerator to deliver stereotactic treatments may therefore require better isocentre accuracy. A conventional machine may have a tolerance allowing the mechanical isocentre of the machine to deviate within a sphere of radius 1 mm for gantry rotation and 2 mm for couch rotation. For specialist radiotherapy machines these tolerances should be reduced to ensure the stereotactic accuracy. This is less important if a machine-independent positioning system is used, but will be an issue for systems relying on CBCT images for positioning.

Other methods for improving the mechanical accuracy of the treatment device include the use of dedicated equipment such as the Gamma Knife® or CyberKnife®, as described below.

Radiobiological planning

Radiobiological treatment planning (Niemierko, 1998) is a process that considers the radiobiological effects of the treatment rather than simply the dose delivered so that the different radiosensitivity of organs can be more readily considered. This may be particularly useful in inverse planning where, instead of determining parameters based on physical dose, radiobiological concepts such as tumour control probability (TCP) and normal tissue complication probability (NTCP) are used to set the planning objectives. Optimising the plan using these is perhaps more likely to achieve tumour control and minimise adverse effects. Most treatment planning systems either have a radiobiological planning module or it is near the top of their development list. However, whereas the arguments in determining the likely efficacy of a treatment plan based on radiobiological quantities can easily be made, the uncertainties associated with the quantities used currently prevent its widespread adoption. However, although many centres might want to adopt this technique, the considerable uncertainties about these concepts argue against their widespread use at the moment.

Non-conventional radiotherapy machines

Gamma Knife®

The Gamma Knife (Leksell, 1983) is a dedicated cranial stereotactic machine used for many years in the treatment of non-malignant and malignant tumours and arterio-venous malformations. It consists of a number of cobalt-60 sources in a collimator helmet focused on a fixed point analogous to the isocentre of a linear accelerator. However, the sources remain fixed and doses are delivered by exposing or shielding a predefined number of the sources to build up the dose distribution. The patient is supported on a treatment couch and positioned so that the treatment volume is at the focal point of the radiation. Using an array of fixed sources reduces the spatial uncertainty from using a conventional linear accelerator.

CyberKnife®

The CyberKnife is a small, linear accelerator attached to a robot which moves the accelerator to the correct position to deliver the intended dose distribution. The radiation is collimated by a series of interchangeable collimators that the robot is able to 'pick up' during treatment without operator intervention in accordance with a previously determined treatment plan. Unlike a conventional accelerator, there is no isocentre, which enables the machine to irradiate from an almost infinite number of angles. The patient is positioned using imaging devices in the room and due to the absence of an isocentre the machine must always direct the radiation beam based on patient anatomy. Consequently, the machine inherently accounts for the patient's position. The system can be used to treat tumours anywhere in the body, but due to the small field sizes used and the relatively long treatment times, its use is generally confined to indications conventionally treated with linear accelerator-based stereotactic techniques.

TomoTherapy®

The TomoTherapy machine (Bortfeld and Webb, 2009) consists of a small, linear accelerator positioned on an annulus that rotates around the patient. Its radiation is collimated by a small collimator and exposes the patient to small fields as the patient is moved through the radiation on a treatment couch. Modulated plans are produced by choosing the collimation of the beam as the accelerator rotates around the patient. Indications for the use of TomoTherapy machines are generally similar to those of VMAT.

Vero®

The Vero treatment device consists of a linear accelerator located on a gimbal so that it can be positioned at angles outside those possible with a conventional accelerator. It is equipped with kilovoltage pair imaging and CBCT equipment enabling rapid positioning of the patient. The gimbaled accelerator gantry, enhanced imaging and couch with 6 degrees of freedom enables the tumour to be tracked during treatment to reduce positional uncertainties. Its prime application is in extracranial SBRT.

References

Alvarez-Moret, J., Pohl, F., Koelbl, O., et al. (2010). Evaluation of volumetric modulated arc therapy (VMAT) with Oncentra MasterPlan® for the treatment of head and neck cancer. *Radiother. Oncol.*, **5**, 110.

Bortfeld, T. (2006). IMRT: a review and preview. *Phys. Med. Biol.*, **51**, R363–R379.

Bortfeld, T. and Webb, S. (2009). Single-Arc IMRT? *Phys. Med. Biol.*, **54**(1), N9–20.

Herman, M. G., Balter, J. M., Jaffray, D., et al. (2001). Clinical use of electronic portal imaging: Report of AAPM Radiation Therapy Committee Task Group 58. *Med. Phys.*, **28**, 712.

Jaffray, D. A, Siewerdsen, J. H., Wong, J. W., et al. (2002). Flat-panel cone-beam computed tomography for image-guided radiation therapy. *Int. J. Radiat. Oncol. Biol. Phys.*, **53**, 1337–1349.

Kagawa, K., Lee, W. R., Schultheiss, T. E., et al. (1997). Initial clinical assessment of CT-MRI image fusion software in localization of the prostate for 3D conformal radiation therapy. *Int. J. Radiat. Oncol. Biol. Phys.*, **38**, 319–325.

Kubo, H. D. and Hill, B. C. (1996). Respiration gated radiotherapy treatment: a technical study. *Phys. Med. Biol.*, **41**, 83.

Leksell, L. (1983). Stereotactic radiosurgery. *J. Neurol. Neurosurg. Psy.*, **46**, 797–803.

Miralbell, R., Bleher, A., Huguenin, P., et al. (1997). Pediatric medulloblastoma: radiation treatment technique and patterns of failure. *Int. J. Radiat. Oncol. Biol. Phys.*, **37**, 523–529.

NRIG. (2012). *National Radiotherapy Implementation Group Report. Image Guided Radiotherapy (IGRT). Guidance for Implementation and Use.* London: National Cancer Action Team.

Niemierko, A. (1998). Radiobiological models of tissue response to radiation in treatment planning systems. *Tumori*, **84**, 140–143.

Norihisa, Y., Nagata, Y., Takayama, K., et al. (2008). Stereotactic body radiotherapy for oligometastatic lung tumors. *Int. J. Radiat. Oncol. Biol. Phys.*, **72**, 398–403.

Rao, M., Yang, W., Chen, F., et al. (2010). Comparison of Elekta VMAT with helical tomotherapy and fixed field IMRT: plan quality, delivery efficiency and accuracy. *Med. Phys.*, **37**, 1350.

UK SBRT Consortium. (2011). *UK SBRT Consortium. Stereotactic Body Radiation Therapy (SBRT) for Patients with Early Stage Non-small Cell Lung Cancer: A Resource. 2nd update Oct 2010.*

van Elmpt, W., McDermott, L., Nijsten, S., et al. (2008). A literature review of electronic portal imaging for radiotherapy dosimetry. *Radiother. Oncol.*, **88**, 289–309.

Webb, S. (2003). The physical basis of IMRT and inverse planning. *Br. J. Radiol.*, **76**, 678.

Research in cancer

Robert Hills

Introduction

It is the responsibility of clinicians to provide the best possible care for their patients. However, this simple statement masks a much more complex issue. How does one know precisely what the best care is for a particular patient? In particular, how does one balance the likely benefits and risks for a particular course of treatment? A new drug may appear promising, but can one really be sure that it represents a real improvement on current practice? Generally speaking, unless the action of a particular treatment is both immediate and breathtaking (such as insulin for diabetic coma), we cannot be absolutely certain which treatment is best for which people. Historical comparisons, or other database-dependent methods, can prove misleading. What is required is a method that will provide reliable, convincing evidence that can be used to inform future practice.

Fortunately, there is such a tool: the randomised controlled trial (RCT). At its heart are two principles. First, through randomisation, any differences between patients receiving one treatment and those receiving another are purely down to chance; therefore, if a sufficiently large difference is detected, then it must be due to the only factor that is systematically different between the two groups, namely the treatment. Second, with large numbers of patients, it becomes easier to detect smaller treatment effects and to conclude that any differences are not the result of chance. This, the statistical aspect of RCTs, is effectively a formalisation of common sense. If one tosses a coin 10 times and gets 6 heads and 4 tails, it is not out of the ordinary; but if one saw 6000 heads and 4000 tails from 10,000 tosses, then one would be concerned that the coin may be biased. The proportion of heads is the same, but larger numbers give stronger evidence of an unfair coin.

This chapter will concentrate on obtaining reliable evidence on the efficacy (whether the treatment works under ideal conditions, usually in a highly selected population) and effectiveness (whether a treatment will be beneficial in a real-life setting) of treatments for cancer. In particular, it will look at the factors that constitute a successful clinical trial, how the ideas can be extended to look at the weight of evidence provided by a number of clinical trials (meta-analysis) and how additional laboratory studies can help assess more modern targeted therapies. Much excellent literature (e.g. Altman, 1991; Pocock, 1996; Duley and Farrell, 2002) has already been devoted to the theory of the RCT (and much that is less excellent). Likewise, medical statistics has been well covered in a number of books and articles (Altman *et al.*, 2000; Swinscow and Campbell, 2002). This chapter will concentrate on the underlying principles, with particular emphasis on their applications in cancer. This chapter is intended to provide useful information for researchers planning to conduct an RCT, and also provides useful pointers for clinicians wanting to critically appraise a trial for reliability.

Clinical trials

Introduction

The path taken by a new treatment before it comes into common use is typically a long one. Initially, a compound may well be developed based on an association seen in a laboratory and backed up by early research involving animals. However, while this avenue may identify promising treatments, it does not tell us the proper dose to give for treatment (or even if it is safe at all to use in humans), whether promising laboratory results translate into activity in humans, and, most

Practical Clinical Oncology, Second Edition, ed. Louise Hanna, Tom Crosby and Fergus Macbeth. Published by Cambridge University Press. © Cambridge University Press 2015.

important, whether the treatment gives better results when used in clinical practice compared to current best care. Increasingly, too, health-care providers are interested in determining whether new treatments represent sufficiently good value for money.

Thus, a new treatment (typically, but not always, a drug) will go through four stages of development, and at each stage a clinical trial will be run to ascertain that the treatment still remains sufficiently promising to proceed:

Phase I represents the first trials performed in humans; it determines that the treatment is safe and identifies the target dose. Such trials can involve either healthy volunteers or patients with the condition in question. The treatment dose starts off quite low, at a point where no real toxicity is expected, and is increased until the maximally tolerated dose (MTD), defined according to the proportion of patients experiencing significant toxicity, is found. A number of different designs for phase I trials have been proposed, ranging from the traditional Fibonacci design to more sophisticated techniques based on modelling the predicted toxicity levels based on all available data (Storer and DeMets, 1987; Storer, 1989).

Phase II trials identify whether the treatment, at a safe dose, demonstrates sufficient evidence of activity. These studies can be considered as small screening studies, typically with a few dozen patients, and they weed out treatments that are unlikely to be of any benefit in clinical practice. There is little point in going to the considerable effort and expense of setting up a large RCT if there is only a small likelihood of success. Typically, such trials use short-term surrogate endpoints, such as tumour shrinkage or remission induction, which are correlated with more clinically relevant endpoints such as overall survival. Historically, phase II studies were uncontrolled studies, where all enrolled patients received the study drug, but recently, a randomised design has increasingly been used. Such trials are still relatively small, and tend to use short-term surrogate endpoints, but can be an efficient way of evaluating new treatments and can form the basis of a larger phase III study if the treatment appears sufficiently promising.

Phase III trials tend to be relatively large and randomised. These identify whether the treatment, given either in addition to or instead of current therapy, gives improved clinical outcomes. The phase III RCT is dealt with in more detail in the next section.

After a new drug has been identified and demonstrated to provide worthwhile benefit in a phase III trial, it is studied further in **phase IV** trials. The entirety of the phase I to III process may have meant that only a few hundred patients have been given the drug, and that rare or long-term side effects may not have become apparent. Phase IV trials allow the study of the drug in standard clinical care in a large number of patients to identify any important safety issues, and to look at the long-term balance of risks and benefits.

This four-stage process of treatment development is not set in stone; indeed, for many non-pharmaceutical treatments, the earlier phases of development may not be directly relevant. Also, some of the phases may be performed simultaneously. For example, identifying the ideal dose for a new drug may not be a factor of toxicity alone: similar efficacy may be obtained at drug doses lower than the MTD, with a corresponding reduction in toxicity levels. Thus, it may make sense to perform a phase I/II trial in which both activity and toxicity are considered simultaneously (see, for example, Yin *et al.*, 2006). Likewise, a phase II/III trial could be designed in which a small, randomised pilot is assessed and the preliminary results of this pilot can be used, either to make a Stop/Go decision (as in the Pick-A-Winner design in leukaemia: Hills and Burnett, 2011, or other Multi-Arm Multi-Stage designs), or to further refine the larger phase III trial in the light of the results (for example, to change the sample size, as in Mehta and Pocock, 2011).

Randomised controlled trials

The main idea underlying the RCT is the need to distinguish between effects that are moderate but still clinically meaningful, and those that are too small to be of any real clinical interest (Yusuf *et al.*, 1984). Often, early reports of a treatment tend to be extremely positive and raise the possibility of major clinical advances. Yet, only a few treatments in current practice tend to work overwhelmingly well; the history of improvements in outcomes in cancer is one of incremental progress, and many of the drugs taken for granted today (e.g. tamoxifen in breast cancer) produce only moderate benefits, yet, owing to the worldwide prevalence of the conditions being treated, save many hundreds of thousands of lives annually. The actual likelihood

Box 7.1 SAB in acute myeloid leukaemia

When comparing SAB with DAT treatment for acute myeloid leukaemia, the following results were obtained (Wheatley, 2002).

Treatment	Period	Number of patients	CR rate	Induction death	Resistant disease
DAT	1984–90	167	47%	30%	23%
SAB	1990–98	284	61%	15%	24%
p-value			0.006	0.00007	0.2

DAT, daunorubicin + Ara-C + thioguanine; SAB, same as before (i.e. DAT).

of a new intervention having a big treatment effect, or being vastly superior to an existing therapy, is fairly low. It is more realistic to expect a moderate difference between interventions, or a moderate effect compared with placebo.

Therefore, it is important to provide reliable evidence about moderate benefits and to be able to reduce as far as possible any systematic biases that might affect the results. For this reason, non-randomised studies do not typically provide robust enough evidence. Case studies, in particular, may be seriously misleading. A potentially serious risk of selection bias exists: it is impossible to tell whether only the most promising patients are selected for the new treatment, and without a comparator group, the true scale of any 'breakthrough' cannot be gauged. Similarly, historically controlled studies, in which care involving the new treatment is compared to previous outcome rates before the new care was introduced, can provide unreliable estimates of a treatment's effectiveness. For example, a comparison of today's A-level results with those of 1980 show an improved pass rate. Students sitting A levels in 1980 received free school milk while at primary school; those sitting them today do not. So, are we to conclude that free milk makes you less intelligent? More seriously, the general improvement in cancer outcomes over time means that one cannot be sure if any improvements are due to the drug, to the generally improving prognosis, to differences in case mix over time or to a combination of all three. In acute myeloid leukaemia, a historically controlled study of standard DAT therapy for patients over age 60 against the SAB regimen showed a statistically significant benefit for SAB (Wheatley, 2002; Box 7.1). This appears promising until one realises that SAB stands for 'same as before'; in other words, the improvement has nothing to do

with the treatment, but is likely instead to be a result of better supportive care. Likewise, if clinicians are more likely to give a treatment to patients with more severe symptoms, then those who receive therapy are of worse prognosis than those who do not. A straight comparison could therefore show that the treatment appeared worse (Green and Byar, 1984).

The only way to reduce such selection biases as much as possible is to randomise patients: allocate treatments in a way that produces equivalent groups and precludes the chance that the next treatment allocation can be predicted. Allocation by date of birth, for example, may not produce equivalent groups because it is easy to predict what a person's treatment is going to be and then make a decision on whether to enter the trial based on this knowledge.

A number of ways of allocating patients can produce equivalent groups (Altman and Bland, 1999, 2005). The simplest method is to use so-called simple randomisation in which the chance of receiving a given treatment is the same, irrespective of previous entries into the trial. Simple randomisation can be achieved using a random number list, a computer-generated random number or even tossing a coin. This method, however, can lead to chance imbalances in the numbers allocated to different treatment groups, so some trials use permuted block randomisation in which the number of patients in each group is required to be in balance at various stages through the trial (e.g. after every 4 or 6 patients). Some more sophisticated methods also ensure balance across important prognostic factors. It is possible to extend permuted block randomisation to this scenario or to use allocation algorithms such as minimisation, which generally require the use of a computer. In all except simple randomisation, where previous allocations do not influence the next, it is important

Box 7.2 Good practice in randomisation

- Use third-party randomisation.

  An independent randomisation service with a degree of separation between clinician and patient provides more security. Envelopes containing the treatment allocation may appear an attractive option, but need to be policed to stop clinicians from opening several envelopes until they find the preferred treatment. A secure computer database held at a central trials office is a good way to ensure allocation concealment.
- Collect all important prognostic factors prior to randomisation.

  The recorded value of a prognostic factor may change or be influenced by treatment allocation.
- Balance prognostic groups by stratification or minimisation.

  Similar numbers of different types of patient are ensured to be in each group. At its simplest, this could be achieved by a randomisation list for each category, but for more than a few variables this becomes cumbersome and a computerised system is preferable and allows simultaneous minimisation across many variables.

to ensure that there are no patterns that could allow the next allocation to be predicted. (For example, in permuted block randomisation with a block length of 2, after an even number of patients the treatments will be in balance – in a single-centre trial, the allocation of every other patient could be predicted precisely (Hills *et al.*, 2009)). It is a fallacy that strict random allocation is required: far more important is concealment of the treatment allocation until the patient is irreversibly committed to the trial. Furthermore, patients who did not receive their preferred treatment cannot be re-randomised. Clinicians can and do attempt to subvert some randomisation approaches, and care needs to be taken to ensure that this is made as difficult as possible (Schulz, 1995). Box 7.2 gives some thoughts on good practice in randomisation.

Choice of endpoints

Generally speaking, the choice of a suitable endpoint in cancer is less tricky than for many other chronic conditions. In many cases, the main aim is to prolong life, so the primary measured outcome in a trial is mortality. However, in certain instances, the outcome measure may be different. For example, in conditions that are relatively rare and where outcomes are already very good (e.g. acute promyelocytic leukaemia and increasingly other cancers such as breast cancer), a trial assessing mortality may have to be very large and also run for a long time, making such a study impractical. In these circumstances, it may be more relevant to assess quality of life – can one achieve as-good outcomes with less toxicity. Indeed, this approach has been used in recent UK National Trials in Acute Promyelocytic Leukaemia, such as AML15

(Burnett *et al.*, 2013) and AML17 (http://aml17.cardiff.ac.uk/aml17/, accessed October, 2014). Similarly, the primary aim of some trials may not be to directly improve mortality, but to reduce the incidence of adverse events, as in the SIGNIFICANT trial of prophylactic antibiotics, which measured the number of febrile episodes (Cullen *et al.*, 2005).

The choice of outcome measure influences both the type of statistical test being performed and the size a trial needs to be. In choosing a suitable outcome measure, it is important to choose a measure that is of clinical relevance and that can be used to help guide future practice. When assessing the results of a clinical trial, it is important to consider its clinical as well as its statistical significance. One may consider outcomes relevant to patients, clinicians, and to organizations such as the National Institute for Health and Care Excellence (NICE). Generally, the simplest outcomes are often the best – they are easy to interpret and the clinical relevance of a given size of treatment effect is clear. It is important, however, not to try and collect too many outcome measures: the trial will then lack focus, and, by chance, one outcome may indicate that one particular treatment is better, while for another outcome, the reverse is the case. Given enough outcomes, it is usually possible to find a significant result for one of them even in trials of the most unpromising treatments. Therefore, it is crucial to identify a small number of primary and secondary outcomes, which are considered the most important. These may be clinical outcomes obtained from notes or patient-centred outcomes collected through questionnaires. If a questionnaire is being used, then it is worthwhile to ensure that it is validated – to make sure that the results are meaningful and reproducible and, if possible, to define how big a difference is relevant.

Sometimes, the real outcome of interest occurs a long time in the future. Because it is impractical to wait many years for an answer, it is tempting instead to use a surrogate outcome, which predicts this future outcome (e.g. recurrence to predict survival benefit). However, this approach can be fraught with difficulties. For example, there may be a difference in recurrence-free survival, but this difference is not necessarily translated into a significant survival benefit (Specht *et al.*, 1998).

Blinding

To create comparable groups for analysis, it is important that there is no foreknowledge of treatment allocation. This concept is known as allocation concealment. However, even after randomisation there are occasions when knowledge of which treatment group a patient is in can influence their treatment or their outcomes. For example, one treatment may require additional follow-up visits, so that supportive care or additional treatments could be provided preferentially to one group or another. Alternatively, if outcomes are dependent on clinician or patient rating of health state (e.g. in quality-of-life trials) then knowledge of a patient's treatment may influence the perception of health status (especially if one option is to offer no treatment).

There are a number of ways of combating this problem. Standardised treatment protocols can be introduced, so that all patients receive equivalent supportive care and clinician contact. Also, the use of objective outcome measures, such as mortality, tends to minimise the effect of knowledge of treatment allocation on outcome. Another alternative is to blind the trial treatments. Trials are typically referred to as either single-blind or double-blind. In the former, either the patient or the clinician/assessor is unaware of the treatment allocation; generally, the person recording the outcome is the one who needs to be blinded. In double-blind trials, both the patient and the clinician/assessor are unaware of which treatment was given. This way, any beliefs about the intervention, negative or positive, should not be expected to influence the outcome. The use of a matching placebo can ensure blinding; alternatively, pharmacists can make up drug solutions that are indistinguishable irrespective of the treatments actually contained. For other trials, some degree of blinding can be achieved with imagination: in trials of surgical techniques, the use of sham surgery has been advocated, although sometimes this will require the participant's acceptance of an additional, clinically unnecessary procedure. It has been argued that sham procedures are methodologically necessary to produce valid results; therefore, as long as the participant is informed that they will receive either a real or a sham intervention and that the sham procedure will be indistinguishable from the real treatment under investigation, there is no deception involved (Miller and Kaptchuk, 2004). Alternatively, if the procedure would be performed after a surgical examination to establish eligibility, some trials have randomised the patient 'on the table' (Daniels *et al.*, 2009) – although, again, care needs to be taken concerning consent.

Choice of subjects, and how many

In a randomised trial, because the different treatment groups are equivalent, it follows that any observed differences must be the result either of chance or of a genuine difference between the treatments. The probability that observed differences (or ones that are more extreme) are the result only of chance differences between groups is given by the *p*-value, which tells you how often a trial of an ineffective treatment would be expected to produce this type of result. If the *p*-value is sufficiently small, then one can conclude that the data are inconsistent with the treatment being ineffective, rather in the same way that a jury starts with the presumption of innocence and asks whether there is enough evidence to overturn it beyond reasonable doubt. Alternatively, one can determine an estimate of the size of the treatment effect, together with a measure of a likely range, based on the natural variability between patients.

Clearly, to detect moderate differences, one must discriminate between the signal and the ambient noise: although one cannot reduce differences between people, larger numbers enable one to improve the signal-to-noise ratio. However, for relatively uncommon conditions, the number of patients required in a study to detect moderate treatment effects may perhaps be more than it is feasible to recruit. The smaller the treatment effect one wishes to detect, the larger the number of patients one needs to recruit. To have a 90% chance of detecting whether a treatment increases the proportion of patients entering remission from 50% to 75% requires only about 150 participants (Machin *et al.*, 1997). However, to detect an improvement from 50% to 60%, which would still be worthwhile, a study needs about 1000 patients; to detect a 5% improvement would require about 4000 participants. A corollary of this is that a non-significant result does not automatically mean that there is no treatment difference: the trial could simply have been too small to detect a moderate, but worthwhile, treatment effect (Altman and Bland, 1995). The use of effect sizes and confidence intervals overcomes this problem. The 95% confidence interval contains the true treatment effect 95% of the time; only if this does not include a clinically relevant treatment effect is it fair to conclude that a worthwhile difference is unlikely.

The number of patients required to answer a question reliably depends on a number of factors. First, the sample size depends on the type of outcome being measured: dichotomous outcomes (e.g. entered remission, experienced grade 3 or 4 toxicity), continuous outcomes (e.g. quality-of-life scores, size of a laboratory measure) and time-to-event outcomes (e.g. survival time, duration of remission) all need different calculations. Second, the size of treatment effect one wishes to detect needs to be specified (e.g. from 50% to 60% entering remission, a difference of 10 points on a scale with a standard deviation of 25, etc.). Finally, it is important to specify the level at which statistical testing will be performed (typically set at a significance level of $p \leq 0.05$) and how certain one wants to be of detecting a treatment effect if it really is there. This latter concept is known as the power and is typically set at 80% or 90%, representing a 1-in-5 or 1-in-10 chance of missing a real treatment effect. The smaller the effect one wishes to detect and the smaller the significance level, or the higher the power, the larger the number of patients required. It may seem attractive to aim at detecting a large treatment effect, or to set the power low, but this means that one runs the risk of the estimate of treatment effect to be sufficiently imprecise as to include both no treatment effect and a clinically relevant effect, thus making the trial inconclusive.

When considering the required number of patients, it is also important to determine how these patients are likely to be found. Extending a trial over a number of centres will increase the relevant pool of potential participants. However, it is important to identify precisely who is eligible for the trial. Patients who could be at risk from one of the trial interventions need to be excluded. However, when deciding which patients to include in a potential trial, it is possible to have selection criteria that are too rigid and exclusive. Not only does restricting the population too much reduce the pool of potential participants, making it more difficult to achieve target recruitment,

but the results of the trial may not be immediately generalisable to other important groups of patients. For example, age can be applied as an exclusion criterion on arbitrary grounds.

For this reason, it has been argued that it is preferable to avoid prescriptive inclusion and exclusion criteria and aim for a representative sample from which generalisable results can be obtained (Collins et al., 1996). For a given patient, there may be uncertainty about the relative merits of different courses of action. Presented with the same circumstances, clinicians may have differences in opinion. The ethical imperative then would be to try to reduce uncertainty by contributing to the evidence, and the most appropriate way of achieving this would be to recruit the patient into a well-designed clinical trial. It would be unethical for a patient to have their treatment chosen at random if either they or their doctor are certain about what treatment they prefer.

However, randomisation can be considered when both doctor and patient are uncertain about which treatment is preferable. No further restrictions, other than diagnostic and safety-related criteria, would then be applied, allowing a wide range of patients to be recruited. This sort of wide, pragmatic entry condition has an added benefit. If a wide range of patients is randomised, it is possible to examine, albeit cautiously, whether different groups of participants respond differently to the treatment. Of course, it is important to collect data to identify precisely what type of patient has been entered, but only by running large-scale randomised trials with wide entry criteria can questions of which treatment is best for which patient be answered with any confidence.

Collecting data

As pointed out earlier, it is important to choose a small number of primary and secondary outcomes to assess the effectiveness of a new treatment. It is also important to determine exactly how these data will be collected. Can, for example, national records (e.g. of mortality) be used to determine outcomes? If so, then this means that one is not reliant on clinicians completing forms, and there can be (virtually) complete ascertainment of the primary outcome measures. Alternatively, it may be preferable to ask clinicians or patients to complete forms at predetermined time points. In this way, additional patient information can be captured. It is often tempting to include extra 'nice-to-know' data, perhaps, with a view to using them for analyses, additional to the main paper. However, before becoming committed to extra work, not only for the statisticians and data managers but also for clinicians, one needs to be sure that the data are really relevant. Data that can be collected only on a minority of patients are unlikely to influence the trial's conclusions. If it is unclear how, or indeed whether, data are to be analysed, they should not be collected. Collecting data that will not be analysed puts an extra burden, without any ultimate purpose, on participants and clinicians. Keeping data collection to a minimum also increases the likelihood of it being collected.

Data should be collected on simple, well-designed forms. It is helpful for trial organisers to liaise with the statistician and the person designing the database for storing information to ensure that forms are clear and unambiguous and that data are coded wherever possible because coded answers are easier to analyse than free text fields, which may require extensive recoding before analysis. Forms that are well designed and as short as possible increase the likelihood of completion (Edwards *et al.*, 2002).

To obtain good follow-up:

- **keep it short** – don't ask for unnecessary data;
- **keep it simple** – don't add unnecessary extra tests; and
- **keep it seldom** – don't repeat assessments too many times.

Analysing data: the intention-to-treat principle

Once patients are randomised into a trial, they should remain in the analyses, even if they stop taking the treatment or, indeed, never even receive it. The main idea behind randomisation is the creation of equivalent groups of patients; if patients are left out of the analysis, the groups cease to be equivalent. Intention-to-treat (ITT) analysis analyses every patient according to the treatment to which they were allocated rather than what they received. In cases in which there are protocol deviations, then ITT analyses tend to be conservative: they underestimate the treatment effect. So, if one sees a difference, then one can be reasonably sure that it really is there. Other sorts of analysis may look attractive because they compare what actually happened, not what was meant to happen. However, as can be seen in Box 7.3, these other analyses can lead to misleading results, making ineffective therapies appear

worthwhile. What ITT really measures is the effect of introducing the policy of giving the treatment: what is the effect of introducing a new treatment in the real world?

Inevitably, there will be circumstances in which patients who have committed to the trial do not complete treatment and follow-up. Sometimes this is treatment-related, for example, if side effects are distressing or if there is no perceived benefit from the treatment. These drop-outs are not random and may appear more frequently in one arm of the study than another, so it is crucial to note the reason for non-compliance or withdrawal, especially if no further follow-up information is obtainable. Failure to do this will introduce a systematic difference between the groups (known as attrition bias). Ideally, however, patients who withdraw from treatment should still be encouraged to contribute to data collection; it is a common misconception that a deviation from the protocol necessitates withdrawal. In cancer trials in which the outcome is mortality, this is less of a problem because simple follow-up should be available from clinicians or from national records, but it can cause serious problems in quality-of-life studies. For such studies, where direct patient contact may be required, a meta-analysis of methods of improving the response rate to postal questionnaires identified a number of successful strategies (Edwards *et al.*, 2002), such as a pre-contact before the questionnaire is sent, provision of a pre-paid reply envelope and using a short, interesting questionnaire, in addition to obvious monetary incentives.

Perils of subgroups

A clinical trial sets out to answer whether a particular treatment is effective, on an average, for a wide range of patients. Although a trial can give some evidence on what treatment to give an individual patient, it does so by considering the population as a whole, and not each separate individual. It is tempting to try and identify subgroups of patients that benefit from an intervention. However, note that a significant result ($p < 0.05$) will be seen by chance 5% of the time. So, in a trial of an ineffective treatment, if one looks at 20 different subgroups of patients, there is likely to be on average a significant result in one subgroup. It is laughable to say that, for people born on one particular day of the month, putting brown sugar in their coffee is any better (or worse!) in controlling febrile neutropenia than using white sugar. However, it is possible that, if one

Box 7.3 Intention to treat

Consider a trial of chemotherapy with associated toxicity.

The trial is performed in two types of patients, who are recruited in equal numbers: 'fit' patients who have 70% survival, and 'unfit' patients who have a 30% survival probability. These survival probabilities are unaffected by the new treatment.

Because the treatment is toxic but potentially curative, some clinicians are not happy to give unfit patients the more-toxic treatment, and they give the less-toxic existing therapy instead. Likewise, fit patients who draw control treatment may receive the new therapy because they are thought to be fit enough to withstand the side effects. In the trial, 20% of each group receives the opposite chemotherapy.

It is possible to derive two tables of the proportions of patients surviving. First, for the ITT analysis,

	Allocated new treatment (%)	Allocated control treatment (%)
Fit	50	50
Unfit	50	50
Survival rate[a]	50	50

And second, for the as-treated analysis,

	Receiving new treatment (%)	Receiving control treatment (%)
Fit	60	40
Unfit	40	60
Survival rate[a]	54	46

[a] The survival rate is calculated as 70% times the proportion who are 'fit' plus 30% times the proportion who are 'unfit' for each group.

Whereas an ITT analysis correctly shows that the new chemotherapy is no better in prolonging survival (and, hence, it is more toxic and less attractive than the original option), the as-treated analysis produces an 8% survival benefit, which may be enough to change clinical practice. The difference arises because fewer poor-risk patients receive the new treatment. This sort of analysis tends to show an artificial benefit for the treatment received by the better-risk patients.

runs a large RCT and 'data dredges' through data from enough subgroups, one will get this kind of spurious result, which will appear purely by chance. If one looks hard enough, it is likely that one will find a statistically significant result – but it is also possible that the result is a fluke.

There are statistical techniques to test whether observed effects are real (Assmann *et al.*, 2000), but trials that look at subgroups usually need to be much bigger. As a rule of thumb, to detect a difference reliably within subgroups of the same size as a treatment effect that you have decided is clinically meaningful would require four times as many trial participants as it would to detect an overall effect. Subgroup analyses are therefore typically designed to detect qualitative differences in treatment effects (treatment works in one group, but not in another) as opposed to smaller, quantitative differences in effect size (treatment works in both groups, but gives greater benefit in one group than another).

If there are subgroups in which there are legitimate reasons for anticipating a different response to treatment (e.g. oestrogen receptor status in trials of hormonal treatments for breast cancer), then these should be specified in the trial protocol in advance, together with a justification of the underlying mechanism and the influence it may have on the outcome. In any case, one should not conclude, simply because a treatment provides a significant effect in one subgroup and not in another, that the treatment works only for one subgroup of patients. (There are a number of examples of this erroneous reasoning in the literature: Cascinelli, 1994; Cascinelli *et al.*, 1994; Creutzig *et al.*, 2001; Wheatley and Hills, 2001.) When significant subgroup differences exist, they should always be viewed in the context of the overall findings. It is unlikely that, if the overall result is positive, a subgroup finding of significant harm is to be relied on. Again, such qualitative effects need to be viewed with scepticism unless there is some

Table 7.1 A typical 2 × 2 factorial design. One-quarter of patients receives both treatments A and B, one-quarter receives A only, one-quarter B only and one-quarter receives control

	Drug B	Control
Drug A	A + B	A
Control	B	Control

plausible, prespecified reason why some subgroups should behave differently.

Additional topics

A common theme in the preceding sections is the need to provide reliable evidence that is likely to influence future clinical practice. This means providing evidence on patients similar to those one would meet in everyday clinical practice and ensuring that the level of evidence is sufficiently strong to enable the making of a decision on treatment. The necessary corollary of this is that trials need to be large. With only a finite population of patients from which to choose, recruiting enough participants can be difficult.

For this reason, there are a number of techniques that can help trials be run more efficiently. In particular, two design features are widely used in cancer clinical trials so that advances can be made as rapidly as possible. The first is the factorial design. Factorial designs allow more than one research question to be answered simultaneously. If two different drugs are available and no interactions are expected between them, then if both drugs were shown to work, it would be reasonable to give them both together. To test both treatments, one can randomise patients in a 2 × 2 factorial trial design to receive drug A or control, in addition to receiving either drug B or control (Table 7.1). Then, to assess the effect of treatment A, one can compare patients receiving A + B with patients receiving B, and those receiving A with control. Because a similar procedure can be done to assess treatment B, every patient is contributing to two comparisons. Thus, two research questions can be answered at once. This method is more complicated if there is evidence of interaction between the treatments, but it is only in a factorial design that such interactions can reliably be investigated.

Factorial designs are common in cancer. For example, the MRC/NCRI trials in acute myeloid leukaemia (AML) typically use factorial designs (e.g. the AML14 trial; see Box 7.4; Burnett *et al.*, 2005).

Other methods can be used to ensure that trials recruit a large, clinically representative group of patients. One such approach is the pragmatic design adopted by the MRC QUASAR trial of chemotherapy for colorectal cancer, which considered the effectiveness of 5-FU/folinic acid-based chemotherapy as well as two different doses of folinic acid and the effect of adding levamisole to chemotherapy (QUASAR Collaborative Group, 2000). To recruit widely, clinicians were able to specify if a patient had a clear indication for chemotherapy (in which case patients were randomised in a 2 × 2 factorial design, between two doses of folinic acid and the addition or not of levamisole), or an uncertain indication, in which case they were randomised either to receive chemotherapy (randomised in the same 2 × 2 design) or not. The trial recruited more than 7000 participants to help provide reliable evidence, not only on whether to give 5-FU/FA chemotherapy but also to provide evidence on the dose of folinic acid and the role of levamisole.

In rarer conditions, the challenge is perhaps a little different. In such conditions, a large trial may take many years to complete, meaning that many treatments compete for the same small pool of patients. Therefore, it is important to identify as efficiently as possible those treatments that are likely to be the most promising. For conditions with a poor prognosis, one possible way forward is the so-called 'Pick-A-Winner' design (Hills and Burnett, 2011) for patients where the outcome is sufficiently poor for data to be available quite early on to determine whether there is likely to be a meaningful treatment effect. This is a version of a Multi-Arm Multi-Stage (or MAMS) design (Royston *et al.*, 2003). Its efficiency comes from requiring the minimum clinically important difference to be large, meaning that if no evidence of benefit is seen early on in the trial, then it is very unlikely that the looked-for large benefit will materialise if recruitment continues, and the arm can reasonably be closed with a low risk of rejecting a treatment that could ultimately prove worthwhile. The approach was used in the NCRI AML16 trial of non-intensive therapy for older patients with AML (see www.aml16.bham.ac.uk, accessed December, 2014). The initial aim was to double survival at 2 years from 11% to 22%, by inducing remission in twice as many patients (increasing the rate from 15% to 30%). This meant that, although a full trial would require about 200 patients per arm, it was possible to look at the data after only 50 patients per arm had been recruited, and reject all treatments which failed to improve remission

Box 7.4 The AML14 trial

The AML14 trial was intended for patients with AML over the age of 60 and ran in two parts depending on whether patients were deemed fit for intensive chemotherapy. For those receiving intensive treatment, the design was a 3 × 2 factorial design for induction, with a further randomisation to either 3 or 4 courses of treatment, giving a total of 12 treatment options (3 × 2 × 2).

Two courses of induction treatment				
Daunorubicin 50 mg/m^2 vs Daunorubicin 35 mg/m^2 vs Daunorubicin 35 mg/m^2 + PSC-833	with	Ara-C 200 mg/m^2 b.d. vs Ara-C 100 mg/m^2 b.d.	and treatment lasting in total for	three courses vs four courses

rates by 2.5%. A further examination after 100 patients had been recruited to the arm could be used further to identify unpromising treatments. In all cases, the comparison was a truly randomised one, to reduce bias: but, one of the advantages of the Pick-A-Winner approach is that it enables new treatments to be introduced to replace those which have failed, giving a rolling programme of drug evaluation. Those treatments which pass the first two hurdles proceed to a full evaluation, powered on overall survival. In AML, the approach is continuing in the LI-1 Programme of drug evaluation.

Ethical considerations

Introduction

Most clinical research can be carried out only with the cooperation of patients who enter clinical trials, agree to be treated according to study protocols, who are followed up and whose information used to assess the value of a new treatment. It is therefore paramount that the rights and well-being of participants are considered. In particular, it is important that patients are aware of any potential risks, and that there is not already good evidence that one or the other treatment is better. There is a considerable body of literature on good clinical practice (GCP) in clinical trials, as well as a growing body of guidance and legislation, including the data protection act, various handbooks on GCP, and the 2001 European Union directive, which is currently going through the process of revision. The directive sets down certain legal responsibilities for investigators in drug trials, including the process of

gaining approvals from both ethics committees and the competent authority, how to approach amendments to studies, and ensuring timely reporting of safety information. The legislation also requires all trials of investigational medicinal products to have a Sponsor, usually either a pharmaceutical company, university or hospital trust. All investigators need to have up-to-date GCP. One area of debate that arose from the signing into law of the EU directive was how to strike the correct balance between protecting the interests of participants and excessive bureaucracy, which may tend to reduce the number and size of clinical trials (Burman *et al.*, 2001) and this debate has to an extent continued.

Study protocol

Perhaps the most important way of achieving good-quality clinical research is by having a well-written trial protocol. Such a protocol is not only a justification for the research being performed, it is the trial 'bible'. It should contain all relevant information and instructions about the trial, including treatment schedules, reporting methods and quality assurance. During a trial, protocols may be modified as new information becomes available, or for more practical reasons, such as alterations in drug supply, doses or route of administration. The protocol needs to be updated with this information and approved by the same authorities who approved the original protocol: all investigators are provided with a copy of the new protocol. For this reason, it can be helpful to store trial documentation on a website so that clinicians can download all the necessary information to fulfil their legal obligation to keep their own site files up to date.

Informed consent

All participants in a clinical trial have the right to be adequately informed about the benefits and risks involved. Participation must be voluntary, and informed consent of participants needs to be taken. Information about the trial is typically given using a *patient information sheet*, which explains the research, the possible treatments, what data are being collected and how data will be used. If tissue samples are to be taken, consent needs to be obtained for this too. Generally, potential participants need to be given time to digest the information they have been given and to ask questions; thus, the taking of participants' consent can involve a period of time. Strategies may need to be considered to allow participants the time they need (e.g. ensuring that a research nurse is present during clinics to help with the process and provide a point of contact for participants).

Good clinical practice (GCP) and ethics committees

The aims of GCP in clinical trials are twofold: to protect the participants and to provide assurance that the trial has been carried out to a sufficiently high standard that results are credible. Various aspects of GCP ensure: the trial is, and remains, ethical; treatments are safe and used appropriately; data collection is adequate and reliable; and data are stored securely. In the UK, the principles of Good Clinical Practice or GCP are enshrined in law. Generally, trials now adhere to International Committee on Harmonisation (ICH) guidelines (see www.ich.org, accessed December, 2014). These guidelines stress the importance of having well-written protocols, independent Trial Steering Committees (TSC) and set roles and responsibilities of the different people taking part in the study. There are also guidelines on on-site monitoring, and other methods which can be used to ensure the integrity of the data provided by the study.

All trials require ethical approval, which involves submitting the study protocol and supporting documentation, such as patient information sheets, to a Research Ethics Committee. The ethics application process has been streamlined and paperwork for ethics committee applications can be found centrally at www.myresearchproject.org.uk (accessed December, 2014).

The ethics committee will assess the protocol and make a judgement. Additionally, each centre is required to undergo a *site-specific assessment* to ensure that the centre and its staff are capable of supporting the protocol. The integrated research application system (IRAS) also allows submission of trials involving investigational medicinal products (IMPs) for clinical trial authorisation from the relevant medicines agency (see https://eudract.ema.europa.eu/, accessed December 2014).

Perhaps one of the most important consequences of the EU Directive is that the reporting of adverse events has now been standardised. All serious adverse events (SAEs) need to be reported to the sponsor, who determines whether or not the SAE is expected. Suspected unexpected serious adverse reactions need to be reported to the ethics committee, and to the Medicines and Healthcare Products Regulatory Agency within 7 days of receipt.

In terms of monitoring, it is often said that excessive on-site monitoring is not cost-effective. It is argued that central monitoring can detect anomalies and errors in data more cost-effectively than on-site monitors (Buyse *et al.*, 1999) and that occasionally monitors in centres have failed to detect problems identified using central checks (Enserink, 1996). Clearly, the issues are complex. However, since the coming of the EU directive, a number of helpful websites have been set up to guide trialists through the increasing maze of regulation, notably the Clinical Trials Toolkit (www.ct-toolkit.ac.uk, accessed December, 2014).

Data monitoring committees: is the trial still ethical?

As discussed earlier, a clinical trial remains ethical only while the question being addressed remains relevant. If there is good evidence that one treatment is better than another, then clearly, one group of patients will be receiving care that is known to be suboptimal, making the trial unethical.

In some clinical trials, the strength of evidence in favour of one treatment over another may be such that an answer is known well before the scheduled end of the trial. Alternatively, the safety profile of one treatment may make it unacceptable. In both cases, there is an argument to abandon the clinical trial. This is one of the roles of the Data Monitoring Committee (DMC). This group should be independent of the trial organisers, and its job is to look at the accumulating data from the trial in light of other external evidence (e.g. other trial reports and new references). If the evidence is sufficiently strong and likely to change clinical practice were it revealed to clinicians and participants, then they can recommend closing the trial. The definition of 'sufficiently strong' needs to be determined before the trial starts. There have been a number of different statistical stopping rules proposed (Ellenberg *et al.*, 2002), but all of them realise that periodically looking at the data increases the chance of a chance positive result, and they therefore require a stronger level of evidence than $p < 0.05$. Some stopping rules set an extreme level of significance (such as $p \leq 0.002$) throughout the trial, whereas others adapt depending on how close the trial is to completion. Increasingly, trials can be stopped for futility when there is strong evidence that the treatments being compared are not materially different. Alternatively, trials can be closed because of safety concerns if the incidence of adverse events in one group is unacceptably high, or, on occasion, if study recruitment is so slow that a reliable answer is unlikely. DMCs have another useful purpose: because interim analyses need to be performed, the preparation of a DMC report (which needs to be kept secret from the trial organisers, clinicians and participants) can identify problems with data collection methods or compliance with treatment.

Research networks

As discussed, to provide reliable results, clinical trials in cancer often need to be large. This poses a challenge for researchers: how does one recruit enough patients? One option would be to recruit over an extended period, but by the time the results are published, the question may no longer be relevant. A better approach is to foster the creation of a collaborative group to enable widespread recruitment. For example, the NCRI/MRC trials in AML recruit widely both in the UK and abroad. Typically, up to 200 clinicians take part in these trials, and annual recruitment is about 1000 patients, out of an incident population of around 2000. Such commitment to recruitment enables trials to recruit and report quickly, thereby advancing knowledge and practice.

Recent initiatives in the UK have recognised the importance of collaboration, and a number of clinical research networks have recently been introduced. In particular the National Cancer Research Network (NCRN) was set up in 2001 to improve the level of recruitment to trials and other well-designed research. In England, the National Institute for Health Research (NIHR) has set up Clinical Research Networks and

employs data managers, nurses and other staff who can provide help and support to clinical trials. These important resources are available for trials that have been funded through the NIHR and CRUK, as well as for other trials that have been formally reviewed and adopted as part of the NCRN trials portfolio. Other NCRN initiatives include the development of a computer infrastructure for clinical trials management and the identification of areas where systematic reviews of current evidence are required.

Health economics

There is an increasing need for research to provide evidence of cost-effectiveness as well as clinical effectiveness. This is something specifically required by NICE both in approving individual interventions for the NHS and in its clinical guidelines programme. Therefore, clinical trials often now include health economic outcomes, or a parallel study may be set up in a subset of patients or participating centres. Typically, this will involve trying to identify and record all the contacts that study participants have with the health services during the trial. These can then be costed, and the information used in combination with the effectiveness outcomes to provide information on cost-effectiveness. Quality-of-life data may also be collected using a standardised instrument and these data may be used to provide a utility estimate, such as the 'quality-adjusted life-year.'

Translational research

There is an increasing amount of laboratory cancer research being carried out and with it comes the need to determine whether novel findings in the laboratory can translate into testable hypotheses in patients and ultimately improved outcomes. This 'bench-to-bedside' approach should lead ultimately to the development of targeted therapies for a wide range of conditions. This approach can be challenging. Trials need to be designed to collect additional disease markers to identify patients who are likely to benefit from targeted therapies, and a concentration on specific subgroups of patients brings with it the problem of recruiting enough patients to provide reliable and meaningful results. Ethically, participants in trials will need to know what samples will be taken, how these will be stored, and how results from any samples will be used.

Additionally, gene array technology has dramatically increased the number of markers available for analysis and is a source of hope for identifying prognostic markers that can then be used to help develop targeted therapies. Of course, the challenge, when there are a large number of potential markers and combinations of markers, is to identify which markers are genuinely prognostic and which are merely artefactual. This new area of laboratory research has led to the development of methods for testing which avenues are the most promising for future research. In the UK, the network of Experimental Cancer Medicine Centres helps facilitate translational research in cancer.

Synthesising research results: systematic reviews and meta-analysis

When deciding the best treatment for a particular patient, it is important to consider all the available research evidence. Whereas one RCT may show a significant benefit for a new treatment, others may not; therefore, it is important to be able to put trial results in context. Additionally, new trials need to be designed with reference to the findings of a systematic review of previous research. This will reduce the chance of repeating previous mistakes and will also stop unnecessary (and therefore unethical) trials from being conducted when there is already enough evidence about the effectiveness of a given treatment. As the editors of the *Lancet* have said: 'Unnecessary and badly presented clinical research injures volunteers and patients as surely as any other form of bad medicine, as well as wasting resources and abusing the trust placed in investigators by their trial participants' (Young and Horton, 2005). The journal now requires authors to include a clear summary of previous research findings.

Of course, to summarise previous research findings, the previous research must be in the public domain. In the past, trials with negative or inconclusive results were considered uninteresting and were much less likely to be published (so-called 'file drawer' or publication bias; Dickersin *et al.*, 1987). Such problems have led to the setting up of a number of online journals where such results can be published and put into the public domain. Otherwise, a search of the published literature would tend only to identify trials that showed significant benefits, giving an unduly optimistic view of a treatment's effectiveness. The issue of 'file drawer bias' is very much a hot topic at present with the launch of campaigns such as AllTrials calls

for all past and present clinical trials to be registered and their full methods and summary results reported (http://www.alltrials.net/, accessed January 2015). Only by having all of the data available can a full picture of treatment benefits (or disbenefits) be seen, and future research can then build on the totality of knowledge at that point in time, rather than reinventing the wheel.

Once relevant research has been identified and systematically reviewed for its quality, it is important to be able to synthesise and summarise the results. In most cases this may just be a narrative summary that describes and comments on all the available evidence; but it may be possible to carry out a statistical synthesis. Meta-analysis is a powerful tool for doing this: it provides quantitative estimates of a treatment's effectiveness by combining data from a number of RCTs. One advantage of doing such an analysis is that it can identify important treatment benefits which previous trials had been too small to detect reliably. One such example comes from the Early Breast Cancer Trialists' Collaborative Group meta-analysis of tamoxifen in breast cancer (Early Breast Cancer Trialists Collaborative Group, 1990). Of the 28 randomised trials of tamoxifen versus no treatment analysed in the first cycle of the overview, only 4 showed a statistically significant survival benefit. Yet, a meta-analysis of their findings demonstrated a highly statistically significant ($p < 10^{-6}$) 16% proportional reduction in mortality achieved with tamoxifen. Previous trials had been too small to detect such an improvement reliably. Only by using a meta-analysis was it possible to demonstrate the utility of a treatment that has since annually saved many thousands of lives.

There are, however, dangers in carrying out an inappropriate meta-analysis. If there is a large amount of heterogeneity between trials, then merely reporting the total treatment effect can give misleading results. For this reason it is important to explore sources of heterogeneity (e.g. different endpoints, doses, dosing regimens, or different patient groups) to determine whether such heterogeneity materially affects the results of the meta-analysis and the estimate of effectiveness.

A meta-analysis or other review is only as good as the data that go into it and needs to be continually updated in light of new results. After a new clinical trial has been completed, the data need to be looked at in relation to previous trials and the impact of the results discussed. This is best achieved by adding the trial into

Box 7.5 Trials in context

- When developing the research question, conduct a systematic review or identify a relevant review done by someone else.
- Learn from the achievements (and mistakes) of past trials, but read critically.
- Discuss the findings of your study in the context of an updated systematic review.

the existing meta-analysis and interpreting any effect that it has on the overall result. It is, after all, the totality of trial data that provides the best evidence, and overemphasis on any particular trial, even the one you conducted, can give misleading findings. Box 7.5 gives guidelines for putting results in context.

Assessing published reports of research

All the ideas presented in this chapter apply equally well to designing one's own clinical trial as they do to assessing other people's research. The obvious questions that one needs to ask when reading research are whether the results appear believable and whether the methodology is sound. Few pieces of research are without some methodological flaws (Altman, 1994), but do these flaws invalidate the findings?

In assessing the merits of different treatments we have already seen that different types of study carry different weight when making evidence-based decisions on health care. There is a generally accepted order of precedence (Guyatt et al., 1995).

1. Systematic reviews and meta-analyses.
2. RCTs with definitive results (based on confidence intervals).
3. RCTs with non-definitive results.
4. Cohort studies.
5. Case-control studies.
6. Cross-sectional studies.
7. Case reports.

As can be seen, for the results of an assessment of a treatment to be reliable, a study needs to be randomised and of sufficient size to provide reliable evidence. Results need to be reported fairly, with no undue emphasis on particular subgroups or endpoints. Faced with a paper, it can sometimes be quite difficult to check whether the report matches the original design of the study. However, a number of journals now allow (and encourage) trialists to publish their study protocols online, allowing readers to make a direct comparison

between the results obtained and the originally proposed methodology. Additionally, some of the larger medical journals require trials to be reported according to the CONSORT guidance (Moher et al., 2001). Perhaps the most important aspect of the CONSORT guidance, and the one that will be most familiar, is the requirement to include in a paper a flowchart showing the journey of the patient population through the trial, showing how many patients did not receive their treatment according to the protocol and how many patients dropped out from (or were lost to) follow-up. However, the CONSORT statement makes a number of other recommendations, including the use of confidence intervals rather than merely p-values, and reporting of eligibility criteria, adverse events, the method of randomisation and the generalisability of findings.

However, even with perfect reporting, not all randomised trials are of equal quality (and, hence, equal reliability). The trial report may demonstrate that the randomisation sequence could have been subverted, but CONSORT is not a device for improving the design of trials; and a poorly designed trial may well lead to misleading results. There are many methods of assessing the quality of trials, from simple checklists to quality scores. Meta-analyses can then be performed with reference to these quality scores to determine whether the quality of the trial affects the result. A recent monograph (Moher et al., 1999) concluded that more research was needed in this area to determine the effect that trial quality, and different assessments of trial quality, have on systematic reviews and, ultimately, on evidence-based practice.

Conclusions

Without proper evidence, evidence-based practice is impossible. In assessing the effects of new treatments, it is impossible to overstate the importance of RCTs, and meta-analyses of such trials. However, randomisation alone is not enough. Trials need to be well designed, use appropriate endpoints and be properly analysed before their results can be fed into clinical practice. This chapter has identified important aspects of researching new treatments in cancer; and applying these guidelines, together with a healthy scepticism and one's innate common sense, should help produce better research and more reliable interpretations of research. It is often said that learning from one's mistakes is fruitful. It is also true that learning from others' mistakes is less painful, so critical reading of existing research is a very good way of starting to design one's own trial.

References

Altman, D. G. (1991). *Statistical Methods for Medical Research*, 2nd edn. London: Chapman and Hall.

Altman, D. G. (1994). The scandal of poor medical research. *Br. Med. J.*, **308**, 283–284.

Altman, D. and Bland, J. M. (1995). Absence of evidence is not evidence of absence. *Br. Med. J.*, **311**, 485.

Altman, D. and Bland, J. M. (1999). How to randomise. *Br. Med. J.*, **319**, 703–704.

Altman, D. and Bland, J. M. (2005). Treatment allocation by minimisation. *Br. Med. J.*, **330**, 843.

Altman, D. G., Machin, D., Bryant, T. N., *et al.* (2000). *Statistics with Confidence*. London: BMJ Books.

Assmann, S. F., Pocock, S., Enos, L. E., *et al.* (2000). Subgroup analysis and other (mis)uses of baseline data in clinical trials. *Lancet*, **355**, 1064–1069.

Burman, W. J., Reves, R. R., Cohn, D. L., *et al.* (2001). Breaking the camel's back: multicenter clinical trials and local institutional review boards. *Ann. Intern. Med.*, **134**, 152–157.

Burnett, A. K., Milligan, D. W., Prentice, A. G., *et al.* (2005). Modification or dose or treatment duration has no impact on outcome of AML in older patients: preliminary results of the UKNCRI AML14 trial. *Blood*, **106**(162A), Abstr. 543.

Burnett, A. K., Russell, N. H., Hills, R. K., *et al.* (2013). Optimization of chemotherapy for younger patients with acute myeloid leukaemia: results of the medical research council AML 15 trial. *J. Clin. Oncol.* **31**, 3360–3368.

Buyse, M., George, S. L., Evans, S., *et al.* (1999). The role of biostatistics in the prevention, detection and treatment of fraud in clinical trials. *Statist. Med.*, **18**, 3435–3451.

Cascinelli, N. (1994). Adjuvant interferon in melanoma – reply. *Lancet*, **343**, 1499 (letter).

Cascinelli, N., Bufalino, R., Morabito, A., *et al.* (1994). Results of adjuvant interferon study in WHO melanoma programme. *Lancet*, **343**, 913–914.

Collins, R., Peto, R., Gray, R., *et al.* (1996). Large-scale evidence: trials and overviews. In *Oxford Textbook of Medicine, Vol. 1*, ed. D. Weatherall, J. G. G. Ledingham and D. A. Warrell, 3rd edn. Oxford: Oxford University Press.

Creutzig, U., Ritter, J., Zimmermann, M., *et al.* (2001). Idarubicin improves blast cell clearance during induction therapy in children with AML: results of study AML-BFM 93. *Leukemia*, **15**, 348–354.

Cullen, M., Steven, N., Billingham, L., *et al.* (2005). Antibacterial prophylaxis after chemotherapy for solid tumors and lymphomas. *N. Engl. J. Med.*, **353**, 988–998.

Daniels, J., Gray, R., Hills, R. K, *et al.* (2009). Laparoscopic uterosacral nerve ablation for alleviating chronic pelvic pain: a randomized controlled trial. *J. Am. Med. Ass.*, **302**, 955–961.

Dickersin, K., Chan, S., Chalmers, T. C., *et al.* (1987). Publication bias and clinical trials. *Contr Clin Trials*, **8**, 343–353.

Duley, L. and Farrell, B. (2002). *Clinical Trials*. London: BMJ Books.

Early Breast Cancer Trialists Collaborative Group. (1990). *Treatment of Early Breast Cancer: Volume 1, Worldwide Evidence 1985–90*. Oxford: Oxford University Press.

Edwards, P., Roberts, I., Clarke, M., *et al.* (2002). Increasing response rates to postal questionnaires: systematic review. *Br. Med. J.*, **324**, 1183.

Ellenberg, S., Fleming, T. and DeMets, D. (2002). *Data Monitoring Committees in Clinical Trials: A Practical Perspective*. Chichester: Wiley.

Enserink, M. (1996). Clinical trials: fraud and ethics charges hit stroke drug trial. *Science*, **274**, 2004–2005.

Green, S. B. and Byar, D. P. (1984). Using observational data from registries to compare treatments – the fallacy of omnimetrics. *Stat. Med.*, **3**, 361–370.

Guyatt, G. H., Sackett, D. L., Sinclair, J. C., *et al.* (1995). Users' guides to the medical literature IX: A method for grading healthcare recommendations. *J. Am. Med. Ass.*, **274**, 1800–1804.

Hills, R. K. and Burnett, A K. (2011). Applicability of a "Pick a Winner" trial design to acute myeloid leukemia. *Blood*, **118**(9), 2389–2394.

Hills, R., Gray, R. and Wheatley, K. (2009). Balancing treatment allocations by clinician or center in randomized trials allows unacceptable levels of treatment prediction. *J. Evid. Based Med.*, **2**(3), 196–204.

Machin, D., Campbell, M. J., Fayers, P. M., *et al.* (1997). *Sample Size Tables for Clinical Research*, 2nd edn. Oxford: Blackwell.

Mehta, C. R. and Pocock, S. J. (2011). Adaptive increase in sample size when interim results are promising: a practical guide with examples. *Statist. Med.*, **30**, 3267–3284.

Miller, F. G. and Kaptchuk, T. J. (2004). Sham procedures and the ethics of clinical trials. *J. R. Soc. Med.*, **97**, 576–578.

Moher, D., Cook, D. J., Jadad, A. R., *et al.* (1999). Assessing the quality of reports of randomised trials: implications for the conduct of meta-analyses. *Health Technol. Assess.*, **3** 12), i–iv, 1–98.

Moher, D., Schulz, K. F. and Altman, D. G. for the CONSORT group. (2001). The CONSORT statement: revised recommendations for improving the quality of reports of parallel-group randomised trials. *Lancet*, **357**, 1191–1194.

Pocock, S. J. (1996). *Clinical Trials: A Practical Approach.* London: John Wiley and Sons.

QUASAR Collaborative Group. (2000). Comparison of fluorouracil with additional levamisole, higher-dose folinic acid, or both, as adjuvant chemotherapy for colorectal cancer: a randomised trial. *Lancet*, **355**, 1588–1596.

Royston, P., Parmar, M. K. and Qian, W. (2003). Novel designs for multi-arm clinical trials with survival outcomes with an application in ovarian cancer. *Stat. Med.*, **22**, 2239–2256.

Schulz, K. F. (1995). Subverting randomization in controlled trials. *J. Am. Med. Ass.*, **274**, 1456–1458.

Specht, L., Gray, R. G., Clarke, M. J., *et al.* for the International Hodgkins Disease Collaborative Group. (1998). Influence of more extensive radiotherapy and adjuvant chemotherapy on long-term outcome of early-stage Hodgkin's disease: a meta-analysis of 23 randomised trials involving 3,888 patients. *J. Clin. Oncol.*, **16**, 830–843.

Storer, B. E. (1989). Design and analysis of Phase I clinical trials. *Biometrics*, **45**, 925–937.

Storer, B. and DeMets, D. (1987). Current Phase I/II designs: are they adequate? *J. Clin. Res. Drug Devel.*, **1**, 121–130.

Swinscow, T. D. V. and Campbell, M. J. (2002). *Statistics at Square One.* London: BMJ Books.

Wheatley, K. (2002.) SAB: a promising new treatment for AML in the elderly? *Br. J. Haematol.*, **118**, 432–433.

Wheatley, K. and Hills, R. K. (2001). Inappropriate reporting and interpretation of subgroups in the AML-BFM 93 study. *Leukemia*, **15**, 1803–1804.

Yin, G., Li, Y. and Ji, Y. (2006). Bayesian dose-finding in phase I/II clinical trials using toxicity and efficacy odds ratios. *Biometrics*, **62**(3), 777–784.

Young, C. and Horton, R. (2005). Putting clinical trials into context. *Lancet*, **366**, 107–108.

Yusuf, S., Collins, R. and Peto, R. (1984). Why do we need some large, simple randomized trials? *Stat. Med.*, **3**, 409–422.

Further reading

There are many excellent books and articles on different aspects of clinical trials, notably those by Altman (1991), Assmann *et al.* (2000), Collins *et al.* (1996), Duley and Farrell (2002) and Yusuf *et al.* (1984). Additionally, the following references are valuable resources.

Chalmers, I. (1993). The Cochrane Collaboration: preparing, maintaining and disseminating systematic reviews of the effects of health care. *Ann. N. Y. Acad. Sci.*, **703**, 156–163.

The DAMOCLES Study Group. (2005). A proposed charter for clinical trial data monitoring committees: helping them do their job well. *Lancet*, **365**, 711–722.

Greenhalgh, T. (2006). *How to Read a Paper*, 3rd edn. Oxford: Blackwell.

Peto, R. (1987). Why do we need systematic overviews of randomized trials? *Stat. Med.*, **6**, 233–244.

Peto, R., Pike, M. C., Armitage, P., *et al.* (1976). Design and analysis of randomized clinical trials requiring prolonged observation of each patient. Part I: introduction and design. *Br. J. Cancer*, **34**, 585–612.

Peto, R., Pike, M. C., Armitage, P., *et al.* (1977). Design and analysis of randomized clinical trials requiring prolonged observation of each patient. Part II: analysis and examples. *Br. J. Cancer*, **35**, 1–39.

Acute oncology 1: oncological emergencies

Betsan Mai Thomas and Paul Shaw

Introduction

An oncological emergency is an acute medical problem related to cancer or its treatment which may result in serious morbidity or mortality if not treated quickly. It may be secondary to a structural/obstructive, metabolic or treatment-related complication (Cervantes and Chirivella, 2004). The emergency may be the first manifestation of malignant disease, particularly for superior vena cava obstruction (SVCO) and malignant spinal cord compression (MSCC).

Around 20–30% of all cancer patients suffer from hypercalcaemia. Spinal cord compression is the commonest neurological complication of cancer, occurring in approximately 5–10% of all cancer patients. Thrombotic events are the second leading cause of death in cancer patients after death from cancer itself.

Types of emergency

Metabolic emergencies include:

- hypercalcaemia,
- syndrome of inappropriate antidiuretic hormone (SIADH).

Structural/obstructive emergencies include:

- MSCC and cauda equina compression,
- SVCO,
- raised intracranial pressure,
- acute airway obstruction,
- bleeding,
- urinary obstruction,
- cardiac tamponade,
- pain: this has been named the 'fifth vital sign' following pulse, blood pressure, temperature and respiration; when pain is present it should evoke an immediate response. Treatment of pain is considered in Chapter 10.
- thromboembolic disease.

Treatment-related emergencies include:

- neutropenic fever/sepsis,
- anaphylaxis related to a chemotherapeutic agent,
- tumour lysis syndrome,
- extravasation of a chemotherapeutic agent.

Treatment overview

As with any acute medical emergency, resuscitation measures may be needed to ensure that airway, breathing and circulation are maintained. Adequate hydration, oxygen and monitoring of fluid balance are particularly important in patients with sepsis or tumour lysis syndrome. Steroids are used in patients with SVCO and suspected spinal cord compression, although the evidence base supporting their use is poor. Mannitol infusions may be needed for severe symptomatic raised intracranial pressure that does not respond to steroids. Pain, breathlessness and distress should be treated as priorities, especially in patients presenting with end-stage cancer and an oncological emergency. The WHO pain ladder is a suitable framework to guide appropriate analgesic use. Some seriously ill patients may need to be transferred to a high-dependency unit (HDU) or intensive therapy unit (ITU), especially those with a treatable malignancy and a good prognosis and those who develop complications of curative chemotherapy. Liaison with specialist colleagues at an early stage is recommended.

An oncological emergency, like any other emergency, requires prompt assessment and action by appropriately experienced staff. Sometimes the emergency situation may be predictable, in which case a previously agreed plan of action will be helpful. Thought must be given to the appropriateness and value of investigations and treatment, because some patients will be in the terminal

Practical Clinical Oncology, Second Edition, ed. Louise Hanna, Tom Crosby and Fergus Macbeth. Published by Cambridge University Press. © Cambridge University Press 2015.

phase with progressive and treatment-refractory disease. End-of-life care should be instituted rapidly as a priority to relieve unnecessary distress.

Metabolic emergencies

Hypercalcaemia

Definition

Hypercalcaemia occurs when corrected calcium is greater than 2.6 mmol/L. Hypercalcaemia of malignancy is the commonest cause of hypercalcaemia in inpatients. In patients with osteolytic metastases, hypercalcaemia is primarily due to increased bone resorption and release of calcium from bone. In patients without bone metastases, hypercalcaemia is secondary to circulating factors such as parathyroid hormone-related peptide (PTH-RP) or 1,25-dihydroxyvitamin D (calcitriol). However, it is important also to remember that patients with cancer may also have incidental primary hyperparathyroidism (Stewart, 2005). Hypercalcaemia of malignancy carries a poor prognosis.

Presentation

Hypercalcaemia occurs in 20–30% of patients with advanced solid tumours. Symptoms are fatigue, anorexia, nausea, vomiting, abdominal pain/constipation, polyuria, polydipsia and confusion. If left untreated it leads to somnolence, coma and death.

Investigations

Serum-corrected calcium level, electrolytes, renal biochemistry, phosphate and magnesium levels and PTH. An ECG may show increased PR interval or widened QRS.

Treatment if corrected calcium is less than 3.0 mmol/L

Asymptomatic patients with a corrected calcium of less than 3.0 mmol/L who are about to have chemotherapy or radiotherapy should be rehydrated, kept mobile and monitored regularly. Patients who are symptomatic or who are expected to have a slow response to anti-cancer treatment should be treated as follows.

Treatment if corrected calcium is greater than or equal to 3.0 mmol/L or patient is symptomatic

Fluid replacement:

- Give at least 3 L NaCl 0.9% in 24 hours. Correct hypokalaemia and hypomagnaesia if present. Be

careful to watch for fluid overload if the patient has evidence of cardiac or renal failure. Aim for a urine output of 100–150 mL/h.
- Stop thiazide diuretics.
- Furosemide does increase calcium excretion but should not be given until dehydration has been treated.

Bisphosphonates:

Bisphosphonates inhibit calcium release by interfering with osteoclast-mediated bone resorption.

- Zoledronic acid has a fast onset and a long duration of action. Ensure adequate hydration, and then give a dose of 4 mg in at least 50 mL of either NaCl 0.9% or glucose 5% over 15 minutes.
- Monitor renal function and serum calcium, phosphate and potassium. Be careful if there is known renal impairment, which may require a reduced dose or slower infusion rate.
- The side effects of bisphosphonates include gastrointestinal upset, flu-like symptoms and exacerbation of metastatic bone pain. Osteonecrosis of the mandible can occur after chronic use.
- Hypocalcaemia occurs in 50% of patients, but it rarely causes symptoms because of a compensatory increase in PTH levels secondary to the decreased calcium levels.

Other drugs used less frequently for hypercalcaemia include the following.

- Calcitonin increases renal calcium excretion and decreases bone resorption. Salcatonin has a very rapid onset and may be used in patients with dangerously high serum calcium levels, regardless of fluid status. Tachyphylaxis develops, so the effectiveness of salcatonin is limited.
- Gallium nitrate inhibits osteosclastic bone resorption and inhibits PTH secretion.
- Mithramycin.
- Consider dialysis in patients with severe hypercalcaemia if the prognosis is good but adequate hydration cannot be administered because of cardiac or renal failure.

Syndrome of inappropriate antidiuretic hormone (SIADH)

SIADH is caused by excess levels of antidiuretic hormone (ADH), normally secondary to ectopic hormone production from the tumour. SIADH will lead to failure to excrete dilute urine, and so water retention and low serum sodium levels occur. It is most commonly associated with small-cell lung cancer (SCLC). It occasionally occurs in a wide variety of other cancers and can also be caused by chest infections, hypothyroidism and drugs such as antidepressants, anticholinesterase (ACE) inhibitors, cyclophosphamide and cisplatin.

Presentation

Hyponatremia is commonly defined as a serum sodium concentration below 135 mmol/L. Patients are often asymptomatic but may experience fatigue, lethargy, nausea, anorexia, muscle cramps, depression and behavioural changes; it may also be an incidental finding. The presence of symptoms will depend on the speed of onset and the severity of the hyponatremia. If the serum sodium is less than 110 mmol/L, somnolence, depressed deep tendon reflexes, pseudobulbar palsy, seizure, coma and death may occur.

Investigation

In patients with normal blood volume, hyponatremia and reduced plasma osmolarity (< 270 mmol/kg) in the presence of inappropriately concentrated urine (urine osmolarity > 100 mmol/kg) is diagnostic of SIADH (Bartter and Schwartz, 1967). Urinary sodium will be high. Renal failure, hypothyroidism and adrenal insufficiency are excluded by checking biochemistry, thyroid function tests and a short synacthen test.

Treatment

- Fluid restriction to 0.5–1 L/day usually results in symptomatic and biochemical improvement.
- Demeclocycline (600–1200 mg/day) should be given if the patient does not respond to fluid restriction alone. Demeclocycline causes a nephrogenic form of diabetes insipidus, thereby decreasing urine concentration. Treatment must be continued for several days to achieve maximal diuretic effects and renal function will need to be monitored.
- The underlying malignancy should be treated to reverse the cause of electrolyte imbalance.
- In an emergency situation, such as altered consciousness or fitting, cautious administration of intravenous 1.8% NaCl may be considered. However, a rapid rise in sodium may cause osmotic demyelination syndrome and therefore the infusion should be reduced or stopped as soon as the patient's neurological condition improves or a safe level of plasma sodium is reached (> 120 mmol/L). Serum sodium levels must be carefully monitored at frequent intervals (2–4 hourly) during infusion of hypertonic saline.
- Tolvaptan, a selective vasopressin V2 receptor antagonist, has been licensed in the UK since 2009 for the treatment of adults with hyponatremia secondary to SIADH (15–60 mg daily). Therapeutic effects are mediated through increased loss of free water without altering sodium excretion. Serum sodium should be closely monitored, especially with levels below 120 mmol/L at baseline, as rapid elevation of sodium has led to reports of demyelination syndromes.

Structural/obstructive emergencies

Malignant spinal cord and cauda equina compression

This condition is caused by pressure from a tumour (growing directly between vertebral bodies or growing from bone metastases) or a collapsed vertebral body on the spinal cord or cauda equina. This may then cause paraparesis, or paraplegia, loss of sensation and bladder or bowel dysfunction. It is particularly associated with breast cancer, lung cancer, prostate cancer and multiple myeloma. Patients at increased risk of developing bone metastases or patients with diagnosed bone metastases should be informed about the symptoms of metastatic cord compression (NICE, 2008).

Presentation

Symptoms and signs will depend on the level of compression. Because the spinal cord ends at about the L1 level, compression above this point will give an upper motor neurone pattern of weakness and below this point, a lower motor neurone pattern. Muscle weakness often occurs before sensory loss or autonomic dysfunction (impotence, urinary or faecal incontinence or retention). Approximately 60% of patients will have pain, which may be radicular. Asymptomatic cord compression is estimated to occur in one-third of patients with prostate cancer and bone metastases (Bayley et al., 2001).

Investigation

NICE guidance recommends performing an MRI of the whole spine within 24 hours of presentation to detect the level of compression (NICE, 2008). Multiple levels of compression may be found. Intravenous contrast improves the detection of intradural and intramedullary tumours.

In patients who have not been previously diagnosed with cancer it is important to establish a tissue diagnosis if possible (e.g. by needle biopsy or during surgical decompression).

Initial treatment

Initial treatment includes the following.

- Give dexamethasone 16 mg (unless contraindicated) daily in divided doses with proton pump inhibitor protection, reducing the dose after a few days to avoid toxicity. If neurological function deteriorates at any time the dose should be reconsidered. Blood sugar levels should be monitored.
- Prescribe adequate analgesia.
- Consider thromboprophylaxis if mobility is reduced.
- Nurse the patient in the supine position if there is any possibility of spinal instability.
- Patients require a multidisciplinary team approach including specialist physiotherapy and nursing care.

Surgery

In selected patients with a single area of MSCC from a solid tumour, the benefit of immediate circumferential decompression of the spinal cord followed by 10×3 Gy fractions of radiotherapy has been shown to be superior to radiotherapy alone (Patchell *et al.*, 2005). This study was closed early after the accrual of 123 patients when the surgical arm was superior at interim analysis, with the percentage of patients retaining the ability to walk after surgery being greater than those receiving radiotherapy alone (84% versus 57%; $p = 0.001$). In addition, 10 out of 16 paraplegic patients gained the ability to walk following surgery as opposed to only 3 of 16 in the radiotherapy-only group. It is important that patients need to be carefully selected for this approach. In this study patients were included if they had a good performance status, predicted survival greater than 3 months and had not been paraplegic for more than 48 hours.

Table 8.1 A revised scoring system for pre-operative evaluation of metastatic spinal tumour progression

Tokuhashi scoring criteria	
General condition	
Poor	0 points
Moderate	1 point
Good	2 points
Number of extraspinal bone metastases	
≥ 3	0 points
1–2	1 point
1	2 points
Number of metastases in vertebral body	
≥ 3	0 points
2	1 point
1	2 points
Metastases to the major internal organs	
Inoperable	0 points
Operable	1 point
None	2 points
Primary site of cancer	
Lung, osteosarcoma, stomach, bladder, oesophagus, pancreas	0 points
Liver, gallbladder, unknown	1 point
Others	2 points
Kidneys, uterus	3 points
Rectum	4 points
Thyroid, breast, prostate, carcinoid tumour	5 points
Neurological deficit	
Complete paraplegia	0 points
Weakness	1 point
None	2 points.
Total score	**Prognosis**
0–8	85% of people will live less than 6 months
9–11	73% of people will live greater than 6 months, and 30% of people will live more than 1 year
12–15	95% of people will live more than 1 year

Adapted from Tokuhashi *et al.*, 2005.

The Tokuhashi scoring system as shown in Table 8.1 can be helpful in making a decision for spinal surgery. Spinal surgery should also be considered if there is a need to obtain histology, if there is spinal instability or if pain has not been controlled despite adequate analgesia (NICE, 2008).

Role of radiotherapy

Radiotherapy is the most commonly used treatment of MSCC. Patients should receive radiotherapy as soon as is practically possible after arrival in the oncology unit. Referrals occur most frequently on Friday afternoons, as confirmed by a retrospective review of 443 patients treated over 10 years (Poortmans et al., 2001). A radiotherapy technique is as follows.

- Patient preparation, positioning and immobilisation: patient lies prone or supine, with arms by the side. Polystyrene knee support and/or head support may be used.
- Localisation and target volume: simulator films are taken at the level of spinal cord compression. After cross-sectional imaging, the target volume includes the level of compression and one vertebral body above and below this level, usually ensuring that the inferior and superior limits cross an intervertebral space. Typically, the field borders are defined at the time of simulation. The centre of the field is in the midline along the spinous processes and is usually 8 cm wide.
- Plan: a single posterior field is used most often. However, upper cervical cord compression can be treated using opposed lateral fields to avoid having the exit beam pass through the throat and mouth. A typical field length for a posterior treatment field would be 10–15 cm.
- Dose, fractionation and energy: for patients with metastatic disease, typical doses include 20 Gy in 5 daily fractions or 30 Gy in 10 daily fractions given as either an applied dose or prescribed at the depth of the spinal cord (which is determined using the MRI scan) using 6 MV photons. A single fraction of 8 Gy may be appropriate for a patient with poor prognosis and established neurological deficit (see below). If opposed lateral beams are used then the same dose may be given, but it is prescribed to the ICRU reference point (centre of the intersecting beams). For patients with primary tumours, such as solitary plasmacytoma of bone, a higher dose may be required with the aim of achieving a cure.

Areas of current interest

There is no standard fractionation schedule. The SCORAD trial is a randomised phase III trial of single fraction radiotherapy compared to multi-fraction radiotherapy in patients with metastatic spinal cord compression. Patients are randomised to receive either 20 Gy over 5 fractions or 8 Gy in a single fraction. The results of this trial are awaited.

A recent retrospective study of radiotherapy dose has compared 8 Gy in a single fraction, 20 Gy in 5 fractions over 1 week, 30 Gy in 10 fractions over 2 weeks, and 40 Gy in 20 fractions over 4 weeks in patients with non-small-cell lung cancer (NSCLC; Rades et al., 2006). The functional outcome was equivalent for short-course regimens (8 and 20 Gy) and for long-course treatment, and the authors concluded that 8 Gy in a single fraction is an appropriate dose in patients with NSCLC who generally have a poor prognosis. The outcome was related to the length of time over which the motor deficit developed before radiotherapy, with more than 14 days being better than a shorter time interval. Overall there was an improvement in motor function in 14% of patients, no change in 54%, and deterioration in 32%.

Superior vena cava obstruction

SVCO is caused by compression, invasion of or, occasionally, intraluminal thrombus in the superior vena cava (SVC). It is most often associated with carcinoma of the bronchus (75%) and lymphomas (15%). Thymoma and germ cell cancer are rarer causes.

Presentation

The onset is typically insidious over weeks and results in the development of compensatory collateral venous channels in the territory of the SVC. The symptoms are worse on bending forwards and they include neck and face swelling, conjunctival suffusion, headache, nasal congestion, epistaxis, dizziness and syncope. Examination reveals a non-pulsatile raised jugulo-venous pressure, venous collaterals, arm oedema and plethora. Occasionally sudden occlusion occurs and the patient becomes acutely unwell.

Investigation

SVCO is rarely an acute emergency, unless there is associated airway obstruction and stridor, and so there is usually time for further investigation aimed at making a histological diagnosis (Ostler *et al.*, 1997). A chest X-ray often shows a widened mediastinum. A CT scan will give information about both the site and the cause of the obstruction, by distinguishing external compression from intravascular thrombosis. It can also give staging information about the underlying tumour. An attempt should be made to establish a histological diagnosis before starting treatment, either by CT-guided fine-needle aspiration or biopsy or by bronchoscopy, sputum cytology or biopsy of enlarged neck nodes. Sometimes mediastinoscopy or thoracoscopy may be required (Ostler *et al.*, 1997).

Treatment

Treatment includes the following.

- Initial management: sit the patient up, giving oxygen as required and steroids (e.g. dexamethasone 12–16 mg daily in divided doses), with proton pump inhibitor protection.
- Give oxygen if required.
- A superior vena caval stent can be a useful holding measure in patients who require urgent symptom relief, and this will often allow time to establish a tissue diagnosis.
- Thrombosis should be appropriately treated if present.
- Treat the underlying tumour as appropriate. Chemotherapy is indicated for patients with chemosensitive tumours such as lymphoma, germ cell tumour or SCLC. Radiotherapy is the mainstay of treatment for patients with other solid tumours.

A Cochrane systematic review concluded that chemotherapy and radiotherapy were equally effective at relieving SVCO secondary to lung cancer, whereas stent insertion provided higher rates of response more rapidly (Rowell and Gleeson, 2001). It seems appropriate that highly responsive tumours (NHL, HL, SCLC) should be treated with chemotherapy first, whereas patients with NSCLC and severe SVCO should be offered a stent first.

A radiotherapy technique is as follows.

- Patient preparation, positioning and immobilisation: the patient lies supine, with a headrest and arms by the side. If the patient is unable to lie flat, the sitting position can be used, with arms by the side.
- Localisation and target volume: simulated treatment fields or, where available, CT planning is used with the target volume to cover the SVC, tumour and mediastinum.
- Dose, energy and fractionation: short palliative fractionation regimens may be used (e.g. 10 Gy in single fraction or 16 Gy in 2 fractions) if the patient's performance status and prognosis are poor and if the field size is limited to 12×12 cm. This may result in quick symptom relief with minimal visits to the radiotherapy department. Patients with localised disease and better performance status may benefit from a higher dose (e.g. 36 Gy in 12 fractions over 2.5 weeks) in the hope that the tumour and symptomatic control will be prolonged. Occasionally radiotherapy may be given with radical intent in appropriately selected patients such as those with NSCLC whose disease can be encompassed in a radical volume (as described in Chapter 31).

Raised intracranial pressure

Raised intracranial pressure (ICP) results from the space-occupying effect of intracranial tumours, which are most often metastatic. Other possible causes of raised ICP in malignancy include intracranial haemorrhage, cerebral oedema following intracranial surgery or radiotherapy, venous sinus thrombosis or intracranial infection in an immunosupressed patient.

Presentation

Patients present with headache, nausea, vomiting, visual disturbance, seizure, ataxia and changes in personality and behaviour. Clinical findings may include visual field loss, loss of spontaneous retinal venous pulsations, papilloedema and sixth cranial nerve palsy. There may be a reduced consciousness level. The Cushing's response (bradycardia and hypertension) is a pre-terminal sign due to impending herniation of the brainstem. Herniation of the cerebral peduncle can result in hemiplegia. Focal signs may present depending on the site of the tumour.

Investigation

A CT scan of the brain will detect most brain metastases. MRI has a greater sensitivity for detecting small metastases, meningeal disease and fourth ventricle obstruction. In most patients who have not been previously diagnosed with cancer, efforts should be made to obtain a histological diagnosis, especially if there is a single brain tumour. Such cases should be discussed with the neurosurgical team. A biopsy might not be appropriate in frail patients who have multiple cerebral metastases and other possible sites of metastatic disease.

Treatment

Treatment is as follows.

- Assess and manage airway, breathing and circulation. Provide high-flow oxygen.
- Document the Glasgow Coma Score (GCS) initially and reassess regularly.
- Give dexamethasone 12–16 mg daily in divided doses with proton pump inhibitor cover.
- If severe (rapidly falling GCS or moribund state), give mannitol 0.5–1 g/kg i.v. over 15 minutes.
- Avoid fluid overload.
- Provide analgesia for headache (paracetamol with or without NSAID or stronger analgesia as documented in WHO pain ladder).
- Prescribe antibiotics ± antivirals ± antifungals if any suspicion of infection.
- Request platelets for transfusion if there is a possibility of thrombocytopenia.
- Ensure i.v. maintenance fluids are not hypotonic, i.e. use 0.9% NaCl initially.
- For specific anti-cancer treatment, if three or fewer brain metastases are found, consider seeking a neurosurgical opinion. Stereotactic radiotherapy may also be considered. If there are multiple metastases, patients who are most likely to benefit from whole-brain radiotherapy are those who are mobile and have had a good symptomatic benefit from steroids. A randomised controlled trial has shown that 12 Gy in 2 fractions on consecutive days is not inferior to 30 Gy in 10 fractions over 2 weeks in patients with symptomatic cerebral metastases and poor performance status who need treatment (Priestman *et al.*, 1996).

Special case: obstructive hydrocephalus

Patients presenting *de novo* with tumours causing obstruction to the flow of cerebrospinal fluid and resulting in obstructive hydrocephalus should be considered for neurosurgical intervention. Immediate resuscitation with mannitol and steroids should be started.

Acute airway obstruction

Acute airway obstruction is blockage of the main-stem bronchi, carina, trachea or larynx and is commonly caused by direct tumour extension from lung cancer or head and neck cancer.

Presentation

The patient presents with dyspnoea and stridor.

Investigation

Patients with upper airway obstruction should have direct visualisation, laryngoscopy, bronchoscopy, nasendoscopy or mediastinoscopy according to the level of obstruction. Clinical clues as to the level of obstruction include the presence of neck swelling and stridor with upper obstruction or monophonic wheeze (on auscultation) with lower airway obstruction. Chest X-ray or CT scan of neck and thorax or both should be considered. Check full blood count (FBC) because anaemia may exacerbate the dyspnoea.

Treatment

Treatment is as follows.

- Heliox (79% He, 21% O2) contains helium, which has a lower density and therefore lower specific gravity than oxygen, nitrogen or air. As a result, during turbulent flow, the flow velocity will be higher when heliox is used. This reduces the work required to breathe when the upper airway is obstructed.
- Consider high-dose steroids (with gastroprotection) although there is no good evidence of its effectiveness.
- Give nebulised bronchodilators if there is any evidence of bronchospasm.
- If the upper airway is severely compromised, emergency tracheostomy or endotracheal intubation may be required.
- Specific interventions should aim to diagnose and treat the obstruction.

Interventional bronchoscopy

For the majority of patients, external beam radiotherapy is all that is required. However, Table 8.2 shows the options available (adapted from Freitag, 2004), which can be combined with chemotherapy and/or

Table 8.2 Endobronchial intervention in lung cancer

Lung pathology	Endoscopic intervention
Bleeding from central airway tumour	Argon plasma coagulator
Intraluminal tumour	Nd-YAG laser
	Electrocautery
	Argon plasma coagulator
	Cryotherapy
	Photo-dynamic therapy
Intramural tumour	HDR endobronchial brachytherapy (^{192}Ir)
Extrinsic compression/ airway wall destruction	Airway stent

Adapted from Freitag (2004).

radiotherapy. These endobronchial treatments have been reviewed by Morris *et al.* (2002), who concluded that 'good to excellent short term palliation' may be achieved.

External beam radiotherapy

Patients are usually treated with 20 Gy in 5 fractions to reduce the chance of larger single fractions increasing oedema.

Bleeding

Bleeding is more likely to occur in patients treated with anticoagulants.

Examples

Massive haemoptysis is most commonly associated with lung cancer, but can also occur in patients with endobronchial metastases from carcinoid, breast, kidney, sarcoma and colon cancers. It is defined as expectoration of more than 100 mL of blood in a single episode during 24–48 hours. It may be associated with respiratory difficulty and can lead to rapid deterioration with airway obstruction, anaemia and hypovolaemic shock. It may also be associated with coagulation disorder, thrombocytopenia or fungal infection.

In haematemesis, approximately 2–5% of upper GI bleeding is related to malignancy. Even in patients with cancer, haematemesis may be caused by benign disease (peptic ulcer disease, oesophagitis, gastritis, duodenitis). Mallory–Weiss tears may be secondary to vomiting induced by chemotherapy, renal failure or advanced malignancy (Palmer, 2004). With the move from surgical treatment towards chemotherapy with or without radiotherapy for the treatment of primary gastric lymphoma (the commonest extranodal site of NHL), the incidence of GI haemorrhage is estimated at 5% (Maisey *et al.*, 2004). Oesophagogastric tumours rarely present with acute GI haemorrhage.

The Rockall score is a risk assessment tool for GI haemorrhage (Rockall *et al.*, 1996: see Table 8.3). Patients with a Rockall score of 6 or more have a predicted mortality of around 50%. Multivariate analysis identifies shock, age, comorbidity and specific endoscopic findings as independent variables predicting re-bleeding and death (Palmer, 2004).

Haematuria may occur with malignant tumours involving the genitourinary tract, but it occurs most commonly in renal, bladder and prostate cancer. Patients may present with asymptomatic haematuria, associated symptoms related to the underlying cancer, or severe pain caused by clot retention.

Assessment and investigation

Secure the airway, breathing, and circulation first. Then:

- perform a full blood count, clotting screen and renal and liver profile;
- perform a CT scan or endoscopy (e.g. bronchoscopy, upper or lower GI endoscopy, cystoscopy) to establish diagnosis and identify the site of bleeding. These tests also provide prognostic information in the case of upper GI bleeding to direct the appropriate level of care (Palmer, 2004);
- perform a urine or sputum microscopy and culture as appropriate.

Treatment

For patients who require active resuscitation/ intervention:

- secure airway, breathing and circulation;
- use fluid resuscitation with 0.9% NaCl or colloid to restore blood pressure and urine output, which can be monitored by measuring the central venous pressure (CVP);
- patients with haemoglobin below 100 g/L should receive a blood transfusion;

Table 8.3 The Rockall scoring system

Variable	Score 0	Score 1	Score 2	Score 3
Age (years)	< 60	60–79	≥ 80	–
Shock	None	Pulse > 100 bpm, normal BP	Pulse > 100 bpm, systolic BP < 100 mmHg	–
Comorbidity	None	–	Cardiac failure, ischaemic heart disease, other major co-morbidity	Renal failure, liver failure, disseminated malignancy
Diagnosis	Mallory–Weiss tear, no lesion seen, no SRH	All other diagnoses	Malignancy of upper GI tract	–
Major SRH	None	–	Blood in upper GI tract, adherent blood clot, visible or spurting vessel	–

BP, blood pressure; bpm, beats per minute; SRH, stigmata of recent haemorrhage. Three clinical variables (age, shock and comorbidity) and two endoscopic variables (diagnosis and major SRH) are each categorised as shown in the table. A score of 0 to 3 points is awarded for each category, giving a maximum total score of 11. Patients with a Rockall score of 6 or more have a predicted mortality of around 50%. Adapted from Rockall *et al.* (1996).

- recognise and treat underlying renal impairment, and cardiovascular or cerebrovascular disease, because comorbid conditions can decompensate in the presence of acute haemorrhage;
- consider tranexamic acid (with caution in haematuria because of the risk of clot retention) or specific measures for a bleeding disorder (e.g. platelet transfusion, vitamin K, fresh frozen plasma);
- actively bleeding and shocked patients should be managed in a high-dependency unit, assuming this is appropriate for the individual patient.

Site-specific interventions include the following.

- Haemoptysis – bronchoscopy/radiotherapy as discussed earlier.
- Haematemesis options:
  drug therapy (e.g. proton pump inhibitors, somatostatin);
  endoscopic therapy (e.g. direct injection of adrenaline into bleeding ulcers, effective in 90%), fibrin glue and human thrombin (Palmer, 2004) and heat and mechanical devices;
  radiotherapy to the tumour bed, single fraction of 8 Gy or 20 Gy in 5 fractions over 1 week.
- Haematuria options:
  radiotherapy to the prostate or bladder with a single fraction of 8 Gy (or a planned volume for radical treatment);
  cystoscopy with electrocautery/laser;
  renal artery embolism for renal tumours bleeding into the urogenital tract.

For patients in the terminal phase of advanced malignancy who experience massive and uncontrollable bleeding such as carotid blow-out or massive haemoptysis, intravenous midazolam and diamorphine provides rapid sedation and palliation.

Urinary obstruction

This is associated with urological or gynaecological tumours, especially carcinoma of prostate or cervix. Recurrent rectal cancer or pelvic metastases may result in bilateral ureteric dilatation and hydronephrosis. Constipation is a reversible cause.

Presentation

The patient may be asymptomatic or present with flank pain, anuria and raised creatinine. Partial obstruction may present with alternating polyuria and oliguria. Urinary tract infection may occur because of the obstruction.

Investigation

A renal tract ultrasound may show bilateral hydronephrosis. A CT scan of the pelvis can be used to identify the site and the cause of obstruction, especially a retroperitoneal or pelvic mass.

Treatment

Renal failure should be managed by correcting life-threatening electrolyte abnormalities. Bladder outflow obstruction will be relieved by insertion of a urethral or suprapubic catheter. If the obstruction is secondary to ureteric compression, the decision whether to place stents should take into account the patient's performance status, stage of disease, and chance of response to anti-cancer treatment. Ureteric stents may be placed under local anaesthetic or, if this is not feasible, by percutaneous nephrostomy. Pain and urinary tract infection should be treated. Consider haemofiltration or dialysis if the patient has severe uraemia or if hyperkalaemia has not responded to treatment, depending on the patient's performance status and prognosis.

Cardiac tamponade

Increased intrapericardial pressure results from excess pericardial fluid, which reduces cardiac filling and leads to impaired blood circulation. Cardiac tamponade is most commonly associated with a malignant pericardial effusion from lung cancer, ovarian cancer and primary cardiac tumours.

Presentation

Two-thirds of patients are asymptomatic. Symptoms include breathlessness, chest pain, orthopnoea and weakness. There are signs of haemodynamic compromise – raised jugulo-venous pressure (JVP), tachycardia, hypotension, increased pulsus paradoxus and oedema.

Investigation

Two-dimensional echocardiography should be used to diagnose the effusion, assess the haemodynamic impact and assist with obtaining fluid for cytological examination.

Treatment

- Oxygen therapy.
- Volume expansion with blood, plasma or isotonic sodium chloride solution, as necessary, to maintain adequate intravascular volume.
- Pericardiocentesis under ultrasound guidance.

- A surgical pericardial window should be created if fluid re-accumulates.
- In patients for whom a pericardial window is not thought suitable, radiotherapy to the pericardium could be considered: 30 Gy in 10 fractions over 2 weeks.

Thromboembolic disease

The pro-coagulant activity of tumour cells and treatments such as chemotherapy and surgery increase the risk of thromboembolism. If renal function is adequate, treatment with low molecular weight heparin (LMWH) should be administered for at least three to six months provided there are no significant complications. LMWH reduces the rate of recurrent VTE compared with warfarin for longer term anticoagulation in patients with cancer (Lee *et al.*, 2003). The placement of a vena cava filter may be considered in patients with recurrent VTE when anticoagulation has been optimised or is associated with bleeding complications (Farge *et al.*, 2013).

Treatment-related emergencies

Neutropenic sepsis

Neutropenic sepsis may occur after almost any chemotherapy regimen, but is mainly associated with cancers that have been treated with intensive myelosuppressive regimens (e.g. lymphoma or leukaemia). Neutropenia with sepsis or severe sepsis is a very serious problem and needs to be managed as an acute emergency.

The risk factors for developing neutropenic sepsis include age (greater than 65 yrs), poor performance status, previous episodes of febrile neutropenia, combined chemotherapy and radiotherapy, poor nutrition, advanced disease, comorbidities and open wounds or active infections.

The prevention and management of neutropenic sepsis in cancer patients is outlined in NICE clinical guideline 151 (NICE, 2012).

Patient education

Patient education is essential, and should be provided in oral and written form. Patients receiving chemotherapy should be advised of the importance of recognising infective symptoms and how to monitor their temperature. They should inform the cancer centre immediately if they develop signs of an infection or have a temperature of > 37.5°C.

Table 8.4 The MASCC scoring system

Characteristic	Score
No hypotension	5
Symptoms related to this infective neutropenic episode	3 for moderate symptoms 5 for severe symptoms
No chronic obstructive pulmonary disease	4
Solid tumour or no previous fungal infection	4
No dehydration	3
Outpatient status	3
Age < 60 yrs	2

Note: The variable 'burden of illness' is a subjective assessment of the degree of symptoms experienced by the patient. Points attributed to 'burden of illness' are not cumulative. The maximum theoretical score is therefore 26. Adapted from Klastersky *et al.* (2000).

Presentation

Patients usually present with a raised temperature, a history of recent cytotoxic chemotherapy and a low neutrophil cell count. Sepsis-induced vasodilation and hypotension can rapidly cause end-organ (renal, hepatic, cerebral) damage that can be fatal.

NICE recommends diagnosing neutropenic sepsis in patients having anti-cancer treatment whose neutrophil count is 0.5×10^9/L or lower and who have either a temperature higher than 38°C or other signs or symptoms consistent with clinically significant sepsis.

Risk of complications

Patients with neutropenic sepsis can be stratified into those with a low or high risk of serious complications according to their MASCC score (Multinational Association for Supportive Care in Cancer; Klastersky *et al.*, 2000). Age (over 60 yrs), evidence of dehydration, hypotension, coexisting chronic obstructive pulmonary disease (COPD), haematological malignancies with previous fungal infections, moderate to severe symptoms or current in-patient status at time of febrile neutropenia are all considered to be risk factors for developing serious complications. A well, low-risk patient such as with a MASCC score of ≥ 21 can be considered for early discharge on oral antibiotics provided they are supported at home, have a telephone, are registered with a GP and live near a hospital (see below). Table 8.4 shows the MASCC

scoring system. Patients who have signs of sepsis but whose neutrophil count lies outside of the NICE criteria may also be at risk of complications of sepsis or a falling neutrophil count and should be treated according to local antimicrobial policies.

Initial assessment and treatment

All patients suspected of having neutropenic sepsis should be assessed promptly, to allow the administration of intravenous antibiotics within one hour. Whenever possible, patients should be assessed within a cubicle. A full history and examination should be undertaken and patients should have 15-minute observations initially. Investigations should include FBC, urea and electrolytes (U+E), liver function tests (LFT), bone profile, coagulation screen, c-reactive protein (CRP), blood cultures (from lines and peripherally), blood sugar, lactate and an MSU (mid-stream urine). If indicated, sputum samples, stool samples, wound swab ± chest X-ray (CXR) should be requested.

Signs of sepsis include a temperature of < 36°C or >38°C, tachycardia, tachypnoea, an altered mental state, hyperglycaemia (in the absence of diabetes) or a white cell count (WCC) >12 or $< 4 \times 10^9$/L.

Identify any patients with severe sepsis or septic shock immediately. Septic shock is sepsis with hypotension, despite adequate fluid resuscitation. It is often accompanied by perfusion abnormalities that may include lactic acidosis, oliguria or an acute alteration in mental state. Hypotension is a systolic blood pressure of less than 90 mmHg or a reduction of greater than 40 mmHg from baseline in the absence of other causes. Patients may develop clotting disorders or become thrombocytopenic and they need prompt resuscitation, possibly including transfer to ITU/HDU. Timely contact with intensive care specialists may help decide whether they need intensive organ support.

Initial management of septic shock

Immediate measures include the following.

- Intravenous access with medium- to wide-bore cannula.
- Start 1 L 0.9% NaCl or 500 mL colloid over 30 minutes.
- If there is evidence of hypoxia, give oxygen (24% if COPD or previous bleomycin).
- Investigate serum lactate, FBC, U+E, creatinine and LFTs, clotting, glucose, line cultures, blood cultures, blood gases and MSU.

- Give intravenous antibiotics according to local hospital policy within 1 hour.
- Record vital signs every 15 minutes.
- Request a CXR if signs suggest a chest infection.
- If serum lactate is greater than 4 mmol/L consider transfer to ITU/HDU.

After 30 minutes, if the patient is still hypotensive, start 1 L 0.9% NaCl or colloid over 1 hour (but use caution if there is a history of cardiac disease) and consider transfer to ITU/HDU. If there is evidence of renal impairment, monitor urine output via indwelling catheter.

After 1 hour, urine output should be 0.5–1 mL/kg per hour. If it remains below this level, consider transfer to ITU.

Management of neutropenic sepsis

Patients may be categorised as being high-risk or low-risk of septic complications to determine the most appropriate management.

Always follow the local hospital policy

For high-risk patients intravenous antibiotics should be given within one hour according to the local protocol. For patients without an allergy to penicillin, start with a first line agent such as meropenem 1 g i.v. t.d.s. For patients with a penicillin allergy, use vancomycin 1 g b.d. and gentamicin 6 mg/kg i.v. o.d. For those with specific localising signs, additional antibiotics may be added; for example, clarithromycin for chest infection. It is important to follow local guidelines and consult the bacteriologist. If the fever settles within 48–72 hours, the intravenous antibiotics should be continued for an additional 24 hours. Oral antibiotics are then given for 5 days, similar to the low-risk protocol. If the fever persists beyond 48–72 hours, advice should be sought from the microbiologist.

If patients have a proven intravenous line infection, are very unwell and have a central or peripheral line *in situ*, or are known to be colonised with MRSA, consider adding vancomycin. Consider removing the catheter, and contact the microbiology department to discuss test results and possible antifungal therapy. If a pathogen has not been isolated, additional cultures and serology are needed, along with a CT scan of the chest and broncho-alveolar lavage. The use of amphotericin B or antiviral agents or non-infectious causes of fever should also be considered.

Low-risk patients who are well with a neutrophil count greater than 0.5×10^9/L should be treated with oral antibiotics according to hospital guidelines and can be considered for early discharge. Ideally these patients should not live alone, have a telephone, live less than 30 minutes away from a hospital and be registered with a GP.

Low-risk patients with a neutrophil count less than 0.5×10^9/L should be admitted and observed for at least 24 hours. For patients without an allergy to penicillin, start oral ciprofloxacin 750 mg b.d. and co-amoxiclav 625 mg t.d.s. for 7 days. For those with a penicillin allergy, use oral levofloxacin 500 mg b.d. for 7 days. Patients should take the first dose under supervision and can subsequently be discharged with an information sheet.

Patients with epilepsy should not be given ciprofloxacin or levofloxacin, and patients on sodium valporate should not be given meropenem as it can increase the risk of seizures.

Use of granulocyte-colony stimulating factor (G-CSF)

G-CSF is not used routinely in patients with neutropenic sepsis, but can be considered in those with a high risk of complications (Smith *et al.*, 2006). Such patients include those with the following:

- profound neutropenia (ANC < 0.1×10^9/L);
- prolonged neutropenia (> 10 days);
- pneumonia;
- hypotension;
- multiorgan dysfunction;
- uncontrolled primary disease;
- invasive fungal infections;
- age > 65 years;
- hospital inpatients at the time of developing the fever.

Prophylaxis of neutropenic sepsis

Primary and secondary prophylaxis using G-CSF is discussed in Chapter 1.

Prophylactic antibiotics

- A randomised double-blind placebo controlled trial in patients receiving cyclic chemotherapy for solid tumours and lymphoma and who are at risk of neutropenia (< 0.5×10^9/L) compared the use of prophylactic levofloxacin or placebo for 7 days during the period of neutropenia. Levofloxacin significantly reduced the incidence of clinically documented infection (3.5% versus 7.9%; $p < 0.001$) and hospitalisation for the treatment of neutropenic infection (15.7% versus 21.6%; $p < 0.004$) with few adverse effects (Cullen *et al.*, 2005).
- A recent meta-analysis of trials of prophylactic antibiotics in neutropenic patients has shown

a decrease in the risk of death with their use compared to placebo or no treatment (RR = 0.67; 95% CI 0.55 to 0.81). Fluoroquinolone prophylaxis reduced the risk for all-cause mortality (RR = 0.52; 95% CI 0.35 to 0.77) as well as infection-related mortality, fever, clinically documented infections and microbiologically documented infections. The authors concluded that antibiotic prophylaxis, preferably with a fluoroquinolone, should be considered for neutropenic patients (Gafter-Gvili *et al.*, 2005).

- Patients receiving chemotherapy for solid tumour or lymphoma and who are at risk of bacterial infection and severe neutropenia ($< 0.5 \times 10^9$/L) without G-CSF support should be considered possible candidates for prophylactic levofloxacin.

Anaphylaxis related to anti-cancer drugs

Anaphylaxis is associated particularly with paclitaxel, carboplatin and docetaxel. L-asparaginase may cause anaphylaxis in 10% of patients treated for acute lymphoblastic leukaemia. When first used, taxanes resulted in major hypersensitivity reactions in 30% of patients, with 40% suffering mild symptoms. These reactions were associated with fast infusion rates and usually occurred after the second infusion, often in the first few minutes of treatment, resolving 15–20 minutes after stopping the infusion. Carboplatin sensitivity is unpredictable and reactions may occur following a prolonged course of treatment – at any time during the infusion or indeed days following its administration. Monoclonal antibodies such as rituximab and cetuximab may cause a cytokine release syndrome.

Presentation

Patients may present with agitation, hypotension, bronchospasm and rash. Angioedema and urticaria, abdominal pain, rash, chest tightness, laryngeal oedema and tongue swelling may also occur.

Prevention

Prophylactic steroids and antihistamines reduce the incidence of hypersensitivity reactions to taxanes and carboplatin.

Treatment

Treat for anaphylaxis as follows.

- Stop the drug infusion.
- Secure airway, breathing and circulation.
- Give oxygen, lie the patient flat and elevate the legs if he/she is hypotensive.
- If there is stridor, wheeze, respiratory distress or clinical signs of shock, give adrenaline (epinephrine; 1:1000 solution) 0.5 mL i.m. and repeat the dose after 5 minutes if there is no improvement.
- Give 10 mg i.v. chlorphenamine.
- For all severe or recurrent reactions give 200 mg i.v. hydrocortisone.
- If shock fails to respond to drug measures, give 1–2 L of i.v. crystalloid.
- Most deaths due to anaphylaxis are associated with giving adrenaline too late.

Tumour lysis syndrome

Tumour lysis syndrome (TLS) is caused by sudden tumour necrosis either due to treatment or occurring spontaneously. It causes metabolic abnormalities, particularly hyperkalaemia, hyperuricaemia, hyperphosphataemia and secondary hypocalcaemia.

TLS is associated with chemosensitive, bulky tumours such as high-grade lymphoma, acute leukaemia and Burkitt lymphoma. It is rarely seen in low-grade lymphomas or solid tumours. Pre-existing renal failure may be a contributory factor.

Patients with lymphoma who have a raised lactate dehydrogenase (LDH) (> 1500 IU/L) are likely to have a high tumour burden and are at increased risk.

Presentation

Patients present with the following.

- Non-specific symptoms of weakness, nausea, vomiting, myalgia and dark urine.
- Electrolyte imbalance which can result in arrhythmias, neuromuscular irritability, seizure and death. Arrhythmias are a common cause of death if left untreated.
- Renal failure, which occurs frequently, secondary to hyperuricaemia.

Investigation

- Check levels of serum electrolytes, phosphate and calcium; uric acid; acid/base balance; and renal function.
- Monitor ECG.

- The typical biochemical picture is of hyperuricaemia, hyperkalaemia, hyperphosphataemia, hypocalcaemia, lactic acidosis and renal failure.

Prevention

- Early diagnosis requires a high level of suspicion. In patients at particular risk, routine uric acid and electrolyte measurements are sensible. Correct any pre-existing electrolyte abnormalities.
- Hydrate the patient with at least 3 L of normal saline per 24 hours to maintain urine output greater than 100 mL per hour with or without a loop diuretic to maintain urate clearance.
- Give oral sodium bicarbonate to alkalise the urine and prevent urate nephropathy in acidic conditions.
- If low-risk, give allopurinol 100 mg/m^2 every 8 hours to prevent hyperuricaemia.
- If high-risk (pre-existing hyperuricemia or renal impairment, high tumour burden, high sensitivity to chemotherapy), give rasburicase 200 μg/kg o.d.
- Unfortunately, despite these treatments, 14% of patients will still develop renal problems (Bessmertny *et al.*, 2005).

Treatment

- Aggressive hydration is required.
- Therapy for hyperkalaemia includes cation exchange resins binding potassium (sodium polystyrene sulphonate), calcium gluconate, sodium bicarbonate to correct acidosis and dextrose/insulin injection.
- Therapy for hyperphosphataemia and hypocalcaemia involves oral phosphate binders (aluminium hydroxide 30 mL q.d.s.) and calcium gluconate (10 mL i.v. injection).
- Therapy for hyperuricaemia involves sodium bicarbonate to maintain urine pH > 7.0 and allopurinol 600–800 mg/day.
- When severe TLS develops, intensive care support and continuous monitoring are necessary.
- Renal dialysis is required if hyperphosphataemia, symptomatic hypocalcaemia, persistent hyperkalaemia, hyperuricaemia and anuria/oligouria, acidosis or volume overload develops.

Table 8.5 Cytotoxic agents classified according to the type of reaction they typically produce

Class of drug	Definition	Examples
Vesicant	Capable of causing pain, inflammation, blistering, necrosis	Anthracyclines Vinca alkaloids Paclitaxel Streptozocin Mechlorethamine Oxaliplatin Mitomycin
Irritant	Capable of causing irritation and inflammation	Platinum compounds Etoposide Irinotecan Topotecan Flurouracil
Non-irritant	Non-irritant	Cyclophosphamide Ifosfamide Bleomycin Fludarabine Gemcitabine Methotrexate

Adapted from Goolsby and Lombardo (2006).

Rasburicase is the first recombinant uricolytic agent (urate oxidase) and it metabolises uric acid to allantoin, which is 5–10 times more soluble in urine than uric acid. It has a role in the prevention and treatment of TLS and is licensed for use immediately before and during the start of chemotherapy. Rasburicase has been shown to provide control of plasma uric acid more rapidly than allopurinol in adults at high risk of tumour lysis syndrome (Cortes *et al.*, 2010).

The safety and efficacy of rasburicase is currently being assessed and compared with allopurinol in a phase III clinical trial (Rampello *et al.*, 2006).

Extravasation of chemotherapy

Extravasation is leakage of intravenous drugs from a vein into the surrounding tissue.

Presentation

Extravasation may present during the administration of chemotherapy or later, with pain and swelling at the site

109

Table 8.6 Risk factors for extravasation

Factor	Description
Vein physiology	Fragile, small, sclerosed
Pharmacological	Duration and chemotherapy dosage exposure to tissue
Physiological	SVCO, lymphoedema, peripheral neuropathy, phlebitis
Radiotherapeutic	Previous local radiotherapy, radiation recall reactions
Mechanical	Needle insertion technique, multiple venepuncture sites

Adapted from Goolsby and Lombardo (2006).

Table 8.7 Antidotes for extravasation

Drug	Antidote/treatment
Anthracyclines	Topical DMSO 50% Topical hydrocortisone cream 1% Cold compress
Mitomycin	As for anthracyclines
Vinca alkaloids	Infiltrate the site with hyaluronidase (1500 units of hyaluronidase in 1 mL of water for injection) using 0.2 mL injections over and around the affected area Warm compress Topical NSAID cream
Platins and Taxanes	Infiltrate site with hyaluronidase Warm compression
Anti-metabolites	Topical hydrocortisone cream Cold compress

DMSO, dimethyl sulfoxide. For more details see Allwood and Stanley (2002).

of the intravenous cannula. Most commonly, it causes pain and localised tissue inflammation. More seriously, it can result in ulceration, necrosis, sloughing of the skin, damage to underlying structures and permanent disability. Table 8.5 shows cytotoxic agents classified according to the type of reaction they produce. The severity of an extravasation will depend on the infusion site, the concentration and volume of the chemotherapy drug and the treatment given for the extravasation. Table 8.6 shows the risk factors for extravasation.

Treatment

Experience from case reports and small series has resulted in the publication of guidelines for the prevention and treatment of extravasation (Goolsby and Lombardo, 2006). There are some general principles for the management of extravasation, together with specific measures for each chemotherapy drug. Initial management should include the following.

- Stop infusion, disconnect tubing, but leave i.v. cannula *in situ*.
- Attempt aspiration of vesicant and administer antidote (see Table 8.7) if appropriate.
- Keep limb elevated with either cold or warm compression as indicated (see Table 8.7 for examples).
- Ensure adequate analgesia is provided.
- Provide full documentation and monitoring (consider using a photograph record).
- Estimate the amount of extravasated drug.
- Consider immediate surgical opinion in cases of extravasation of a vesicant drug or when conservative treatment fails to improve symptoms or tissue damage occurs.
- Arrange appropriate follow up: telephone contact or day case review.

References

Allwood, M. and Stanley, A. (2002). *The Cytotoxics Handbook*. Oxford: Radcliffe Medical Press.

Bartter, F. and Schwartz, W. B. (1967). The syndrome of inappropriate secretion of antidiuretic hormone. *Am. J. Med.* **42**, 790–806.

Bayley, A., Milosevic, M., Blend, R., *et al.* (2001). A prospective study of factors predicting clinically occult spinal cord compression in patients with metastatic prostate carcinoma. *Cancer*, **92**, 303–310.

Bessmertny, O., Robitaille, L. M. and Cairo, M. S. (2005). Rasburicase: a new approach for preventing and/or treating tumour lysis syndrome. *Curr. Pharm. Des.*, **11**, 4177–4185.

Cervantes, A. and Chirivella, L. (2004). Oncological emergencies. *Ann. Oncol.*, **15** (Suppl. 4), S299–306.

Cortes, J., Moore, J. O., Maziarz, R. T., *et al.* (2010). Control of plasma uric acid in adults at risk for tumor lysis syndrome: efficacy and safety of rasburicase alone and rasburicase followed by allopurinol compared with allopurinol alone – results of a multicenter phase III study. *J. Clin. Oncol.*, **28**, 4207–4213.

Cullen, M., Steven, N., Billingham, L., *et al.* (2005). Antibacterial prophylaxis after chemotherapy for solid tumours and lymphomas. *N. Engl. J. Med.*, **353**, 988–998.

Farge, D., Debourdeau P., Beckers, M., *et al.* (2013). International clinical practice guidelines for the treatment and prophylaxis of venous thromboembolism in patients with cancer. *J. Thromb. Haemost.*, **11**, 56–70.

Freitag, L. (2004). Interventional endoscopic treatment. *Lung Cancer*, **45** (Suppl. 2), S235–238.

Gafter-Gvili, A., Fraser, A., Paul, M., *et al.* (2005). Meta-analysis: antibiotic prophylaxis reduces mortality in neutropenic patients. *Ann. Intern. Med.*, **142**, 979–995.

Goolsby, T. V. and Lombardo, F. A. (2006). Extravasation of chemotherapeutic agents: prevention and treatment. *Semin. Oncol.*, **33**, 139–143.

Klastersky, J., Paesmans, M., Rubenstein, E. B., *et al.* (2000). The Multinational Association for Supportive Care in Cancer risk index: a multinational scoring system for identifying low-risk febrile neutropenic cancer patients. *J. Clin. Oncol.*, **18**, 3038–3051.

Lee, A. Y., Levine, M. N., Baker, R. I., *et al.* (2003). Low-molecular-weight heparin versus a coumarin for the prevention of recurrent venous thromboembolism in patients with cancer. *N. Engl. J. Med.*, **349**, 146–153.

Maisey, N., Norman, A., Prior, Y., *et al.* (2004). Chemotherapy for primary gastric lymphoma: does in-patient observation prevent complications? *Clin. Oncol. (R. Coll. Radiol.)*, **16**, 48–52.

Morris, C. D., Budde, J. M., Godette, K. D., *et al.* (2002). Palliative management of malignant airway obstruction. *Ann. Thorac. Surg.*, **74**, 1928–1932.

NICE. (2008). *Metastatic Spinal Cord Compression. Diagnosis and Management of Adults At Risk Of and With Metastatic Spinal Cord Compression. NICE Clinical Guideline 75.* Manchester: National Institute for Health and Clinical Excellence.

NICE. (2012). *Neutropenic Sepsis: Prevention and Management of Neutropenic Sepsis in Cancer Patients. NICE Clinical Guideline 151.* Manchester: National Institute for Health and Clinical Excellence.

Ostler, P. J., Clarke, D. P., Watkinson, A. F., *et al.* (1997). Superior vena cava obstruction; a modern management strategy. *Clin. Oncol. (R. Coll. Radiol.)*, **9**, 83–89.

Palmer, K. (2004). Management of haematemesis and melaena. *Postgrad. Med. J.*, **80**, 399–404.

Patchell, R. A., Tibbs, P. A., Regine, W. F., *et al.* (2005). Direct decompressive surgical resection in the treatment of spinal cord compression caused by metastatic cancer: a randomised trial. *Lancet*, **366**, 643–648.

Poortmans, P., Vulto, A. and Raaijmakers, E. (2001). Always on a Friday? Time pattern of referral for spinal cord compression. *Acta Oncol.*, **40**, 88–91.

Priestman, T. J., Dunn, J., Brada, M., *et al.* (1996). Final results of the Royal College of Radiologists' trial comparing two different radiotherapy schedules in the treatment of cerebral metastases. *Clin. Oncol. (R. Coll. Radiol.)*, **8**, 308–315.

Rades, D., Stalpers, L. J., Schulte, R., *et al.* (2006). Defining the appropriate radiotherapy regimen for metastatic spinal cord compression in non-small cell lung cancer patients. *Eur. J. Cancer*, **42**, 1052–1056.

Rampello, E., Fricia, T. and Malaguarnera, M. (2006). The management of tumour lysis syndrome. *Nat. Clin. Pract. Oncol.*, **3**, 438–447.

Rockall, T. A., Logan, R. F., Devlin, H. B., *et al.* (1996). Risk assessment after acute upper gastrointestinal haemorrhage. *Gut*, **38**, 316–321.

Rowell, N. P. and Gleeson, F. V. (2001). Steroids, radiotherapy, chemotherapy and stents for superior vena caval obstruction in carcinoma of the bronchus. *Cochrane Database Syst. Rev.*, **4**, CD001316.

Smith, T. J., Khatcheressian, J., Lyman, G. H., *et al.* (2006). 2006 update of recommendations for the use of white blood cell growth factors: an evidence-based clinical practice guideline. *J Clin Oncol.*, **24**, 3187.

Stewart, A. F. (2005). Hypercalcemia associated with cancer. *N. Eng. J. Med.*, **352**, 373–379.

Tokuhashi, Y., Matsuzaki, H., Oda, H., *et al.* (2005). A revised scoring system for preoperative evaluation of metastatic spine tumor prognosis. *Spine*, **30**, 2186–2191.

Chapter

9

Acute oncology 2: cancer of unknown primary

Najmus Sahar Iqbal and Paul Shaw

Introduction

Cancer of unknown primary origin is a condition in which a patient has metastatic tumour without an identified primary source (NICE, 2010). Cancer of unknown primary is an imprecise term, and it is often applied to patients in whom limited investigations have been performed. To clarify this, NICE clinical guideline CG104 has used the terms 'metastatic malignancy of uncertain origin' (MUO), 'provisional carcinoma of unknown primary' (provisional CUP) and 'confirmed carcinoma of unknown primary (confirmed CUP)' as summarised in Table 9.1 (NICE, 2010).

For those patients whose primary tumour is identified, treatment should continue as for that individual tumour site. But if a primary tumour is not identified after the initial investigation, treatment has to be empirical and based on research in patients whose primary tumour is known. This chapter focuses on the investigation of patients presenting with malignancy of unidentified primary origin (MUO) and the treatment possibilities for those whose primary tumour is not identified after initial investigation.

Incidence and epidemiology

Cancer of unknown primary accounts for 3–5% of all invasive malignancies in the western world (Greco and Hainsworth, 2001; Pavlidis and Pentheroudakis, 2012) and ranks in the top 10 most common cancer diagnoses. In 2011, there were 9762 new cases of cancer of unknown primary diagnosed in the United Kingdom (http://www.cancerresearchuk.org/cancer-info/cancerstats/, accessed December 2014). The age-standardised rate in the UK is 10.2 per 100,000 population. The rate is higher in men than women. The incidence of cancer of unknown primary has halved in the last 20 years and most of this decrease is likely to be due to improved detection of the primary site using techniques such as histopathology, immunohistochemistry and cross-sectional imaging, which have resulted in patients not being registered as having cancer of unknown primary.

Hospital Episode Statistics (HES) data for England (06–07) recorded a total of 25,318 episodes of care for patients with a diagnosis of cancer of unknown primary representing 308,359 NHS bed-days. The majority of patients were first admitted as an emergency.

Deaths from CUP account for 7% of all cancer deaths (http://www.cancerresearchuk.org/cancer-info/cancerstats/, accessed December 2014). However, in the absence of a standard definition, the true rate may be underestimated.

The median age at diagnosis is 65–70 years, but patients presenting with a midline distribution of poorly differentiated carcinoma have a median age of 39 years (Casciato, 2006; and Kramer *et al.*, 2008).

In patients whose primary site is subsequently identified, the commonest primary sites are the pancreas (20–26%), lung (17–23%), liver (3–11%), large bowel (4–10%), stomach (3–8%), kidney (4–6%), ovary (3–4%), prostate (3–4%) and breast (2%) (Kramer *et al.*, 2008).

It is important to consider the possibility of potentially curable malignancies, such as germ cell tumours or lymphoma, and the investigation of patients with cancer of unknown primary is therefore likely to include biopsy with immunohistochemistry to identify the cell lineage, if possible. Investigations are determined by the site of cancer, the patient's symptoms, and the general condition of the patient; however, an exhaustive diagnostic work-up is not usually justified because it is unlikely to influence the outcome of treatment.

Practical Clinical Oncology, Second Edition, ed. Louise Hanna, Tom Crosby and Fergus Macbeth. Published by Cambridge University Press. © Cambridge University Press 2015.

Table 9.4 Standardised treatments for 'favourable' CUP patients

CUP subgroup	Recommended treatment
Poorly differentiated carcinoma in midline (extragonadal germ cell syndrome)	Platinum-based regimen (germ cell)
Woman with papillary serous or serous adenocarcinoma of peritoneal cavity	As for FIGO stage III ovarian cancer
Woman with adenocarcinoma involving axillary nodes	As for breast cancer
Squamous cell carcinoma of cervical nodes	Radical radiotherapy/surgery/adjuvant chemotherapy
Adenocarcinoma with colon cancer profile (CK20, CK7, CDX2+)	As for metastatic colon cancer
Isolated inguinal lymphadenopathy (squamous cell carcinoma)	Surgical dissection ± radiotherapy
Poorly differentiated neuroendocrine carcinoma	Platinum-based regimen (e.g. platinum/etoposide)
Man with blastic bone metastases and elevated PSA	Endocrine treatment as for prostate cancer
Single metastasis only	Definitive local treatment (surgery or radiotherapy)

Adapted from Pavlidis and Pentheroudakis (2012), NICE (2010) and Fizazi *et al.* (2011).

management of isolated brain metastases or be used for palliation of specific problems (e.g. prophylactic surgery for bone metastases or epidural spinal cord decompression). Patients with solitary tumour in the liver, bone, brain, skin or lung should be referred to the appropriate MDT for consideration of local treatments because what appear to be metastases could be an unusual primary tumour. There has been no direct comparison of different treatments for solitary metastases (NICE, 2010). Close collaboration between medical and surgical specialists is important to ensure the most appropriate patient management.

Radiotherapy

Radiotherapy treatment may be indicated in a number of circumstances including:

- as part of standard treatment for a probable primary cancer in patients with CUP;
- to treat squamous cell cancer of cervical lymph nodes or isolated inguinal lymphadenopathy, following surgical excision. The management of squamous cancer of unknown primary in cervical lymph nodes is discussed further in Chapter 11;
- as palliative treatment (e.g. bone pain, epidural spinal cord compression, SVCO).

Chemotherapy

A wide variety of chemotherapy regimens for CUP has been reported in phase II studies, with an overall response rate of less than 20%, and so it is not surprising that an audit showed that 18 different chemotherapy regimens were used to treat 37 patients with CUP (Shaw *et al.*, 2007). Platinum-based chemotherapy regimens seem to give a higher response rate than others (Kramer *et al.*, 2008). Of the few published randomised studies, one showed an improved response rate of 55% when patients were treated with cisplatin and gemcitabine (Culine *et al.*, 2002). A meta-analysis comparing 10 randomised phase II trials showed no significant survival benefit from the different chemotherapy regimens (Golfinopoulos *et al.*, 2009).

For patients in one of the more favourable CUP subgroups, specific chemotherapy is suggested in Table 9.4 and Figure 9.1.

Unfortunately, 80% patients with CUP are in the unfavourable subgroup (Pavlidis and Pentheroudakis, 2012). Treatment in this group is palliative and may include chemotherapy if the patient is fit enough and is prepared to accept treatment. There is little evidence to suggest that any particular regimen has a survival advantage or a positive effect on the quality of life; the choice of regimen will therefore be influenced by local experience and practice, as well as the likely site of primary disease. Commonly used regimens include epirubicin, cisplatin and 5-FU (ECF) or other infusional 5-FU-based regimens. More recent combinations include newer agents such as capecitabine, gemcitabine and the taxanes.

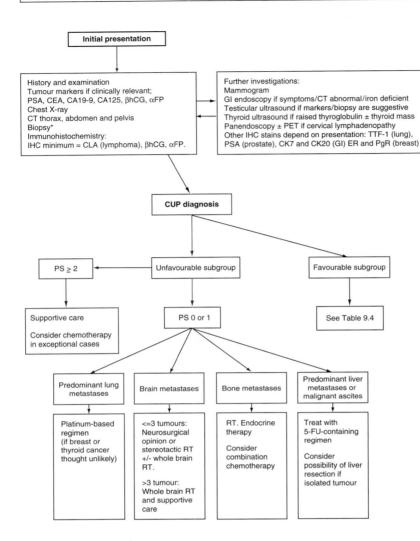

Figure 9.1 Diagnostic and treatment algorithm for CUP. *Consider the value of obtaining a tissue diagnosis if epithelial markers are positive with radiological evidence of malignancy, PS > 2, more than three metastatic sites and liver metastases. 5-FU, 5-fluorouracil; αFP, alpha feto-protein; βhCG, beta human chorionic gonadotrophin; CA, cancer antigen; CEA, carcino-embryonic antigen; CK, cytokeratin; CLA, common leukocyte antigen; CT, computed tomography; ER, oestrogen receptor; GI, gastrointestinal; IHC, immunohistochemistry; PET, positron emission tomography; PgR, progesterone receptor; PS, WHO performance status; PSA, prostate-specific antigen; RT, radiotherapy; TTF-1, thyroid transcription factor 1.

Table 9.5 'Unfavourable' CUP subgroups

Metastatic adenocarcinoma in liver or multiple sites
Malignant ascites (non-papillary serous adenocarcinoma)
Multiple cerebral metastases (adeno- or squamous carcinoma)
Multiple lung/pleural metastases (adenocarcinoma)
Multiple metastatic bone metastases (adenocarcinoma)
Squamous cell carcinoma of the abdomino-pelvic cavity

Adapted from Pavlidis and Pentheroudakis (2012).

Patients with unfavourable CUP and performance status 0 or 1 who fall into certain subgroups may be treated as follows.

1. Brain metastases – consider whole brain radiotherapy ± stereotactic boost for patients with two to three brain metastases. Systemic chemotherapy has not been shown to improve survival in patients with multiple metastases including brain involvement (NICE, 2010).
2. Predominant liver metastases or malignant ascites – consider a 5-FU-based regimen, e.g. epirubicin, oxaliplatin and capecitabine.
3. Predominant lung metastases – consider a platinum-based treatment regimen (assuming breast or thyroid cancer thought unlikely).
4. Bone metastases – consider radiotherapy for painful sites and a trial of hormone treatment (breast or prostate cancer) or possible combination chemotherapy. Bisphosphonates can be useful to palliate widespread bone pain when there is no

single site amenable to radiotherapy (National Cancer Institute, www. cancer.gov/cancertopics/types/unknownprimary, accessed December 2014).

Palliation

Early involvement of an oncologist, palliative care physician and key worker has been strongly recommended by NICE. There is evidence that such involvement leads to improved patient care and avoidance of unnecessary investigations or treatment. There is an overlap between CUP and the acute oncology service.

Unfortunately, the majority of patients with CUP have incurable disease at diagnosis, and the focus of treatment should be to ensure useful palliation with the least toxicity. Patients with unfavourable CUP and poor performance status with either liver metastases or more than three metastatic sites of disease are probably best treated with supportive care alone, with palliative radiotherapy for local symptom control.

Prognosis

One-year and 5-year survival is 16% and 8%, respectively. There has been no significant change in survival of cancer of unknown primary between 1992 and 2006. This is in contrast with all cancer mortality in the UK, which has reduced by 15% for men and 11% for women in the above-mentioned time period.

The overall median survival in a study of 657 cancer of unknown primary patients in whom just fewer than 50% underwent chemotherapy was 11.0 months with only 1.5% alive at 5 years (Abbruzzese et al., 1994). Patients in a good prognostic group (PS 0 or 1 without liver metastases), intermediate prognostic group (PS > 1 or liver metastases) or poor prognostic group (PS > 1 and liver metastases) had a median survival of 10.8, 6 and 2.4 months, respectively (Culine et al., 2002; van de Wouw et al., 2004). Perhaps not surprisingly, patients treated with radiotherapy do not have a significantly better survival (median survival = 3.0 months (95% CI 1.8–4.2)) than those who had no radiotherapy (median survival = 2.0 months; (95% CI 1.2–2.7) months, $p = 0.135$; Shaw et al., 2007).

Prognostic factors

Poor prognostic factors include the following (Pasterz et al., 1986; Culine et al., 2002; van de Wouw et al., 2004; Pavlidis and Pentheroudakis, 2012):

- more than three metastatic sites;
- PS 2 or more;
- male;
- non-lymph node metastases;
- raised LDH, lymphopaenia, low serum albumin;
- 'unfavourable' CUP subgroup (see Table 9.4).

Current trials

CUP-One trial is a phase II multicentre UK-based trial which prospectively analysed new tools in diagnosis such as molecular profiling, metabonomics of blood and urine for response and toxicity prediction and a proposed immunohistochemistry classifier. The second part of the trial is to establish the effectiveness of ECX (epirubicin, cisplatin and capecitabine) chemotherapy. This trial has recently closed and will set the scene for future research in CUP.

Areas of current interest

In the future, the treatment for patients with cancer of unknown primary is likely to move away from that based on the most likely anatomical site of origin to one based on molecular profiling predicting treatment response.

Acknowledgements

The authors would like to acknowledge the contribution of Dr Tom Crosby to this chapter.

References

Abbruzzese, J. L., Abbruzzese, M. C., Hess, K. R., et al. (1994). Unknown primary carcinoma: natural history and prognostic factors in 657 consecutive patients. J. Clin. Oncol., **12**, 1272–1280.

Casciato, D. A. (2006). In Manual of Clinical Oncology, ed. D. A. Casciato, 5th edn. Philadelphia, PA: Lippincott Williams and Wilkins, pp. 402–14.

Culine, S., Kramar, A., Saghatchian, M., et al. (2002). Development and validation of a prognostic model to predict the length of survival in patients with carcinomas of an unknown primary site. J. Clin. Oncol., **20**, 4679–4683.

Fizazi, K., Greco, F. A., Pavlidis, N., et al. (2011). Cancers of unknown primary site: ESMO Clinical Practice Guidelines for diagnosis, treatment and follow-up. Ann. Oncol., **22**(Suppl 6), vi64–vi68.

Greco, F. A. and Hainsworth, J. D. (2001). In Cancer: Principles and Practice of Oncology, ed. V. T.

DeVita Jr., S. Hellman and S. A. Rosenberg, 6th edn. New York: Lippincott Williams and Wilkins, pp. 2537–2560.

Golfinopoulos. V., Pentheroudakis. G., Salanti. G., *et al.* (2009). Comparative survival with diverse chemotherapy regimens for cancer of unknown primary site: multiple-treatments meta-analysis. *Cancer Treat. Rev.*, **35**, 570–573.

Hainsworth, J. D. and Greco F. A. (1993). Treatment of patients with cancer of an unknown primary site. *N. Engl. J. Med.*, **329**, 257–263.

Hainsworth, J. D., Rubin, M. S., Spigel, D. R., *et al.* (2013). Molecular gene expression profiling to predict the tissue of origin and direct site-specific therapy in patients with carcinoma of unknown primary site: a prospective trial of the Sarah Cannon Research Institute. *J. Clin. Oncol.*, **31**, 217–223.

Kramer, A., Hubner, G., Scheeweiss, A., *et al.* (2008). Carcinoma of unknown primary – an orphan disease. *Breast Care*, 3, 164–170.

Neumann, K. H. and Nystrom, J. S. (1982). Metastatic cancer of unknown origin: nonsquamous cell type. *Sem. Oncol.*, **9**, 427–434.

NICE. (2010). *Metastatic Malignant Disease of Unknown Primary Origin: Diagnosis and management of metastatic malignant disease of unknown primary origin. NICE Guidelines [CG104].* Manchester: National Institute for Health and Clinical Excellence.

Nystrom, J. S., Weiner, J. M. Wolf, R. M., *et al.* (1979). Identifying the primary site in metastatic cancer of unknown origin. Inadequacy of roentgenographic procedures. *J. Am. Med. Ass.*, **241**, 381–383.

Oien, K. A. and Dennis, J. L. (2012). Diagnostic work-up of carcinoma of unknown primary: from immunohistochemistry to molecular profiling. *Ann. Oncol.*, **23**(Suppl 10), x271–7.

Pasterz, R., Savaraj, N. and Burgess, M. (1986). Prognostic factors in metastatic carcinoma of unknown primary. *J. Clin. Oncol.*, **4**, 1652–1657.

Pavlidis, N. and Pentheroudakis, G. (2012). Cancer of unknown primary site. *Lancet*, **379**, 1428–1435.

Pavlidis, N., Briasoulis, E., Hainsworth, J., *et al.* (2003). Diagnostic and therapeutic management of cancer of an unknown primary. *Eur. J. Cancer*, **39**, 1990–2005.

Shaw, P., Adams, R., Jordan, C., *et al.* (2007). A clinical review of the investigation and management of carcinoma of unknown primary in a single cancer network. *Clin. Oncol. (R. Coll. Radiol.)*, **19**, 87–95.

Stella, G. M., Senetta, R., Cassenti, A., *et al.* (2012). Cancers of unknown primary origin: current perspectives and future therapeutic strategies. *J. Transl. Med.*, **10**, 12.

UICC. (2009). *TNM Classification of Malignant Tumours*, ed. L. H. Sobin, M. K. Gospodarowicz and C. Wittekind, 7th edn. Chichester: Wiley-Blackwell.

van de Wouw, A. J., Jansen, R. L., Griffioen, A. W., *et al.* (2004). Clinical and immunohistochemical analysis of patients with unknown primary tumour. A search for prognostic factors in UPT. *Anticancer Res.*, **24**, 297–301.

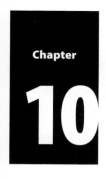

Chapter 10

Palliative care

Siwan Seaman and Simon Noble

Introduction

Changing role of palliative care in oncology

The World Health Organisation (WHO) defines palliative care as 'the active total care of patients whose disease is not responsive to curative treatment, where control of pain, of other symptoms and of psychological, social and spiritual problems is paramount with the achievement of the best possible quality of life for patients and their families as the goal' (World Health Organisation, 1990). Palliative care should now be considered an integral part of service planning and care delivery in oncology.

This chapter covers common problems in symptom control, communication, ethical decision making, and the financial difficulties of patients with advanced cancer.

Changing model of palliative care

In the old model of the cancer journey (Figure 10.1(a)), palliative care services would only be involved at the end of life when no further oncological or supportive treatments were available. This was a 'terminal care' service for those clearly at the end of life. However, the symptoms that were being controlled occur not only at the end of life but also to different degrees throughout the cancer journey. The new model (Figure 10.1(b)) attempts to dovetail palliative care with active treatment, gradually increasing its involvement as active treatment becomes less appropriate. Some patients, such as those with carcinoma of the pancreas, are likely to need palliative care input early in their illness.

Pain control

Pain is an unpleasant sensory and emotional experience associated with actual or potential tissue damage. It is experienced by up to 70% of patients with

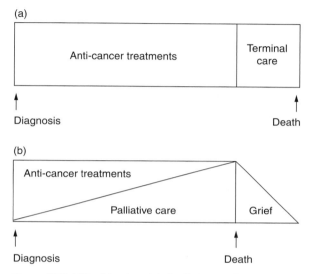

Figure 10.1 (a) Traditional model of palliative care showing set point at which active treatment ceases and comfort-only begins. (b) Current model of palliative care showing the gradual introduction of increasing palliative care as active treatment becomes less appropriate.

advanced cancer and of these, one-third have a single pain, one-third have two pains and one-third have three or more pains (Royal College of Physicians, 2000). Pain may be:

- related to the cancer itself (e.g. metastatic bone pain);
- treatment-related (e.g. neuropathy secondary to chemotherapy);
- related to cancer and debility (e.g. constipation);
- unrelated to the cancer (due to another coexisting condition) e.g. osteoarthritis.

Pharmacological methods

The WHO analgesic ladder (World Health Organisation, 1990) is very useful in managing cancer

Practical Clinical Oncology, Second Edition, ed. Louise Hanna, Tom Crosby and Fergus Macbeth. Published by Cambridge University Press. © Cambridge University Press 2015.

Table 10.1 The World Health Organisation (WHO) analgesic ladder

Step	Severity of pain	Analgesia	Examples
Step 1	Mild	Non-opioid ± adjuvant	Paracetamol
Step 2	Mild to moderate	Weak opioid ± non-opioid ± adjuvant	Codeine Dihydrocodeine
Step 3	Moderate to severe	Strong opioid ± non-opioid ± adjuvant	Morphine Fentanyl Oxycodone Hydromorphone

Table 10.2 Adjuvant analgesics

Drug type	Indication – examples
Non-steroidal anti-inflammatory drugs (e.g. diclofenac 50 mg t.d.s.)	Bone metastases Liver capsule pain Soft tissue infiltration
Corticosteroids (e.g. dexamethasone 8–16 mg daily)	Raised intracranial pressure Soft tissue infiltration Liver capsule pain Nerve compression
Anticonvulsants/antidepressants (e.g. gabapentin 100–300 mg nocte, amitriptyline 25 mg nocte)	Nerve compression or infiltration Paraneoplastic neuropathies
Bisphosphonates (e.g. pamidronate, zoledronate)	Malignant bone pain

pain. It can alleviate pain in more than 80% of patients by starting at a level most appropriate to the patient's pain and increasing in steps until adequate analgesia is achieved (Table 10.1). Adjuvant analgesics may be used at any point depending on the type of pain the patient is experiencing; an adjuvant analgesic is a drug whose primary indication is for something other than pain but which has an analgesic effect for certain types of pain (Table 10.2).

When starting someone on an opioid, it is important to prescribe regular laxatives and a suitable anti-emetic (such as haloperidol 1.5 mg nocte). Patients should also be written up for adequate breakthrough analgesia, which amounts to one-sixth of the total dose of morphine prescribed for 24 hours (Fallon and McConnell, 2006; see Tables 10.3 and 10.4 for breakthrough doses and conversions to other opiates).

Opioid toxicity

Morphine undergoes glucuronidation in the liver and is then excreted through the kidneys. Renal impairment and/or dehydration may lead to accumulation of opioid metabolites and opioid toxicity, which commonly results in cognitive impairment and confusion (Hall and Sykes, 2004). Other causes of confusion such as hyponatraemia, cerebral disease, infection and hypercalcaemia should be considered and excluded.

The other features of opioid toxicity include the following:

- pinpoint pupils;
- myoclonus/metabolic flap;
- visual hallucinations. Patients typically see dark spots in the periphery of their vision and may think they have seen animals run under the bed;
- drowsiness (severe toxicity);
- respiratory depression (severe toxicity).

Non-pharmacological methods

Wherever possible, non-pharmacological methods of analgesia should be considered. There are many options available and their use is likely to depend on:

Table 10.3 Morphine doses and conversion

Breakthrough dose of morphine = total dose of morphine in 24 hours, divided by 6 e.g. for someone on MST 60 mg b.d. (i.e. total 24-hour dose = 60 mg × 2 = 120 mg):

Breakthrough dose = {60 mg × 2} ÷ 6 = 120 mg ÷ 6 = 20 mg p.r.n.

Converting oral morphine to subcutaneous diamorphine via syringe driver

Take the total 24-hour dose of morphine and divide by 3 (subcutaneous diamorphine is three times as potent as oral morphine), e.g. for someone on MST 60 mg b.d.:

Subcutaneous diamorphine dose = {60 mg × 2} ÷ 3 ≈ 40 mg diamorphine s.c. over 24 hours

Table 10.4 Morphine potencies

Oxycodone is twice as potent as oral morphine (e.g. 10 mg oxynorm ≈ 20 mg oromorph)

Tramadol is stronger than you think! 100 mg tramadol q.d.s. ≈ 80 mg oral morphine = 40 mg MST b.d.

Co-codamol 30/500 2 tabs. q.d.s ≈ 24 mg morphine

Table 10.5 Non-pharmacological methods of pain control for cancer patients

Procedure	Indication	Other important issues
Radiotherapy	Commonly used for pain from bone metastases	Useful for opioid-sparing Need for transfer to oncology department
Transcutaneous electrical nerve stimulation	Used as an adjuvant to other analgesics	Requires expertise of physiotherapist
Nerve blocks	For neuropathic pain in clearly identifiable nerve distribution	Anaesthetic involvement required
Epidural/intrathecal analgesia	For complex cord-related pains and plexopathies	Anaesthetic involvement essential. Ongoing care difficult if an indwelling catheter is used
Orthopaedic stabilisation	Useful for incident pain (pain on movement), e.g. vertebral disease or prophylaxis of fracture in long bones with metastases	Orthopaedic opinion required
Vertebroplasty	Useful for stabilisation and analgesia of pain related to vertebral metastatic disease	Radiological expertise required

- the needs and views of the patient and carers,
- the experience of the referring physician,
- the availability of the procedure,
- available expertise (e.g. nursing staff) to manage the intervention.

Table 10.5 shows examples of non-pharmacological methods of pain control.

Anti-emetic prescribing

Numerous neurotransmitter receptors are involved in transmitting the impulses connected with nausea and vomiting to the vomiting centre (VC) and chemoreceptor trigger zone (CTZ) in the midbrain (Mannix, 2006).

Chemical triggers (such as drugs, metabolites and toxins) are detected at the CTZ, whereas the VC receives input from stretch receptors on nerve terminals (e.g. from the liver capsule being stretched by metastases or bowel dilatation due to obstruction (Baines, 1997)) as well as input from higher mental centres (e.g. pain, fear memory) and integrates these with input from the CTZ.

Different anti-emetics block different receptors and the choice of anti-emetic should be guided by the underlying cause of vomiting (Glare *et al.*, 2004; Rhodes and McDaniel, 2001; Tables 10.6 and 10.7).

When managing a patient with nausea and vomiting:

Table 10.6 Different anti-emetics

Drug	Mechanism of action	Clinical uses
Metoclopramide	Prokinetic, weak dopamine (D_2) antagonist	Gastric outflow obstruction
		Upper GI bleed
		Liver metastases
		Carcinoma head of pancreas
Haloperidol	Dopamine (D_2) antagonist. Good central anti-emetic effect	Metabolic causes of nausea:
		Hypercalcaemia
		Uraemia
		Antibiotics
		Opioids
Cyclizine	Histamine (H_1) antagonist. Anti-muscarinic (ACh_m). Centrally acting	Central causes
		Raised intracranial pressure
		Motion sickness/vestibular problems
Ondansetron or granisetron	Serotonin (5-HT_3) antagonist (Very constipating)	Chemotherapy-induced nausea
Aprepitant	Neurokinin I (NK_1) antagonist	Chemotherapy-induced nausea

Table 10.7 Choices of anti-emetics

Cause of vomiting	Choice of anti-emetic
Drug/toxin/metabolic	Haloperidol, levomepromazine
Radiotherapy	Haloperidol
Chemotherapy	Ondansetron, dexamethasone, metoclopramide, aprepitant
Bowel obstruction	Cyclizine, hyoscine butylbromide, octreotide, corticosteroids
Delayed gastric emptying	Metoclopramide, domperidone
Raised intracranial pressure	Cyclizine, dexamethasone

- identify possible causes;
- consider the probable pathways and neurotransmitters involved to choose the most appropriate anti-emetic;
- use an anti-emetic regularly and titrate the dose, considering alternatives to the oral route if necessary;
- when using combinations of drugs, remember potential interactions (e.g. metoclopramide and cyclizine may have an antagonistic effect; using haloperidol and metoclopramide together increases the risk of extrapyramidal side effects);
- consider non-pharmacological measures such as relaxation, acupuncture, and providing small frequent meals that do not have extremes of taste or smell.

Constipation

Constipation is a common symptom facing cancer patients and should be prevented because it can cause:

- abdominal pain and colic;
- intestinal obstruction;
- confusion;
- urinary retention;
- overflow diarrhoea.

Consider and, if appropriate, treat the cause of the constipation:

- drugs (e.g. opioids, tricyclics, antacids, phenothiazines);
- dehydration;
- abdominal wall muscle paresis (e.g. from spinal cord compression);

Giving too much information too quickly

The main task in breaking bad news is taking a patient from a point where he or she knows nothing to a point where he or she understands everything, if he or she wants to. The skill is in slowing down the transition of information so that the patient can handle it. Too much too soon will lead to psychological disturbance and possibly denial. The 'warning shot' technique helps test the water and find out how much the patient will allow you to tell. Sometimes the patient will make it quite clear that they do not want any more information; this wish should be respected.

When talking to relatives, the principles of communication are the same as talking with patients. However, it is important to acknowledge that their agenda or concerns may differ from those of the patient. Anger and distress are frequently encountered and should be handled sensitively and calmly. Listening to and addressing each of their concerns is essential, although your duty of care must always remain with the patient. Don't forget that you must respect the patient's right to confidentiality and discuss his or her care only if given permission to do so.

Not allowing for silence

If there is an uncomfortable pause, we may feel that we have to fill the silence with more information or an inappropriate comment – this should always be avoided. Silence is a valuable tool in communicating. It helps by showing that you are listening and by giving the patient time to assimilate the news, to react to it and to ask questions. As a patient once explained, 'When you give me bad news, you will pause and all you can hear is silence. Well, all I hear is noise; it's just that it is internal. When you speak you are interrupting me getting my head together.'

Discomfort with patient distress

BAD NEWS IS BAD NEWS! YOU CAN'T TURN IT INTO GOOD NEWS!

By definition, bad news is going to upset the receiver. If a patient cries, he or she is expressing an appropriate emotion in response to devastating news, and we need to be comfortable with that. The problem is that we may feel guilty that we have made them cry and may feel compelled to say something to 'make it better'. What happens in practice is that we end up giving patients false hope or reassurance, which often makes it harder for them to come to terms with their illness later on. Sometimes it will pave the way for a highly complicated bereavement.

Financial considerations

The impact of advanced cancer is not limited to the physical and emotional. Patients and families commonly experience financial difficulties, especially when the patient or main carer is self-employed. The role of the welfare rights adviser as part of the MDT is important in ensuring that financial aspects of the patient's life are addressed. Simple things like accessing critical illness payments and pension plans, and arranging mortgage payment holidays, can all contribute to making life more manageable. Most patients will be entitled to financial assistance in the form of benefits. In assessing someone for benefits, there are several things that must be considered:

- the patient's age (i.e. whether he or she is younger or older than 65);
- the patient's prognosis (i.e. whether his or her prognosis is less than 6 months).

Commonly claimed benefits follow below.

Attendance allowance is paid to individuals over the age of 65 who have 'care' needs, although they do not need to be receiving care. An individual may also be eligible for this benefit without having any care needs if this benefit is claimed under the special rules with a DS1500 report.

Personal Independent Payment (PIP) which has now replaced disability living allowance is paid to people under the age of 65 who need help looking after themselves; this benefit is split into two components: the daily living component and the mobility component. An individual without care needs may be eligible for PIP with a DS1500 report under the special rules.

Employment and Support Allowance (ESA) has replaced incapacity benefit and is paid to people who are too unwell to work. They usually claim it once the *statutory sick pay* (SSP) has ended or if they do not qualify for SSP.

Carer's allowance is not claimable by the patient; it is claimable by an individual providing the care. The claimant needs to be over the age of 16 and providing at least 35 hours of care a week. The carer may work, but they cannot earn more than £100 a week after certain deductions.

The *DS-1500* form is a route of claiming disability benefits for patients under 'special rules', usually when the patient has a terminal condition with a prognosis of less than 6 months; these benefits are processed without delay.

There are many more benefits and tax credits and grants that patients with advanced cancer may be eligible for. An award of Attendance Allowance or Personal Independence Payment may increase entitlement or bring about a new entitlement to benefit. Therefore, it is important that these patients are offered access to independent welfare advice.

Ethical decision-making

The management of cancer patients is not solely guided by evidence-based guidelines. Sometimes decisions will need to be made for which there is no clear-cut answer. In weighing up the pros and cons of a decision, it is useful to base it around the following ethical domains.

- Autonomy.
- Beneficence.
- Non-maleficence.
- Justice.

Autonomy

Autonomy gives the patient the opportunity to make known his or her wishes and to make an informed decision. For a patient to do this, he or she needs the 'capacity' to make such a decision. The Mental Capacity Act (2005) sets out how to assess capacity and the steps that should be taken when caring for patients who lack capacity. For a patient to have capacity, he or she must be able to:

- understand the information given to them;
- retain that information long enough to be able to make the decisions;
- weigh up all the information available to make a decision;
- communicate their decision by any means (writing, talking, sign language, etc.).

If a patient has the capacity to make a decision, teams should respect his or her wishes, even if they consider it to be an unwise decision. However, doctors are not obliged to give a treatment against their better clinical judgement if they feel it is futile. When a patient is deemed to lack capacity to make a particular decision then a best-interest decision should be made by the treating clinician.

Beneficence

Professionals should make decisions with the intention of doing what is most likely to benefit the patient – the intention to do good.

Non-maleficence

Conversely, non-maleficence dictates that when making a decision it should be done with the intention of doing no harm.

Justice

Justice guides us to do what is fair, not only for the patient in question but also for other patients as a whole. It also ensures that we practice within what is legal within our society.

Areas of current interest

By the nature of medical advances resulting in more people experiencing cancer as a chronic disease, the field of palliative care has expanded to play a critical role not only at diagnosis and through treatment but also in cancer survivorship and late-effects of treatment.

Other areas of current interest include the importance of advance care planning (ACP) and tied in with ACP is exploring patients' preferred place of care and preferred place of death to establish the support they will require in order to achieve their goals. Another area of interest is the role of artificial hydration at the end of life; there is currently lack of evidence of when artificial hydration should be used at the end of life, but the issue will continue to be debated.

Another contentious area of palliative care relates to physician-assisted suicide and euthanasia. Both acts remain illegal in the UK. The impact of physician-assisted suicide or euthanasia in countries where it has become legal is the subject of much research.

Ongoing research

There is increased focus on research into the supportive needs of patients during oncological treatment. In addition, the importance of treatments on overall quality of life is being recognised as well as the importance of early referral to palliative care for patients with advanced stage disease (Temel *et al.*, 2010).

References

Baines, M. J. (1997). ABC of palliative care: nausea, vomiting, and intestinal obstruction. *Br. Med. J.*, **315**, 1148–1150.

Barraclough, J. (1997). ABC of palliative care: depression, anxiety, and confusion. *Br. Med. J.*, **315**, 1365–1368.

Breitbart, W., Marotta, R., Platt, M. M., *et al.* (1996). A double-blind trial of haloperidol, chlorpromazine, and lorazepam in the treatment of delirium in hospitalized AIDS patients. *Am. J. Psych.*, **153**, 231–237.

Candy, B., Jackson K. C., Jones, L., *et al.* (2012). Drug therapy for symptoms associated with anxiety in adult palliative care patients. *Cochrane Database of Systematic Reviews 2012, Issue 10.* Chichester: John Wiley and Sons.

Candy, B., Jones, L., Larkin, P. J., *et al.* (2015) Laxative for the management of constipation in people receiving palliative care. *Cochrane Database of Systematic Reviews 2015. Issue 5.*

Cathcart, F. (2006). Psychological distress in patients with advanced cancer. *Clin. Med.*, **6**, 148–150.

Endicott, J. (1984). Measurement of depression in patients with cancer. *Cancer*, **53**, 2243–2249.

Fallon, M. and McConnell, S. (2006). The principles of cancer pain management. *Clin. Med.*, **6**, 136–139.

Glare, P., Pereira, G., Kristjanson, L. J., *et al.* (2004). Systematic review of the efficacy of antiemetics in the treatment of nausea in patients with far-advanced cancer. *Support. Care Cancer*, **12**, 432–440.

Greer, S., Moorey, S., Baruch, J. D., *et al.* (1992). Adjuvant psychological therapy for patients with cancer: a prospective randomized trial. *Br. Med. J.*, **304**, 675–680.

Hall, E. J. and Sykes, N. P. (2004). Analgesia for patients with advanced disease: 1. *Postgrad. Med. J.*, **80**, 148–154.

Lawlor, P. G., Fainsinger, R. L. and Bruera, E. D. (2000). Delirium at the end of life: critical issues in clinical practice and research. *J. Am. Med. Ass.*, **284**, 2427–2429.

Lloyd-Williams, M., Friedman, T. and Rudd, N. (1999). A survey of antidepressant prescribing in the terminally ill. *Pall. Med.*, **13**, 243–248.

Lloyd-Williams, M., Spiller, J. and Ward, J. (2003). Which depression screening tools should be used in palliative care? *Pall. Med.*, **17**, 40–43.

Mannix, K. (2006). Palliation of nausea and vomiting in malignancy. *Clin. Med.*, **6**, 144–147.

Meyer, T. J. and Mark, M. M. (1995). Effects of psychosocial interventions with adult cancer patients: a meta-analysis of randomized experiments. *Health Psychol.*, **14**, 101–108.

Rhodes, V. A. and McDaniel, R. W. (2001). Nausea, vomiting, and retching: complex problems in palliative care. *CA Cancer J. Clin.*, **51**, 232–248. Erratum in: *CA Cancer J. Clin.*, 51, 320.

Royal College of Physicians. (2000). *Principles of Pain Control in Palliative Care for Adults. Working Party Report.* London: Royal College of Physicians.

Temel, J. S., Greer, J. A., Muzikansky, A., *et al.* (2010). Early palliative care for patients with metastatic non-small-cell lung cancer. *N. Engl. J. Med.*, **363**, 733–742.

World Health Organisation. (1990). *Cancer Pain Relief and Palliative Care.* WHO Technical Report Series, 804. Geneva: World Health Organisation.

Further reading

Department of Constitutional Affairs (DCA). (2007) *Mental Capacity Act 2005 Code of Practice (2007 Final Edition)* London: The Stationary Office.

Watson, M., Lucas, C., Hoy, A., *et al.* (2005). *Oxford Handbook of Palliative Care.* Oxford: Oxford Medical University Press.

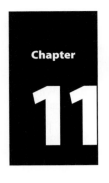

Chapter

11

Management of cancer of the head and neck

Nachi Palaniappan, Waheeda Owadally and Mererid Evans

Introduction

This chapter focuses on the practical aspects of managing tumours arising in the head and neck region and highlights the principles of treatment. The major sites with respective subsites are detailed in Table 11.1. Tumours arising from the thyroid gland and skin of the head and neck region are addressed in Chapters 38 and 36.

Epidemiology and aetiology of head and neck cancers

The incidence of head and neck cancer in the UK is increasing, predominantly due to an increase in oropharyngeal cancers, with approximately 8800 new cases diagnosed in 2010; the crude incidence rate was 14/100,000 in males and 7/100,000 in females. Almost half of all cancers are diagnosed in patients between 45 and 64 years of age (Cancer Research UK, 2010).

The major risk factors for head and neck squamous cell carcinomas (HNSCC) in the UK are tobacco smoking and alcohol consumption. Viral infections have an established relationship with head and neck cancers, including Epstein Barr virus (EBV) and human papilloma virus (HPV). EBV is associated with the pathogenesis of nasopharyngeal carcinoma, and HPV infection is most commonly associated with oropharyngeal carcinoma (tonsils and tongue base), mostly in the middle-aged population who are non/minimal users of tobacco and alcohol. Fewer than 5% of tumours of oral cavity and larynx are associated with HPV.

The other less-common risk factors include: wood dust (adenocarcinoma of nasal cavity and paranasal sinus); nitrosamines (nasopharyngeal carcinoma); poor oral hygiene and periodontal disease; genetic factors (Fanconi anaemia); and betel nut chewing, which

Table 11.1 Major sites and subsites of the head and neck

Major site	Subsites
Oral cavity	Lips, buccal mucosa, anterior tongue, floor of mouth, hard palate, upper and lower gingiva/alveolus and retromolar trigone
Pharynx	Nasopharynx
	Oropharynx – tonsil, tongue base, soft palate, vallecula and posterior pharyngeal wall
	Hypopharynx – pyriform fossa, post cricoid and posterior pharyngeal wall below the level of hyoid
Larynx	Supraglottis, glottis and subglottis
Nasal cavity	Septum, lateral wall, floor and vestibule
Paranasal sinuses	Maxillary, frontal, sphenoid and ethmoid
Salivary glands	Major (parotid, submandibular, sublingual) and minor salivary glands

is common in South Asian countries and increases the risk of oral cavity cancers.

Anatomy

Anatomical details relevant to radiotherapy planning will be covered in the subsite sections. This section will focus on the lymph node levels in the neck.

The consensus guidelines for delineating the neck node levels for radiation treatment incorporate all

---

Practical Clinical Oncology, Second Edition, ed. Louise Hanna, Tom Crosby and Fergus Macbeth. Published by Cambridge University Press. © Cambridge University Press 2015.

Table 11.2 Boundaries of cervical lymph node levels

Level	Cranial	Caudal	Anterior	Posterior	Lateral	Medial
Ia Submental LN	Mylo-hyoid m.	Caudal edge of ant. belly of digastric m.	Symphysis menti	Body of hyoid bone/mylo-hyoid m.	Medial edge of ant. belly of digastric m.	n.a.
Ib Submandibular LN	Cranial edge of submandibular gland; anteriorly mylo-hyoid m.	Caudal edge of hyoid/mandible/submandibular gland, whichever is lower	Symphysis menti	Posterior edge of submandibular gland (caudally) and posterior belly of digastric m. (cranially)	Medial aspect of mandible up to lower border and then platysma m and medial pterygoid m. (posteriorly)	Lateral edge of ant. belly of digastric m. (caudally)/post. belly of digastric m. (cranially)
II Upper jugular group	Caudal edge of lateral process of C1	Caudal edge of the body of hyoid bone	Posterior edge of submandibular gland (caudally) and posterior belly of digastric m. (cranially)	Posterior edge of sternocleidomastoid m.	Deep (medial) surface of sternocleido-mastoid m/platysma m/parotid gland/post belly of digastric m.	Medial edge of internal carotid artery/scalenius m.
III Mid jugular group	Caudal edge of the body of hyoid bone	Caudal edge of cricoid cartilage	Ant. edge of sterno-cleido-mastoid m/posterior third of thyro-hyoid m.	Posterior edge of sternocleidomastoid m.	Deep (medial) surface of sternocleido-mastoid m.	Medial edge of common carotid artery/scalenius m.
IVa Lower jugular group	Caudal edge of cricoid cartilage	2 cm cranial to sternal manubrium	Anterior edge of sternocleido-mastoid m. (cranially)/body of sternocleido-mastoid m. (caudally)	Posterior edge of sternocleido-mastoid m. (cranially)/scalenius mm (caudally)	Deep (medial) surface of sternocleido-mastoid m. (cranially)/lateral edge of sternocleidomastoid m. (caudally)	Medial edge of common carotid artery/lateral edge of thyroid gland/scalenius mm (cranially)/medial edge of sternocleido-mastoid m. (caudally)
IVb Medial supraclavicular group	Caudal border of level IVa (2 cm cranial to sternal manubrium)	Cranial edge of sternal manubrium	Deep surface of sternocleido-mastoid m./deep aspect of clavicle	Anterior edge of scalenius m. (cranially)/apex of lung, the brachio-cephalic vein, the brachio-cephalic trunk (right side) and the common carotid artery and subclavian artery on the left side (caudally)	Lateral border of scalenius m.	Lateral border of level VI (pre-tracheal component)/medial edge of common carotid artery
V (Va and Vb) posterior triangle group	Cranial edge of the body of hyoid bone	Plane just below transverse cervical vessels	Posterior edge of sternocleido-mastoid m.	Anterior border of trapezius m.	Platysma m./skin	Levator scapulae m./scalenius m. (caudally)

Table 11.2 (cont.)

Level	Cranial	Caudal	Anterior	Posterior	Lateral	Medial
Vc Lateral supraclavicular group	Plane just below transverse cervical vessels (caudal border of level V)	2 cm cranial to sternal manubrium, i.e. caudal border of level IVa	Skin	Anterior border of trapezius m. (cranially)/±1 cm anterior to serratus anterior m. (caudally)	Trapezius m (cranially)/clavicle (caudally)	Scalenius m./lateral edge of sternocleido-mastoid m, lateral edge of level IVa
VIIa Retropharyngeal nodes	Upper edge of body of C1/hard palate	Cranial edge of the body of the hyoid bone	Posterior edge of the superior or middle pharyngeal constrictor m.	Longus capitis m. and longus colli m.	Medial edge of the internal carotid artery	A line parallel to the lateral edge of the longus capiti muscle
VIIb Retrostyloid nodes	Base of skull (jugular foramen)	Caudal edge of the lateral process of C1 (upper limit of level II)	Posterior edge of prestyloid para-pharyngeal space	Vertebral body of C1, base of skull	Styloid process/deep parotid lobe	Medial edge of the internal carotid artery
VIII Parotid group	Zygomatic arch, external auditory canal	Angle of the mandible	Posterior edge of mandibular ramus and posterior edge of masseter m. (laterally) medial pterygoid muscle (medially)	Anterior edge of sternocleido-mastoid m. (laterally), posterior Belly of digastric m. (medially)	SMAS layer in subcutaneous tissue	Styloid process and styloid m.
IX Bucco-facial group	Caudal edge of the orbit	Caudal edge of the mandible	SMAS layer in subcutaneous tissue	Anterior edge of masseter m. and corpus adiposum buccae (Bichat's fat pad)	SMAS layer in subcutaneous tissue	Buccinator m.
Xa Retroauricular nodes	Cranial edge of external auditory canal	Tip of the mastoid	Anterior edge of the mastoid (caudally)/posterior edge of the external auditory canal (cranially)	Anterior border of occipital nodes – posterior edge of sternocleido-mastoid m.	Subcutaneous tissue	Splenius capitis m. (caudally)/temporal bone (cranially)
Xb Occipital nodes	External occipital protuberance	Cranial border of level V	Posterior edge of sternocleido-mastoid m.	Anterior (lateral) edge of trapezius m.	Subcutaneous tissue	Splenius capitis m.

m., muscle; SMAS, superficial musculo-aponeurotic system. Adapted from Grégoire et al., 2014.

nodes in the head and neck region (superficial and deep) without anatomic differentiation and classify them into ten levels (Grégoire *et al.*, 2014). Some levels are further divided into sublevels. Level II is subdivided into IIa and IIb by an artificial horizontal line at the posterior edge of the internal jugular vein. Level IVb (medial supraclavicular group) and level Vc (lateral supraclavicular group) together constitute the supraclavicular fossa (SCF). Level VIII, IX and X lymph nodes are most commonly involved by tumours arising in the skin of the head and neck region or if the skin is involved by cancers of the head and neck.

The boundaries of each lymph node level are described in relation to the cross-sectional anatomy to facilitate accurate delineation and are detailed as per the consensus guidelines in Table 11.2.

Pathology of head and neck cancer

Premalignant conditions

Leukoplakia, erythroplakia and dysplasia graded as mild, moderate and severe are common premalignant lesions seen in head and neck. Severe dysplasia is also known as carcinoma *in situ* (CIS). Leukoplakia and erythroplakia are commonly seen in the oral cavity; epithelial dysplasia is demonstrated in 25% of biopsies of leukoplakia and in most cases of erythroplakia. Dysplasia can occur in most subsites of the head and neck. Systematic reviews of oral (992 patients) and laryngeal (942 patients) dysplasia showed malignant transformation in 12.1% and 14% after a mean interval of 4.3 and 5.8 years, respectively (Mehanna *et al.*, 2009; Weller *et al.*, 2010).

Benign and malignant tumours

The common benign pathologies include: pleomorphic adenoma of salivary glands; hemangioma; glomus tumour; juvenile angiofibroma (commonly seen in the nasopharynx in the adolescent age group); ameloblastoma (commonly arising from the mandible) and chondromas.

Squamous cell carcinoma (SCC) is the commonest malignancy constituting over 90% of cancers arising from the mucosal lining of the head and neck. Other malignant tumours include:

- adenocarcinoma (of unknown origin);
- tumours of the salivary gland: adenocarcinoma, mucoepidermoid carcinoma; adenoid cystic carcinoma; acinic cell carcinoma;

- mucosal melanoma;
- neuroendocrine carcinoma including olfactory neuroblastoma mostly arising from the nasal cavity and Merkel cell carcinoma arising from the skin;
- lymphoma (Hodgkin and non-Hodgkin);
- sarcoma (soft tissue sarcoma including Kaposi's and rhabdomyosarcoma; osteosarcoma; chondrosarcoma);
- metastatic deposits in cervical lymph nodes (breast, prostate, lung, renal cell carcinoma, melanoma of skin, thyroid and from the gastrointestinal tract).

Natural history of head and neck cancer

Head and neck cancers spread locally to involve adjacent subsites involving soft tissues, muscles, nerves and bone leading to destruction and loss of function. Tumours can spread through lymphatics to regional lymph nodes on one or both sides of the neck, depending upon the site of primary. Lateralised tumours (e.g. buccal mucosa, tonsil, lateral border of tongue) generally metastasise to ipsilateral lymph nodes in the neck, while tumours arising from midline structures (tongue base, soft palate, pharyngeal wall) can metastasise to both sides of the neck. Distant metastasis is generally less common and occurs via the blood stream to the lungs, liver and bone either at presentation (less than 10%) or after definitive treatment (15–20%).

Clinical presentation of head and neck cancer

The most common presenting symptom is a painless neck mass with or without other symptoms relating to the site of the primary. Site-specific symptoms are detailed under each subsite. Systemic symptoms are uncommon at presentation, but may be due to metastatic disease and include weight loss, failure to thrive, bone pain and rarely hypercalcemia-related symptoms.

Clinical examination in head and neck cancer

Examination includes inspection, palpation and assessment of the local extent of disease using either an indirect laryngoscope or flexible nasendoscope. A systematic approach is advised.

Start the examination by inspecting the oral cavity (gums, floor of mouth, tongue) and oropharynx and pay specific attention to assess the mucosal extent of disease (e.g. in a tonsil tumour, assess the involvement of the anterior pillar, soft palate, glosso-tonsillar sulcus and how close to midline the extent of disease is). With the aid of a flexible nasendoscope, examine the nasal cavity, nasopharynx, oropharynx, hypopharynx and larynx for abnormal lumps, mucosal irregularity, pooling of secretions and bleeding. Assess vocal cord movement, involvement of the anterior commissure and subglottic extension in all laryngeal and hypopharyngeal tumours. The extent of involvement of the tongue base is best assessed by digital palpation. Complete the examination by palpating the neck to assess neck node involvement. Most patients undergo examination under anaesthesia to assess the extent of disease, to look for second primaries at other sites and biopsy to confirm the diagnosis.

Investigations in head and neck cancer: general considerations

The following investigations are recommended to diagnose and assess the extent of disease in most patients.

- Ultrasound of the neck.
- Fine-needle aspiration cytology (FNAC) of abnormal neck nodes with or without ultrasound guidance has high sensitivity and specificity (94% and 97%, respectively) for diagnosing pathologically involved nodes (Tandon et al., 2008). FNAC of neck nodes is mostly done under ultrasound guidance.
- Contrast-enhanced CT scan of head and neck region to assess the local extent of disease. Bone involvement is best assessed using CT.
- MRI scan of the craniofacial region provides better soft tissue definition compared to CT and is most useful in patients with dental amalgam due to the artefacts on CT scan and in patients where there is skull base involvement, as it provides information regarding perineural invasion and intracranial extension. MRI also helps to differentiate tumour from mucous membrane and bone marrow involvement.
- CT scan of chest to assess for distant metastasis.
- PET-CT: ^{18}F-FDG PET-CT is not routinely used in the UK for staging purposes. All patients with metastatic squamous cancer in cervical neck nodes with no obvious primary on clinical and radiological (CT and MRI) examination should undergo a PET-CT scan to identify the possible site of the primary. Other indications include assessment of possible tumour recurrence where conventional imaging fails to differentiate between tumour and fibrosis.

Staging in head and neck cancer: general principles

The AJCC Cancer Staging Manual, seventh edition, is currently used to stratify tumours in the head and neck region. This takes into account the size and extent of primary tumour (T); involvement of regional lymph node (N) and the presence or absence of distant metastasis (M) (AJCC, 2009).

Primary tumour (T): the size of the primary tumour along with extent is taken into account only in oral cavity, oropharynx, hypopharynx and major salivary gland tumours. The T stage for the rest of the subsites of the head and neck is primarily based on the extent of the disease. The details of the T stage are described in the respective subsites. There is no subclassification of T4 in nasopharynx into T4a and T4b.

Regional nodes (N): nodal staging for all sites in the head and neck region are similar apart from the nasopharynx, as shown in Table 11.3.

Distant metastasis (M): stratified according to the presence (M1) or absence (M0) of distant metastasis.

Stage grouping also remains similar for all sites in the head and neck region apart from the nasopharynx, as shown in Table 11.4.

Treatment overview for head and neck cancer

The choice of treatment depends on a number of patient, tumour and treatment factors, the aim being to maximise the chance of cure/local control and minimise the resulting functional compromise.

- Patient factors: age, performance status, comorbidity and patient's choice/preference.
- Tumour factors: site of primary, stage and pathology.
- Treatment factors: morbidity associated with treatment, functional outcome, cosmetic result and local resource and expertise.

Table 11.3 Nodal staging of head and neck cancers

N stage	All sites – description	Nasopharynx – description
N1	Ipsilateral single node ≤ 3 cm	Unilateral metastasis in lymph nodes above SCF, all ≤ 6 cm; and/or unilateral or bilateral retropharyngeal nodes all ≤ 6 cm
N2	N2a – Ipsilateral single node > 3 cm and ≤ 6 cm	Bilateral lymph nodes above SCF all ≤ 6 cm
	N2b – Ipsilateral multiple lymph nodes, all ≤ 6 cm	–
	N2c – Bilateral or contralateral lymph nodes all ≤ 6 cm	–
N3	Nodes > 6 cm	N3a – Nodes > 6cm
		N3b – Extension to the SCF

SCF, supraclavicular fossa. Adapted from AJCC, 2009.

Table 11.4 Stage groupings for head and neck cancers

Stage group	All sites			Nasopharynx		
	T	N	M	T	N	M
Stage 0	Tis	N0	M0	Tis	N0	M0
Stage I	T1	N0	M0	T1	N0	M0
Stage II	T2	N0	M0	T2	N0	M0
				T1–2	N1	M0
Stage III	T3	N0	M0	T3	N0–N2	M0
	T1-3	N1	M0	T1–2	N2	M0
Stage IVA	T4a	N0–N2	M0	T4	N0–N2	M0
	T1–3	N2	M0			
Stage IVB	T4b	Any N	M0			
	Any T	N3	M0	Any T	N3	M0
Stage IVC	Any T	Any N	M1	Any T	Any N	M1

Adapted from AJCC, 2009.

In general, patients with early-stage (I and II) disease should be managed with a single modality treatment, either surgery or radiotherapy and those with advanced stage (III, IVA and IVB) disease managed with multi-modality treatment with the aim of organ and function preservation.

Patients with metastatic, local and/or regional recurrent disease are considered for palliative chemotherapy and/or best supportive care. Patients with recurrent disease confined to the head and neck region may benefit from salvage surgery and/or re-irradiation and will depend upon a number of factors.

Role of surgery in head and neck cancer

Surgery plays a key role in the management of both primary head and neck cancers and neck nodes. The main aim of surgery is to achieve complete microscopic clearance of tumour with appropriate margins according to type, site and stage of cancer. One of the most important recent advances in the surgical field is the use of transoral laser microsurgery (TLM) and transoral robotic surgery (TORS) to resect primary tumours.

Table 11.5 Neck dissections for head and neck cancer management

Category	Type of neck dissection	Structures removed
Comprehensive	Radical neck dissection	Lymph nodes in levels I–V, accessory nerve, internal jugular vein and sternocleido-mastoid muscle
	Modified radical neck dissection	Lymph nodes in levels I–V, and preservation of one or more of the accessory nerve, internal jugular vein and sternocleido-mastoid muscle (Type I, II and III, respectively)
	Extended radical neck dissection	Removal of one or more additional lymphatic and/or non-lymphatic structures relative to radical neck dissection, e.g. spinal muscles due to involvement; lingual or hypoglossal nerve or other lymph node levels apart from level I–V
Selective	Supra-omohyoid neck dissection	Nodes in levels I–III; also called extended when level IV is included, mostly done in oral cavity cancers
	Lateral neck dissection	Nodes in levels II–IV
	Central compartment dissection	Nodes in level VI, mostly done in thyroid cancers

Surgery for primary tumours generally involves wide local excision with or without reconstruction to close the defect. Minimal access techniques (TLM or TORS) are most commonly employed for early-stage oropharyngeal and glottic/supraglottic tumours and can also be used for advanced-stage disease in selected patients. Patient selection remains crucial and depends on factors such as access to surgery, need for adjuvant treatment, local expertise and availability of resources.

The details of surgical management of various subsites are discussed in the relevant sections and for neck nodes are discussed in detail in the next section.

Management of neck nodes

The management of the neck can be broadly considered for the node-negative (clinically and radiologically uninvolved neck nodes) and node-positive neck (clinically and/or radiologically involved neck nodes) for all subsites in head and neck.

Management of the node-negative neck

The optimal management is debated constantly and the options include either prophylactic selective neck dissection/radiation or observation, with the option of therapeutic neck dissection in patients who develop disease subsequently.

The agreed level of risk in the head and neck community beyond which all node negative necks are treated is 15–20%, based on risk–benefit analysis in the late 1970s, whereby the morbidity associated with radical neck dissection was considered to outweigh the benefit for patients with risk of neck node involvement of less than 20%.

Local control rates achieved by prophylactic surgery or prophylactic radiation to neck nodes are similar. When observation is chosen, patients should be on regular ultrasound surveillance to ensure early detection.

Surgery involves removal of nodes at all levels (I to V) in the neck either on one or both sides and is influenced by the site of primary and presence or absence of neck node metastases. A comprehensive neck dissection is usually done for a node-positive neck and a selective neck dissection for a node-negative neck. The common types of neck dissections are detailed in Table 11.5.

Management of the node-positive neck

This depends upon the stage of neck disease and is influenced by the treatment of choice for the primary. For early-stage (N1) neck disease, single modality treatment is sufficient and is often the same as that used to treat the primary site.

Neck nodes larger than 3 cm or multiple lymph nodes (N2a and above) may require combined modality treatment due to increased risk of recurrence associated with either surgery or radiotherapy alone and is influenced by the treatment of choice for the primary tumour. The options are either a modified radical neck dissection along with resection of primary followed by adjuvant treatment depending on histology or chemoradiotherapy along with the primary followed by a surveillance PET CT scan at 10 to 12 weeks post completion of treatment and neck dissection only in patients with equivocal or persistent uptake in neck node/s as per the UK PET Neck randomised study results, presented at ASCO 2015 (Mehanna *et al.*, 2015). This approach has shown to result in similar survival rates and less morbidity. It is cost effective compared with routine planned neck dissection and is likely to become the standard of care for this group of patients.

Role of radiotherapy in head and neck cancer

Radiotherapy is used with or without chemotherapy in approximately 60–70% of patients with head and neck cancer, either as a definitive treatment or as an adjuvant treatment following surgery. The delivery of radiation treatment has improved significantly in the last decade due to advances in technology, leading to improved local control and reduced late morbidity, particularly xerostomia. The most commonly used forms of radiation in the head and neck are high-energy photons and electrons. Protons are used rarely for treatment of skull base lesions in order to limit dose to critical normal structures.

Radiotherapy pretreatment evaluation

All patients for radical radiotherapy should undergo the following assessments before starting treatment.

- Dental assessment: dentulous patients should have a dental assessment (orthopantomogram (OPT) and a review) if their upper or lower jaw is likely to be in the radiation field. Dental treatment, particularly extraction, should be done prior to the start of radiotherapy (ideally two weeks before) to reduce the risk of osteoradionecrosis.
- Nutritional assessment: most patients should be reviewed by the dietetic team prior to the start of treatment; those with significant weight loss (> 10%) should be started on supplement feeding prior to the start of treatment. Patients planned for curative intent radiotherapy/chemoradiotherapy are assessed for the need for a feeding tube to support their nutritional requirements during and after treatment. The choice between feeding gastrostomy tube (proactive or reactive) or

nasogastric tube depends upon each centre's preference, expertise and availability of resources.
- Speech and swallowing assessment: most patients should be assessed by the speech therapist prior to the start of treatment for baseline speech and swallowing function. Patients are educated on proactive swallowing exercise and are advised to repeat the exercise daily (2 or 3 times) prior to and during treatment in an attempt to minimise swallowing difficulties both in the short and long term.

Radiotherapy energy, fractionation and dose

Radiation treatment is given to cure or control disease and/or symptoms. The dose and fractionation vary with the intent and also between different institutions. The commonly used dose fractionation regimens are detailed below according to the intent of treatment.

Energy

Photons with energies in the range of 4–6 MV are typically used. Electrons are used for lateralised and superficial lesions; energy depends upon the depth of the lesion and varies from 4 to 20 MeV.

Kilovoltage X-rays (90–300 KV) are used to treat superficial skin lesions and or fungating neck nodes with skin involvement in a palliative setting.

Fractionation

The current standard is conventional fractionation with a dose of 1.8–2.2 Gy per fraction given 5 days a week. Several altered fractionation regimens have been studied in head and neck cancer, most commonly hyperfractionation and accelerated fractionation. A meta-analysis of altered fractionation in head and neck cancer showed improved overall survival of 2% and 8% at 5 years for accelerated and hyperfractionation, respectively (Bourhis *et al.*, 2006). Despite this, these regimens have not been widely accepted. There are no trials that have directly compared hyperfractionated radiotherapy with concurrent chemotherapy and conventional radiotherapy with concurrent chemotherapy, the current standard of care for locoregionally advanced tumours. The addition of chemotherapy concurrently with accelerated fractionation showed no

Table 11.6 Examples of radical dose fractionation regimens for the treatment of head and neck cancers

Prescription dose and fractionation	Number of dose levels	Dose and fractionation	Regions included
66/30	2	66/30	Primary and involved node (GTV) + 1 cm margin and all involved nodal levels – radical dose
		54/30	Low-risk regions (uninvolved nodal levels at risk of involvement) – treated to prophylactic dose
	3	66/30	Primary and involved node (GTV) + 1 cm margin and all involved nodal levels – radical dose
		60/30	High-risk regions adjacent to gross disease (e.g. involved nodal levels; including entire oropharynx when the tumour is at one subsite (tongue base))
		54/30	Low-risk regions (uninvolved nodal levels at risk of involvement) – treated to prophylactic dose
70/35	2	70/35	Primary and involved node (GTV) + 1 cm margin and all involved nodal levels – radical dose
		56/35	Low-risk regions (uninvolved nodal levels at risk of involvement) – treated to prophylactic dose
	3	70/35	Primary and involved node (GTV) + 1 cm margin and all involved nodal levels – radical dose
		60/35	High-risk regions adjacent to gross disease (e.g. involved nodal levels; including entire oropharynx when the tumour is at one subsite (tongue base))
		56/35	Low-risk regions (uninvolved nodal levels at risk of involvement) – treated to prophylactic dose

difference in overall survival when compared with conventional radiotherapy with concurrent chemotherapy (Ang *et al.*, 2010).

Moderate acceleration using DAHANCA regimen of 6 fractions per week with a total dose in 70 Gy given over 6 weeks showed a 12% improvement of local control at the primary site and 7% improvement in disease-specific survival with no improvement in overall survival and was associated with increased acute toxicity (Overgaard *et al.*, 2003).

Dose

Curative/radical intent

Most patients are treated with curative intent either with radiotherapy alone or in combination with chemotherapy/targeted agents. The following dose fractionation regimens are typical examples of curative intent that applies to all subsites.

- 65–66 Gy in 30# over 6 weeks,
- 70 Gy in 35# over 7 weeks.

Shorter fractionation regimens are used when the irradiated volume is small. Typical fractionation schedules include:

- 55 Gy in 20# over 4 weeks,
- 50 Gy in 15# over 3 weeks.

Currently, most centres use a simultaneous integrated boost technique to treat head and neck cancers, where multiple dose levels are delivered to different regions in a single phase. Normally two or three dose levels are used to treat different regions. Examples of 2- and 3-dose level radical intent dose fractionation regimens are given in Table 11.6.

Palliative intent

Patients are treated with palliative intent mostly due to poor performance status and/or advanced inoperable disease where a cure is not possible. There is no agreed consensus regarding dose and fractionation. Typical palliative dose fractionation regimens include:

- 20 Gy in 5# over 1 week,

Table 11.7 Pathological risk factors for recurrence following head and neck cancer surgery

Factor	Intermediate-risk factors	High-risk factors
Primary tumour factors	Advanced tumour (T) stage (T3/T4) Close margin (defined as tumour present < 5 mm and > 1 mm from resection margin) Perineural invasion Lymphovascular space invasion	Positive margin (defined as tumour present at or < 1 mm from resection margin)
Lymph node factors	Two or more positive lymph nodes Nodes greater than 3 cm Multiple lymph node level involvement	Extracapsular spread (ECS) of nodal disease

- 30 Gy in 10# over 2 week,
- 40 Gy in 15# over 3 weeks,
- 30 Gy in 5–6# over 5–6 weeks depending on the patient's tolerance, for patients who are unable to attend daily for treatment.

Some patients with very advanced disease (T4b) but with good performance status are treated to curative doses, but the intent is control of disease rather than cure.

Adjuvant/postoperative radiotherapy

The aim of adjuvant radiotherapy is to improve locoregional control and survival following surgical resection. The addition of radiotherapy following surgery compared with surgery alone has shown improved locoregional control rates (Mishra *et al.*, 1996; Lavaf *et al.*, 2008). Studies have identified a number of primary tumour and lymph node pathological features which are associated with increased risk of locoregional recurrence; these may be classified as 'intermediate' and 'high' risk features as shown in Table 11.7.

Most centres in the UK currently use a total dose of 60 Gy in 30 fractions given over 6 weeks. A boost dose (typically of 5–6 Gy) is used at some centres in patients with either positive primary tumour margins and/or extracapsular spread (ECS) of nodal disease. Adjuvant radiotherapy should start within 5 weeks of surgery, as overall treatment time from the date of surgery to completion of adjuvant radiotherapy (< 11 weeks versus > 13 weeks) has been shown to reduce local control from 76% to 38% (Ang *et al.*, 2001).

Concurrent cisplatin with postoperative radiotherapy showed 12% and 10% improvement in locoregional control, 11% and 9% improvement in disease-free survival for patients with positive margins and/or extracapsular extension, respectively, compared with postoperative radiotherapy alone. Combined analysis also confirmed an improvement in overall survival. There was a significant increase in acute mucosal toxicity (77% versus 34%), but late toxicity was similar in both groups (Bernier *et al.*, 2004; Cooper *et al.*, 2004).

Postoperative concurrent chemoradiotherapy with cisplatin is now the current standard of care for patients with high-risk features (positive margin and ECS) and good performance status. Carboplatin may be used instead if cisplatin is contraindicated. Patients with intermediate-risk factors are treated with postoperative radiotherapy alone. An ongoing phase III study (RTOG 0920) is evaluating the benefit of cetuximab in the adjuvant setting, but currently this has not been established.

Radiotherapy planning

This section focuses on immobilisation, target volume delineation and planning common to all subsites.

Immobilisation

Patients with head and neck tumours require custom-made thermoplastic immobilisation shells in a reproducible position for accurate radiotherapy delivery. Prior to this, the following need to be considered:

- Mouth bite: a spacer device to limit/minimise unnecessary radiation to adjacent normal structures used when treating oral cavity, nasal cavity and maxillary sinus tumours.
- Bolus: required when skin and superficial tissue need to be treated to prescription dose.
- Skin marking: to identify the extent of scar or when treating skin lesions usually with the aid of a lead wire that can be visualised on the planning CT scan.

141

Patients lie supine with appropriate head rest and knee support. A five-point immobilisation system is normally used which includes head, neck and both shoulders. The position of the chin is normally neutral and the shoulders are kept as low as possible. Patients undergo a planning CT scan in the treatment position with the thermoplastic shell usually with intravenous contrast to aid accurate delineation of targets. CT slice thickness varies between 2 and 4 mm.

Target volume delineation

Target delineation requires a detailed knowledge of cross-sectional anatomy. With the use of multiple dose levels to treat different regions, it is important to name each volume according to an agreed departmental protocol. The delineation process can be staged in five steps both in the definitive and postoperative setting. The steps detailed here are for two dose levels, CTV1 (high dose) and CTV2 (prophylactic dose).

Target delineation in the primary/definitive setting

Step 1: Delineate gross tumour volume (GTV)

This includes outlining both primary tumour (GTVp) and all involved nodes (GTVn). The primary is outlined with the knowledge of all available information (diagnostic imaging (CT, MRI and PET-CT if available) and clinical examination findings including pan endoscopy, the best modality to assess the mucosal extent of disease.

Co-registration of diagnostic images (CT, MRI or PET-CT) with planning CT aids in delineating the GTV accurately.

Step 2: Delineate clinical target volume (CTV1)

This CTV includes the GTVp and GTVn with a 1 cm isotropic expansion in all directions, adjacent high-risk regions and whole involved nodal level(s) in the neck and is delineated using the following steps.

- Add a 1 cm isotropic margin in all directions to GTV primary and GTV nodes. A 1.5 cm margin may be used around poorly defined primary tumours (e.g. in the tongue base).
- Edit out natural tissue planes (bone, air cavities and fasciae).
- Include the entire involved nodal level(s) according to the consensus guidelines as in Table 11.3.
- CTV1 may be extended to include adjacent high-risk regions (e.g. parapharyngeal spaces; remaining oropharynx/larynx, etc.) if an

Table 11.8 Prophylactic neck irradiation for head and neck cancers

Level involved	Levels to include in prophylactic dose
Any level (I to IVa)	Level Va and Vb
II	Ib and VII b (retrostyloid nodes)
IVa and/or V (Va and Vb)	IVb (medial supraclavicular group) and Vc (lateral supraclavicular group)

anatomical approach to outlining is used. Alternatively, these regions can be included in CTV2 and/or can be omitted altogether if a purely geometric (or volumetric) approach to outlining is used.

Step 3: Delineate elective clinical target volume (CTV2)

This volume varies with the site of the primary and the status of the neck and usually consists of uninvolved at-risk nodal levels in the neck (unilateral or bilateral) to be treated to a prophylactic dose. Levels Ib to Vb are irradiated in most node-positive cases and other lymph node levels are included in CTV2 depending on which nodal level(s) are involved, as shown in Table 11.8. In a node-negative neck, selective neck irradiation is considered when the risk of involvement is more than 15–20% and usually includes level II–IV in most subsites, but can vary with site of primary.

Step 4: Delineate organs at risk (OAR)

The OARs are classified as serial and parallel organs. Serial organs such as spinal cord and brainstem are routinely outlined in all head and neck tumours with others (optic chiasm, optic nerves) outlined as required depending upon the site of the primary and the extent of treatment fields. Parallel organs such as parotids and mandible are routinely outlined with other areas/structures (oral cavity, larynx, oesophagus, lacrimal gland, retina) on a patient-by-patient basis.

Step 5: Create planning target volume (PTV) and planning risk volume (PRV)

The PTV/PRV is generated geometrically by the planning system and the margin used varies from centre to centre to ensure adequate CTV coverage. The magnitude of this volume depends upon accuracy of the immobilisation systems, day-to-day set-up

Table 11.9 Radiation dose constraints for organs at risk

OAR	Dose	Endpoint
Spinal cord PRV	Max 48 Gy	Myelopathy
Brainstem PRV	Max 54 Gy	Necrosis
Optic nerve PRV	Max 50 Gy	Neuropathy
Optic chiasm PRV	Max 50 Gy	Visual loss
Retina PRV	Max 45 Gy	Scotomas/visual field loss
Lens PRV	Max 8 Gy	Cataract
Parotid gland	Mean < 26 Gy	> Grade 2 xerostomia

variation and is normally between 3 and 5 mm, grown isotropically in all directions. Each CTV is grown to create respective PTV and all serial OAR are grown to create respective planning risk volume (PRV).

Target delineation in the postoperative setting

The following steps are a guide to delineate target volumes in this setting and are based on the general principles of radiotherapy in the definitive setting. The postoperative histology report and intraoperative findings aid in outlining the at-risk regions accurately.

Step 1: Re-create preoperative primary and nodal gross tumour volume ('GTVp' and 'GTVn')

The position of the primary and involved node(s) is re-created on the planning CT scan. The accuracy of this step is improved with the aid of co-registration of diagnostic scans (CT, MRI and/or PET-CT). The volumes are labeled 'GTVp' and 'GTVn'.

- Edit 'GTVp' and 'GTVn' as necessary, based on the postoperative change in anatomy.
- Add 1- to 1.5-cm isotropic margin in all directions to 'GTVp' to create CTVp.
- Add 1-cm isotropic margin in all directions to 'GTVn' to create CTVn.

Step 2: Delineate clinical target volume (CTV1)

This clinical target volume includes the primary and nodal tumour bed with a margin and all pathologically involved nodal levels.

- Edit the volumes CTVp and CTVn for anatomical barriers such as bone, fascia and air.
- Extend CTVn to include all pathologically involved nodal levels according to the consensus guidelines.
- Extend this volume to include seromas and any other postoperative changes.

Step 3: Delineate elective clinical target volume (CTV2)

This includes all uninvolved nodal levels in the dissected neck and other at-risk nodal levels as in Table 11.9.

Steps 4 and 5 are the same as those in the definitive setting described above.

Setting objectives/constraints and order of priorities

This step is essential for inverse planning and is required to achieve an optimal plan. An objective is a parameter desired to be met where compromise may be an option, while a constraint is a parameter that must be met where compromise is not an option. A planning risk volume is added to all OARs, and priorities are individualised for each patient.

Normally constraints to serial OARs are set at the highest priority and the maximum dose to these organs cannot exceed a predetermined level, even to achieve PTV coverage (there are exceptions to this). The next priority is to achieve PTV coverage, followed by objectives for dose to the parotid gland and other OARs. On occasions, the dose to the parotid gland on the uninvolved contralateral neck is prioritised at the expense of the PTV coverage. Table 11.9 shows the dose constraints for various OARs in the head and neck region with the respective endpoints. The accepted standard level of risk is 5% complication rate at 5 years (TD-5/5).

Planning

All patients undergoing radical radiotherapy are conformally planned usually in a single phase (forward or inverse planned) and most centres in the UK now use intensity-modulated radiotherapy (IMRT) to treat a majority of curative intent head and neck cancer patients. Intensity modulation is delivered using a step

Table 11.10 PTV objectives for head and neck radiotherapy planning

Volume of PTV (%)	% Prescribed dose
99	> 90
95	> 95
50	100
5	< 105
2	< 107

and shoot technique or more recently using dynamic volumetric-modulated arc therapy (VMAT).

Table 11.10 shows an example of PTV objectives that are normally used to assess a plan quantitatively.

Radiotherapy side effects

Radiation treatment-induced reactions are divided into acute and late side effects. Acute side effects are defined as events that happen during radiotherapy or within 90 days after starting treatment. The following steps at the start of radiation treatment help to minimise the reactions.

- Avoiding sun exposure, wet shaving and perfumed soap and toiletries.
- Twice daily application of skin moisturiser to the head and neck region.
- Maintaining oral hygiene by using regular mouth wash three to four times a day.

Patients are closely monitored on a weekly basis during treatment to provide support and to grade the acute toxicities using either RTOG or common toxicity criteria (CTCAE) grading systems.

Acute radiation reactions: typically start to manifest during the third week of radiation therapy and continue to intensify as treatment progresses, with the worst reactions often seen during the week after the end of treatment.

Late radiation reactions: these occur many months to years after completion of treatment. Concurrent chemoradiotherapy is associated with significant late toxicities in 43% of patients (Machtay et al., 2008). The most common late toxicities in long-term survivors are xerostomia and swallowing dysfunction, with a small proportion experiencing trismus, subcutaneous fibrosis and osteoradionecrosis. Swallowing dysfunction has the most profound impact on long-term quality of life (Langendijk et al., 2008). A significant proportion of patients (approximately 24% at 1 year, 14% at 2 years

and 12% at 3 years) experience long-term feeding tube dependence after treatment, which has reduced considerably in the current IMRT era to less than 5% at 2 years.

Increasing treatment conformality, reducing radiotherapy dose and substituting chemotherapy with biological agents are all being investigated as ways to reduce the long-term consequences of treatment on swallowing.

Management of acute reactions

Skin: unguentum is used for the affected areas (patchy moist desquamation) while continuing with regular moisturising cream (e.g. Epaderm®) to the unaffected regions. Confluent desquamation needs a moist wound management system such as Intrasite Gel®, a topical application that helps to maintain the moisture and aids in wound debridement or alternatively a polymer dressing when there is a large area of skin ulceration.

Mucous membrane: all patients develop mucositis (oral and/or pharyngeal) during the course of radiotherapy, the severity varying from patient to patient. The management consists of:

- maintaining scrupulous oral hygiene by brushing the teeth twice with soft brush and rinsing the mouth regularly with saline;
- Caphosol® mouth rinse (calcium and phosphate ions) can prevent and reduce the duration and pain of oral mucositis;
- benzydamine mouth wash, a topical, non-steroidal anti-inflammatory drug with analgesic and anaesthetic properties to control pain;
- systemic analgesics according to the WHO pain ladder;
- topical mucoprotectant such as Gelclair®, MuGard®, Episil®;
- treat super-added infection (bacterial or fungal) if present;
- avoid smoking, alcohol and certain foods (citrus, spicy, hot and hard);
- avoid chlorhexidine mouth wash, as this may inhibit the re-growth of the mucosa.

Xerostomia: artificial saliva preparations can be used to help with this symptom (AS Saliva Orthana®, Gladosane®, Biotène® oral balance gel).

Odynophagia: analgesics according to the WHO pain ladder and the use of soft, pureed diet and supplements (given orally or via nasogastirc and/or gastrostomy tubes) to maintain nourishment during treatment.

Role of systemic therapy in head and neck cancer

Systemic therapy plays an important role in the management of HNSCC and includes chemotherapy and biotherapy, both in the curative and palliative setting.

Chemotherapy as part of radical treatment

The timing of chemotherapy in combined modality approaches may be as follows.

- Neoadjuvant or induction chemotherapy followed by radiotherapy.
- Concurrent chemoradiotherapy.
- Sequential therapy (neoadjuvant chemotherapy followed by concurrent chemoradiotherapy).

The optimal combination of chemotherapy drugs and the timing with radiation are yet to be determined. The results of the Meta-Analysis of Chemotherapy on Head and Neck Cancer (MACH-NC) updated in 2009 confirmed the following benefits (Pignon *et al.*, 2009).

- Concurrent chemoradiotherapy improved overall survival by 6.5% at 5 years compared to radiotherapy alone. A statistically significant decrease in benefit was observed with increasing age with no benefit over 70 years.
- Induction chemotherapy with cisplatin and 5-FU resulted in significant improvement in overall survival compared with local therapy alone. There was no benefit with other chemotherapy regimens.
- There was no improvement in overall survival when concurrent chemotherapy and radiotherapy were compared with induction chemotherapy followed by radiotherapy alone. However, concurrent chemoradiotherapy was more effective in preventing locoregional failure, while induction chemotherapy provided a relatively more pronounced effect on distant metastasis.
- There was no improvement in overall survival following adjuvant chemotherapy compared with definitive local therapy alone.

Chemotherapy regimens

The most common drugs with proven activity in HNSCC include cisplatin, 5-flurouracil (5-FU) and taxanes (docetaxel and paclitaxel) and are used in a combination regimen of either two (cisplatin and 5-FU) or three (cisplatin, 5-FU and docetaxel) drugs in the neoadjuvant setting.

Neoadjuvant chemotherapy

Neoadjuvant chemotherapy with three drugs (docetaxel, cisplatin and 5-FU; TPF) compared to a two drug (cisplatin and 5-FU; PF) regimen has shown improved outcomes. A meta-analysis of five studies that used taxanes (neoadjuvant) confirmed significant reductions in progression, locoregional failure, distant failure and improved overall survival compared with PF (Blanchard *et al.*, 2013). This regimen is associated with higher acute toxicity (12% experiencing neutropenic sepsis and the non-haematological toxicities include mucositis, oesophagitis, nausea and anorexia) and should be offered only to patients with good performance status with little or no comorbidity.

The benefit of TPF over PF chemotherapy prior to radical cisplatin-based concurrent chemoradiotherapy is still not fully established (see sequential therapy below).

Concurrent chemotherapy

The MACH-NC meta-analysis demonstrated a survival benefit for concurrent chemoradiotherapy compared with radiotherapy alone for all chemotherapy regimens and a greater benefit for cisplatin-based regimens.

The most common regimen used in the UK is high-dose bolus cisplatin given at 100 mg/m^2 on days 1 and 22 along with curative radiotherapy (RTOG 0129 and RTOG 91-11). This regimen is associated with significantly higher mucosal toxicity compared with radiotherapy alone (82% versus 61%) and therefore should be used only in patients with good performance status.

Other regimens include weekly cisplatin at 40 mg/m^2 for 6 weeks; carboplatin at AUC 5 on Days 1 and 22 or weekly at AUC 1.5–2 may be used in patients who are not suitable for cisplatin. None of these regimens have been compared with high-dose bolus cisplatin for efficacy, but are considered reasonable alternative options.

Sequential therapy

Based on the results of the meta-analysis, the optimal way to incorporate chemotherapy with locoregional therapy would be sequential therapy with induction chemotherapy followed by concurrent chemoradiotherapy. Studies thus far showed conflicting results with some favouring sequential therapy while others suggested no added benefit of induction therapy for a number of reasons (choice of chemotherapy regimens, trial design, and difference in patient population).

An Italian phase II/III study randomised 421 patients with locally advanced squamous cell carcinoma to induction chemotherapy with TPF followed by radiotherapy alone or concurrent chemoradiotherapy alone. The sequential therapy significantly improved survival (at 3 years, 58% versus 46%, median 54 versus 30 months) and progression-free survival (47% versus 37%, median 30 versus 19 months) compared to concurrent chemoradiotherapy alone (Ghi et al., 2014).

While the long-term outcome of these studies are still awaited, the use of sequential therapy in clinical practice should be individualised and offered to a select group of patients with good performance status (0, 1), limited or no comorbidity and high risk of locoregional and distant recurrence.

Biological treatments as part of radical treatment

Epidermal growth factor receptor (EGFR) is overexpressed in HNSCC and is associated with poor prognosis. The role of EGFR inhibitors in the management of patients with locally advanced squamous cell carcinoma has been tested (cetuximab, panitumumab and erlotinib) either alone or in combination with concurrent chemotherapy with curative intent radiotherapy.

The combination of cetuximab and radiotherapy improved the median locoregional control (24.4 versus 14.9 months) and median duration of overall survival (at median follow up of 54 months, 49 versus 29.3 months) compared to radiotherapy alone (Bonner et al., 2006). The addition of cetuximab along with concurrent chemoradiotherapy did not improve outcome compared to chemoradiotherapy alone (Ang et al., 2014).

Studies comparing the benefit of cetuximab and radiotherapy against concurrent chemotherapy, the current standard of care for patients with locally advanced squamous cell carcinoma, have not yet reported. The use of cetuximab in the UK is therefore limited to patients who have good performance status and have contraindications for the use of cisplatin-based chemotherapy.

Systemic treatment with palliative intent

Patient groups for palliative intent treatment include inoperable locoregionally recurrent disease, distant metastatic disease, or a combination of both. Systemic therapy improves quality of life and overall survival compared with best supportive care, but is associated with side effects and should be considered only in suitable patients.

The commonly used active agents include platins (cisplatin, carboplatin), taxanes (paclitaxel, docetaxel), 5-FU, methotrexate and cetuximab. The prognostic factors for favourable and poor outcomes following treatment are listed in Table 11.11 (Argiris et al., 2004).

First-line systemic treatment with palliative intent

Single agent versus combination regimen

Single-agent treatment (cisplatin, carboplatin, methotrexate) results in a response rate of approximately 10–15%, while a combination regimen (cisplatin plus 5-FU or carboplatin plus 5-FU) significantly improves the response rate to around 25–35%, with a median duration of response of 4–5 months, but is associated with an increased incidence of acute haematological and non-haematological toxicities and does not improve overall survival (median survival 5–7 months; Forastiere et al., 1992). The selection of regimen will therefore depend on the patients' performance status and comorbidity.

The addition of taxane (paclitaxel or docetaxel) with cisplatin or carboplatin has been studied in various combinations. None of these have demonstrated a better response or survival compared to the cisplatin and 5-FU regimen. The ECOG group studied the combination of platin plus taxane versus platin plus 5-FU in a phase III trial. The response rate (27 versus 26) and median overall survival (8.7 versus 8.1 months) were not statistically significant (Gibson et al., 2005).

A platin doublet with 5-FU or taxane is the preferred regimen in this setting in patients with good performance status.

Combination of biological therapy with chemotherapy

The most commonly studied biotherapy agents in combination with cisplatin and 5-FU in the palliative setting are the EGFR monoclonal antibodies cetuximab and panitumumab. The addition of cetuximab to

Table 11.11 Factors associated with favourable and poor outcome following palliative chemotherapy

Factors	Favourable outcome	Poor outcome
Performance status	0	1
Comorbidity	None	Significant comorbidity
Prior chemotherapy	Good response	Poor or no response
Prior radiotherapy	None	Radiation treatment
Weight loss	No weight loss	Presence of weight loss

cisplatin and 5-FU significantly prolonged overall survival (10.1 versus 7.4 months), progression-free survival (5.6 versus 3.3 months) and objective response rates (36% versus 20%) when compared to cisplatin and 5-FU alone in a randomized trial (Vermorken *et al.*, 2008). This regimen is now used in UK centres as the first-line systemic therapy in the palliative setting where funding is available.

Panitumumab in combination with cisplatin and 5-FU improved progression-free survival (5.8 versus 4.6 months) but did not improve overall survival (median survival 11.1 versus 9 months) when compared with cisplatin and 5-FU alone (Vermorken *et al.*, 2013).

Second-line systemic treatment with palliative intent

Second-line treatment results in objective response rates of less than 10% with no improvement in overall survival and its use should be considered in a very select group of patients with good performance status, good response to prior treatment and longer treatment-free interval.

The choice of treatment depends upon the prior treatment regimen and associated toxicities. Drugs include a combination regimen of carboplatin and paclitaxel when cisplatin and 5-FU were used initially or single agents such as cetuximab, methotrexate or gemcitabine.

Prognosis in head and neck cancer

Prognosis depends upon the stage and site/subsite, discussed in respective sites later in the chapter. The term 'relative survival' is used which accounts for differences in the risk of dying from causes other than the disease under study. It is the ratio of observed survival rate to the expected rate for a group of people in the general population similar to the patient group with respect to race, sex and age.

Carcinoma of the oral cavity

Anatomy

The boundaries extend from the vermilion border of lips anteriorly to the junction of the soft and hard palate (above) and to the circumvallate papillae of the tongue (below) posteriorly. The glosso-tonsillar sulcus and anterior pillars of the tonsil form the lateral boundaries between the oral cavity and the oropharynx.

Risk factors

Tobacco and alcohol are the most common risk factors for oral cavity cancers; sun exposure is an important risk factor for lower lip carcinoma; tobacco and betel nut chewing, most widely practised in Asia and India, is an important risk factor for buccal mucosa cancers.

Subsites

Table 11.1 details the subsites. The commonest subsites for cancers in the Western world are the floor of mouth, the oral tongue and lip cancers, while the buccal mucosa is more common in Asia and India.

Clinical presentation

The commonest clinical presentation is a non-healing ulcer with or without associated symptoms of pain, difficulty in chewing, swallowing or speaking, and/or swelling in the neck.

Investigations and staging

Investigations are detailed in an earlier section. Primary T staging is summarised in Table 11.12 and

Table 11.12 T staging of oral cavity cancers

T1	Tumour ≤ 2 cm
T2	Tumour > 2 cm but ≤ 4 cm
T3	Tumour > 4 cm
T4a	Moderately advanced local disease Lip: tumour invades through cortical bone, inferior alveolar nerve, floor of mouth or skin of face (chin or nose) Other subsites: tumour invades through adjacent structures only (through cortical bone, deep extrinsic muscles of tongue, maxillary sinus and skin of face)
T4b	Very advanced local disease Tumour invades through masticator space, pterygoid plates or skull base and/or encases internal carotid artery

Adapted from AJCC, 2009.

nodal staging is summarised in Table 11.3. All patients are staged as in Table 11.4.

Treatment

Early-stage (I and II)

Single modality treatment with surgery is the treatment of choice. Surgery involves wide local excision. The extent of the defect determines the nature of closure and ranges from primary closure where possible, local flap mobilisation to fill the defect when primary closure is not possible and to achieve better cosmesis or microvascular flap reconstruction, when there is a large defect to achieve better cosmesis and function.

The management of a node-negative neck depends upon the primary subsite. A prophylactic neck dissection (unilateral for lateralised tumour and bilateral for midline tumours) is routinely recommended for floor of mouth and tongue primary tumours due to the higher incidence of occult metastasis (25–45%), while observation or neck dissection are options for other subsites, as the incidence of occult metastasis is less than 10–15%.

Radiotherapy

Radiotherapy is considered in patients who decide not to have surgery or are not able to have surgery due to comorbidities. Radiotherapy is planned using the general principles outlined earlier including target volume delineation. For buccal mucosa cancers a 2-cm margin around the gross tumour volume is recommended to create a clinical target volume. Elective nodal irradiation depends upon subsite and is recommended in oral tongue and floor of mouth cancers.

For patients with lip cancer, radiation treatment using electrons (9–15 MeV) or kilovoltage X-rays (170–300 KV) is an option. The following steps ensure optimal treatment using electrons.

- Assess the dimension of tumour including depth.
- Add 1 cm for microscopic spread and a further 5 mm for penumbra.
- Use internal shielding (lead covered in wax) to protect deep normal tissues (teeth and gums). The thickness of lead depends upon the energy of the electrons used (general rule – energy/2 in mm of lead).
- Exclude the uninvolved lip from the radiation field by using a mouth bite.
- Use a custom-made end plate cut-out to shape the field.
- Use a bolus of 5–10 mm thickness to ensure the prescription dose to the surface of the tumour.

When kilovoltage X-ray is used, the above steps ensure optimal treatment with the following exceptions: the additional 5 mm for penumbra and bolus are not required and a lead cut-out is used to shape the field.

Locally advanced stage (III and IV)

Patients with advanced disease have tumours more than 4 cm and/or invasion of adjacent structures (extrinsic muscles of tongue, bone) and/or involvement of regional lymph nodes. A combined modality approach is normally recommended to treat this group of patients due to the high risk of locoregional recurrence. Surgery is the treatment of choice for all subsites followed by adjuvant radiotherapy with or without concurrent chemotherapy based on postoperative pathology.

Surgery to the primary site involves wide local excision to achieve clear resection margins and reconstruction with either a composite free flap (soft tissue and bone, usually fibula) or soft tissue free flap (usually radial forearm) or a pedicle flap to improve functional and cosmetic outcome. The type and extent of surgery varies with the subsite of the primary tumour. All patients will undergo either unilateral or bilateral neck dissection according to the subsite of primary tumour; the types of dissections

Table 11.13 Five-year relative survival for oral cavity cancers

Stage	Oral cavity (%)	Lip (%)
I	71.5	89.6
II	57.9	83.5
III	44.5	54.6
IV	31.9	47.2

Adapted from AJCC, 2009.

are described earlier and will depend on the status of the neck nodes.

Radiotherapy

Radiotherapy with or without concurrent chemotherapy is an alternative in patients who refuse surgery, are medically unfit, would have an unacceptable functional outcome with surgery, or in patients with inoperable disease. Adjuvant radiotherapy with or without chemotherapy following surgery is recommended when pathological risk factors for recurrence are present as described earlier.

Radiotherapy planning

All patients needing radiotherapy (definitive and adjuvant) are immobilised, scanned and outlined as detailed before. The decision to treat the unilateral or bilateral neck depends on the site and extent of the primary tumour. The ipsilateral neck is treated for primary tumours arising from the buccal mucosa, alveolus, retromolar trigone and the lateral border of the oral tongue and the lateralised floor of mouth. The bilateral neck is treated in all patients when the primary tumour crosses the midline.

Prognosis

The five-year relative survival by combined (clinical and pathological) AJCC stage for oral cavity squamous cell carcinoma and lip are shown in Table 11.13.

Carcinoma of the nasopharynx

Introduction

Nasopharyngeal carcinoma (NPC) is rare in the Western world, but is much more common in parts of Asia, such as southern China. In the West, the adjusted incidence is around 1 per 100,000 per annum compared to 20–30 per 100,000 in Hong Kong (British Association of Otorhinolaryngology, 2011).

Anatomy

The nasopharynx is a narrow tubular space situated behind the nasal cavity and is bound by the following.

1. Superior – the floor of the sphenoid sinus and clivus.
2. Inferior – the caudal edge of C1 or nasal aspect of the soft palate.
3. Anterior – the junction with the nasal choanae.
4. Posterior – the posterior pharyngeal wall.
5. Lateral – the lateral pharyngeal wall and the medial border of the parapharyngeal space.

The retropharyngeal lymph nodes are the first echelon nodes draining the nasopharynx. The nasopharynx also drains to level II nodes and upper level V nodes.

The lateral wall or roof of the nasopharynx is the commonest site of origin of carcinoma. Approximately 60–90% of patients present with ipsilateral palpable lymphadenopathy and 50% have bilateral enlarged nodes. The skull base is involved in about 30% of cases.

Risk factors

The commonest risk factors are Epstein Barr virus (EBV) and nitrosamines, which are present in salt-cured fish and meat and released during the cooking process. Other risk factors include genetic predisposition and heavy alcohol intake.

Clinical presentation

The clinical symptoms are non-specific and include:
- painless neck lump in the posterior triangle;
- unilateral otitis media, conductive deafness and tinnitus;
- nasal obstruction, epistaxis;
- sore throat;
- cranial nerve dysfunction (II–VI or XI–XII).

Investigations and staging

Investigations are detailed in an earlier section. Primary T staging is summarised in Table 11.14 and nodal staging is summarised in Table 11.3. All patients are assigned an overall stage as in Table 11.4.

Histology

Squamous cell carcinoma (SCC) is the commonest carcinoma affecting the nasopharynx, and the World

Table 11.14 T staging of nasopharyngeal cancers

T1	Tumour confined to the nasopharynx or tumour extending to oropharynx and/or nasal cavity without parapharyngeal extension
T2	Tumour with parapharyngeal extension
T3	Tumour involves bony structures of skull base and/or paranasal sinuses
T4	Tumour with intracranial extension and/or involvement of cranial nerves, hypopharynx, orbit, or with extension to the infratemporal fossa/masticator space

Adapted from AJCC, 2009.

Health Organisation (WHO) histopathological grading system divides these tumours into three types (Shanmugaratnam *et al.*, 1978):

- type I or keratinising SCC is more common in the West and accounts for about 20% of NPC. Local control is harder;
- type II or non-keratinising SCC is common in endemic cases and is associated with EBV. It accounts for about 30% of NPC. This type is more responsive to radiotherapy and chemotherapy and has a higher predilection for distant metastases;
- type III or undifferentiated carcinoma is also common in endemic cases and associated with EBV. It accounts for about 50% of NPC.

Other histological subtypes include adenocarcinoma and lymphoma (T cell).

Treatment

Overview

Non-surgical treatment with radiotherapy with or without concurrent chemotherapy remains the treatment of choice for all stages of disease. Intensity-modulated radiotherapy (IMRT) should be used for all patients with NPC due to its close proximity to critical structures and complex target volumes. IMRT also results in less xerostomia and improved quality of life when compared to conventional 3D radiotherapy (Pow *et al.*, 2006).

The role of surgery is limited to diagnosis (biopsy) and salvage neck dissection for recurrent or persistent positive nodes after chemoradiotherapy.

The addition of chemotherapy (neoadjuvant, adjuvant or concurrent) to radiotherapy improves outcomes with the largest benefit seen with concurrent

chemotherapy and radiotherapy, leading to a survival benefit of 20% at 5 years (Langendijk *et al.*, 2004). The Cochrane individual patient meta-analysis of 1753 NPC patients in 8 randomised trials comparing chemotherapy plus radiotherapy versus radiotherapy alone showed an absolute overall survival benefit of 6% at 5 years and an absolute event-free survival benefit of 10% at 5 years with the addition of chemotherapy (Baujat *et al.*, 2006). The optimal combination of chemotherapy and radiation in the treatment of NPC is yet to be determined.

Commonly used chemotherapy strategies include the following:

- Neoadjuvant chemotherapy – often 2 cycles of PF for fit patients with bulky nodal disease prior to chemoradiotherapy with cisplatin.
- Concurrent chemoradiotherapy alone with cisplatin.
- Concurrent chemoradiotherapy with cisplatin followed by 3 cycles of adjuvant PF (Al-Sarraf *et al.*, 1998).

The most commonly used strategy in many centres in the UK is neoadjuvant chemotherapy: 2 cycles of PF followed by concurrent chemoradiotherapy (single agent cisplatin at 100 mg/m² given at 3-weekly intervals for 3 doses).

There is no evidence to date for the use of docetaxel or cetuximab in the treatment of NPC.

Treatment of early-stage (I)

Patients with stage I disease should be treated with radical radiotherapy alone.

Treatment of intermediate stage (II)

Concurrent chemoradiotherapy is recommended for this group of patients due to the higher incidence of distant failure with radiotherapy. The Intergroup Study 0099 comparing radiotherapy alone and chemoradiotherapy included patients with stage II disease (Al-Sarraf *et al.*, 1998).

Treatment of locally advanced stage

Most patients present with locally advanced disease and should be offered concurrent chemoradiotherapy or radiotherapy alone in patients unfit for chemotherapy.

Radiotherapy planning

The general principles of target delineation as outlined in the earlier section are followed to delineate the targets. All lymph node levels on both sides of the neck are at risk and are included in the treatment volume in virtually all patients. The practice varies across different centres regarding clinical target volume (CTV) delineation, dose prescription, dose constraints and acceptance criteria. Most centres use a three-dose volume with the high-dose volume receiving 70 Gy over 35 fractions and the dose to the intermediate and prophylactic dose volumes as in Table 11.6.

CTV1 should include GTV + 1 cm, the whole nasopharynx and all involved lymph node levels. Following induction chemotherapy, post-chemotherapy residual volumes are outlined as GTV.

CTV2 includes the following regions.

- Posteriorly – the bilateral retropharyngeal nodes when not involved.
- Anteriorly – the posterior third nasal cavity, posterior ethmoid and posterior third maxillary antrum anteriorly.
- Laterally – the bilateral parapharyngeal spaces, pterygoid plates ± pterygoid muscles.
- Superiorly – skull base and floor of the sphenoid sinus superiorly including bilateral foramen ovale, carotid canal and foramen spinosum, clivus and petrous tips.

CTV3 includes:

- the upper half of the sphenoid sinus;
- the infraorbital fissure, orbital apex and supraorbital fissure;
- uninvolved nodal levels at risk of harbouring microscopic disease. The at-risk lymph node levels include bilateral levels Ib–Va, Vb, the retrostyloid space and the supraclavicular fossa.

Treatment is planned and delivered using IMRT. Most patients in the UK are treated with external beam radiotherapy, but intracavitary and interstitial brachytherapy boosts are alternative treatment options to improve dose delivery to the primary tumour in the nasopharynx.

The incidence of acute mucositis increases by 30% with the addition of chemotherapy (Lee et al., 2012). Tumour control in NPC is highly correlated with radiation dose, and a high dose of at least 70 Gy equivalent is needed for gross tumour eradication.

Prognosis

The five-year relative survival by combined (clinical and pathological) AJCC stage for nasopharynx squamous cell carcinoma is shown in Table 11.15.

Table 11.15 Five-year relative survival for nasopharyngeal cancer

Stage	Five-year relative survival (%)
1	71.5
2	64.2
3	62.2
4	38.4

Adapted from AJCC, 2009.

Historically, local control rates for patients with NPC who receive conventional radiotherapy range from 64% to 95% for T1–2 tumours and 44–68% for T3–4 tumours (Lee et al., 2009). Most contemporary IMRT series report excellent local control results exceeding 90% at 2–5 years, but with distant metastases remaining as high as 44% at 4 years (Lee et al., 2009, 2012). Patients with metastatic disease have a median survival of about 6 months.

Carcinoma of the oropharynx

Introduction

The incidence of oropharyngeal carcinoma (OPC) in the UK doubled over the last decade to 2.3 per 100,000 (National Cancer Intelligence Network, 2010), mostly attributed to human papillomavirus (HPV) infection and affecting younger patients, while the incidence related to smoking and drinking is decreasing and affects older patients.

Current HPV prevalence in OPC in the West is reported to be as high as 72% (Mehanna et al., 2013), with HPV 16 being the predominant subtype. The most common subsites are the tonsil and tongue base. HPV-positive patients typically present with early T stage and more advanced N stage with lymph nodes that are often cystic in nature.

Anatomy

The oropharynx extends from the palate to the hyoid. The boundaries are:

- superior – the junction of the hard and soft palate;
- inferior – the vallecula/hyoid;
- anterior – the circumvallate papillae;
- posterior – the posterior pharyngeal wall;
- lateral – the lateral pharyngeal wall.

151

Subsites of the oropharynx include:

- tonsil;
- tongue base;
- vallecula;
- soft palate;
- posterior pharyngeal wall.

Level II nodes are the first echelon nodes draining the oropharynx. Approximately 60–80% of patients present with involved lymph nodes and between 15% and 40% of clinically node-negative patients have occult nodal disease. The tongue base, soft palate and posterior pharyngeal wall are midline structures with a high risk of contralateral neck node involvement.

Risk factors

The principal risk factors are tobacco and alcohol use. Despite the reducing use of tobacco, there is an increasing incidence of these cancers in younger adults caused by HPV infection. HPV 16 is the commonest subtype.

Clinical presentation

The majority of patients present with sore throat and/ or painless neck swelling and/or occasionally foreign body sensation in the throat. Patients with advanced stage present with:

- difficulty in swallowing and odynophagia;
- referred otalgia;
- trismus;
- impaired tongue movement and altered speech.

Investigations and staging

Investigations are detailed in an earlier section. Primary T staging is summarised in Table 11.16 and nodal staging is summarised in Table 11.3. All patients are staged as in Table 11.4.

Histology

Squamous cell carcinoma is the commonest histology. Other histological subtypes include adenocarcinoma, small cell carcinoma, lymphoma and mucosal melanoma.

Treatment overview

The treatment of choice depends upon the subsite, stage, morbidity associated with treatment modality and local expertise. Early-stage disease can often be

Table 11.16 T staging of oropharyngeal cancers

T1	Tumour ≤ 2 cm
T2	Tumour > 2 cm but ≤ 4 cm
T3	Tumour > 4 cm or extension into lingual surface of epiglottis
T4a	Moderately advanced local disease: the tumour invades the larynx, extrinsic muscle of tongue, medial pterygoid, hard palate or mandible
T4b	Very advanced local disease: the tumour invades the lateral pterygoid muscle, pterygoid plates, lateral nasopharynx or skull base or encases the carotid artery

Adapted from AJCC, 2009.

treated by transoral surgery and neck dissection or radiotherapy as a single modality achieving comparable control and survival rates. Locally advanced stage disease is treated using multimodality to improve outcomes, usually a combination of chemotherapy and radiotherapy with surgery limited to neck dissection, either prior to or following definitive treatment.

Tumours of the oropharynx are broadly classified into lateralised and non-lateralised tumours based on the primary site of the tumour in order to determine the treatment of the uninvolved contralateral neck.

Lateralised tumour

- Tumour confined to the tonsillar fossa or extending onto or into the adjacent tongue base and/or soft palate by less than 1 cm.

Non-lateralised tumour

- Tonsillar tumour that involves the adjacent tongue/soft palate by more than 1 cm.

OR

- A tumour that arises from a midline structure (tongue base/soft palate/posterior pharyngeal wall, vallecula).

A contralateral N0 neck should be treated prophylactically in non-lateralised tumours.

Surgery

Early-stage (I and II)

Surgery involves wide local excision using a transoral approach (TLM or TORS) with selective neck dissection (ipsilateral or bilateral) based on the lateralisation of the tumour.

Patient selection is crucial and is based on examination findings under anaesthesia (mobile tumour not fixed to constrictors) and imaging, with the anticipation that surgery will achieve clear resection margins and would avoid adjuvant treatment where possible. The most common subsite for transoral resection is the tonsil, although a small proportion of early tongue base tumours can also be resected using TORS. Results from TLM and TORS studies show good oncologic and functional outcomes (Moore and Hinni, 2013).

Open surgery with lip split mandibulotomy, resection of primary tumour and reconstruction with a free flap is not recommended due to the associated morbidity of poor long-term swallowing function affecting quality of life.

Locally advanced stage (III and IV)

The role of surgery in advanced stage disease is limited to neck dissection (prior to or following chemoradiotherapy) in the definitive setting or as a salvage for patients who have persistent or relapsed disease following definitive treatment. Salvage surgery for locoregional disease offers a small chance of long-term survival and usually involves a total glosso-pharyngo-laryngectomy and reconstruction.

Radiotherapy and systemic therapy

Early-stage (I and II)

Primary radiotherapy is an alternative treatment option for all subsites with early-stage disease and includes ipsilateral elective nodal treatment for lateralised tumours and bilateral elective nodal treatment for non-lateralised tumours. The outcomes (locoregional control and survival) are comparable to surgery with lower rates of complications (Parsons et al., 2002).

Adjuvant radiotherapy with or without chemotherapy following surgery is based on the histology. The indications for adjuvant treatment are detailed in an earlier section of this chapter.

Locally advanced stage (III and IV)

Concurrent chemoradiotherapy remains the treatment of choice for locally advanced OPC and involves a given combination of radiotherapy and chemotherapy as below.

- Concurrent chemoradiotherapy.
- Radiotherapy with concomitant cetuximab (where chemotherapy is contraindicated).
- Radiotherapy alone.
- Induction chemotherapy followed by radiotherapy or concurrent chemoradiotherapy.

The additional benefit of concurrent chemotherapy decreases with age with no significant benefit in patients over 70 years of age as a whole. The addition of chemotherapy in patients over 70 years of age should be carefully considered on an individual basis.

Patients with a high risk of systemic metastasis (T4, N2c and N3 neck disease) and those who are symptomatic due to large-volume primary tumours are considered for neoadjuvant chemotherapy. There is an increasing trend to use TPF in this group of patients with good performance status, following a recent meta-analysis (Blanchard et al., 2013).

Patients with bulky resectable neck disease (N2a and above), particularly those not suitable for systemic therapy, are considered for neck dissection, either before or after completion of radiotherapy.

Radiotherapy planning

All patients needing radiotherapy (definitive and adjuvant) are immobilised, scanned and outlined as detailed previously. Two outlining protocols for oropharyngeal tumours are commonly used in the UK: anatomical and volumetric (or geometric).

CTV1 (Step 2) with these different approaches includes:

- anatomic – the entire oropharynx from the soft palate to the bottom of the hyoid for all subsites;
- volumetric – the GTV and 1 cm around the tumour (edited for bone, air and natural barriers): this method relies on accurately identifying the tumour on the planning CT scan.

CTV2 (Step 3) includes:

- all at-risk uninvolved lymph node levels as per Table 11.17.

All curative intent patients should be routinely planned using intensity modulation to spare the parotids (contralateral) in order to reduce the incidence of long-term xerostomia because forward planned conformal treatment is associated with a higher incidence of severe xerostomia (83% versus 29% at 24 months; Nutting et al., 2011). Figure 11.1 shows a radiotherapy

Table 11.17 Nodal levels at risk for oropharyngeal cancers

Neck node status	Lateralised tumours	Non-lateralised tumours
Node-negative	Ipsilateral level Ib to IVa Level VIIa (retropharyngeal)	Ipsilateral level Ib to IVa Level VIIa Contralateral level II to IVa
Node-positive	Ipsilateral Level Ib to IVa Level VIIa Other lymph node levels as per Table 11.8	Ipsilateral level Ib to IVa Level VIIa Contralateral level II to IVa Other lymph node levels as per Table 11.8

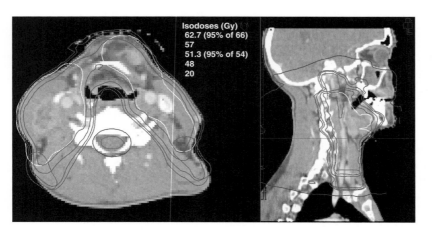

Isodoses (Gy)
62.7 (95% of 66)
57
51.3 (95% of 54)
48
20

Figure 11.1 Axial and sagittal views of a patient with stage T4a N2c squamous carcinoma of the tonsil planned using VMAT showing the prescription isodose lines conforming to the target volumes and sparing the posterior pharyngeal wall and spinal cord. The involved regions receive a dose of 66 Gy and at-risk regions receive a dose of 54 Gy.

plan for a patient with locally advanced, node-positive carcinoma of the tonsil.

Prognosis

The five-year relative survival by combined (clinical and pathological) AJCC stage for oropharynx squamous cell carcinoma is shown in Table 11.18. This is not stratified by HPV or smoking.

As well as being dependent on disease stage, the prognosis of oropharyngeal carcinoma is strongly influenced by HPV status and smoking history. The 3-year overall survival for HPV-positive OPC is 82.4% compared to 57.1% in patients with HPV-negative OPC (Ang *et al.*, 2010), with a 3-year overall survival of 93% in HPV-positive patients with a low smoking history.

Carcinoma of the hypopharynx

Anatomy

The hypopharynx lies posterior and inferior to the oropharynx, extending below the oropharynx to the oesophageal inlet inferiorly. It is divided into three subsites: pyriform sinus, posterior pharyngeal wall and post cricoid region.

The hypopharynx has an extensive lymphatic drainage pattern which commonly involves:

- levels II to V and retropharyngeal lymph nodes (pyriform sinus);
- levels II, III and retropharyngeal lymph nodes (posterior pharyngeal wall);
- levels III, V and para tracheal nodes (post cricoid region).

Approximately two-thirds of patients are lymph node-positive at presentation, and occult lymph node metastases are found in approximately 30–50% of clinically node-negative patients.

Subsites

Pyriform sinus: bounded medially and superiorly by the aryepiglottic fold, anterosuperiorly by the pharyngoepiglottic fold and laterally by the superior edge of the thyroid cartilage. Inferiorly the apex opens into the

Table 11.18 Five-year relative survival of oropharyngeal cancer

Stage	Five-year relative survival (%)
1	73
2	58
3	45
4	32

Adapted from AJCC, 2009.

Table 11.19 T staging of hypopharyngeal cancers

T1	Tumour limited to one subsite and/or ≤ 2 cm
T2	Tumour invades more than one subsite, or > 2 cm but ≤ 4 cm without fixation of hemilarynx
T3	Tumour > 4 cm or with fixation of hemilarynx or extension to oesophagus
T4a	Moderately advanced local disease Tumour invades thyroid/cricoid cartilage, hyoid bone, thyroid gland, or central compartment soft tissue (prelaryngeal strap muscles and subcutaneous fat)
T4b	Very advanced local disease Tumour invades prevertebral fascia, encases carotid artery or involves mediastinal structures

Adapted from AJCC, 2009.

oesophagus. Approximately 65–75% of hypopharyngeal carcinomas arise from this subsite.

Posterior pharyngeal wall: extends from a plane drawn from the tip of the epiglottis to the plane drawn at the inferior border of the cricoid. Approximately 10–20% of hypopharyngeal carcinomas arise from here.

Post cricoid region: extends from the posterior surface of the arytenoids to the inferior border of the cricoid cartilage. About 5–10% of hypopharyngeal tumours arise from this subsite.

Risk factors

Smoking and alcohol use are the main risk factors. Other environmental risk factors include iron and vitamin C deficiency, occupational exposure to asbestos, wood and coal dust.

Clinical presentation

Patients are often asymptomatic during the early stages of the disease and usually present late with:

- odynophagia, difficulty in swallowing, weight loss;
- referred otalgia, haemoptysis;
- difficulty in breathing;
- painless neck swelling.

Investigations and staging

Investigations are detailed in the earlier section. The primary T staging for hypopharyngeal cancer is given in Table 11.19 and nodal staging as in Table 11.3. Patients are assigned an overall stage as in Table 11.4.

Histology

The most common histological subtype is squamous cell carcinoma. Others include basaloid SCC, spindle cell carcinoma and minor salivary gland adenocarcinoma.

Treatment overview

The treatment of choice is influenced by stage, subsite and the ability to preserve laryngeal function in patients with a functioning larynx and maximising the chance of achieving locoregional control and long-term survival. Elective treatment of the bilateral neck is recommended for all stages, even in a clinically node-negative neck due to the high incidence of occult lymph node metastasis (30–50%).

Early-stage disease is usually treated with a single modality (surgery or radiotherapy). The treatment of choice for locally advanced disease with functioning larynx (minimal extralaryngeal disease and no obvious cartilage or bone involvement) is concurrent chemoradiotherapy, aiming to preserve laryngeal function, and surgery followed by adjuvant treatment for patients with evidence of cartilage/bone invasion and large-volume extralaryngeal disease.

Surgery

Early-stage (I and II)

Selected patients are suitable for transoral resection (TLM or TORS). This depends on the subsite (pyriform sinus or posterior pharyngeal wall), access to resection and local expertise. Open surgical procedures (partial pharyngolaryngectomy) are not recommended routinely for early-stage patients due to poor functional outcome (swallowing and speech).

Locally advanced stage (III and IV)

Surgery usually involves total laryngectomy, partial or total pharyngectomy, permanent tracheostomy, bilateral neck dissection and reconstruction. The reconstruction varies from primary closure to free flap to gastric pull-up when a total oesophagectomy is done due to upper oesophageal involvement.

Bilateral neck dissection (selective in a node-negative neck and modified radical in a node-positive neck) is recommended for all stages.

Adjuvant treatment depends on the final postoperative histology and involves radiotherapy with or without chemotherapy as discussed in an earlier section.

Radiotherapy and systemic therapy

Early-stage (I and II)

Primary radiotherapy is an alternative for early-stage tumours, achieves comparable outcomes to radical or larynx preserving surgery (Takes *et al.*, 2012) and remains the treatment of choice for patients where larynx-preserving surgery is not possible. There are no randomised trials comparing surgery and radiotherapy for early hypopharyngeal cancers.

Locally advanced stage (III and IV)

A combined modality treatment is advocated for advanced-stage disease with the aim of organ and function preservation and/or local control, and the various options include:

- concurrent chemoradiotherapy;
- radiotherapy with concomitant cetuximab (where chemotherapy is contraindicated);
- induction chemotherapy with TPF followed by radiotherapy or concurrent chemoradiotherapy, in selected patients to improve organ and function preservation;
- radiotherapy alone;
- surgery followed by adjuvant treatment based on histology.

Radiotherapy planning

Patients are immobilised and scanned as detailed before. The general principles of outlining (definitive and postoperative) as detailed before are followed. For hypopharyngeal tumours, CTV1 (Step 2) includes the following.

- The GTV is grown asymmetrically (1 cm in anterior, posterior, right and left and by 2 cm in the superior and inferior directions).
- The whole hypopharynx (all subsites) and larynx (tip of epiglottis to bottom of cricoid or lower as dictated by lower extent of tumour plus 1 cm below) are included.
- The parapharyngeal space on the ipsilateral side in patients with gross disease involving the space.

CTV2 (Step 3) includes the following.

- The posterior pharyngeal wall outside of the GTV + 2 cm in the superior and inferior direction from the skull base to the cricoid is included for tumours arising from the posterior pharyngeal wall or when it is involved by tumours from other subsites.
- All at-risk uninvolved lymph node levels (all subsites) as per Table 11.20.

Prognosis

The five-year relative survival by combined (clinical and pathological) AJCC stage for hypopharyngeal squamous cell carcinoma is shown in Table 11.21.

Carcinoma of the larynx

Introduction

The incidence of laryngeal cancer has been decreasing since the 1990s (from 7 to 5 per 100,000) and is more common in men than women. The commonest subsite is the glottis followed by the supraglottis and the subglottis. Glottic cancers present early while other subsites generally present late. Bilateral lymph node metastasis is more common in supraglottic cancers (approximately 50% of cases) due to the rich lymphatic supply.

Anatomy

The larynx is subdivided into three subsites, the supraglottis, glottis and subglottis.

- Supraglottis: epiglottis (suprahyoid and infrahyoid), aryepiglottic folds, arytenoids and false cords.
- Glottis: vocal cords, anterior and posterior commissure.
- Subglottis: from below the vocal cords to the bottom of the cricoid.

Table 11.20 Nodal levels at risk for hypopharyngeal cancers

Node-negative neck	Node-positive neck
• Ipsilateral levels II to Va and Vb	• Ipsilateral levels Ib to Va and Vb
• Level VIIa (retropharyngeal)	• Level VIIa (retropharyngeal)
• Contralateral levels II to IVa	• Contralateral level IIs to IVa
• Ipsilateral Ib – in patients with extralaryngeal disease	• Ipsilateral Ib – in patients with extralaryngeal disease
• Level VI – in patients with subglottic extension, apex of pyriform sinus involvement, post cricoid extension and upper oesophageal involvement	• Level VI – in patients with subglottic extension, apex of pyriform sinus involvement, post cricoid extension and upper oesophageal involvement
	• Other lymph node levels as per Table 11.8

Table 11.21 Five-year relative survival of hypopharyngeal cancers

Stage	Hypopharynx (%)
I	53.0
II	39.3
III	36.0
IV	24.4

Adapted from AJCC, 2009.

The lymphatic drainage is to levels II and III cervical lymph nodes.

Risk factors

The use of tobacco and alcohol are the commonest risk factors.

Clinical presentation

A hoarse voice is the commonest symptom in patients with glottic cancer and is often diagnosed at an early stage. Other symptoms include:

- sore throat, odynophagia, difficulty in swallowing;
- difficulty in breathing and stridor;
- painless neck swelling.

Investigations and staging

Investigations are detailed in the earlier section. The primary T staging for the subsites of larynx cancer are detailed in Table 11.22 and nodal staging as in Table 11.3. Patients are staged as in Table 11.4.

Histology

Squamous cell carcinoma is the commonest histology. Other histological subtypes include adenocarcinoma, neuroendocrine carcinoma, small cell carcinoma, chondrosarcoma and lymphoma.

Treatment overview

The treatment of choice depends on stage, access to surgery, local expertise and the ability to preserve the larynx and maintain its function (airway, swallowing and speech). Early-stage disease can be treated either by surgery or radiotherapy alone as a single modality resulting in similar local control and survival outcomes. The choice of modality is influenced by location of the primary, access to surgical resection and functional outcome. Locally advanced disease is treated using a combined modality approach, aiming to preserve laryngeal function. Patients not suitable for larynx preservation are treated using a combination of surgery followed by adjuvant treatment.

Surgery

Early-stage (I and II)

Surgery usually involves transoral laser resection in supraglottic and glottic cancers. Open partial laryngectomy/cordectomy is rarely considered in patients with poor access to laser surgery. Neck nodes are routinely treated in patients with supraglottic cancer (selective neck dissection considered in N0 patients), but are observed in glottic cancer due to the low risk of nodal metastasis.

Patients with recurrent/persistent disease following radiotherapy usually require a salvage laryngectomy, but in carefully selected cases with small-volume disease, a larynx preservation approach of partial laryngectomy may be considered.

Table 11.22 T staging for subsites of larynx

Supraglottis	
T1	Tumour limited to one subsite of supraglottis with normal vocal cord mobility
T2	Tumour invades the mucosa of more than one adjacent subsite of the supraglottis or glottis or the region outside the supraglottis (mucosa of tongue base, vallecula, medial wall of pyriform sinus) without fixation of the larynx
T3	Tumour limited to the larynx with vocal cord fixation and/or invades any of the following: postcricoid area, pre-epiglottic space, paraglottic space and/or the inner cortex of thyroid cartilage
T4a	Moderately advanced local disease Tumour invades through the thyroid cartilage and/or invades tissues beyond the larynx (trachea, soft tissues of the neck including deep extrinsic muscle of the tongue, strap muscles, thyroid or oesophagus)
T4b	Very advanced local disease Tumour invades prevertebral space, encases carotid artery or invades mediastinal structures
Glottis	
T1	Tumour limited to the vocal cords (may involve anterior or posterior commissure) with normal mobility
T1a	Tumour limited to one vocal cord
T1b	Tumour involves both vocal cords
T2	Tumour extends to the supraglottis and/or subglottis and/or with impaired vocal cord mobility
T3	Tumour limited to the larynx with vocal cord fixation and/or invasion of paraglottic space, and/or the inner cortex of the thyroid cartilage
T4a	Moderately advanced local disease Tumour invades through the outer cortex of the thyroid cartilage and/or invades tissues beyond the larynx (trachea, soft tissues of the neck including deep extrinsic muscle of the tongue, strap muscles, thyroid, or oesophagus)
T4b	Very advanced local disease Tumour invades the prevertebral space, encases the carotid artery, or invades the mediastinal structures
Subglottis	
T1	Tumour limited to subglottis
T2	Tumour extends to vocal cords with normal or impaired mobility
T3	Tumour limited to larynx with vocal cord fixation
T4a	Moderately advanced local disease Tumour invades the cricoid or thyroid cartilage and/or invades tissues beyond the larynx (trachea, soft tissues of the neck including deep extrinsic muscle of the tongue, strap muscles or oesophagus)
T4b	Very advanced local disease Tumour invades the prevertebral space, encases the carotid artery, or invades the mediastinal structures

Adapted from AJCC, 2009.

Locally advanced stage (III and IV)

Surgery for patients with advanced-stage disease, not suitable for larynx preservation, involves a total laryngectomy and bilateral neck dissection. Patients presenting with stridor usually require a tracheostomy to maintain their airway. However, in selected cases the tumour can be debulked, thereby avoiding a tracheostomy.

Salvage surgery following chemoradiotherapy for locally advanced disease usually requires a total laryngectomy with or without neck dissection.

Radiotherapy and systemic therapy

Early-stage (I and II)

Primary radiotherapy is an alternative treatment option for early-stage disease at all subsites and is the treatment of choice in patients with poor access to surgery. Radiotherapy is usually delivered over 4 weeks and neck nodes are selectively irradiated in supraglottic cancers.

Patients with carcinoma *in situ* (CIS) of the glottis may be offered radical radiotherapy when there is persistence of symptoms and progression of clinical abnormalities despite multiple biopsies failing to confirm invasive disease.

Locally advanced stage (III and IV)

The patients in this group are broadly classified into those with minimal/no extralaryngeal disease with useful laryngeal function and those with poor function and/or gross cartilage destruction and/or extralaryngeal disease. For patients in the latter group, surgery (total laryngectomy and neck dissections) and adjuvant radiotherapy or chemoradiotherapy should be recommended. For the others, treatment options include:

- concurrent chemoradiotherapy with the aim of preserving the larynx and its function (Forastiere *et al.*, 2003);
- patients with large-volume disease (primary and nodes) may benefit from neoadjuvant chemotherapy with TPF followed by concurrent chemoradiotherapy in selected patients (Pointreau *et al.*, 2009);
- radiotherapy alone in patients over the age of 70 or who are not suitable for concurrent systemic therapy;
- radiotherapy with concurrent cetuximab in patients with contraindications to systemic chemotherapy.

Radiotherapy planning

Patients are immobilised and scanned as detailed before. The general principles of outlining (definitive and postoperative) as detailed before are followed. For laryngeal tumours, CTV1 (Step 2) includes:

- the GTV is grown asymmetrically (1 cm in the anterior, posterior, right and left and 2 cm in the superior and inferior directions);
- the whole larynx (the tip of the epiglottis to the bottom of the cricoid or lower as dictated by the lower extent of the tumour plus 1 cm below) is included;
- a 2-cm wide midline bolus (1-cm thick) anteriorly is used when anterior commissure is involved.

Table 11.23 Nodal levels at risk for laryngeal cancers

Node-negative neck	Node-positive neck
• Bilateral levels II to IVa • Ipsilateral Ib – in patients with extralaryngeal disease • Level VI – in patients with subglottic extension, post cricoid extension and upper oesophageal involvement	• Ipsilateral levels Ib to Va and Vb • Contralateral levels II to IVa • Ipsilateral Ib – in patients with extralaryngeal disease • Level VI – in patients with subglottic extension, post-cricoid extension and upper oesophageal involvement • Other lymph node levels as per Table 11.9

CTV2 (Step 3) for locally advanced stage disease includes:

- all at-risk uninvolved lymph node levels as per Table 11.23.

Prognosis

The five-year larynx preservation rate for locally advanced stage III/IV disease following concurrent chemoradiotherapy is 84%, neoadjuvant chemotherapy and radiotherapy is 71% and following radiotherapy alone is 66%.

The five-year relative survival by combined (clinical and pathological) AJCC stage for squamous cell carcinoma of the larynx and its subsites are shown in Table 11.24.

Carcinoma of the paranasal sinuses

Introduction

Paranasal sinus malignancies are rare in the Western world and affect less than 1 in 100,000 people each year in the UK (British Association of Otorhinolaryngology, 2011). They represent 3% of all head and neck cancers.

The majority of paranasal sinus tumours (approximately 60–70%) arise in the maxillary sinus, followed by the nasal cavity, especially the lateral wall (20–30%) and ethmoid sinuses (10–15%). Tumours of the frontal and sphenoid sinuses are rare.

Anatomy

The boundaries of the maxillary sinus are:

- superior wall: floor of the orbit;
- inferior wall: the alveolar process of the maxilla;

Table 11.24 Five-year relative survival for laryngeal cancer

Stage	Larynx (%)	Supraglottis (%)	Glottis (%)	Subglottis (%)
I	84.3	59.1	89.8	65.3
II	66.0	59.7	74.0	55.9
III	52.1	52.8	55.7	47.2
IV	35.5	34.3	44.4	31.5

Adapted from AJCC, 2009.

Table 11.25 T staging for maxillary sinus tumours and nasal cavity/ethmoid sinus tumours

Maxillary sinus	
T1	Tumour limited to maxillary sinus mucosa with no erosion or bone destruction
T2	Tumour causing bone erosion or destruction including extension into the hard palate and/or middle nasal meatus, except extension to posterior wall of maxillary sinus and pterygoid plates
T3	Tumour invades any of the following: bone of posterior wall of maxillary sinus, subcutaneous tissues, floor or medial wall of orbit, pterygoid fossa, ethmoid sinus
T4a	Moderately advanced local disease – tumour invades anterior orbital contents, skin of cheek, pterygoid plates, infratemporal fossa, cribriform plate, sphenoid or frontal sinus
T4b	Very advanced local disease – tumour invades any of the following: orbital apex, dura, brain, middle cranial fossa, cranial nerves other than maxillary division of trigeminal nerve (V2), nasopharynx, clivus
Nasal cavity and ethmoid sinus tumours	
T1	Tumour restricted to any one subsite, with or without bony invasion
T2	Tumour invading two subsites in a single region or extending to involve an adjacent region within nasoethmoidal complex with or without bony invasion
T3	Tumour extends to invade the medial wall or floor of the orbit, maxillary sinus, palate or cribriform plate
T4a	Moderately advanced local disease – tumour invades any of the following: anterior orbital contents, skin of nose or cheek, minimal extension to anterior cranial fossa, pterygoid plates, sphenoid or frontal sinuses
T4b	Very advanced local disease – tumour invades any of the following: orbital apex, dura, brain, middle cranial fossa, cranial nerves other than maxillary division of trigeminal nerve (V2), nasopharynx, clivus

Adapted from AJCC, 2009.

- medial wall: the nasal cavity;
- anterior wall: the anterior wall of the maxilla;
- posterior wall: the pterygoid and pterygopalatine fossa;
- Ohngren's line connects the medial canthus of the eye to the angle of the mandible. This line is used to divide the maxillary antrum into the antero-inferior portion (which is associated with earlier presentation and good prognosis) and the supero-posterior portion (which is associated with a worse prognosis due to early involvement of adjacent critical structures including the orbit, skull base, pterygoids and infratemporal fossa).

The lymphatic drainage of the sinuses is to the retropharyngeal nodes, levels I and II. Regional lymph node spread from cancer of paranasal sinuses is relatively uncommon (less than 5%) with a higher incidence in locally advanced maxillary tumours (10–15%).

Risk factors

Risk factors include occupational exposures (leather, textile, wood dust, and nickel dust), air pollution, tobacco and viruses. Squamous cell carcinoma is associated with nickel dust, and adenocarcinoma is associated with wood dust.

Clinical presentation

Most patients with early stage disease are asymptomatic and patients typically present at a later stage, with symptoms related to invasion of adjacent structures. The symptoms include:

- nasal obstruction, anosmia, nasal discharge, epistaxis;
- facial/cheek swelling;
- eye symptoms – diplopia, watering of eyes, proptosis;
- pain in face, numbness;
- non-healing ulcer in the oral cavity, loosening of tooth, trismus.

Investigations and staging

Investigations are detailed in an earlier section. Primary T staging for maxillary sinus and nasal cavity/ethmoid sinus is summarised in Table 11.25 and nodal staging as in Table 11.3. Patients are staged as in Table 11.4.

Histology

Squamous cell carcinoma (SCC) is the commonest malignant tumour type (50%). Others include adenocarcinoma (22%), mucosal melanoma, olfactory eisthesioneuroblastoma (3%) and adenoid cystic carcinoma (10%) (Jegoux et al., 2013).

Maxillary sinus tumours are SCC in 75% of cases, whereas ethmoid tumours are adenocarcinoma in 75% of cases.

Treatment with surgery

Surgery remains the treatment of choice for early and advanced-stage resectable disease followed by adjuvant treatment (local radiotherapy with or without chemotherapy) based on postoperative pathology. Two-thirds of tumours present at a locally advanced stage (T3–4) due to late presentation with non-specific symptoms that are often ignored.

The extent of resection varies from wide local excision to primary reconstruction with free flap and/or osseo-integrated implants for titanium prosthesis. For maxillary sinus tumours, this varies from partial, total or extended maxillectomy combined with orbital exenteration (in patients with orbital involvement) and reconstruction. Patients must be of good performance status, have limited comorbidity and must be able to manage with the functional and cosmetic alterations that result from surgical resection. Endoscopic surgery is currently being explored as an alternative to standard surgical treatment of sinonasal tumours.

Ipsilateral selective neck dissection is recommended for clinically node-negative advanced-stage maxillary sinus tumours due to higher incidence of occult metastasis.

Radiotherapy and systemic therapy

Radiotherapy with or without chemotherapy is an alternative treatment option for patients with either unresectable disease or in those who are unable to undergo surgery due to comorbidities.

There are no randomised studies for the use of chemotherapy; however, it has been incorporated in the multimodality treatment of inoperable disease both in the neoadjuvant setting and concurrently during radiotherapy in patients with good performance status. The reported outcomes are better for those patients who responded to systemic therapy.

Radiotherapy planning

All patients for radiotherapy undergo pretreatment evaluation and preparation for radiotherapy planning as described earlier in the chapter. The use of mouth bite needs to be considered in patients with maxillary sinus tumours to reduce the dose to the oral tongue. The target volumes are outlined as detailed before.

As well as GTV + 1 cm, the following should be included in the high- or low-dose CTV, according to risk of involvement and proximity to OARs.

- The whole maxillary antrum, bilateral ethmoid sinuses and ipsilateral nasal cavity.
- Pterygopalatine fossa and masticator space in maxillary sinus tumours.
- Sphenoid sinus when the ethmoid sinus is involved.
- Entire orbit when there is gross orbital fat involvement.

Radiotherapy is planned using the inverse planning technique, and may need a non co-planar beam arrangement to reduce dose to critical structures.

Prognosis

Prognosis is poor and is determined by local control. Survival is dependent on histology (78% for adenocarcinoma, 60% for squamous cell carcinoma), site

Table 11.26 Five-year relative survival of paranasal sinus and nasal cavity tumours

Stage	Five-year relative survival (%)
1	63
2	61
3	50
4	36

Adapted from AJCC, 2009.

(62% for maxillary sinus, 48% for ethmoid sinus) and stage (91% for T1, 49% for T4) (Dulguerov *et al.*, 2001). Survival is extremely poor when there is involvement of the orbit and/or brain.

The five-year relative survival by combined (clinical and pathological) AJCC stage for sinonasal carcinomas of all histologies is shown in Table 11.26.

Carcinoma of the nose and nasal cavity

Introduction
Primary tumours of the nasal cavity are rare and account for less than 3% of all tumours. They are more common in males than females and are usually diagnosed in the sixth decade or later in life.

Anatomy
The nasal cavity is divided in the midline by the nasal septum and has the following boundaries.

1. Superior wall: cribriform plate of ethmoid bone and ethmoid sinus.
2. Inferior wall: hard palate.
3. Lateral wall: medial wall of maxillary sinus; it includes the turbinates and nasolacrimal duct.
4. Anterior wall: external nose.
5. Posterior wall: nasopharynx and sphenoid sinus (posterosuperiorly).

The lymphatic drainage of the nasal cavity includes levels I and II. Regional lymph node spread from cancers of the nasal cavity is relatively uncommon.

Risk factors
Tobacco smoke is the major risk factor followed by occupational exposure (wood dust, glues and adhesives). Squamous cell carcinoma is associated with tobacco smoke, while adenocarcinoma is associated with wood dust.

Premalignant lesions such as inverted papillomas, which usually arise in the nasal cavity, have a 2% risk of malignant transformation. They can be easily mistaken for well-differentiated SCC. They are locally aggressive and carry a high risk of recurrence or residual disease after treatment.

Clinical presentation
Most patients present with symptoms of nasal obstruction, nasal discharge or epistaxis. Patients with advanced disease with involvement of adjacent structures may present with facial pain, numbness, proptosis, diplopia, cranial nerve dysfunction and/or palpable neck nodes.

Investigations and staging
Investigations are done as detailed in an earlier section. The T stages for primary tumours of nasal cavity are detailed in Table 11.25 and N stage as in Table 11.3. All patients are staged as in Table 11.4.

Histology
SCC is the commonest histological type. Non-squamous histologies include adenocarcinoma and its variants, mucosal melanoma, olfactory neuroblastoma (Jegoux *et al.*, 2013).

Treatment overview
There are no randomised studies comparing treatment modalities, and treatment recommendations are based on single-centre series. Surgery plays a key role in the treatment of these tumours at all stages. Locally advanced-stage patients are managed with surgery and radiation as there is a significant risk of local recurrence following surgery alone.

Surgery
The goal of surgery is to remove all visible tumours with clear margins, while maintaining function and cosmesis. Clear margins are not achievable in many cases due to close proximity of vital structures.

Surgical techniques include:

- wide local excision for small tumours;
- lateral rhinotomy for larger tumours involving the lateral wall and septum;
- total rhinectomy for tumours involving nasal cartilage and or bone and prosthesis for rehabilitation;

- craniofacial resection and reconstruction for tumours involving the skull base, and may include total maxillectomy and or orbital exenteration when involved;
- endoscopic resection followed by adjuvant radiotherapy.

Patients with pathological nodes in the neck should undergo modified radical neck dissection. A clinically negative neck is monitored closely and is not treated prophylactically because the risk of neck node involvement is less than 10%.

Radiotherapy and systemic therapy

Primary radiotherapy with curative intent is an alternative treatment option for early-stage disease in patients who refuse surgery or in patients not suitable for surgery due to comorbidity. Adjuvant radiotherapy also plays a key role in the curative treatment of nasal cavity tumours following surgery.

Patients with unresectable disease are treated with definitive radiotherapy alone or with the addition of chemotherapy (neoadjuvant and concurrent) in patients with squamous histology and good performance status.

Radiotherapy planning

All patients needing radiotherapy are immobilised, scanned and the target volumes are delineated as described earlier.

Prognosis

The prognosis for sinonasal carcinoma includes the nasal cavity as in Table 11.26.

Carcinoma of salivary glands

Introduction

Salivary gland tumours are rare and represent only 3–7% of all head and neck cancers. Population-based studies report 8–9 cases of malignant salivary gland tumours per 1,000,000 (British Association of Otorhinolaryngology, 2011).

- Of salivary gland tumours, 70% occur in the parotid gland. However, less than half of parotid gland tumours are malignant. Benign diagnoses, such as pleomorphic adenomas and Warthin's tumour, are more common (Adelstein et al., 2012).

- Ten per cent of salivary gland tumours occur in the submandibular glands, where approximately 50% of these tumours are malignant.
- Less than one per cent of salivary gland tumours occur in the sublingual glands.
- The remaining 20% of salivary gland tumours arise from the minor salivary glands and are generally malignant.

Anatomy

Salivary glands are broadly classified into major and minor salivary glands.

- Major salivary glands – paired parotid, submandibular and sublingual glands.
- Minor salivary glands – found throughout the lining membrane of the upper aerodigestive tract with the highest concentration present on the hard palate followed by the oral cavity.

Parotid gland

- Consists of two lobes (superficial and deep) separated by the facial nerve. The parotid boundaries are:
  - anterior – masseter,
  - posterior – mastoid process,
  - medial – styloid process,
  - lateral – skin and subcutaneous tissue,
  - superior – zygomatic arch,
  - inferior – anteromedial border of sternomastoid.
- Most tumours of the parotid gland arise in the superficial lobe. They can invade the facial nerve causing facial nerve palsy and can extend into the pterygopalatine fossa and lateral parapharyngeal space to cause trismus.
- Lymphatic drainage is to the preauricular and intraparotid nodes, spreading subsequently to the subparotid nodes or directly to level II nodes.

Submandibular gland

- Consists of two lobes, a large superficial lobe, lateral to mylohyoid, and a small deep lobe medial to the mylohyoid separated by the posterior border of the mylohyoid.
- Tumours can invade the marginal branch of the facial nerve, the lingual nerve and the hypoglossal nerve, causing tongue weakness.

- The submandibular gland drains to level Ib nodes and then to level II nodes.

Sublingual gland

This is the smallest of the three glands and is situated beneath the mucosa of the floor of mouth on either side of the frenulum. The boundaries include:

- anterior – symphysis mentis,
- posterior – deep lobe of submandibular gland,
- superior – mucosa of floor of mouth,
- inferior – myolohyoid muscle,
- medial – genioglossus muscle,
- lateral – mandible.

Clinical presentation

Patients present with a painless lump over the parotid or submandibular region with or without neck lumps. The duration of the lump, pain, rapid growth, facial nerve involvement and fixity suggest a malignant tumour.

Investigations and staging

Investigations are done as detailed in an earlier section. Open biopsy of major salivary gland tumours is not advisable because of a risk of tumour spillage and seeding. Primary T staging is summarised in Table 11.27 and nodal staging is summarised in Table 11.3. All patients are staged as in Table11. 4.

Histology

Salivary gland tumours constitute a wide range of histological types which can be confirmed following surgical resection. The commonest benign tumour is pleomorphic adenoma. Mucoepidermoid carcinoma, adenoid cystic carcinoma, adenocarcinoma, malignant mixed tumours (or carcinoma-ex pleomorphic adenoma) and acinic cell carcinomas are the most common malignant histological subtypes. Adenoid cystic carcinomas are slow-growing but have a high incidence of perineural invasion. Primary squamous cell carcinomas of the parotid gland are rare and have a very poor prognosis. They are more likely to represent a metastatic intraparotid lymph node from a squamous cell carcinoma of skin.

Treatment overview

Surgery remains the treatment of choice for all salivary gland tumours. Adjuvant treatment with radiotherapy

Table 11.27 T staging of salivary gland tumours

T1	Tumour ≤ 2 cm; without clinical or macroscopic extraparenchymal extension
T2	Tumour > 2 cm to ≤ 4 cm without clinical or macroscopic extraparenchymal extension
T3	Tumour > 4 cm and/or having clinical or macroscopic extraparenchymal extension
T4a	Moderately advanced disease: tumour invades skin, mandible, ear canal and/or facial nerve
T4b	Very advanced disease: tumour invades skull base and/or pterygoid plates and/or encases carotid artery

Adapted from AJCC, 2009.

depends upon final histology. Primary non-surgical treatment with radiotherapy alone is aimed at control of symptoms and disease.

Surgery

The type of surgery depends upon the location and extent of the tumour. Surgery involves either a superficial parotidectomy or total parotidectomy for tumours arising in the parotid gland. The facial nerve is preserved where possible. Facial nerve involvement is more likely with larger and higher-grade tumours and with tumours involving both lobes.

A wide local excision with the aim of achieving a clear margin is done for tumours arising from other glands.

Modified radical or selective neck dissection is done in the following situations:

- Clinical or radiological evidence of node involvement.
- Locally advanced tumours (tumours > 4 cm, T3/T4 disease).
- High-grade tumours such as undifferentiated carcinomas, high-grade mucoepidermoid carcinoma, adenocarcinoma and malignant mixed tumours (Armstrong *et al.*, 1992).

Radiotherapy

Primary radiotherapy is an alternative treatment in patients either with locally advanced, inoperable tumours or where comorbidity precludes surgery to improve symptoms and is aimed at control of disease.

Radiotherapy to the postoperative bed following curative surgery has been shown to improve local control.

Table 11.28 Five-year relative survival of salivary gland tumours

Stage	Five-year relative survival (%)
1	91
2	75
3	65
4	38

Adapted from AJCC, 2009.

Indications for adjuvant radiotherapy include the following.

- Close or positive resection margins.
- Residual disease – microscopic or macroscopic.
- Positive nodes.
- High-grade histology – e.g. high-grade mucoepidermoid, adenoid cystic carcinomas, high-grade adenocarcinoma, malignant mixed tumours, except in small T1 tumours with clear margins.
- Tumours > 4 cm, T3/T4 disease, bone or nerve involvement, skin involvement, perineural spread.
- Close proximity to the facial nerve where the nerve has been preserved.
- Pleomorphic adenomas – with positive or close margin and following excision of recurrent tumours. It is important to weigh the risks of radiotherapy, such as second malignancy in this benign disease in young patients against the risk of recurrence.
- Low-grade tumours – close and/or positive margins.

Radiotherapy planning

Patients undergo planning CT scan with immobilisation as described earlier. Treatment volumes are mostly unilateral and usually two clinical target volumes (CTV1 – high dose; CTV2 – prophylactic dose) are outlined.

CTV1 includes:

- the entire parotid bed, triangular in shape on an axial CT slice, which has the following borders:
  - superior: zygomatic arch;
  - inferior: the lower border of the hyoid;
  - anterior: the anterior border of the masseter to include the parotid duct;
  - posterior: attachment of the pinna or posterior to mastoid air cells;
  - lateral: skin;
  - medial: midline (or as a minimum 2 cm from midline) to include the parapharyngeal space and the deep lobe of the parotid.
- The following are additionally included in patients with adenoid cystic carcinoma.
  - Stylomastoid foramen for tumours in the parotid gland.
  - The lingual nerve up to the foramen ovale and the marginal mandibular branch of the facial nerve up to the stylomastoid foramen for tumours in the submandibular gland.

CTV2 includes:

- uninvolved at-risk nodal levels (levels III–Vb);
- other nodal levels as per Table 11.8.

Neck nodes are routinely treated in all high-grade tumours and are not treated in low-grade or benign tumours.

In patients with parotid tumours, the first echelon nodal levels Ib, IIa, IIb and retropharyngeal nodes are included in the high-dose volume due to close proximity to the parotid bed.

The beam arrangement in the forward planning technique typically includes an anterior and a posterior oblique wedged beam. The beam angles are chosen to avoid the contralateral parotid and spinal cord.

Prognosis

The five-year relative survival by combined (clinical and pathological) AJCC stage for major salivary glands is shown in Table 11.28.

Squamous cell carcinoma (of neck nodes) of unknown primary

Introduction

Among patients presenting with metastatic cervical lymphadenopathy, there are few patients where a primary cannot be identified on detailed examination and investigations, accounting for less than 5% of head and neck cancers. Patients with isolated supraclavicular lymph nodes almost always have metastatic disease, with the site of origin mostly below clavicles.

Clinical presentation

Patients usually present with persistent painless neck swelling and/or associated symptoms of pain and a rapid increase in size.

Investigations and staging

Evaluation includes:

- detailed history;
- clinical examination to identify potential primary source for malignant spread to neck nodes, usually in the oropharynx (tonsil and tongue base);
- flexible nasendoscopy to evaluate the nasal cavity, nasopharynx, pharyngeal walls, tongue base, larynx and hypopharynx;
- examination under anaesthesia, panendoscopy and directed biopsies of:
  - postnasal space,
  - tongue base,
  - hypopharynx,
  - bilateral tonsillectomies;
- ultrasound of neck ± FNAC or biopsy using a cutting needle;
- CT scan of neck and thorax;
- MRI of craniofacial region;
- PET-CT scan should be done for patients who are suitable for radical treatment when other investigations have failed to reveal a primary site and may ideally be performed before panendoscopy to direct the biopsies.

A PET-CT scan identifies a primary in approximately 25% of patients.

There is no specific staging system for unknown primary. However, in common with other defined clinical groups in carcinoma of unknown primary, the neck nodes are staged according to the scheme for the most likely primary site. In this case the staging is shown in Table 11.3.

Histology

The most common histology is squamous cell carcinoma with varying degrees of differentiation. The diagnostic biopsy from the neck node should be examined for p16 immunohistochemistry and/or HPV ISH and/or EBV testing to provide prognostic information and to guide the identification of a primary site.

The majority of primary tumours identified in patients with an unknown primary are in the oropharynx (43% tonsil and 39% tongue base) and most of them are p16-positive.

Treatment overview

The optimum treatment for this group of patients remains uncertain. The aim of treatment remains achieving regional control of neck disease and ensuring that the primary cancer does not develop in potential sites of origin. The treatment options are as follows.

- Modified radical neck dissection followed by adjuvant treatment to the neck depending upon postoperative histology and/or prophylactic treatment to potential primary sites.
- Primary radiotherapy alone in patients with small-volume neck disease.
- Concurrent chemoradiotherapy.

Surgery

Surgery involves a modified radical neck dissection which may be sufficient for a select group of patients with pN1 disease, without pathological risk factors for recurrence.

Patients with intermediate or high-risk (positive margin and/or ECS) pathological features need adjuvant treatment with radiotherapy or chemoradiotherapy, respectively, to improve local control rates.

Radiotherapy and systemic therapy

Concurrent chemoradiotherapy is an alternative, with surgery to neck reserved for residual neck nodes on post-treatment scan.

Radiotherapy planning

Patients are immobilised and scanned as detailed before. The general principles of outlining (definitive and postoperative) as detailed before are followed.

CTV1 (Step 2) includes:

- involved nodal levels are included in the high dose (primary or postoperative) CTV;
- the inclusion of potential primary sites in the treatment volume varies both nationally within the UK across different centres and internationally. Most oncologists either include the entire pharyngeal mucosa (total mucosal irradiation) or mucosa of the ipsilateral pharyngeal wall

and tongue base, excluding nasopharynx and hypopharynx. The latter option is associated with less long-term morbidity.

CTV2 (Step 3) includes:
- all at-risk uninvolved nodal levels (Ib–Vb);
- other lymph node levels as per Table 11.9.

The doses are prescribed accordingly (definitive or postoperative). However, the dose prescribed to the pharyngeal mucosa may vary from a radical dose to a prophylactic dose. There are no randomised studies comparing the doses. Higher doses of greater than 60 Gy are associated with significant long-term swallowing impairment, and increasingly the dose to the pharyngeal axis is now reduced to between 54 and 60 Gy, resulting in lower long-term morbidity and comparable outcomes (Sher *et al.*, 2011; Frank *et al.*, 2010).

Prognosis

The 5-year actuarial locoregional control and overall survival from a small cohort are 94% and 89%, respectively (Frank *et al.*, 2010).

The use of radiotherapy in benign conditions

Thyroid eye disease

Thyroid eye disease results from an autoimmune response in which activated T cells invade the orbit and stimulate the production of glycosaminoglycan in fibroblasts.

The patient is treated with a single lateral field angled 5° away from the lens or with half-beam blocking, or using an anterior field with central-axis beam-blocking. Dose: 20 Gy in 8–10 daily fractions, 5 fractions a week, using 4–6 MV photons.

Of patients treated in this way for thyroid eye disease, 75% report an improvement.

Surgery is indicated in the presence of rapidly progressive optic neuropathy. Steroids are used as an alternative to radiotherapy, but the benefits are short-lived. There is a 10% incidence of cataracts found in long-term follow-up studies. Its use is examined in NICE Interventional Procedure Guidance 148, which supports its use in patients for whom other treatments are inadequate or associated with significant side effects.

The management of thyrotoxicosis is described on page 526.

Macular degeneration

Age-related macular degeneration is a leading cause of blindness in developed countries, affecting up to 28% of patients over 75 years old. Proliferation of choroidal vessels causes subretinal haemorrhages and retinal detachment.

Consider giving the patient 15 Gy in 5 fractions in one week using a unilateral 6-MV field with half-beam blocking. Avoid the contralateral eye and pituitary gland.

Visual acuity is improved or stabilised in 66% cases at 12-month follow-up.

Initial trials are promising, but NICE Interventional Procedure Guidance 49 concludes that there is insufficient evidence to offer outwith clinical trials.

Orbital pseudotumour

An orbital pseudotumour is a benign idiopathic orbital inflammation causing periorbital swelling, decreased orbital mobility and pain.

The recommended radiotherapy dose is 25 Gy in 12 fractions with 4–6 MV photons and half-beam blocking.

Control is achieved in 75% of cases.

CT scanning is helpful, but biopsy is required to exclude lymphoma. Consider steroids first line, and radiotherapy if it fails to respond.

Pterygium

Pterygium is a growth of fibrovascular tissue on the cornea which can impare visual acuity.

Use a beta-emitting ^{90}Sr applicator. An energy of 2.2 MeV gives 50% at about 1 mm and 10% at 3.3 mm. The recommended dose is 7 Gy a week for 3 fractions to start within 24 hours of surgery.

Local recurrence rates vary from 3% to 16% compared with 8% to 50% without postoperative radiotherapy.

Radiation appears to reduce vascularisation at the operative site and so decrease recurrence.

References

Adelstein, D. J., Koyfman, S. A., El-Naggar, A.K., *et al.* (2012). Biology and management of salivary gland cancers. *Semin. Radiat. Oncol.* **22**, 245–253.

AJCC. (2009). *AJCC Cancer Staging Manual*, ed. S. B. Edge, D. R. Byrd, C. C. Compton, *et al.,* 7th edn. Chicago: American Joint Committee on Cancer.

Al-Sarraf, M., LeBlanc, M., Giri, P. G., *et al.* (1998). Chemoradiotherapy versus radiotherapy in patients with advanced nasopharyngeal cancer: Phase III randomised intergroup study 0099. *J. Clin. Oncol.* **16**, 1310–1317.

Ang, K. K., Trotti, A., Brown, B. W., *et al.* (2001). Randomised trial addressing risk features and time factors of surgery plus radiotherapy in advanced head and neck cancer. *Int. J. Radiat. Oncol. Biol. Phys.*, **51**, 571–578.

Ang, K. K., Harris, J., Wheeler, R., *et al.* (2010). Human papillomavirus and survival of patients with oropharyngeal cancer. *N. Engl. J. Med.* **363**, 24–35.

Ang, K. K., Zhang, Q., Rosenthal, D. I., *et al.* (2014). Randomised phase III trial of concurrent accelerated radiation plus cisplatin with or without cetuximab for stage III or IV head and neck carcinoma: RTOG 0522. *J. Clin. Oncol.*, JCO.2013.53.5633, published online on 25 August 2014.

Argiris, A., Li, Y., Forastiere, A., *et al.* (2004). Prognostic factors and long-term survivorship in patients with recurrent or metastatic carcinoma of head and neck. *Cancer* **101**, 2222–2229.

Armstrong, J. G., Harrison, L. B., Thaler, H. T., *et al.* (1992). The indications for elective treatment of the neck in cancer of the major salivary glands. *Cancer* **69**, 615–619.

Baujat, B., Audry, H., Bourhis, J., *et al.* (2006). Chemotherapy as an adjunct to radiotherapy in locally advanced nasopharyngeal carcinoma. *Cochrane Database Syst. Rev.* Issue **4** Art No. CD004329.

Bernier, J., Domenge C., Ozsahin, M., *et al.* (2004). Postoperative irradiation with or without concomitant chemotherapy for locally advanced head and neck cancer. *N. Engl. J. Med.* **350**, 1945–1952.

Blanchard, P., Bourhis, J., Lacas, B., *et al.* (2013). Taxane–cisplatin–fluorouracil as induction chemotherapy in locally advanced head and neck cancers: an individual patient data meta-analysis. *J. Clin. Oncol.* **31**, 2854–2860.

Bonner, J. A., Harari, P. M., Giralt, J., *et al.* (2006). Radiotherapy plus cetuximab for squamous-cell carcinoma of the head and neck. *N. Engl. J. Med.* **354**, 567–578.

Bourhis, J., Overgaard, J., Audry, H., *et al.* (2006). Hyperfractionated or accelerated radiotherapy in head and neck cancer: a meta-analysis. *Lancet*, **368**, 843–854.

British Association of Otorhinolaryngology. (2011). *Head and Neck Cancers: Multidisciplinary Management Guidelines*, 4th edn. London: ENT UK.

Cancer Research UK. (2010). *UK Cancer Incidence (2010) by Country Summary, April 2013.* http://publications.cancerresearchuk.org/downloads/Product/CS_DT_INCCOUNTRIES.pdf (accessed December 2014).

Cooper, J. S., Pajak, T. F., Forastiere, A. A., *et al.* (2004). Postoperative concurrent radiotherapy and chemotherapy for high risk squamous cell carcinoma of the head and neck. *N. Engl. J. Med.* **350**, 1937–1944.

Dulguerov, P., Jacobsen, M. S., Allal, A. S., *et al.* (2001). Nasal and paranasal sinus carcinoma: are we making progress? A series of 220 patients and a systematic review. *Cancer* **92**, 3012–3029.

Forastiere, A. A., Metch, B., Schuller, D. E., *et al.* (1992). Randomized comparison of cisplatin plus fluorouracil and carboplatin plus fluorouracil versus methotrexate in advanced squamous-cell carcinoma of the head and neck: a Southwest Oncology Group study. *J. Clin. Onco.,* **10**, 1245–1251.

Forastiere, A. A., Goepfert, H., Maor, M., *et al.* (2003). Concurrent chemotherapy and radiotherapy for organ preservation in advanced laryngeal cancer. *N. Engl. J. Med.* **349**, 2091–2098.

Frank, S. J., Rosenthal, D. I., Petsuksiri, J., *et al.* (2010). Intensity modulated radiotherapy for cervical node squamous cell carcinoma metastasis from unknown head and neck primary site: M.D. Anderson Cancer Centre outcomes and patterns of failure. *Int. J. Radiat. Oncol. Biol. Phys.* **78**, 1005–1010.

Ghi, M. G., Paccagnella, A., Ferrari, D., *et al.* (2014). Concomitant chemoradiation (CRT) or cetuximab/RT (CET/RT) versus induction docetaxel/cisplatin/5-fluorouracil followed by CRT or CET/RT in patients with locally advanced squamous cell carcinoma of head and neck – A randomised phase III factorial study. *J. Clin. Oncol.* **32**, 5s, suppl; abstr. 6004.

Gibson, M. K., Li, Y., Murphy, B., *et al.* (2005). Randomized phase III evaluation of cisplatin plus fluorouracil versus cisplatin plus paclitaxel in advanced head and neck cancer (E1395): an intergroup trial of the Eastern Cooperative Oncology Group. *J. Clin. Oncol.* **23**, 3562–3567.

Grégoire, V., Ang, K. K., Budach, W., *et al.* (2014). Delineation of the neck node levels for head and neck tumours: A 2013 update, Consensus guidelines. *Radiother. Oncol.* **110**, 172–181.

Jegoux, F., Metreau, A., Louvel, G., *et al.* (2013). Paranasal sinus cancer. *Eur. Ann. Otorhinolaryngol. Head Neck Dis.* **130**, 327–335.

Langendijk, J. A., Leemans, C. R., Buter, J., *et al.* (2004). The additional value of chemotherapy to radiotherapy in locally advanced nasopharyngeal carcinoma: A meta-analysis of the published literature. *J. Clin. Oncol.* **22**, 4604–4612.

Langendijk, J. A., Doornaert, P., Verdonck-de Leeuw, I. M., *et al.* (2008). Impact of late treatment related toxicity on quality of life among patients with head and neck cancer treated with radiotherapy. *J. Clin. Oncol.* **26**, 3770–3776.

Lavaf, A., Genden, E. M., Cesaretti, J. A., *et al.* (2008). Adjuvant radiotherapy improves overall survival for patients with lymph node positive head and neck squamous cell carcinoma. *Cancer* **112**, 535–543.

Lee, N., Harris, J., Garden, A. S., *et al.* (2009). Intensity-Modulated Radiation Therapy with or without chemotherapy for nasopharyngeal carcinoma: Radiation Therapy Oncology Group Phase II Trial 0225. *J. Clin. Oncol.* **22**, 3684–3690.

Lee, A., Lin, J. C. and Ng, W. T. (2012). Current management of nasopharyngeal cancer. *Semin. Radiat. Oncol.* **22**, 233–244.

Machtay, M., Moughan, J., Trotti, A., *et al.* (2008). Factors associated with severe late toxicity after concurrent chemoradiation for locally advanced head and neck cancer; An RTOG Analysis. *J. Clin. Oncol.* **26**, 3582–3589.

Mehanna, H., Rattay, T., Smith, J., *et al.* (2009). Treatment and follow up of oral dysplasia – a systematic review and meta-analysis. *Head Neck* **31**, 1600–1609.

Mehanna, H., Beech, T., Nicholson, T., *et al.* (2013). Prevalence of human papillomavirus in oropharyngeal and nonoropharyngeal head and neck cancer – Systematic review and meta-analysis of trends by time and region. *Head Neck* **35**, 747–755.

Mehanna, H. M., Wong. W. L., McConkey, C. C., *et al.* (2015). PET-NECK: a multi-centre, radomized, phase III, controlled trial (RCT) comparing PETCT guided active surveillance with planned neck dissection (ND) for locally advanced (N2/N3) nodal metastases (LANM) in patients with head and neck squamous cell cancer (HNSCC) treated with primary radical chemoradiotherapy (CRT). *J. Clin. Oncol.*, **33**, 2015 (suppl; abstr 6009).

Mishra, R. C., Singh, D.N., Mishra, T. K., *et al.* (1996). Post-operative radiotherapy in carcinoma buccal mucosa, a prospective randomised trial. *Eur. J. Surg. Oncol.* **22**, 502–504.

Moore, E. J. and Hinni, M. L. (2013). Critical review: Transoral laser microsurgery and robotic assisted surgery for oropharynx cancer including human papillomavirus-related cancer. *Int. J. Radiat. Oncol. Biol. Phys.* **85**, 1163–1167.

National Cancer Intelligence Network. (2010). *Profile of Head and Neck Cancers in England – Incidence, Mortality and Survival.* Oxford: Oxford Cancer Intelligence Unit.

Nutting, C. M., Morden, J. P., Harrington, K. J., *et al.* (2011). Parotid-sparing intensity modulated versus conventional radiotherapy in head and neck cancer (PARSPORT): A phase 3 multicentre randomised controlled trial. *Lancet Oncol.* **12**, 127–136.

Overgaard, J., Hansen, H., Specht, L., *et al.* (2003). Five compared with six fractions per week of conventional radiotherapy of squamous-cell carcinoma of head and neck: DAHANCA 6 and 7 randomised controlled trial. *Lancet* **362**, 933–940.

Parsons, J. T., Medenhall, W. M., Stringer, S. P., *et al.* (2002). Squamous cell carcinoma of the oropharynx: surgery, radiation therapy or both. *Cancer* **94**, 2967–2980.

Pignon, J. P., le Maître, A., Maillard, E., *et al.* (2009). Meta-analysis of chemotherapy in head and neck cancer (MACH-NC): An update on 93 randomised trials and 17,346 patients. *Radiother. Oncol.* **92**, 4–14.

Pointreau, Y., Garaud, P., Chapet, S., *et al.* (2009). Randomised trial of induction chemotherapy with cisplatin and 5FU with or without docetaxel for larynx preservation. *J. Natl. Cancer Inst.* **101**, 498–506.

Pow, E. H., Kwong, D. L., McMillan, A. S., *et al.* (2006). Xerostomia and quality of life after intensity-modulated radiotherapy vs conventional radiotherapy for early-stage nasopharyngeal carcinoma: Initial results on a randomised controlled trial. *Int. J. Radiat. Oncol. Biol. Phys.* **66**, 981–991.

Shanmugaratnam, K., Sobin, L. H. and World Health Organization. (1978). *Histological Typing of Upper Respiratory Tract Tumours. International Histological Classification of Tumours: no. 19.* Geneva: World Health Organization.

Sher, D. J., Balboni, T. A., Haddad, R. I., *et al.* (2011). Efficacy and toxicity of chemoradiotherapy using intensity modulated radiotherapy for unknown primary of head and neck. *Int. J. Radiat. Oncol. Biol. Phys.* **80**, 1405–1411.

Takes, R. P., Strojan, P., Silver, C. E., *et al.* (2012). Current trends in initial management of hypopharyngeal cancer: the declining use of open surgery. *Head Neck* **34**, 270–281.

Tandon, S., Shahab, S., Benton, J. I., *et al.* (2008). Fine needle aspiration cytology in a regional head and neck cancer center: comparison with a systematic review and meta-analysis. *Head Neck* **30**, 1246–1252.

Vermorken, J. B., Mesia, R., Rivera, F., *et al.* (2008). Platinum-based chemotherapy plus cetuximab in head and neck cancer. *N. Engl. J. Med.* **359**, 1116–1127.

Vermorken, J. B., Stöhlmacher-Williams, J., Davidenko, I., *et al.* (2013). Cisplatin and fluorouracil with or without panitumumab in patients with recurrent or metastatic squamous-cell carcinoma of the head and neck (SPECTRUM): an open-label phase 3 randomised trial. *Lancet Oncol.* **14**, 697–710.

Weller, M. D., Nankivell, P.C., McConkey, C., *et al.* (2010). The risk and interval to malignancy of patients with laryngeal dysplasia; A systematic review of case series and meta-analysis. *Clin. Otolaryngol.* **35**, 364–372.

Chapter 2

Management of cancer of the oesophagus

Chapter 12

Carys Morgan and Tom Crosby

Introduction

In the past few decades there has been a dramatic increase in the incidence of adenocarcinoma of the oesophagus, predominantly in the lower oesophagus and gastro-oesophageal junction. This trend has been noted across most patient populations worldwide, but is most noticeable in the younger, white male population, and it appears to be primarily with gastro-oesophageal reflux disease (GORD) and less strongly with alcohol and smoking. Meanwhile, the incidence of squamous cancer worldwide has remained steady or has fallen slightly, although there are large geographical variations.

The majority of patients have developed locally advanced or metastatic disease by the time they present with symptoms and this limits their survival from any treatment. Staging is increasingly more accurate with the routine use of positron emission tomography (PET) and endoscopic ultrasound (EUS) enabling those with advanced disease to be excluded from more intensive treatment options, thus avoiding unnecessary adverse effects on the quality of life.

Combined modality therapy is increasingly used in patients who are suitable for curative treatment. There is evidence that preoperative chemotherapy is superior to surgery alone. There is a continuing controversy about the exact role of surgery combined with chemoradiotherapy (CRT) and which modality should be used first. To date it has not been possible to recruit to a comparative clinical trial.

It is known that CRT is more effective than radiotherapy alone and there is now clear evidence of the effectiveness of definitive chemoradiotherapy (dCRT) in oesophageal cancers. dCRT should therefore be considered a treatment option for selected patients such as those who are unfit for surgery, whose local disease extent precludes surgery or those with squamous cancers.

Optimum radiotherapy and chemotherapy regimens are being defined in the preoperative and definitive setting. Despite this, the majority of patients still present with advanced incurable disease where treatment options are more limited, but palliative chemotherapy has a role in some cases.

Early assessment of response to treatment is becoming an area of interest with early PET scans currently being incorporated into several trial protocols.

Types of oesophageal tumour

The types of oesophageal tumours are shown in Table 12.1.

The oesophagus is a relatively common site for a second primary cancer. For instance, following successful treatment for head and neck cancer, 4% of patients per year develop a second primary, 30% of which are oesophageal, especially squamous cancers. This is likely to be related to a 'field change' effect on the mucosa from common aetiological agents.

Anatomy

The oesophagus is usually measured from the central incisors (it usually extends from 15 to 40 cm) at endoscopy. It is often divided into sections, which are defined in Table 12.2.

The sternal notch is at 18 cm and the carina is usually at 25 cm, but this can vary significantly among patients. The gastro-oesophageal (GO) junction is usually at about 40 cm.

Practical Clinical Oncology, Second Edition, ed. Louise Hanna, Tom Crosby and Fergus Macbeth. Published by Cambridge University Press. © Cambridge University Press 2015.

Table 12.1 Types of oesophageal tumour

Type	Examples
Benign	Leiomyoma
	Haemangioma
	Adenoma
Malignant primary	Adenocarcinoma (65%)
	Squamous (~ 25%)
	Others (~ 5%)
	Small cell
	Lymphoma
	BCC
	Melanoma
	Leiomyosarcoma
	Kaposi's sarcoma
	Adenoid cystic
	Mucoepidermoid
	Gastro-intestinal stromal tumour
	Carcinoid
Malignant secondary	Lung
	Breast
	Melanoma

Siewert described a system to classify tumours involving the GO junction. Type I tumours are predominantly oesophageal and type III predominantly gastric. In type II tumours the disease equally straddles the junction.

Incidence and epidemiology

Tumour incidence in the UK is 11 per 100,000, with approximately 7000 new cases and approximately 6000 deaths per year. There is a large worldwide variation in incidence. Squamous cell carcinoma occurs more often in Iran, China and Transkei (South Africa), with rates as high as 100 per 100,000. In the past three decades, there has been a 3.5-fold increase in men and a 2-fold increase in women in the incidence of adenocarcinoma of the lower oesophagus. During the same period, there has also been an increase in the occurrence of adenocarcinoma of the gastric cardia. The incidence of oesophageal cancer increases with age, although there are also increasing numbers of cases occurring in the young, particularly among male Caucasians.

Carcinoma of the oesophagus

Risk factors and aetiology

The increase in adenocarcinomas (about 10% per year) of the middle and lower oesophagus appears to be more associated with reflux of acid (gastric and possibly bile) than with alcohol intake and smoking. The risk increases with age and it is more common in men, except for those cancers occurring in the upper third of the oesophagus, which are associated with Plummer–Vinson syndrome. Risk factors are as follows.

Physical/chemical

Physical and chemical causes of oesophageal cancer include:

- GORD;
- alcohol;
- smoking;
- corrosives;
- reduced dietary vitamin C;
- malnutrition (e.g. zinc deficiency).

Possible infective causes may be associated with:

- *Helicobacter pylori*;
- human papilloma virus;
- fungally infected cereals.

Associated conditions

An associated condition is Barrett's oesophagus. Of people over 30 years old, 10% have symptomatic reflux disease. In 10% of those with the disease, it will be mild and in 3.5%, severe; 1.5% will have long-segment (> 3 cm) Barrett's oesophagus. Over a period of 2–5 years, 0.35% and 0.12% of these patients will develop low- and high-grade dysplastic change, respectively. Therefore, in patients with Barrett's oesophagus, there is only about a 1% lifetime risk of developing an adenocarcinoma. Significant problems exist with interobserver variation among pathologists when classifying dysplastic changes, and severe dysplasia is synonymous with carcinoma *in situ*.

Other related conditions include:

- achalasia;
- tylosis palmaris;
- coeliac disease;
- Plummer–Vinson syndrome.

Table 12.2 Parts of the oesophagus

Part of oesophagus	Anatomical description	Distance from incisors (cm)	Correlation with vertebral bodies
Cervical oesophagus	Starts below cricopharyngeus to thoracic inlet	15–18	C6–T2/3
Thoracic oesophagus			
Upper	To tracheal bifurcation	18–24	T3 ~ T4/5
Middle	To half-way to GO junction	24–32	T5 ~ T8
Lower	To GO junction	32–40	T8 ~ T10

GO, gastro-oesophageal.

Table 12.3 Pathological features of carcinoma of the oesophagus

	Description
Macroscopic features	*Squamous cell*
	Plaque-like lesion or elevation of mucosa evolving into polypoid fungating lesion or necrotic ulceration
	Adenocarcinoma
	Often nodular and multicentric, arising in Barrett's mucosa. Similar growth to above progressing to circumferential mass
Microscopic features	*Squamous cell*
	Usually moderately to well-differentiated with typical features of squamous cancer (i.e. small cells with/without keratinisation)
	Adenocarcinoma
	Usually moderately to poorly differentiated, divided into intestinal, diffuse or adenosquamous type. Intestinal type shows well-formed glands lined by malignant cells whereas the diffuse type is composed of mucin-producing neoplastic cells

Apart from GORD and Barrett's oesophagus, the afore-mentioned conditions are primarily associated with squamous cell carcinoma.

Pathology

Adenocarcinomas occurring in the lower oesophagus usually arise on the background of Barrett's oesophagus, a columnar epithelialisation of the native squamous mucosa. The sequence from metaplasia through degrees of dysplasia to invasive adenocarcinoma is associated with genetic changes such as loss of TP53 function, loss of heterozygosity (LOH) of the Rb gene, overexpression of cyclins D1 and E, and inactivation of p16 and p27. Amplification of MYC and K- and H-RAS occur late in the transition to adenocarcinoma. A high proportion of adenocarcinomas have foci of gastric- or intestinal-type lining in the immediate vicinity of the tumour and elsewhere in the oesophagus. Pathological features are shown in Table 12.3.

Spread

Spread of primary tumour

Oesophageal tumours are usually locally advanced at presentation because there is no peri-oesophageal serosa to inhibit their growth. They spread circumferentially and longitudinally along submucosal and peri-neural pathways to form skip lesions of up to 5–6 cm from the primary tumour. Infiltration into mediastinal structures occurs, most frequently into the trachea, aorta, pleura, diaphragm and vertebrae.

Lymphatic spread

The first-station lymph nodes (N1) of the oesophagus are supraclavicular; upper, middle and lower para-oesophageal; right and left paratracheal; aorto-pulmonary; subcarinal; diaphragmatic; paracardial; left gastric; common hepatic; splenic artery and coeliac.

- Upper third, cervical oesophagus; 15–18 cm.
- Middle third, slightly arbitrary upper limit; 18–31 cm.
- Lower third, to GO junction; 31–40 cm.

Patients with upper-third tumours can be treated in a similar way to patients with head and neck cancer, such as postcricoid carcinoma. A shell is needed for planning, and anterior and anterior oblique fields are used as part of combined modality therapy. This technique will not be discussed further here.

The radiotherapy technique for the middle and lower thirds of the oesophagus includes patient preparation, positioning and immobilisation. 3D conformal planning is standard, but due to the effect of respiratory motion which can be particularly significant in junctional tumours, there needs to be some consideration of this movement either in the margins applied or in use of 4D planning. There is increasing interest in the use of 4D planning in junctional tumours and this is used in some UK centres and is being incorporated into trials protocols. Respiratory gating techniques are likely to be difficult for most patients to comply with.

Patients should be planned and treated in the supine position with their arms above their heads and immobilisation of the legs (e.g.with knee-fix, anterior and two lateral tattoos used). The planning CT scan should be performed within 2 weeks of starting the neoadjuvant phase of chemotherapy with 3-mm slices. To enable accurate assessment of the doses to organs at risk (OAR), the scan should extend superiorly to at least one CT slice above the apices of the lungs and inferiorly to the iliac crest (L2). Scans for upper-third tumours may need to extend superiorly to the tragus. Intravenous contrast should be used as it helps to distinguish the GTV from surrounding tissues.

Target delineation

- The description below is based on the radiotherapy planning technique described in the SCOPE1 trial planning document (see the SCOPE1 radiotherapy protocol for full details). This trial has helped to standardise radiotherapy planning for oesophageal cancer in the UK, although there will be acceptable variations to the described technique.
- In most cases the GTV (extent of primary and nodal disease) is defined by the information available from the diagnostic CT scan, PET-CT scan and EUS. Disease length/extent can often be most apparent on EUS as submucosal spread is better identified. Overall, the GTV should encompass disease defined on any of the available imaging modalities used (i.e. CT, EUS and PET), even if only apparent on a single modality.
- Practically, the EUS is used to define the disease length with the aid of an EUS-derived reference point, i.e. tracheal carina or aortic arch which is easily seen on CT axial images. The site of the tumour on EUS can then be mapped onto the planning CT scan.
- The CTV is usually extended manually 2 cm craniocaudally along the length of the oesophagus from GTV to allow for the inclination of the oesophagus. This volume is referred to as CTVA. It is then grown by 1 cm radially to form CTVB which should encompass the likely areas of microscopic spread. This can be edited for structures such as vertebrae that do not need to be incorporated in CTV, particularly if there is the potential to impact on organs OARs, e.g. the spinal cord.
- It is important to note that if the tumour involves the GO junction, the gastrohepatic ligament region should be encompassed within the CTV due to the high incidence of nodal metastases (even if negative on imaging). For these junctional tumours the CTV should be extended manually along the oesophagus to the GO junction to form CTVA, the radial margin of 1 cm should be added to form the CTVB and then this volume should be manually edited and extended along the gastrohepatic ligament (for 2 cm below the inferior border of GTV), i.e. along the lesser curve to include the paracardial and left gastric lymph nodes with or without the common hepatic, coeliac and splenic arteries. CTVB can also be edited if extending posteriorly into vertebrae. The PTV is created by the addition of a further 1 cm superior/inferior margin and a 0.5 cm radial margin by the treatment planning system.
- Overall, the maximum length of GTV usually treatable within a radical volume is around 12 cm.

Organs at risk

- The full extent of the right and left lungs should be outlined in order to calculate a combined lung dose volume histogram (DVH). The spinal cord should be outlined with creation of a planning risk volume (PRV) for the cord to account for positioning error. The heart, liver and kidneys should also be outlined.

- The normal tissue tolerances below are based on the SCOPE1 trial and are quite conservative but act as a guide.
  - Spinal cord (PRV) should receive less than 40 Gy; D40 = 0%.
  - Heart: less than 30% of the total heart volume should receive more than 40 Gy; V40 < 30%.
  - Lung: less than 25% of the total lung volume should receive more than 20 Gy, i.e. V20 < 25%.
  - Liver: less than 60% liver should receive more than 30 Gy, i.e. V30 < 60%.
  - Individual kidney: V20 < 25%.

Treatment delivery

- All treatment will be delivered in a single 3D (conformal) CT planned phase. A four-field technique is usually satisfactory, with anterior–posterior parallel opposed and two posterior oblique or lateral fields. Additional fields using gantry orientations as above may improve dose homogeneity across the PTV. Inhomogeneity can occur because of changing body contour, the position of the oesophagus along its length and the different tissues through which radiation must pass to the PTV.

Verification

- The plan should be verified on set to ensure accurate treatment delivery.
- Electronic portal imaging (EPI) taken in the first week of treatment on the linear accelerator (for first 3 fractions) and weekly throughout treatment thereafter is standard. Use of cone beam CT scans is helpful as bony match does not give full picture.
- Figure 12.1 shows a 3D conformal radiotherapy plan for carcinoma of the oesophagus.

Typical radiation doses

- If radiation is the sole treatment, a dose of 60–64 Gy (2 Gy per fraction) should be delivered to the target volume.

- If CRT is the sole curative therapy, reduce the dose to 50 Gy in 25 fractions.
- If CRT is preoperative, give 45 Gy in 25 fractions.
- The dose, treating each field daily Monday to Friday, is prescribed to the ICRU 50 reference point, usually the point of intersection of the central axes. The PTV minimum should be no less than 95% and the PTV maximum should be no more than 107%.

Side effects from radiotherapy are shown in Table 12.5.

Concurrent chemotherapy

Cisplatin and capecitabine or 5-FU are the agents most commonly used concurrently with RT. They both have reasonable single-agent activity and are potent radiosensitisers. A commonly used regimen is four three-weekly cycles, in which radiotherapy is given in cycles 3 and 4. This regimen delivers the same number of planned chemotherapy cycles as used in the RTOG-85–01 study (Cooper *et al.*, 1999) and, because the non-concurrent chemotherapy is given in a neo-adjuvant phase, there is time for careful radiotherapy planning and improving the patient's dysphagia before the radiotherapy starts.

Treatment of recurrent carcinoma of the oesophagus

The prognosis of patients with recurrent disease is very poor. The pattern of recurrent disease varies depending on the initial local therapy given. After surgery, the majority of patients who relapse will do so at distant sites and they should be considered for palliative chemotherapy (as discussed in the next section), depending on their level of fitness. Occasionally if disease relapse is at the anastomosis only (and is confirmed as non-metastatic on PET) then dCRT is an option. After dCRT, the tumour most commonly recurs locally and endoscopic placement of a stent as described in the next section is frequently used to relieve dysphagia.

Palliative treatments and treatment of metastatic carcinoma of the oesophagus

Surgery

Surgical resection has no role in the palliation of patients with oesophageal cancer.

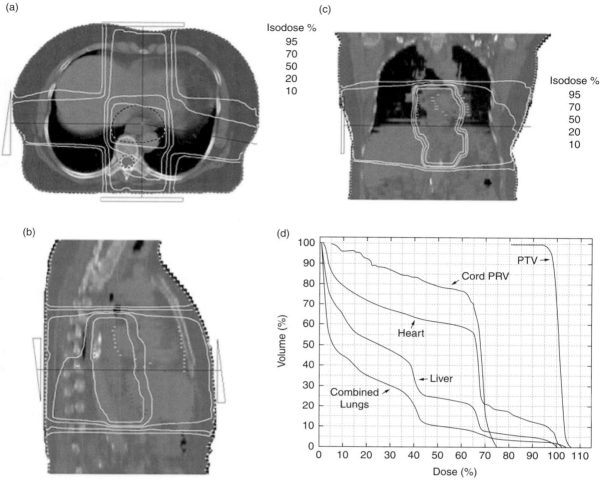

Figure 12.1 A 3D conformal plan for radical radiotherapy for carcinoma of the oesophagus. In this plan, a single-phase treatment has been used with four fields. (a) Transverse section showing how the dose outside the PTV is spread between critical structures. (b) Sagittal section showing the oblique angle of the PTV relative to the horizontal. (c) Coronal section showing how the isodoses have been shaped to conform to the PTV. This has been achieved by the use of multi-leaf collimators. (d) DVHs for the PTV and organs at risk. PRV, planning organ at risk volume; PTV, planning target volume.

Palliative chemotherapy

For patients with advanced GO cancer, chemotherapy has been shown to improve median survival and quality of life. In those who do respond, dysphagia usually improves after about 10 days. The improvement in median survival must be balanced against the effect on quality of life and this requires careful discussion with each patient about the pros and cons of treatment. Those with limited expected survival (< 3 months) or poor performance status will not usually benefit from chemotherapy and are best palliated with endoscopic stenting when required.

For those suitable for chemotherapy, treatment options depend on histological subtype. Over recent years there has been some improvement in survival for specific subgroups, and molecular typing is likely to become increasingly important and will likely be the focus of future clinical trials. Where possible, patients should be offered entry into these studies.

Adenocarcinoma

For those with junctional and gastric adenocarcinomas, HER2 status should be known as this will determine the treatment options. See the gastric cancer

Table 12.5 Side effects of radiotherapy to the oesophagus

Side effect	Management
Acute	
Tiredness	General advice for fatigue: explanation, goal setting, moderate exercise if able
Mucositis	Mucilage
Myelosuppression	Maintain haemoglobin above 120 g/L
Pneumonitis	Usually self-limiting, reducing course steroids if severe
Late	
Benign stricture	Endoscopic evaluation, biopsy, and dilatation; avoid stent if possible
Pulmonary fibrosis	Medical management
Pericarditis	Medical management
Ischaemic heart disease	Medical management
Tracheo-oesophageal fistula	Endoscopic placement of covered stent

chapter for additional details on chemotherapy for this group. A summary follows.

- HER2-negative: for those with HER2-negative adenocarcinoma the optimum combination is unclear. In the UK most regimens contain a combination of platinum (oxaliplatin or cisplatin), fluropyrimidine and an anthracycline (Cunningham *et al.*, 2008). The following is a chemotherapy regimen using epirubicin, oxaliplatin and capecitabine (EOX):
  - epirubicin 50 mg/m^2 day 1;
  - oxaliplatin 175 mg/m^2 day 1;
  - capecitabine 625 mg/m^2 orally b.d., days 1–21);
  - anti-emetics include:
    - dexamethasone 8 mg i.v. and 4 mg p.o. b.d., days 3–7;
    - 5-HT3 antagonist i.v.;
    - metoclopramide 10 mg q.d.s. p.r.n. for 10 days.
- HER2-positive: the results of the ToGA trial (Bang *et al.*, 2010) have changed treatment for this group of patients, and median survival has been seen to

be extended beyond a year for the first time in this group. Trastuzumab, an anti-HER2 monoclonal antibody, given in combination with cisplatin and a fluoropyrimidine, should now be considered standard for those with HER2-positive cancers. The addition of trastuzumab to chemotherapy led to a median survival of 13.8 months versus 11.1 months with chemotherapy alone. The benefit was seen in all HER2-positive patients, but was more marked in those with increased levels of overexpression on immunohistochemical (IHC) testing. In a planned subgroup analysis, those in the IHC 3+ group median survival was further extended to 16 months. This led to a NICE approval for the use of trastuzumab for those with HER2-positive disease with IHC 3+ expression.

- Other molecular targets have been evaluated in advanced disease. No benefit from the addition of bevacuzimab (an anti-VEGF monoclonal antibody) to chemotherapy was seen in the AVAGAST study (Ohtsu *et al.*, 2011) and, disappointingly, the REAL 3 trial showed no benefit from the addition of panitumimab (an anti-EGFR antibody) to EOX chemotherapy (Waddell *et al.*, 2012). These studies were done in unselected populations as opposed to the ToGA trial, where HER2-positive patients alone were treated. Future research is likely to investigate subgroups of patients with targeted agents. At present there is interest around the MET receptor tyrosine kinase which binds hepatocyte growth factor (HGF) and is often amplified in oesophagogastric cancer and several phase III trials are ongoing.

Squamous cancers

- Palliative chemotherapy options in squamous cancers of the oesophagus are similar to those squamous tumours in other sites (e.g. head and neck, cervix.
- Cisplatin-containing regimens usually with a fluoropyrimidine are the most commonly used with response rates of around 35–40%. There may be a role for taxanes in this group and some small trial results are suggestive of higher response rates.
- Consolidation palliative radiotherapy should be considered in patients with responding squamous cancers, particularly in those with tumours of the

cervical oesophagus. Recurrent or progressive dysphagia can be difficult to manage in this group because options for endoscopic stenting are limited in high tumours, and radiotherapy may play a role in preventing or delaying dysphagia and maintaining quality of life. Often a higher dose palliation may be appropriate.

Second-line therapy

Few patients remain fit enough for second-line chemotherapy and they need to be carefully selected. For some, including those with a good response to first-line chemotherapy and a reasonable treatment-free period, it can be an option. Until recently there was little evidence to suggest benefit; however, COUGAR 02 was a UK study comparing docetaxel (75 mg/m²) versus active symptom control in those with metastatic gastroesophageal adenocarcinoma (Ford *et al.*, 2014). The addition of docetaxel to supportive care was associated with a few objective responses (7%), stable disease in 46% and a modest but statistically significant prolongation of median survival (5.2 versus 3.6 months). Despite the high rate of grade 4 toxicity (21%), global and functional quality-of-life scores did not decline and in some areas improved with docetaxel (e.g. pain, dysphagia). This is in keeping with the practice of consideration of second-line therapy for selected individuals with good performance status.

Endoscopic treatment

Stents

In experienced hands, endoscopic stent insertion is usually successful and provides good palliation of dysphagia. Expandable metal stents provide a wider lumen, do not require dilatation to be inserted endoscopically, and are less likely to move than plastic ones. They are, however, more expensive, associated with more pain, and have not been shown to improve survival or quality of life. The role of radiotherapy following endoscopic stenting is unknown but is currently being investigated in the ROCS trial.

Endoscopic laser-thermal Nd-YAG or photodynamic therapy (PDT)

Both of these interventions need two or three sessions to provide worthwhile benefit and often need to be repeated every 4–8 weeks. Laser therapy is better for exophytic, short lesions of the mid or lower oesophagus. PDT is better for submucosal, flat, infiltrating tumours and for repeated treatments, but there may be problems related to the UV sensitiser.

Dilatation

Dilators rarely provide more than a few days of relief from malignant dysphagia.

Alcohol injection

Alcohol injection can be good for tumour overgrowth of stents and bleeding tumours.

Palliative radiotherapy

Both external beam radiotherapy (EBRT) and intraluminal brachytherapy (ILT) are effective in relieving dysphagia.

EBRT has been shown to be effective in 60–80% of cases, although the benefits are not maximal until 4–6 weeks after treatment. It may make dysphagia worse at first because of mucositis. It is most useful for patients with minimal dysphagia and a dose that will control the local disease for the majority of their remaining life should be used.

The dose is 30 Gy in 10 fractions over 2 weeks with anterior–posterior fields or 40 Gy in 15 fractions over 3 weeks either alone or in combination with chemotherapy. Shorter fractionation schedules, such as 20 Gy in 5 fractions over 1 week, may not be effective for long enough.

ILT has the advantage of requiring only a single treatment with fewer systemic side effects and its effect may be seen earlier. The dose is 15 Gy at 1 cm, with high-dose-rate Microselectron®.

Special clinical situations

Small-cell carcinoma of the oesophagus

Small-cell carcinoma of the oesophagus accounts for 0.8–2.4% of all cases of OC. Like pulmonary small-cell carcinoma, it is likely that the cell of origin is a pluripotential stem cell. This may be why the tumours may be mixed with keratin and mucin production, together with small-cell features. Treatment should be similar to that for patients with pulmonary small-cell carcinoma, with combined chemotherapy and radiotherapy. The overall median survival is approximately 12 months for patients with limited disease at presentation. Prophylactic cranial irradiation should also be considered in limited-stage or responding patients based on the data in small cell carcinoma of the lung.

Prognosis of carcinoma of the oesophagus

Results from selected series

For radical surgery, there is a 50% 5-year survival for patients with early tumours (T1 or T2, N0) and 20% 5-year survival for locally advanced tumours. Radical radiotherapy results in 20% 5-year survival, and radical CRT in 30% 5-year survival. In advanced disease, MS is 5 months without treatment versus 11 months with chemotherapy. All cases show ~7% survival at 5 years.

Areas of current interest

Radiation dose escalation

The majority of relapses after dCRT are seen within the treated field which suggest that dose escalation would be of benefit. For example, in the RTOG-85–01 study, which showed a benefit for CRT over radiotherapy alone, there was still a 45% local failure rate. Therefore, INT 0123 was designed to see whether a higher dose of XRT (64.8 Gy) would reduce this finding compared to a modified standard arm (50.4 Gy). There was no difference in the two arms and so the trial closed early (Minsky *et al.*, 2002). However, an overview of trials of CRT has suggested that higher doses are associated with better outcomes (Geh *et al.*, 2000). With modern radiation techniques toxicity may be less significant than in these older studies. Dose escalation is an area of interest and likely to be the basis of future dCRT trials.

Adapting to response to treatment

There is interest in early assessment of response to treatment with the option to change therapy in non-responders or possibly avoid surgery in the 30–50% of those who have a pCR after CRT. However, it is not yet possible to identify such patients preoperatively in a reliable way. We know that even in 41% of patients who are shown by endoscopic mucosal biopsy to be clear of disease, residual disease will be found at surgery (Bates *et al.*, 1996).

Biomarkers

There is increasing interest in using biomarkers to drive treatment decisions particularly in the palliative group where the benefit of trastuzumab has been seen. C-Met is a receptor overexpressed in OG cancer and is currently under investigation in several phase III palliative chemotherapy trials. Additionally, translational components to all major studies are focusing on determining molecular targets for future therapies. The next planned MRC trial for this group (PLATFORM) will be using a biomarker-driven approach to determine maintainence therapy following palliative chemotherapy.

Current trials in oesophageal cancer

The MRC ST03 is a randomised phase II/III trial of perioperative chemotherapy with or without bevacuzimab in operable oesophagogastric adenocarcinoma and (in selected centres) a feasibility study evaluating lapatinib in HER2-positive oesophagogastric adenocarcinomas.

NEOSCOPE is a neoadjuvant randomised phase II study of two preoperative CRT regimens (oxaliplatin and capecitabine followed by radiotherapy with either oxaliplatin and capecitabine or paclitaxel and carboplatin) for resectable oesophageal cancer.

ROCS (Radiotherapy after Oesophageal Cancer stenting) is a study of palliative radiotherapy in addition to a self-expanding metal stent for improving outcomes of dysphagia and survival in advanced oesophageal cancer.

Recent trials in oesophageal cancer

The SCOPE 1 trial was the largest multicentre trial of dCRT in localised oesophageal cancer in the UK and investigated adding cetuximab to standard cisplatin and fluoropyrimidine treatment (Crosby *et al.*, 2013).

Patients received dCRT and were randomised to cisplatin and capecitabine for 4 cycles, cycles 3 and 4 given concurrently with 50 Gy in 25 fractions of RT with or without cetuximab. Two hundred and fifty-eight patients were recruited. The morphology (%) was SCC:ACA 73:27. Patients who received cetuximab had a lower rate of completion of standard therapy due to increased toxicity, reduced median survival (22 versus 25 months,) and 2-year survival (41 versus 56%). However, disease control and survival in the standard dCRT arm was superior to any previous published multicentre studies of dCRT. Cetuximab therefore cannot be recommended in combination with standard dCRT for unselected patients, but strategies to build on these results will now incorporate biomarker-driven technologies to intensify treatment safely and radiation dose escalation is likely to be investigated further.

References

Alderson, D., Langley, R. E., Nankivell, M. G., *et al.* (2015). Neoadjuvant chemotherapy for resectable oesophageal and junctional adenocarcinoma: results from the UK Medical Research Council randomised OE05 trial (ISRCTN 01852072). *J. Clin. Oncol.*, **33**, 2015 (suppl; abstr 4002).

Bang, Y-J., Van Cutsem, E., Feyereislova, A., *et al.* (2010). Trastuzumab in combination with chemotherapy versus chemotherapy alone for treatment of HER2-positive advanced gastric or gastro-oesophageal junction cancer (ToGA): a phase 3, open-label, randomised controlled trial. *Lancet*, **376**, 687–697.

Bates, B. A., Detterbeck, F. C., Bernard, S. A., *et al.* (1996). Concurrent radiation therapy and chemotherapy followed by esophagectomy for localized esophageal carcinoma. *J. Clin. Oncol.*, **14**, 156–163.

Bedenne, L., Michel, P., Bouche, O., *et al.* (2007). Chemoradiation followed by surgery compared with chemoradiation alone in squamous cancer of the esophagus: FFCD 9102. *J. Clin. Oncol.*, **25**, 1160–1168.

Blazeby, J., Farndon, J., Donovan, J., *et al.* (2000). A prospective longitudinal study examining the quality of life of patients with esophageal carcinoma. *Cancer*, **88**, 1781–1787.

Bosset, J. F., Gignoux, M., Triboulet, J. P., *et al.* (1997). Chemoradiotherapy followed by surgery compared with surgery alone in squamous-cell cancer of the esophagus. *N. Engl. J. Med.*, **337**, 161–167.

Cooper, J. S., Guo, M. D., Herskovic, A., *et al.* (1999). Chemoradiotherapy of locally advanced esophageal cancer: long term follow-up of a prospective randomized trial (RTOG 85–01). *J. Am. Med. Ass.*, **281**, 1623–1627.

Crosby, T., Hurt, C. N., Falk S., *et al.* (2013). Chemoradiotherapy with or without cetuximab in patients with oesophageal cancer (SCOPE1): a multicentre, phase 2/3 randomised trial *Lancet Oncol.*, **14**, 627–637.

Cunningham, D., Allum, W. H., Stenning, S. P., *et al.* (2006). Perioperative chemotherapy versus surgery alone for resectable gastroesophageal cancer. *N. Engl. J. Med.*, **355**, 11–20.

Cunningham, D., Starling, N., Rao, S., *et al.* (2008). Capecitabine and oxaliplatin for advanced esophagogastric cancer. *N. Engl. J. Med.* **358**, 36–46.

Earlam, R. and Cunha-Melo, J. R. (1980). Oesophageal squamous cell carcinoma: II. A critical view of radiotherapy. *Br. J. Surg.*, **67**, 457–461.

Ford, H. E., Marshall, A., Bridgewater. J. A., *et al.* (2014). Docetaxel versus active symptom control for refractory oesophagogastric adenocarcinoma (COUGAR-02): an open-label, phase 3 randomised controlled trial. *Lancet Oncol.*, **15**(1), 78–86.

Gebski, V., Burmeister, B., Smithers, B. M., *et al.* (2007). Survival benefits from neoadjuvant chemoradiotherapy or chemotherapy in oesophageal carcinoma: a meta-analysis. *Lancet Oncol.*, **8**(3), 226–234.

Geh, J., Bond, S., Bentzen, S., *et al.* (2000). Preoperative chemoradiotherapy in esophageal cancer: evidence of dose response. *Proc. Am. Soc. Clin. Oncol.*, abstr. 958.

Kelsen, D. P., Ginsberg, R., Pajak, T. F., *et al.* (1998). Chemotherapy followed by surgery compared with surgery alone for localized esophageal cancer. *N. Engl. J. Med.*, **339**, 1979–1984.

Luketich, J. D., Schauer, P. R., Meltzer, C. C., *et al.* (1997). Role of positron emission tomography in staging esophageal cancer. *Ann. Thoracic. Surg.*, **64**, 765–769.

Medical Research Council Oesophageal Cancer Working Group. (2002). Surgical resection with or without preoperative chemotherapy in oesophageal cancer: a randomised controlled trial. *Lancet*, **359**, 1727–1733.

Minsky, B. D., Pajak, T. F., Ginsberg, R. J., *et al.* (2002). INT 0123 (Radiation Therapy Oncology Group 94–05) phase III trial of combined-modality therapy for esophageal cancer: high-dose versus standard-dose radiation therapy. *J. Clin. Oncol.*, **20**, 1167–1174.

Ohtsu, A., Shah, M. A., Van Cutsem, E., *et al.* (2011). Bevacizumab in combination with chemotherapy as first-line therapy in advanced gastric cancer: a randomized, double-blind, placebo-controlled phase III study. *J. Clin. Oncol.*, **29**, 3968–3976.

O'Neill, J. R., Stephens, N. A., Save, V., *et al.* (2013). Defining a positive circumferential resection margin in oesophageal cancer and its implications for adjuvant treatment. *Br. J. Surg.*, **100**, 1055–1063.

Reid, T. D., Chan, D. S., Roberts, S. A., *et al.* (2012). Prognostic significance of circumferential resection margin involvement following oesophagectomy for cancer and the predictive role of endoluminal ultrasonography. *Br. J. Cancer*, **107**, 1925–1931.

Sjoquist, K. M., Burmeister, B. H., Smithers B. M., *et al.* (2011). Australasian Gastro-Intestinal Trials Group (2011). Survival after neoadjuvant chemotherapy or chemoradiotherapy for resectable oesophageal carcinoma: an updated meta-analysis. *Lancet Oncol.*, **12**, 681–692.

Stahl, M., Wilke, H., Fink, U., *et al.* (1996). Combined preoperative chemotherapy and radiotherapy in patients with locally advanced esophageal cancer: Interim analysis of phase II trial. *J. Clin. Oncol.*, **14**, 829–837.

Sykes, A. J., Burt, P. A., Slevin, N. J., *et al.* (1998). Radical radiotherapy for carcinoma of the oesophagus: an effective alternative to surgery. *Radiother. Oncol.*, **48**, 15–21.

UICC. (2009). In *TNM Classification of Malignant Tumours*, ed. L. H. Sobin, M. K Gospodarowicz and Ch. Wittekind, 7th edn. New York: Wiley-Liss, pp. 66–72.

Urba, S. G., Orringer, M. B., Turrisi, A., *et al.* (2001). Randomized trial of preoperative chemoradiation versus surgery alone in patients with locoregional esophageal carcinoma. *J. Clin. Oncol.*, **19**, 305–313.

van Hagen, P., Hulshof, M. C., van Lanschot, J. J., *et al.* (2012). Preoperative chemoradiotherapy for esophageal or junctional cancer. *N. Engl. J. Med.*, **366**, 2074–2084.

Vogt, K., Fenlon, D., Rhodes, S., *et al.* (2006). Preoperative chemotherapy for resectable thoracic esophageal cancer (Cochrane Review). In *The Cochrane Library*, Issue 7. Oxford: Update Software.

Waddell, T., Chau, I., Cunningham, D., *et al.* (2013). Epirubicin, oxaliplatin, and capecitabine with or without panitumumab for patients with previously untreated advanced oesophagogastric cancer (REAL3): a randomised, open-label phase 3 trial. *Lancet Oncol.*, **14**, 481–489.

Walsh, T., Noonan, N., Hollywood, D., *et al.* (1996). A comparison of multimodal therapy and surgery for esophageal adenocarcinoma. *N. Engl. J. Med.*, **335**, 462–467.

Wong, R. and Malthaner, R. (2005). Combined chemotherapy and radiotherapy (without surgery) compared with radiotherapy alone in localized carcinoma of the esophagus (Cochrane Review). In *The Cochrane Library*, Issue 2. Oxford: Update Software.

Chapter

13

Management of cancer of the stomach

Sarah Gwynne, Mick Button and Tom Crosby

Introduction

There has been a steady decline in the incidence of gastric cancer in most countries in the world in the last 50 years. However, gastric cancer remains a major health problem: it is the 13th most common malignancy in the UK, the 7th most common cause of cancer-related death in the UK, and ranks second worldwide. The decline in incidence in the UK has not been in all anatomical locations. The previously most common, distal type, has become less common, but there has been an increase in cancers affecting the gastro-oesophageal junction and cardia, particularly among young Caucasians, reflecting changes in aetiological factors.

The only current curative treatment is surgery, but in the UK most patients present late, with locally advanced or metastatic disease. Only 25–40% of cases are amenable to potentially curative surgery and, even in these, local recurrence may occur in up to 50% and the 5-year survival is 30–40%. Because of this and because response rates to combination chemotherapy are 40–50% in patients with advanced disease, adjuvant therapy is increasingly being used. Perioperative chemotherapy is used most commonly in the UK, while postoperative chemoradiotherapy is more commonly used as standard treatment in the USA.
Each year the outcomes for patients with oesophagogastric cancer are audited in the National Oesophagogastric Audit (https://www.rcseng.ac.uk/media/docs/press_releases/national-oesophago-gastric-cancer-audit-2013, accessed August 2014).

Types of tumour

The types of tumour affecting the stomach are shown in Table 13.1. Adenocarcinoma accounts for 95% of all malignant tumours.

Anatomy

The stomach begins at the gastro-oesophageal junction and ends at the pylorus and is anatomically defined in three parts: the proximal fundus (cardia), the body and the distal pylorus (antrum). Anteriorly it is covered by the peritoneum of the greater sac, posteriorly by the peritoneum of the lesser sac. Proximally it abuts the diaphragm on the left and the left lobe of the liver on the right. Other adjacent organs (and therefore potential sites of direct invasion) are the spleen, the left adrenal gland, the superior portion of the left kidney, the pancreas and the transverse colon.

The vascular supply of the stomach comes from the coeliac axis via the left gastric, right gastric and gastro-epiploeic arteries (from the common hepatic artery) and the left gastro-epiploeic and short gastric arteries (from the splenic artery). The coeliac axis originates at or below the pedicle of T12 in 75% of people and at or above the pedicle of L1 in 25% (Kao *et al.*, 1992).

Lymphatic drainage follows the vascular supply, mostly draining into the coeliac nodal area, although a rich lymphatic plexus means drainage routes are complicated. The nodal stations are shown in Figure 13.1.

Incidence and epidemiology

- UK annual incidence 15–20/100 000.
- Approximately 7500 new cases per year in the UK.
- Approximately 5000 deaths per year in the UK.
- The incidence is falling for endemic distal intestinal-type tumours which are related to environmental factors, but it is rising for proximal tumours and intestinal-type which are related to gastro-oesophageal reflux disease (GORD). Proximal tumours now account for 50% of diagnoses of gastric cancer.

Practical Clinical Oncology, Second Edition, ed. Louise Hanna, Tom Crosby and Fergus Macbeth. Published by Cambridge University Press. © Cambridge University Press 2015.

Table 13.1 Types of stomach tumour

Type	Examples
Benign	Inflammatory fibroid polyp Adenoma (sessile/pedunculated polyps) Leiomyoma Adenoid cystic Hamartoma
Malignant primary	*Carcinomas:* Adenocarcinoma – diffuse/intestinal types Squamous Small cell *Others:* Lymphoma (most common site of primary GI lymphoma) Carcinoid Gastrointestinal stromal tumour
Malignant secondary	Rare, involvement of stomach by lobular carcinoma breast

- In some series, oesophageal cancer is now more common than gastric cancer, but this may reflect diagnostic uncertainties in the classification of tumours around the gastro-oesophageal junction.
- Incidence varies greatly across the world, with an incidence of 26.9 per 100,000 per year in Asian males as opposed to 7.4 per 100,000 per year in their North American counterparts. This is probably due to exposure to environmental factors in early life, because the risk in migrants changes towards that in the host country over several generations.
- Peak incidence age 65 years.
- Male : female ratio 3 : 2.

Carcinoma of the stomach

Risk and protective factors

- Environmental risk factors: diets low in vitamins A and C; diets high in salty/smoked foods or nitrates; smoking; low socioeconomic status (this may be related to the previous factors); radiation exposure at a young age.
- Infection: *Helicobacter pylori* infection gives a three- to sixfold increase in risk, especially for intestinal-type distal carcinoma; the falling incidence of this may be related to improving treatment of *H. pylori*. *H. pylori* has been classified as a class I carcinogen for gastric cancer. Expression of the Cag A virulence factor further increases the risk.
- Inflammation: Barrett's oesophagitis (related to obesity, smoking and GORD) is associated with proximal gastric and gastro-oesophageal cancers. Atrophic gastritis (secondary to *H. pylori*) is associated with distal disease. There is a sevenfold increase in the incidence of malignancy in the five years after diagnosis of a benign gastric ulcer.
- Immunological: pernicious anaemia (threefold increase).
- Genetic: e.g. CDH1 mutation (E-cadherin) which carries a risk of stomach cancer of up to 80% by the age of 80 (V. Blair, conference presentation, ASCO Gastrointestinal Cancers Symposium virtual meeting 2006, www.asco.org); inherited cancer syndromes such as FAP, HNPCC, BRCA2, and Li Fraumeni syndrome; blood group A.
- Benign adenoma: 10–20% of tumours more than 2 cm in size transform into carcinoma.
- Protective factors: the use of aspirin or NSAIDs; diets rich in fruit and vegetables or vitamin C; blood group O.

Pathology

In the past, 50% of tumours started in the pyloric region, 25% in the body and 25% in the cardia; tumours in the lesser curve were three or four times more frequent than those in the greater curve. However, the frequency of proximal tumours is increasing. The two histological variants described in the Lauren classification, *intestinal* and *diffuse*, are both mucin-secreting adenocarcinomas (see Tables 13.2 and 13.3 for pathological features). Environmental factors are thought to be more important in the aetiology of the intestinal variant, and this tumour may arise in a multistage process from chronic active gastritis through gastric atrophy, intestinal metaplasia and dysplasia to frank malignancy (Correa, 1995). Genetic factors are more associated with the diffuse type. However, *H. pylori* infection is associated with both histological types.

The appearance of gastric cancers can also vary. The Borrman classification divides tumours into five types: type I polypoid or fungating, type II ulcerated with elevated borders, type III ulcerated and invading the gastric wall, type IV diffusely infiltrating (linitus plastica) and type V unclassifiable (Borrman, 1926).

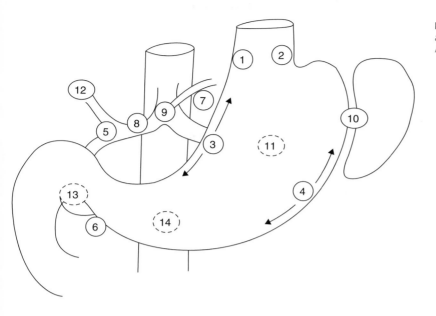

Figure 13.1 Japanese nodal stations as described in Japanese Gastric Cancer Association (1998).

Table 13.2 Pathological features of intestinal-type stomach cancers

	Description
Macroscopic features	Usually exophytic, producing nodular, polypoid or fungating masses which often ulcerate. Often metastasise to the liver
Microscopic features	Glandular formation predominates with varying degrees of differentiation. Associated with intestinal metaplasia in nearly 100% of cases

Table 13.3 Pathological features of diffuse-type stomach cancers

	Description
Macroscopic features	Usually endophytic, growth penetrates the stomach wall and spreads laterally producing marked thickening ('leather bottle stomach' or linitus plastica) with or without ulceration. May include serosal or lymph node involvement
Microscopic features	Diffusely infiltrative with sheets of cells (often 'signet ring' due to nuclear compression by mucin). Often poorly differentiated. Minimal gland formation. Not associated with intestinal metaplasia

Immunohistochemistry with cytokeratin markers CK7 and 20 and mucin (MUC1, 2, 5AC, and 6) are often positive in oesophago-gastric cancers. It is not clear whether differences in the patterns of staining could be used to differentiate tumours of the antrum, cardia and those related to Barrett's oesophagitis.

Approximately 20% of oesophogastric cancers overexpress the type 2 EGFR receptor, HER2. It is more common in proximally situated tumours of intestinal-type. The relationship between HER2 expression and prognosis is not well defined.

Spread

Gastric cancers usually spread either by direct extension, the lymphatic system, the vascular system or by the transperitoneal route. Thirty per cent of patients have liver involvement at presentation, and around

60% have lymph node involvement (see Smalley *et al.*, 2002, for discussion).

Gastric cancer spreads locally to:

- contiguous structures (as described in anatomy section above);
- the anterior abdominal wall.

Once local invasion has occurred, there may be haematogenous or lymphatic spread.

Lymphatic spread:

- The rich submucosal lymphatic plexus helps intramural spread, including proximally into the oesophagus, but not usually into the duodenum ('duodenal block').
- The initial draining lymph nodes sit on the greater and lesser curves but other lymph node groups are often involved (including in the supraclavicular fossa, SCF).
- The patterns of involvement are difficult to predict because of the rich lymphatic network.
- Spread via the falciform ligament can produce subcutaneous, periumbilical tumour deposits (Sister Mary Joseph's nodules).

Haematogenous spread:

- Initially, venous drainage is to the liver (involved in 30% of cases).
- Systemic metastases are seen less commonly – lung, bone and brain in decreasing frequency.

Trans-coelomic spread:

- Peritoneal dissemination after extension through the serosal surface of the stomach, to the ovaries (Krukenberg tumours), rectum or rectal shelf (Blumer's tumour).

Clinical presentation

Symptoms

Anorexia, weight loss, epigastric discomfort, early satiety, dysphagia, vomiting, bleeding (haemetemesis or melaena; 10%).

Examination findings

Epigastric mass, SCF lymph nodes, weight loss (indicator of a poor prognosis), performance status, signs of metastases.

Investigation and staging

- Full history and directed clinical examination.

- FBC (anaemia) and biochemistry (albumin, liver function tests, renal function if chemotherapy contemplated).
- Endoscopy: highly sensitive in experienced hands, but may miss diffuse or intramucosal tumours.
- Barium swallow: may be more sensitive for linitis plastica, which may be missed endoscopically but may show characteristic radiological features.
- CT chest/abdomen/pelvis: to assess primary tumour, lymph nodes and metastases.
- Endoscopic ultrasound (EUS): used for assessing depth of penetration, local lymph node involvement and extension of disease into the oesophagus (important when considering type of surgical procedure) although less sensitive than in the assessment of oesophageal tumours.
- A systematic review of the T staging evaluation by EUS, CT and MRI showed a similar accuracy between these techniques (65–92.1%, 77.1–88.9% and 71.4–82.6%, respectively; Kwee *et al.*, 2007).
- Laparoscopy: assesses peritoneum, liver capsule and mobility of stomach, and is considered a standard investigation before surgical resection.
- Other investigations as clinically indicated (e.g. bone scan).
- CEA has low sensitivity (raised in only 30%) and therefore is not clinically useful.
- PET may have a role, but with 1/3 of gastric cancer being PET-negative (especially in diffuse type), caution is required.

The aim is to stage patients accurately and to reduce the rate of 'open and close' laparotomies.

Stage classification

The TNM classification and stage groupings are shown in Tables 13.4 and 13.5, respectively. It is important to note the total number of nodes examined. Tumours are also graded:

- GX: grade cannot be assessed;
- G1: well-differentiated;
- G2: moderately differentiated;
- G3: poorly differentiated;
- G4: undifferentiated.

Table 13.4 UICC/TNM 7th edition for carcinoma of the stomach (applies to carcinomas only)

Stage	Description
TX	Primary tumour cannot be assessed
T0	No evidence of primary tumour
Tis	Carcinoma *in situ*: intraepithelial tumour without invasion of the lamina propria
T1	Tumour invades lamina propria, muscularis mucosae or submucosa
T1a	Tumour invades lamina propria, muscularis mucosae
T1b	Tumour invades submucosa
T2	Tumour invades muscularis propria
T3	Tumour penetrates subserosa
T4	Tumour perforates serosa or invades adjacent structures
T4a	Tumour perforates serosa
T4b	Tumour invades adjacent structures
NX	Regional lymph nodes cannot be assessed
N0	No regional lymph nodes
N1	Metastases in 1–2 regional lymph nodes
N2	Metastases in 3 to 6 regional lymph nodes
N3	Metastases 7 or more regional lymph nodes
N3a	Metastasis in 7–15 regional lymph nodes
N3b	Metastasis in 16 or more regional lymph nodes
MX	Distant metastases cannot be assessed
M0	No distant metastases
M1	Distant metastases

Adapted from UICC (2009).

Table 13.5 Stage groupings for carcinoma of the stomach

Stage	Description
Stage 0	Tis N0 M0
Stage IA	T1N0M0
Stage IB	T2N0M0
	T1N1M0
Stage IIA	T3N0M0
	T2N1M0
	T1N2M0
Stage IIB	T4aN0M0
	T3N1M0
	T2N2M0
	T1N3M0
Stage IIIA	T4aN1M0
	T3N2M0
	T2N3M0
Stage IIIB	T4bN0/N1M0
	T4aN2M0
	T3N3M0
Stage IIIC	T4aN3M0
	T4bN2/N3M0
Stage IV	Any T Any N M1

Adapted from UICC (2009).

Treatment overview

Surgery is the mainstay of radical treatment, and the type of resection is tailored to the site of the tumour in the stomach. There is debate about the optimal extent of lymph node dissection, and because of this, there are large geographical variations in treatment. Following the publication of the Intergroup 0116 randomised controlled trial, the use of adjuvant chemoradiotherapy has become standard in the USA, but not in Europe. The role of perioperative chemotherapy has been established by the UK MRC ST02 (MAGIC) trial.

In the palliative setting, combination chemotherapy is effective at improving symptoms and offers a survival benefit with improved quality of life. For tumours that overexpress HER2, the addition of trastuzumab to chemotherapy is advantageous.

Surgery

Radical surgery

Complete resection is the only curative treatment (Jansen *et al.*, 2005). However, over two-thirds of patients diagnosed with gastric cancer will have unresectable disease or metastases at presentation. Of those whose disease is resectable, local and/or regional lymph node recurrence occurs in 54% in a second-look laparotomy series (Gunderson and Sosin, 1992), and in up to 90% cases at autopsy (Lim *et al.*, 2005). In the UK, only 5% of patients present with T1 disease.

Total gastrectomy may not be necessary as long as free resection margins can be obtained with a subtotal resection. Distal tumours can be treated by partial gastrectomy (if a 6 cm proximal clearance can be achieved). However, proximal tumours usually require total gastrectomy, because more limited resections tend to produce worse functional outcomes and may result in a higher rate of local recurrence. Surgical

(a) (b)

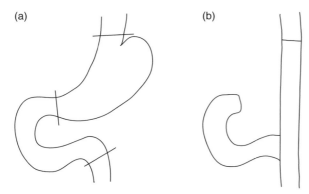

Figure 13.2 Surgical scheme for a total gastrectomy: (a) before and (b) after, with a Roux-en-Y reconstruction.

(a) (b)

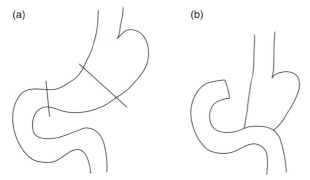

Figure 13.3 Surgical scheme for a Billroth II partial gastrectomy: (a) before and (b) after.

schemes for total and partial gastrectomy are shown in Figures 13.2 and 13.3.

There is controversy about the extent of lymph node resection required. D1 resection includes removal of the perigastric nodes within 3 cm of the tumour. D2 resection involves a more extensive lymph node dissection, with removal of lymph nodes around the left gastric artery, hepatic artery, splenic hilum and also a splenectomy and distal pancreatectomy. D2 resection is more common in Japan, while the more limited D1 resection is more common in Western centres (see Table 13.6). Outcomes from Western centres performing more extensive D2 resections are worse than those obtained in Japan with greater postoperative morbidity and mortality (up to 10% perioperatively). These differences may be related to surgical experience, to the surgery itself, to stage migration, to the fact that patients in Japan are often younger and fitter, or even to a difference in disease biology. At least three randomised trials and a Cochrane review (McCulloch *et al.*, 2003)

have not shown an advantage for more extensive lymph node resection. The majority of specialist upper GI surgeons in the UK perform a modified D2 resection for suitably fit patients.

There has been increasing interest in the potential for laparoscopic resection of gastric cancer, with procedures being either totally laparoscopic or more usually laparoscopically assisted. Studies have confirmed the safety of this approach and that a D2 lymphadenectomy can be performed to the same standard as with an open operation. A meta-analysis of open versus laparoscopically assisted distal gastrectomy yielded only a small number of suitable RCTs with small sample sizes and limited follow-up. It showed no differences between the groups except for a longer operating time and reduced nodal yield in the laparoscopic group along with a trend towards faster postoperative recovery and discharge (Memon *et al.*, 2008).

Despite extensive surgery, locoregional recurrence is common. As a result, the role of adjuvant treatments has been investigated extensively.

Chemotherapy

Adjuvant chemotherapy

Despite gastric carcinomas being the most chemosensitive of gastrointestinal carcinomas with high response rates seen in phase II studies, prospective randomised controlled trials of postoperative adjuvant chemotherapy have not shown a significant effect on survival (Shimada and Ajani, 1999). Several meta-analyses have shown that if there is benefit, it is small and does not seem to justify its routine use (Hermens *et al.*, 1993; Hallisey *et al.*, 1994; Earle and Maroun, 1999). Adjuvant therapy should not be routinely offered to patients with gastric cancer except as part of a clinical trial.

Perioperative chemotherapy

The MRC ST02 (MAGIC) trial (Cunningham *et al.*, 2006) included 503 patients of WHO performance status 0 or 1 with stage II or greater adenocarcinoma of the stomach, lower oesophagus or gastro-oesophageal junction. The extent of resection was not specified and was left to the discretion of the surgeon. Trial accrual was slow and it took over 10 years to complete the study. A protocol change to include patients with adenocarcinoma of the lower third oesophagus was made toward the end of the study. The results showed that perioperative chemotherapy (three cycles of pre- and three cycles

Table 13.6 Patterns of failure following surgery for stomach cancer

Pattern of failure	Incidence (%)		
	Clinical	Reoperation	Autopsy
Locoregional	38	67	80–93
Gastric bed	21	54	52–68
Anastomosis/stumps	25	26	54–60
Abdominal wound		5	
Lymph nodes	8	42	52
Peritoneal seeding	23	41	30–50
Localised		19	
Diffuse		22	
Distant metastases	52	22	49

From Smalley *et al.*, 2002.

of postoperative epirubicin, cisplatin and continuous infusional 5-FU) improved survival compared to surgery alone, with a higher overall survival (HR for death = 0.75; 95% CI = 0.60 to 0.93; p = 0.009; 5-year survival rate, 36% versus 23%) and progression-free survival (HR for progression = 0.66; 95% CI = 0.53 to 0.81; p < 0.001). Resected tumours were smaller and of less advanced T-stage after chemotherapy, and only 10% of patients had local recurrence alone suggesting that this regimen was effective at improving local as well as distant control. A similar benefit for perioperative chemotherapy was noted in a French multicentre trial (Ychou *et al.*, 2011).

Palliative chemotherapy

Randomised trials comparing palliative chemotherapy with best supportive care have shown a significant improvement in median survival (Murad *et al.*, 1993; Pyrhonen *et al.*, 1995; Glimelius *et al.*, 1997) from about 3 to 10 months. It has also been shown to improve quality of life and to be cost-effective (Glimelius *et al.*, 1997). However, it can be toxic and take up a significant amount of the patient's remaining life and so the decision about whether it is appropriate for an individual patient needs to be taken carefully.

It is not clear what combination regimen is the most effective. 5-FU is active as a single agent and is included in most combination regimens. A commonly used regimen in the UK and Europe is a combination of anthracycline (epirubicin), platin (cisplatin/oxaliplatin) and a fluoropyrimidine (5-FU/capecitabine) which has response rates of 40–50%.

Recently published phase III trials have investigated various chemotherapy regimens for advanced disease (Ajani, 2005), all of which are 5-FU-based and give similar median overall survival and two-year survival rates. The TAX-325 trial (the largest to date) compared cisplatin/5-FU with docetaxel/cisplatin/5-FU in 457 chemotherapy-naïve patients and found higher response rates and survival in the docetaxel-containing arm (RR 37 versus 25%; median OS 9.2 versus 8.6 months; 2-year survival 18% versus 9%) at the cost of greater toxicity (Moiseyenko *et al.*, 2005).

The REAL II trial, a phase III trial which evaluated the potential role of oxaliplatin and capecitabine in chemotherapy-naïve patients of ECOG performance status 0 to 2 with histologically proven oesophago-gastric cancer, found equivalence between oxaliplatin and cisplatin and that oral capecitabine could safely replace infusional 5-FU (Cunningham *et al.*, 2008). The median survival was 11.2 months among the patients treated with EOX and 9.9 months among the patients treated with ECF.

ECF regimen

- Epirubicin 50 mg/m² day 1.
- Cisplatin 60 mg/m² day 1.
- 5-FU 200 mg/m² per day, days 1–21 (or capecitabine 625 mg/m² p.o. b.d. days 1–21).

ECX

- Epirubicin 50 mg/m² day 1.
- Cisplatin 60 mg/m² day 1.
- Capecitabine 625 mg/m² days 1–21.

EOX

- Epirubicin 50 mg/m^2 day 1.
- Oxaliplatin 130 mg/m^2 day 1.
- Capecitabine 625 mg/m^2 days 1–21.
- Anti-emetics:
  - dexamethasone 8 mg i.v. then 4 mg p.o. b.d. for 3 days,
  - 5-HT3 antagonist, e.g. ondansetron 8 mg i.v. then 8 mg b.d. for 1 day,
  - metoclopramide 10 mg q.d.s. p.r.n. for 5 days.

After failure of this combination of anti-emetics, the addition of aprepitant can be considered:

- aprepitant 125 mg o.d. then 80 mg for 2 days.

The role of trastuzumab, a therapeutic anti-HER2 monoclonal antibody, in HER2 positive gastric cancer was tested in the phase 3 ToGA trial (Bang *et al.*, 2010). This trial compared standard chemotherapy (six courses of cisplatin plus either infusional 5-FU or capecitabine) with and without trastuzumab (8 mg/kg loading dose and then 6 mg/kg every 3 weeks until disease progression). HER2 overexpression was indicated by either IHC 3+ or FISH positive. The objective response rate was significantly higher with trastuzumab (47% versus 35%). Median OS was significantly better with trastuzumab (13.8 versus 11.1 months). Toxicities in the two arms were comparable, except for slightly higher rates of diarrhoea and asymptomatic decrease in the left ventricular ejection fraction in the trastuzumab arm. Based upon these data trastuzumab, in combination with cisplatin and a fluoropyrimidine, was approved by NICE for use in patients with metastatic HER2 overexpressing gastric or GOJ adenocarcinomas who have not received prior chemotherapy. N.B. HER2 overexpression, for the purpose of therapy with trastuzumab for gastric cancer, is defined by NICE as 3+ on IHC, unlike breast cancer where IHC 2+ and FISH positive is accepted.

In the REAL3 trial, 553 patients with previously untreated advanced unselected oesophagogastric cancer were randomly assigned to EOX (epirubicin 50 mg/m^2 on day 1, oxaliplatin 130 mg/m^2 on day 1, and capecitabine 1250 mg/m^2 per day), or modified EOX (with a reduction in oxaliplatin to 100 mg/m^2 and capecitabine to 1000 mg/m^2 per day) plus panitumumab (Waddell *et al.*, 2012). In a preliminary report presented at the 2012 ASCO meeting, the addition of panitumumab was associated with a similar response rate but a significantly worse overall survival (median

8.8 versus 11.3 months). The authors postulated that the lower chemotherapy doses and/or higher toxicity rates in the panitumumab arm may have compromised outcomes in this group.

Second-line palliative chemotherapy

In general, clinical trials assessing the effectiveness of a variety of second-line chemotherapy regimens after failure of the first-line regimen have shown that response rates are lower than they are in previously untreated patients, and toxicity rates tend to be higher. Regimens used include carboplatin and paclitaxel and docetaxel single agent and irinotecan. A trial comparing single agent irinotecan with best supportive care closed early because of low recruitment but showed a better MS with the use of irinotecan (4 versus 2.4 months) (HR = 0.48, p = 0.023; Thuss-Patience *et al.*, 2009). COUGAR 02 was a UK study comparing docetaxel (75 mg/m^2) with active symptom control (ASC). In a preliminary report presented at the 2013 ASCO GI Cancers Symposium, the addition of docetaxel to supportive care was associated with few objective responses (7%), stable disease in 46% and a modest but statistically significant prolongation of median survival with docetaxel (5.2 versus 3.6 months; Cook *et al.*, 2013). Despite the high rate of grade 4 toxicity (21%), global and functional quality-of-life scores did not decline.

There remains no standard approach for second-line therapy. For patients with adequate performance status, the use of other active agents not tried in the first-line regimen is reasonable. Quality of life and minimisation of side effects are key considerations when choosing the regimen.

Future areas of research

ST03 attempts to assess the benefit of addition of bevacizumab to standard chemotherapy in HER2-negative gastric cancer and lapatinib in HER2-positive gastric cancer (http://public.ukcrn.org.uk/search/StudyDetail. aspx?StudyID=1752, accessed August 2014). Future studies are likely to take a more biomarker-driven approach, using markers such as HER2 and PD-L1, such as the PLATFORM trial.

Radiotherapy and chemoradiotherapy

Adjuvant chemoradiotherapy

The very high local recurrence rates after radical surgery mean that adjuvant radiotherapy is an important option. The US Intergroup Study 0116 (Macdonald *et al.*, 2001) showed significant improvements in disease-free and overall survival for patients treated with adjuvant radiotherapy (45 Gy in 25 fractions over 5 weeks) and concomitant 5-FU/folinic acid compared to surgery alone. As a result, adjuvant chemoradiotherapy has become standard in the USA for high-risk patients. However, only 10% of patients had extensive (D2) resection, 30% did not complete the chemoradiation because of toxicity and more than 40% of the radiotherapy plans had significant errors.

This treatment has not been adopted as standard therapy in the UK or large parts of Europe. Its benefit after more extensive surgery and following preoperative chemotherapy is not known and it should be carried out only in specialist centres with appropriate experience.

Despite its not being used routinely, the principles of radiotherapy planning of gastric tumours should be known. Radiotherapy should start where possible within 10 weeks of surgery.

External beam – technique

- Patient preparation: nutritional support is very important and patients should be consuming over 1500 kcal/day before starting treatment. This is often difficult when over three-quarters of the stomach has been resected. Differential renal function should be measured because one kidney often receives a dose of radiation above tolerance.
- Positioning and immobilisation: supine with arms raised and supported. The planning CT should extend from the sternal notch to L3 to generate adequate dose–volume histograms for organs at risk.
- Localisation and target volume: target volume is defined using preoperative and postoperative CT scans (ideally, diagnostic quality with oral and i.v. contrast as well as non-contrast planning scan), pathology report, operative note and ideally personal discussion with the surgeon to identify areas at highest risk of recurrence. The placing of radio-opaque clips can help. The treatment volume will depend on tumour factors (e.g. proximal or distal location, stage and sites of involved lymph nodes) and type of operation (total or partial gastrectomy), but needs to cover the tumour bed, gastric remnant (if applicable), anastomosis, duodenal stump (distal resection margin) and

regional lymphatics (varying depending on those most at risk). Therefore:

- target volume: the tumour bed, anastomosis and residual gastric remnant should be adequately covered. The nodal areas at risk include the gastric and gastroepiploic (usually resected with primary); coeliac nodes, porta hepatis, subpyloric, gastroduodenal, splenic-suprapancreatic and retropanceaticoduodenal nodes. (For a more detailed discussion about this treatment technique, see Smalley *et al.*, 2002);
- margins of 1 cm around the CTV should usually be adequate to generate a PTV accounting for set-up errors and organ motion.

- Plan: in the Macdonald Intergroup 0116 study, anterior–posterior fields were used throughout. This will give a dose to the cord of approximately 48 Gy and higher doses to small bowel. CT planning and individually-tailored field arrangements may reduce dose to organs outside the PTV.
- Typical size of field: superior–inferior extent: T8/9 or T9/10 interspace to L1/2 interspace (for proximal tumours) or L3/4 interspace (distal tumours), 20 cm × 20 cm maximum.
- Verification techniques: all patients should have a simulator check film prior to starting treatment. Portal images should be obtained on at least the first two days of treatment and thereafter once weekly.
- Dose, fractionation and energy: isocentric treatment, minimum energy 6 MV, source–axis distance 100 cm, giving 45 Gy in 25 fractions over 5 weeks to the entire tumour bed, anastomoses and regional lymph nodes in a single phase, treating all fields each day. MLCs, wedges and dual asymmetric collimators are recommended. Dose-limiting structures:

  - kidneys: at least three-quarters of one kidney should receive < 20 Gy;
  - heart: no more than 30% should receive > 40 Gy;
  - liver: no more than 60% should receive > 30 Gy;
  - spinal cord: no part should receive > 45 Gy.

Table 13.7 Side effects of chemoradiotherapy for gastric cancer

Side effect	Comments
Acute	
Nausea	Anti-emetics including 5-HT3 if required
Fatigue	Advice re: management fatigue, check haemoglobin
Diarrhoea	Low-residue diet, loperamide as required
Myelosuppression	Weekly FBC
Late	
Myelopathy	The risks of these late sequelae should be kept to a minimum with careful planning
Malabsorption	
Radiation enteritis	

Concurrent chemotherapy

A regimen of 5-FU/folinic acid was used in the Intergroup Study 0116, but this regimen is probably suboptimal, and infusional 5-FU, oral fluoropyrimidines or a combination regimen may be better. Clinical trials are under way to confirm this.

Table 13.7 shows the toxicity from chemoradiotherapy.

The future role of chemoradiotherapy in gastric cancer is being explored in two current phase 3 trials. CRITICS (http://www.cirro.dk/assets/files/Protokoller/CIRRO-IP050109-CRITICS.pdf, accessed January 2015) is a Dutch study comparing postoperative chemotherapy with chemoradiotherapy after induction chemotherapy, while the TROG study TOPGEAR (http://meetinglibrary.asco.org/content/99024–114, accessed January 2015) is comparing preoperative chemotherapy and chemoradiotherapy.

Palliative radiotherapy

Palliative radiotherapy 30 Gy in 10 fractions or an 8 Gy single fraction, given by antero-posterior fields, simulated either with barium contrast, or by outlining tumour on virtual CT simulation using radiological information on tumour position can be very effective at controlling pain or bleeding. Treatment is usually well tolerated, but can cause short-lived nausea and vomiting, abdominal cramps or diarrhoea, many of which are prevented by the routine use of 5-HT3 antagonists.

Other palliative treatments

Endoscopic laser photocoagulation can be useful for controlling bleeding or for debulking a large, obstructing tumour. Expandable metal stents may relieve dysphagia due to gastro-oesophageal tumours. Occasionally, palliative surgical bypass may be required for gastric outlet obstruction or even gastrectomy for uncontrollable bleeding. Coeliac plexus block may palliate severe pain.

Prognosis

Because patients usually present late, the overall five-year survival is less than 10%, but it is as high as 70% for early (T1) tumours. The median survival for patients with unresectable (or untreated metastatic) disease is around 4 months. Even in patients with resectable disease, locoregional recurrence and distant metastases are common (see Table 13.6).

Prognostic factors

• Tumour stage at presentation.
• Resectability.
• Morphology – diffuse types have worse prognosis.
• Poor tumour differentiation.

References

Ajani, J. A. (2005). Evolving chemotherapy for advanced gastric cancer. *The Oncol.*, **10** (Suppl. 3), 49–58.

Bang, Y-J., Van Cutsem, E., Feyereislova, A., *et al.* (2010). Trastuzumab in combination with chemotherapy versus chemotherapy alone for treatment of HER2-positive advanced gastric or gastro-oesophageal junction cancer (ToGA): a phase 3, open-label, randomised controlled trial. *Lancet*, **376**, 687–697.

Borrman, R. (1926). Geschwulste des magens und duodenums. In *Handbuch der Speziellen Pathogischen Antomie und Histologie*, ed. F. Henske and O. Lubarsch. Berlin: Julius Springer, IV-L864-71.

Cook, N., Marshall, A., Blazeby, J., *et al.* (2013). Cougar-02: a randomised phase 3 study of docetaxel versus active symptom control in patients with relapsed oesophago-gastric adenocarcinoma. *J. Clin. Oncol.*, **31** (Suppl, abstract 4023).

Correa, P. (1995). *Helicobacter pylori* and gastric carcinogenesis. *Am. J. Surg. Path.*, **19** (Suppl. 1), S37–43.

Cunningham. D., Allum W. H., Stenning S. P., *et al.* (2006). Perioperative chemotherapy versus surgery alone for resectable gastroesophageal cancer. *N. Engl. J. Med.*, **355**, 76–77.

Cunningham, D., Starling, N., Rao, S., *et al.* (2008). Capecitabine and oxaliplatin for advanced esophagogastric cancer. *N. Engl. J. Med.*, **358**, 36–46.

Earle, C. C. and Maroun, J. A. (1999). Adjuvant chemotherapy after curative resection for gastric cancer in non-Asian patients: revisiting a meta-analysis of randomized trials. *Eur. J. Cancer*, **35**, 1059–1064.

Glimelius, B., Ekstrom, K., Hoffman, K., *et al.* (1997). Randomized comparison between chemotherapy plus best supportive care with best supportive care in advanced gastric cancer. *Ann. Oncol.*, **8**, 163–168.

Gunderson, L. L. and Sosin, H. (1992). Adenocarcinoma of the stomach: areas of failure in a re-operation series (second or symptomatic look) clinicopathologic correlation and implications for adjuvant therapy. *Int. J. Rad. Oncol. Biol. Phys.*, **8**, 1–11.

Hallisey, M. T., Dunn, J. A., Ward, L. C., *et al.* (1994). The second British Stomach Cancer Group trial of adjuvant radiotherapy or chemotherapy in resectable gastric cancer: five year follow-up. *Lancet*, **343**, 1309–1312.

Hermans, J., Bonenkamp, J. J., Boon, M. C., *et al.* (1993). Adjuvant therapy after curative resection for gastric cancer: meta-analysis of randomised trials. *J. Clin. Oncol.*, **11**, 1441–1447.

Jansen, E., Boot, H., Verheij, M., *et al.* (2005). Optimal locoregional treatment in gastric cancer. *J. Clin. Oncol.*, **23**, 4509–4517.

Japanese Gastric Cancer Association. (1998). Japanese classification of gastric carcinoma – 2nd English edition. *Gastric Cancer*, **1**, 10–24.

Kao, G., Whittington, R. and Coia, L. (1992). Anatomy of the coeliac axis and superior mesenteric artery and its significance in radiation therapy. *Int. J. Rad. Oncol. Biol. Phys.*, **25**, 131.

Kwee, R. M. and Kwee, T. C. (2007). Imaging in local staging of gastric cancers systematic review. *J. Clin. Oncol.*, **25**, 2107–2116.

Lim, L., Michael, M. Mann, G. B., *et al.* (2005). Adjuvant therapy in gastric cancer. *J. Clin. Oncol.*, **23**, 6220–6232.

Macdonald, J.S., Smalley, S.R., Benedetti, J., *et al.* (2001). Chemoradiotherapy after surgery compared with surgery alone for adenocarcinoma of the stomach or gastro-oesophageal junction. *N. Engl. J. Med.*, **345**, 725–730.

McCulloch, P., Nita, M. E., Kazi, H., *et al.* (2003). Extended versus limited lymph nodes dissection technique for adenocarcinoma of the stomach. *The Cochrane Database Syst. Rev.*, **18**, no. CD001964.

Memon, M., Khan, S., Yunus, R., *et al.* (2008). Meta-analysis of laparascopic and open distal gastrectomy for gastric carcinoma. *Surg. Endosc.*, **22**, 1781–1789.

Moiseyenko, V., Ajani, J., Tjulandin, S., *et al.* (2005). Final results of a randomised phase III trial (TAX 325) comparing docetaxel (T) combined with cisplatin (C) and 5-fluorouracil (F) to CF in patients with metastatic gastric adenocarcinoma. *J. Clin. Oncol.*, **23**, 308s.

Murad, A. M., Santiago, F. F., Petroianu, A., *et al.* (1993). Modified therapy with 5-fluorouracil, doxorubicin, and methotrexate in advanced gastric cancer. *Cancer*, **72**, 37–41.

Pyrhonen, S., Kuitunen, T., Nyandoto, P., *et al.* (1995). Randomised comparison of fluorouracil, epidoxorubicin and methotrexate (FEMTX) plus supportive care with supportive care alone in patients with non-resectable gastric cancer. *Br. J. Cancer*, **71**, 587–591.

Shimada, K. and Ajani, J. A. (1999). Adjuvant therapy for gastric carcinoma patients in the last 15 years: a review of Western and Oriental trials. *Cancer*, **86**, 1657–1668.

Smalley, S., Gunderson, L., Tepper, J., *et al.* (2002). Gastric surgical adjuvant radiotherapy consensus report: rationale and treatment implication. *Int. J. Radiat. Oncol. Biol. Phys.*, **52**, 283–293.

Thuss-Patience, P., Deist, T., Hinke, A., *et al.* (2009). Irinotecan versus best supportive care (BSC) as second line therapy in gastric cancer: a randomised phase 3 study of the Arbeitsgemeinschaft Internistische Onkologie (AIO). *J. Clin. Oncol.*, **27**(15 Suppl.; abstract 4520).

UICC. (2009). *TNM Classification of Malignant Tumours*, ed. L. H. Sobin, M. K. Gospodarowicz and Ch. Wittekind, 7th edn. Chichester: Wiley-Blackwell.

Waddell, T. S., Chau, I., Barbachano, Y., *et al.* (2012). A randomized multicenter trial of epirubicin, oxaliplatin, and capecitabine (EOC) plus panitumumab in advanced esophagogastric cancer (REAL3). *J. Clin. Oncol.*, **30** (Suppl.; abstract LBA4000).

Ychou, M., Boige, V., Pignon, J. P., *et al.* (2011). Perioperative chemotherapy compared with surgery alone for resectable gastroesophageal adenocarcinoma: an FNCLCC and FFCD multicenter phase III trial. *J. Clin. Oncol.*, **29**, 1715.

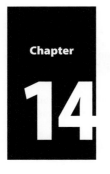

Chapter

14

Management of cancer of the liver, gallbladder and biliary tract

Emma Harrett, Seema Safia Arif and Somnath Mukherjee

Introduction

Primary liver cancer is one of the commonest cancers worldwide, and it predominantly affects people in developing countries. It is often associated with chronic liver infections and it is more common in males. Patients usually present with advanced disease, and treatment options are influenced, and often limited, by comorbidities, especially poor function of the rest of the liver.

Tumours of the gallbladder and biliary tract are relatively rare. Patients often present late with symptoms of biliary obstruction, which, together with cholangitis, is a common cause of morbidity and death and the main target for palliative therapies. Gallbladder and biliary tract tumours are moderately chemosensitive. Cytological or histological confirmation of disease is often difficult, and specialist multidisciplinary teams with expert radiologists and pathologists should be involved in the diagnosis and staging. Radical surgery should be carried out only by tertiary surgical teams, and patients should be managed, whenever possible, within clinical trials.

Tumours of the liver

Types of tumour affecting the liver are shown in Table 14.1.

Anatomy of the liver

The liver is divided into right and left lobes by the falciform ligament, but more importantly, in terms of surgical resection, a segmental division can be made and seen with imaging, which is based upon the relationship to the hepatic and portal veins. There are four segments in both the left and the right liver. The left liver consists of the caudate lobe (segment I), the lateral segments II and III (superior and inferior lateral, respectively, seen extending to the left surface on CT) and the medial segment IV. The division between the lateral and medial segments is the gall bladder and IVC and not the falciform ligament. The right part of the liver is made up anteriorly of segments V and VIII (inferior and superior, respectively) and posteriorly of segments VI and VII (inferior and superiorly, respectively). The latter is the right lateral surface as seen on CT scan. Contrast in the portal, hepatic and inferior caval veins on CT allows distinct segmental definition.

Hepatocellular carcinoma

Incidence and epidemiology

Primary hepatocellular carcinoma (HCC) is the sixth most common solid tumour worldwide. Although the incidence is low in the UK and other developed countries, it is rising because of the increase in viral hepatitis.

- The UK annual incidence rate is 1.8/100,000 with 3000 new cases per year.
- The number of deaths may be higher than the incidence. This anomaly is probably due to the poor long-term survival and misdiagnosis of secondary malignancies as primary disease.
- Male : female ratio is 3 : 1.
- There is a varied incidence of hepatocellular carcinoma throughout the world and this is due to variations in the incidence of risk factors associated with development of HCC.
- High-risk areas worldwide are East and Southeast Asia and Sub-Saharan Africa.
- Countries such as Taiwan, China, Malaysia, those in middle Africa and Japan have the highest rates (up to 36/100,000) because of the high incidence of hepatitis B.

Practical Clinical Oncology, Second Edition, ed. Louise Hanna, Tom Crosby and Fergus Macbeth. Published by Cambridge University Press. © Cambridge University Press 2015.

Table 14.1 The range of tumours affecting the liver

Type	Examples
Benign	Haemangioma
	Focal nodular hyperplasia
	Nodular regenerative hyperplasia
	Hepatic adenoma
	Hepatic cystadenoma
	Lipoma
	Hamartoma
	Bile duct cystadenoma
Malignant primary	Hepatocellular (conventional; fibrolamellar)
	Cholangiocarcinoma (intrahepatic)
	Mixed hepatocellularcholangio-carcinoma
	Hepatoblastoma
	Hepatic angiosarcoma
Malignant secondary	Any tumour
	Adenocarcinoma e.g. bowel, breast, lung
	Sarcoma
	Lymphoma
	Carcinoid

Table 14.2 Pathological features of hepatocellular carcinoma

	Description
Macroscopic features	Yellowish-white nodules with areas of haemorrhage or necrosis. Background features of cirrhosis
Microscopic features	Large cells similar to hepatocytes with clear cytoplasm cf. renal cell carcinoma
	In the fibrolamellar variant the tumour forms cords with collagen strands

Risk factors and aetiology

The main causative factors in developing HCC appear to be both chronic liver-cell injury and inflammation due to a variety of causative agents.

Infective

HCC is associated with hepatitis B and C virus infections (HBV and HCV). Chronic hepatitis B and C, with or without cirrhosis infection, increases the risk of HCC 100 times. In Europe the main factor is HCV infection.

Inflammatory

HCC is also associated with other causes of cirrhosis, such as hereditary haemochromatosis, Wilson's disease and type 1 glycogen storage disease.

Chemical injury

Exposure to a number of chemical agents increases the risk of HCC. Alcohol is the commonest, but others are nitrites, hydrocarbons, solvents and PVC, which is particularly associated with hepatic angiosarcoma.

Aflatoxins, hepatotoxic agents produced by fungi *Aspergillus flavus* and *parasiticus*, are causative factors in Africa and Asia.

These factors can be additive or synergistic. For instance, chronic HCV infection is more commonly associated with HCC in chronic alcohol drinkers. Aflatoxin interacts with HBV infection to increase the risk of HCC threefold.

Pathology

Tumours may appear as a large solitary lesion (30%) or be multicentric (60%). Even what appear to be solitary tumours may have multiple satellite lesions around a central tumour. The pathological features of hepatocellular carcinoma are shown in Table 14.2.

Many signalling pathways responsible for cell survival and proliferation are involved in the pathogenesis of HCC. TP53 can be mutated in 25–40% of HCC cases and the β catenin gene CTNNB1 in 25% of cases. Oncogenes and tumour suppressor genes can be affected by amplifications and deletions. The EGFR and RAS signalling pathways can be activated, as well at the WNT pathway and MTOR pathways. Therefore, molecular profiling of HCC may lead to more targeted therapies for this disease (Forner *et al.*, 2012).

Clinical presentation

HCC is usually asymptomatic. It is often an incidental finding in chronic liver disease (hepatitis or cirrhosis) and it may be picked up on imaging or with a sudden rise in alpha feto-protein (αFP), although as many as 30% of tumours do not produce αFP.

Patients may present with liver decompensation with features such as ascites, jaundice, anorexia, GI bleeding, weight loss and encephalopathy.

Occasionally, patients may have paraneoplastic syndromes such as hypoglycaemia, hypercalcaemia, erythrocytosis and ectopic gonadotrophic or adrenocorticotrophic hormones.

Metastases to lung, bones, adrenal and lymph nodes are rare.

Diagnostic and staging investigations

Radiology is important in the diagnosis and staging of hepatocellular carcinoma, and in selected cases, specific CT/MRI criteria may be able to establish the diagnosis of HCC without the need for formal histology. These radiology criteria apply only to cirrhotic patients. They require multiphase multidetector CT or dynamic contrast-enhanced MRI and are based on typical vascular hallmarks of HCC (hypervascularity in the arterial phase with washout in the portal venous phase). Currently, FDG-PET is not recommended for the diagnosis of HCC.

Biopsy confirmation of HCC is required in patients where a radiological diagnosis cannot be established. There is a risk of needle-track seeding from liver biopsy of between 0% and 10%, and median time to seeding is 17 months. Biopsy should be avoided if the patient is not a candidate for therapy due to poor performance status, in cases where resection of the tumour can be carried out with acceptable morbidity/mortality, or in patients with decompensated disease awaiting liver transplant.

As well as diagnosis and staging, investigations are aimed at assessing the patient's suitability for treatment, in particular the level of function of the 'normal' or non-malignant liver.

- Medical and family history (previous liver disease, drug exposure, symptoms) and examination for signs of chronic liver disease, performance status and nutritional state.
- Full blood count, renal, liver and bone profile.
  - HBV, HCV serology and αFP. Blood clotting tests and serum albumin.
- Assessment for portal hypertension including upper GI endoscopy (for varices and/or hypertensive gastropathy) with/without transjugular measurement of hepatic-venous pressure gradient.

Staging classification

The TNM staging system has been upated (UICC, 2009). The TNM and stage groupings are shown in Tables 14.3 and 14.4, respectively.

The Barcelona Clinic Liver Cancer (BCLC) strategy can also be employed to stage patients in a way

Table 14.3 TNM staging classification of hepatocellular carcinoma

Stage	Description
T1	Solitary tumour without evidence of vascular invasion
T2	Solitary tumour with evidence of vascular invasion; or multiple tumours none more than 5 cm in greatest dimension
T3	Multiple tumours more than 5 cm or tumour involving a major branch of the portal or hepatic vein(s) T3a Multiple tumours any more than 5 cm T3b Tumour involving a major branch of the portal or hepatic vein(s)
T4	Tumour(s) with direct invasion of adjacent organs other than the gallbladder or with perforation of visceral peritoneum
NX	Regional lymph nodes cannot be assessed
N0	No regional lymph node metastasis
N1	Regional lymph node metastasis
MX	Distant metastasis cannot be assessed
M0	No distant metastasis
M1	Distant metastasis

The regional lymph nodes are the hilar, hepatic (along the proper hepatic artery), periportal (along the portal vein) and those along the abdominal inferior vena cava above the renal veins (except the inferior phrenic nodes). Adapted from UICC, 2009.

Table 14.4 Stage groupings for hepatocellular carcinoma

Stage	Description
I	T1 N0 M0
II	T2 N0 M0
IIIA	T3a N0 M0
IIIB	T3b N0 M0
IIIC	T4 N0 M0
IVA	Any T N1 M0
IVB	Any T Any N M1

Adapted from UICC, 2009.

that indicates appropriate treatment strategies and prognosis. This strategy encorporates tumour size, performance status, vascular invasion, extrahepatic spread and extent of cirrhosis in patients with hepatocellular carcinoma. Figure 14.1 shows this algorithm.

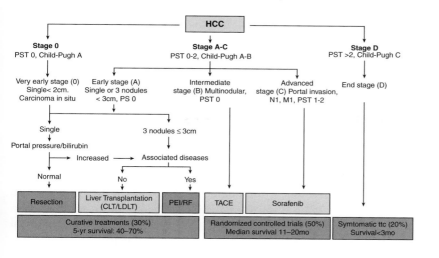

Figure 14.1 The Barcelona Clinic Liver Cancer Strategy. Adapted from Aitken and Hawkins, 2014. PST, performance status based on Eastern Cooperative Oncology Group Score; HCC, hepatocellular carcinoma; CLT, cadaver liver transplant; LDLT, living donor liver transplant; PEI, percutaneous ethanol injection; RF, radiofrequency ablation; TACE, transarterial chemoembolisation; ttc, treatment; N, nodal stage; M, metastases stage.

Surveillance

Patients at high risk of developing HCC should be entered into a surveillance programme and the European Societies of Medical Oncology and Digestive Oncology have published guidelines for the surveillance of HCC (Verslype *et al.*, 2012). Surveillance should be offered to patients with established cirrhosis, non-cirrhotic HBV patients with high viral load or HCV patients with bridging fibrosis. The current recommendation for surveillance is abdominal ultrasound every 6 months.

For patients who develop new nodules during the surveillance, the following approach is recommended.

- For nodules < 1 cm:
  - Repeat US at 4 months. If the nodule grows, further investigation is warranted depending on the size of the nodule. If it remains stable, a further 4-monthly US is recommended for 1 year and then 6-monthly USs.
- For nodules 1–2 cm:
  - 4-phase CT and/or dynamic contrast-enhanced MRI;
  - if hallmarks of HCC are not seen then a biopsy should be obtained. A second biopsy should be obtained if the first is inconclusive. If HCC is still not confirmed then 4-monthly interval US should be performed and repeat biopsy if lesion changes.
- For nodules >2 cm:
  - 4-phase CT or dynamic contrast-enhanced MRI;

- if radiologically not characteristic of HCC, then biopsy is recommended;
- if biopsy is inconclusive, 4-monthly interval US should be performed.

Treatment overview

A large proportion of these patients are very complex due to underlying liver disease and therefore they should be discussed and managed by specialist multidisciplinary teams which should include a liver surgeon, pathologist, hepatologist, radiologist and oncologist. Surgical resection, liver transplantation and ablative therapies are curative options, but there are no randomised controlled trials comparing these therapies directly.

Patients who have unresectable tumours or who are unsuitable for curative options may be suitable for palliative systemic treatment, although response rates are poor.

Curative options

Surgery

Local resection

Local resection of small isolated tumours is possible, but because hepatitis or chronic liver cell injury or cirrhosis is multicentric, further tumours in the liver are often seen. Local resection is the treatment of choice for patients with non-cirrhotic livers and for patients with Child class A cirrhosis who have a small solitary tumour and minimal portal hypertension (hepatic venous pressure gradient less than 10 mmHg). The

Table 14.5 The Child–Pugh grading system for cirrhosis. Scores of 1–3 are given for clinical investigations and features and summated: Child class A, score 5–6; Child class B, score 7–9; Child class C, score > 9

Score	Bilirubin (µmol/L)	Albumin (g/L)	Prothrombin time (sec)	Hepatic encephalopathy[a]	Ascites
1	< 34	> 35	< 4	None	None
2	34–50	28–35	4–6	1–2	Mild
3	> 50	< 28	> 6	3–4	Severe

[a] Encephalopathy score determined by degree of consciousness, intellectual/personality impairment, neurological signs and EEG changes. Adapted from Pugh *et al.*, 1973.

Child–Pugh grading system for cirrhosis is shown in Table 14.5.

Liver transplantation for HCC

The risk of multicentric recurrence is significantly reduced by the use of liver transplantation (Llovet *et al.*, 1999). Risk factors for recurrence are the presence of HBV infection, multiple tumours, tumour size and vascular invasion (Mazzaferro *et al.*, 1996).

- Rationale: liver transplantation treats hepatoma, as well as the underlying problem (cirrhosis).
- Selection (Milan criteria): one tumour between 2 and 5 cm or two or three tumours, all ≤ 3 cm; selected patients with HCC > 5 cm size have been treated with multimodal therapy (chemoembolisation, surgery, systemic chemotherapy) with a report of a 4-year survival rate of 75% (Mazzaferro *et al.*, 1996).
- A significant problem with liver transplantation is a lack of donor organs and many patients progress while awaiting a donor. Local therapies may 'bridge' the gap between diagnosis and transplantation.

Local non-surgical therapy

Image-guided tumour ablation

Radiofrequency ablation, microwave, cryoablation, ethanol or acetic acid injections are all options for patients with early-stage hepatocellular carcinoma. There have been reports of survival similar to surgical studies and their use often reflects local experience and expertise. Radiofrequency ablation (RFA) has been shown to be more effective than percutaneous ethanol injection (PEI), and for tumours up to 2 cm in diameter, an 85% complete response has been reported. RFA is now the first-line technique for image-guided tumour ablation. If tumours are greater than 5 cm or near large blood vessels, RFA is not recommended.

A recent Cochrane review summarised that two clinical trials showed that hepatic resection had a better overall survival and progression-free survival compared to RFA. However, hepatic resection was associated with an eight-times greater risk of complications. The review concluded that there was insufficient evidence due to low patient numbers to draw valid conclusions, and further randomised controlled trials are needed (Weis *et al.*, 2013).

Palliative treatments

Transarterial chemo-embolisation (TACE) combines intra-arterial chemotherapy, often doxorubicin and lipiodol, an oily iodised contrast agent administered under direct vision, with embolisation of the arterial blood supply. This exploits the fact that HCCs are highly vascular and predominantly take their blood supply from the hepatic arteries. This can be used for large or multifocal tumours that are not appropriate for curative options. Contraindications for TACE include thrombosis in the main portal vein, encephalopathy, biliary obstruction and Child class C cirrhosis of the liver. A meta-analysis that included seven randomised trials of arterial embolisation has shown that TACE is more effective than conservative therapy or 5-FU chemotherapy, with a significant improvement in two-year survival (OR = 0.53, 95% CI = 0.32 to 0.89) and a median survival of more than 2 years (Llovet and Bruix, 2003). However, a more recent Cochrane meta-analysis of three randomised controlled trials concluded that there is insufficient evidence to support or dismiss TACE as a treatment for HCC and more robust clinical trials are needed (Oliveri *et al.*, 2011).

Radiotherapy

Toxicity from radiotherapy to the liver has been the major limiting factor in the advancement of radiotherapy techniques for HCC. Radiation-induced liver

Table 14.7 Bismuth classification for perihilar tumours

Type	Description
Type I	Tumour is below confluence of right and left ducts
Type II	Confined to the confluence
Type III	Extension into right or left hepatic ducts
Type IV	Extension into right and left hepatic ducts or multicentric

Adapted from Bismuth and Corlette, 1978.

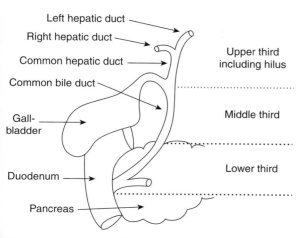

Figure 14.2 Locations of the upper, middle and lower thirds of the extrahepatic biliary tree (as described in Chamberlain and Blumgart, 2000). Perihilar tumours are classified further according to the Bismuth classification (see Table 14.7).

- Constitutional: weight loss (> 50% cases), anorexia, fatigability.
- Hepatomegaly and right upper quadrant pain (especially hilar tumours, carcinoma gallbladder).
- Palpable, non-tender gallbladder: obstructive tumour below the level of cystic duct (Courvoisier's law); gallbladder carcinoma.
- Symptoms/signs of metastasis: ascites, pleural effusion.
- Carcinoma of the gallbladder: presentation as acute or chronic cholecystitis, incidental diagnosis made at surgery.

Investigations

Blood tests

Full blood count, renal and liver profiles and CA19-9 tumour marker: LFT derangement consistent with obstructive jaundice (raised alkaline phosphatase, gamma-glutamyl transferase, bilirubin) and persistent elevation of CA19-9 despite decompression of biliary tree suggests biliary duct/pancreatic malignancy. It is raised in up to 85% of patients with cholangiocarcinoma.

Imaging

- Ultrasonography is the first-line investigation for suspected biliary tract obstruction. Findings: intrahepatic duct dilatation. Extrahepatic ducts may be dilated in carcinoma of the distal bile duct/pancreatic head tumours. Useful in ruling out choledocholithiasis.
- CT scan is useful in assessing the extent of local disease and regional lymphadenopathy (gallbladder, intrahepatic and perihilar cholangiocarcinoma) and to look for metastatic disease. It can establish resectability in approximately 60% of cases.
- Endoscopic retrograde cholangiopancreatogram (ERCP) and percutaneous transhepatic cholangiograph (PTC) are used to image the intra- and extrahepatic bile ducts and to localise the site of obstruction. PTC is useful for proximal tumours (perihilar cholangiocarcinomas), whereas ERCP is most useful for distal bile duct tumours. Although invasive, the procedure allows a cytological diagnosis (positive in 30%), biopsy and insertion of endobiliary stents.
- EUS is useful for imaging the gallbladder, distal extrahepatic bile duct and lymph nodes, and it facilitates a guided biopsy.
- Laparoscopy rules out peritoneal metastases before curative surgery.
- MRI and magnetic resonance cholangiopancreaticogram (MRCP) are non-invasive investigations to evaluate the biliary tree in suspected cholangiocarcinoma.

Advantages

Noninvasive.
Shows the extent of duct involvement (MRCP).
Local staging (invasion of adjacent liver, vessels, lymph nodes).
Detects liver metastasis.

Disadvantages

Does not give histological/cytological diagnosis.

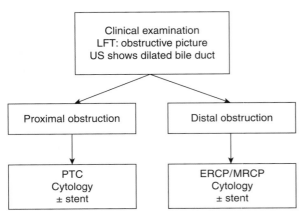

Figure 14.3 Investigation strategy for a patient with obstructive jaundice. ERCP, endoscopic retrograde cholangiopancreatogram; LFT, liver function tests; MRCP, magnetic resonance cholangiopancreatogram; PTC, percutaneous transhepatic cholangiograph; US, ultrasound.

- PET scan is investigational, but has been shown to detect cholangiocarcinomas more than 1 cm diameter and metastases in 30% of cases (Anderson *et al.*, 2004). Figure 14.3 shows an investigation strategy for a patient with obstructive jaundice.

Treatment overview

Fewer than 20% of the patients have resectable tumours at the time of diagnosis and there is a high risk of recurrence after surgery. Adjuvant treatment is unproven and should be considered only in the context of a clinical trial. Radiotherapy and chemoradiotherapy, both as adjuvant and primary therapy, should be regarded as investigational, and are not widely practised in the UK. The median survival of patients without treatment is about 3 months. Palliative chemotherapy is an option for fitter patients (performance status 0–2) with incurable disease. A plastic or metallic stent is useful in palliating obstructive jaundice, which is often a common feature of the disease. Given these uncertainties about management, patients should always be considered for clinical trials.

Surgery

Radical surgery for carcinoma of the gallbladder

Carcinoma of the gallbladder is found incidentally in fewer than 1% of cases of routine cholecystectomies for cholelithiasis; carcinoma *in situ* and tumours limited to the muscle layer may be effectively treated by this

alone. Advanced stages require radical cholecystectomy, which involves nodal dissection and may entail excision of adjacent liver tissue. Laparoscopic procedures are contraindicated in patients with known carcinoma because of the high risk of needle-track seeding.

Radical surgery for carcinoma of the bile duct

Hepaticojejunostomy is usually possible for tumours below the first division of the left or right main duct with uninvolved vessels. There is a high risk of local recurrence at the porta hepatis and of distant metastases.

Surgical options include:

- Perihilar tumours:
  - Bismuth I and II: *en bloc* resection of the bile duct, gallbladder, lymph nodes, Roux-en-Y hepatico-jejunostomy;
  - Bismuth III: as above, plus right or left hemi-hepatectomy;
  - Bismuth IV: as Bismuth I–II, plus extended right or left hemi-hepatectomy.
- Lower third: pancreatico-duodenectomy.
- Intrahepatic cholangiocarcinoma: resection of involved segments/lobes.

Patients who achieve R0 resection at surgery have better survival compared to patients who have positive margins.

Systemic treatment

Adjuvant treatment

There are not many prospective clinical trials for adjuvant therapy. One randomised trial has shown that there is no survival advantage from giving adjuvant chemotherapy using infusional 5-FU and mitomycin followed by a prolonged course of oral fluoropyramidine compared to surgery alone (Takada *et al.*, 2002). ESPAC-3 showed no survival advantage using 5-FU and leucovorin or gemcitabine as adjuvant therapy over observation alone following resection for peri-ampullary cancers (Neoptolemos *et al.*, 2012). The results of the BILCAP trial investigating the role of adjuvant capecitabine versus clinical follow-up in patients with completely resected biliary tract cancer are awaited. Two other European trials are evaluating adjuvant strategies in resected biliary tract cancer. The PRODIGE 12 trial is evaluating the role of adjuvant gemcitabine-oxaliplatin chemotherapy over observation alone, and the ACTICCA-01 trial is evaluating the role of gemcitabine-cisplatin (compared to observation alone).

There is no well-established evidence for postoperative chemoradiotherapy due to a lack of randomised clinical controlled trials, although there is some evidence of a survival advantage in retrospective studies.

Despite the lack of evidence, the European Society of Medical Oncology (ESMO) recommends postoperative chemoradiotherapy after surgical resection and the National Comprehensive Cancer Network (NCCN) recommends adjuvant chemotherapy with fluoropyrimidine or gemcitabine except in T1N0 tumours. The current standard UK practice is not to offer adjuvant therapy (chemotherapy or chemoradiotherapy) for resected biliary tract cancer.

Palliative chemotherapy

Palliative chemotherapy has demonstrated a survival advantage over active supportive care and should be considered for all patients who are well enough to receive treatment (WHO performance status 0–2) (Glimelius et al., 1996; Sharma et al., 2010).

The ABC-02 trial, a randomised phase III trial comparing gemcitabine–cisplatin combination to single-agent gemcitabine, demonstrated significant overall survival advantage for the combination treatment (median OS = 11.7 months versus 8.1 months; PFS 8 months versus 5 months; Valle et al., 2010). The results have been replicated in a Japanese randomised trial, BT-22 (median OS = 11.2 months versus 7.7 months) (Okusaka et al., 2010) establishing gemcitabine-cisplatin as the standard for this condition. Patients not fit for combination chemotherapy (including patients who are WHO PS 2) should be offered single-agent gemcitabine.

Other chemotherapy regimens

Single-agent 5-FU (modified by leucovorin) has been reported to produce response rates of up to 32% (Choi et al., 2000). Other drugs that seem to be active in cholangiocarcinoma include epirubicin, mitomycin, gemcitabine, oxaliplatin, docetaxel, interferon and the novel tumour antibiotic rebeccamycin. The combination of 5-FU and mitomycin has been reported to give a response rate of 26% (Chen et al., 2001) and one randomised phase II trial showed superior survival and response rate for the addition of cisplatin to 5-FU (median survival 7.8 months versus 5.3 months; 19% versus 7%; Mitry et al., 2002). The combination

of gemcitabine and oxaliplatin has demonstrated a response rate of 35.5% (Maindrault-Goebel et al., 2003). Oral capecitabine has also shown activity in biliary tract tumours either as a single agent or in combination with cisplatin (Kim et al., 2003), gemcitabine (Cho et al., 2005) and mitomycin (Kornek et al., 2004).

Acceptable treatment options include the following.

- Gemcitabine and cisplatin combination therapy: gemcitabine 1000 mg/m^2 and cisplatin 25 mg/m^2 on days 1 and 8 of a 21-day cycle. Rescan after 4 cycles, continue to 8 cycles.
- Gemcitabine (for patients not fit for combination chemotherapy): 1000 mg/m^2 days 1, 8 and 15 of a 28-day cycle; rescan after 3 cycles, continue to 6 cycles.

Alternative regimens (e.g. if gemcitabine intolerance):

- 5-FU (modified by leucovorin) with or without mitomycin C. Although most trials have used bolus 5-FU, an infusional regimen through a central access device is more commonly used in the UK;
- cisplatin and 5-FU.

Molecular therapy

Cetuximab, erlotinib, bevacizumab and many other novel agents have been tested in biliary tract cancers. The BINGO trial, a randomised phase II trial, compared gemcitabine/oxaliplatin chemotherapy ± cetuximab, and failed to show a survival advantage for the latter combination (Malka et al., 2014). Similarly, a phase III study of gemcitabine/oxaliplatin with or without erlotinib failed to demonstrate benefit for addition of erlotinib over conventional chemotherapy (Lee et al., 2012). The ABC-03 trial evaluated efficacy of the pan-VEGF inhibitor, cediranib, over and above gem–cis chemotherapy – although the response rate was higher, there was no difference in survival for the novel combination.

Second-line chemotherapy

The role of second-line chemotherapy in biliary tract cancers is not established (Lamarca et al., 2014). A subgroup of patients who remain of good PS following progression on first-line chemotherapy may benefit from second-line treatment. Patients who achieve a longer progression-free interval following first-line chemotherapy are more likely to respond to second-line treatment. For patients who have received gem–cis combination as first-line, a fluoropyrimidine-based regimen may be active. Patients should be encouraged to enter clinical trials.

Radiotherapy and SIRT

Adjuvant radiotherapy/chemoradiotherapy has been mentioned previously. For locally advanced and unresectable disease, radiotherapy may also be a possibility, but current evidence is limited. SABR may also be a therapeutic option and the ABC-07 trial will evaluate the role of SABR following induction gem–cis chemotherapy. Small retrospective series and prospective studies have demonstrated some activity of SIRT in localised inoperable intrahepatic cholangiocarcinoma, but this procedure remains largely experimental (Khanna *et al.*, 2009; Saxena *et al.*, 2010; Hoffmann *et al.*, 2011; Rafi *et al.*, 2011).

Photodynamic therapy (PDT)

This involves injection of a photosensitiser followed by direct illumination of the tumour endoscopically using light of a specific wavelength. This causes activation of the photosensitising compound, release of oxygen-free radicals and tumour death. Ortner *et al.* (2003) carried out a randomised prospective trial that showed a median survival of 493 compared to 93 days ($p < 0.0001$) for patients treated with stenting followed by PDT compared to stenting alone. A second study of 32 patients showed a median survival of 21 months in patients treated with PDT compared to 7 months in patients treated with stenting alone (Zoepf *et al.*, 2005). However, a large randomised study evaluating the role of PDT over and above conventional stenting (PHOTOSTENT 2) was terminated by the independent data monitoring committee after 98 patients were recruited due to inferior survival in the PDT arm (6.1 months versus 9.2 months). The worse survival may have been caused by fewer patients having palliative chemotherapy in the PDT arm (Pereira *et al.*, 2010).

Stent insertion

Biliary obstruction and cholangitis are a common cause of morbidity and death. Plastic stents are placed if surgery is planned or if the prognosis is poor. Metallic stents have a lower complication rate (infection, blockage) but are more expensive. Patients should be prescribed ursodeoxycholic acid in an attempt to keep the stent open. If the obstruction cannot be relieved endoscopically from below, percutaneous transhepatic cholangiography (PTC) can be attempted for providing external biliary drainage and thereafter by placing the stent internally across the stricture.

Prognosis

Prognosis after surgery

One-year survival is 22% and 5YS is 5–10%. Lymph node metastasis, perineural invasion, positive resection margin and perihilar tumours are all associated with a poorer prognosis. In one series a 5-year survival of 43% has been reported for patients who have resected intrahepatic cholangiocarcinoma (Nakagohri *et al.*, 2003).

Ongoing trials in biliary tract cancer

PRODIGE 12: a randomised trial is evaluating the role of adjuvant gemcitabine and oxaliplatin chemotherapy compared to observation alone in resected biliary tract cancers.

ACTICCA-01: a randomised trial is evaluating the role of adjuvant gemcitabine and cisplatin chemotherapy compared to observation alone in resected biliary tract cancers.

SWOG 0202: a phase II study of gemcitabine and capecitabine in patients with unresectable locally advanced or metastatic gallbladder cancer or cholangiocarcinoma.

ABC05: a first-line trial for advanced biliary tract cancers. Patients are randomised to gemcitabine and cisplatin chemotherapy or to same chemotherapy plus the MEK inhibitor, selumitinib.

ABC06: a second-line trial for advanced biliary tract cancer, for patients who have progressed on first-line chemotherapy. Patients are randomised to ASC or ASC plus FOLFOX.

ABC07: SABR for locally advanced biliary tract cancer. A randomised phase II study of induction gemcitabine and cisplatin chemotherapy (4 cycles) followed by randomisation to SABR or continuing further chemotherapy in patients whose disease remains localised following induction chemotherapy.

Further details on current clinical trials can be found from http://www.ncri.org.uk/ (accessed January 2015).

References

Aitken, K. L and Hawkins, M. A. (2014). The role of radiotherapy and chemoradiation in the management of primary liver tumours. *Clin. Oncol. (R. Coll. Radiolol.)*, **26**, 569–580.

Anderson, C. A., Rice, M., Pinson, C. W. *et al.* (2004). FDG PET imaging in the evaluation of gallbladder carcinoma and cholangiocarcinoma. *J. Gastrointest. Surg.*, **8**, 90–97.

Bismuth, H. and Corlette, M. B. (1975). Intrahepatic cholangioenteric anastomosis in carcinoma of the hilus of the liver. *Surg. Gynecol. Obstet.*, **140**, 170–178.

Bismuth, H., Majno, P. E. and Adam, R. (1999). Liver transplantation for hepatocellular carcinoma. *Semin. Liver Dis.*, **19**, 311–322.

Bujold, A., Masey,C. A., Kim, J. J., *et al.* (2013). Sequential phase I and II trials of stereotactic body radiotherapy for locally advanced hepatocellular carcinoma. *J. Clin. Oncol.*, **31**, 1631–1637.

Chamberlain, R. S. and Blumgart, L. H. (2000). Hilar cholangiocarcinoma: a review and commentary. *Ann. Surg. Oncol.*, **7**, 55–66.

Chen, J. S., Lin, Y. C., Jan, Y. Y., *et al.* (2001). Mitomycin with weekly 24-h infusion of high dose 5-fluorouracil and leucovorin in patients with biliary tract and periampullar carcinomas. *Anticancer Drugs*, **12**, 339–343.

Cheng, A. L., Kang, Y.K., Chen, Z., *et al.* (2009). Efficacy and safety of sorafenib in patients in the Asia–Pacific region with advanced hepatocellular carcinoma: a phase III randomised, double-blind, placebo-controlled trial. *Lancet Oncol.*, **10**, 25–34.

Cho, J. Y., Paik, Y. H., Chang, Y. S., *et al.* (2005). Capecitabine combined with gemcitabine (CapGem) as first-line treatment in patients with advanced/metastatic biliary tract carcinoma. *Cancer*, **104**, 2753–2758.

Choi, B. O., Jang, H. S., Kang, K. M., *et al.* (2006). Fractionated stereotactic radiotherapy in patients with primary hepatocellular carcinoma. *Jpn. J. Clin. Oncol.*, **36**, 154–158.

Choi, C. W., Choi, I. K., Seo, J. H., *et al.* (2000). Effects of 5-fluorouracil and leucovorin in the treatment of pancreatic-biliary tract adenocarcinomas. *Am. J. Clin. Oncol.*, **23**, 425–428.

Fong, Y., Sun, R. L., Jarnagin, W., *et al.* (1999). An analysis of 412 cases of hepatocellular carcinoma at the Western center. *Ann. Surg.*, **229**, 790–800.

Forner, A., Llovet, J. M. and Bruix, J. (2012). Hepatocellular carcinoma. *Lancet*, **379**, 1245–1255.

Glimelius, B., Hoffman, K., Sjödén, P. O., *et al.* (1996). Chemotherapy improves survival and quality of life in advanced pancreatic and biliary cancer. *Ann. Oncol.*, **7**, 593–600.

Hoffmann, R. T., Paprottka, P. M., Schön, A., *et al.* (2011). Transarterial hepatic yttrium-90 radioembolization in patients with unresectable intrahepatic cholangiocarcinoma: factors associated with prolonged survival. *Cardiovasc. Intervent. Radiol.*, **35**, 105–106.

Khanna, V., Dhanasekaran, R., Barron, B. J., *et al.* (2009). Yttrium-90 radioembolization (SIR-Spheres) for cholangiocarcinoma: preliminary study. *J. Vasc. Intervent. Radiol.*, **26** (2 Suppl.), S116–S117.

Kim, T. W., Chang, H. M., Kang, H. J., *et al.* (2003). Phase II study of capecitabine plus cisplatin as first-line chemotherapy in advanced biliary cancer. *Ann. Oncol.*, **14**, 1115–1120.

Kornek, G. V., Schuell, B., Laengle, F., *et al.* (2004). Mitomycin C in combination with capecitabine or biweekly high-dose gemcitabine in patients with advanced biliary tract cancer: a randomised phase II trial. *Ann. Oncol.*, **15**, 478–483.

Lamarca, A., Hubner, R. A., Ryder, W. D., *et al.* (2014). Second-line chemotherapy in advanced biliary cancer: a systematic review. *Ann. Oncol.*, **25**, 2328–2338.

Lau, W. Y., Leung, W. T., Ho, S., *et al.* (1994). Treatment of inoperable hepatocellular carcinoma with intrahepatic arterial yttrium-90 microspheres: a phase I and II study. *Br. J. Cancer*, **70**, 994–999.

Lau, W. Y., Leung, T. W., Ho, S. K., *et al.* (1999). Adjuvant intra-arterial iodine-131-labelled lipiodol for resectable hepatocellular carcinoma: a prospective randomised trial. *Lancet*, **353**, 797–801.

Lau, W. Y., Leung, T. W., Lai, B. S., *et al.* (2001). Pre-operative systemic chemoimmunotherapy and sequential resection for unresectable hepatocellular carcinoma. *Ann. Surg.*, **233**, 236–241.

Lee, J., Park, S. H., Chang, H. M., *et al.* (2012). Gemcitabine and oxaliplatin with or without erlotinib in advanced biliary-tract cancer: a multicentre, open-label, randomised, phase 3 study. *Lancet Oncol.*, **13**, 181–188.

Leung, T. W. T., Patt, Y. Z., Lau, W. Y., *et al.* (1999). Complete pathological remission is possible with systemic combination chemotherapy for inoperable hepatocellular carcinoma. *Clin. Cancer Res.*, **5**, 1676–1681.

Llovet, J. M. and Bruix, J. (2003). Systematic review of randomized trials for unresectable hepatocellular carcinoma: chemoembolization improves survival. *Hepatology*, **37**, 429–442.

Llovet, J. M., Furster, J. and Bruix, J. (1999). Intention to treat analysis of surgical treatment for early hepatocellular carcinoma: resection versus transplantation. *Hepatology*, **30**, 1434–1440.

Llovet, J. M. Ricci, S., Mazzaferro, V., *et al.* (2008). Sorafenib in advanced hepatocellualr carcinoma. *N. Engl. J. Med.*, **359**, 378–390.

Lozano, R. D., Patt, Y. Z., Hassan, M. M., *et al.* (2000). Oral capecitabine (Xeloda) for the treatment of hepatobiliary cancers (hepatocellular carcinoma, cholangiocarcinoma, and gallbladder cancer). *Proc. Am. Soc. Clin. Oncol.*, **19**, abstr. 1025.

Maindrault-Goebel, F., Selle, F., Rosmorduc, O., *et al.* (2003). A phase II study of gemcitabine and oxaliplatin (GEMOX) in advanced biliary adenocarcinoma (ABA). Final Results. *Proc. Am. Soc. Clin. Oncol.*, **22**, abstr. 1178.

Malka, D., Cervera, P., Foulon, S., *et al.* (2014). Gemcitabine and oxaliplatin with or without cetuximab in advanced biliary-tract cancer (BINGO): a randomised, open-label, non-comparative phase 2 trial. *Lancet Oncol.* **15**, 819–828.

Mazzaferro, V., Regalia, E., Doci, R., *et al.* (1996). Liver transplantation for the treatment of small hepatocellular carcinomas in patients with cirrhosis. *N. Engl. J. Med.*, **334**, 693–699.

Mitry, E., van Custem, E., Van Laethem, J., *et al.* (2002). A randomised phase II trial of weekly high-dose 5FU with and without folinic acid and cisplatin in patients with advanced biliary tract adenocarcinoma: the EORTC 40955 trial. *Proc. Am. Soc. Clin. Oncol.*, **21**, abstr. 696.

Mornex, F., Girard, N., Beziat, C., *et al.* (2006). Feasibility and efficacy of high-dose three-dimensional-conformal radiotherapy in cirrhotic patients with small-size hepatocellular carcinoma non-eligible for curative therapies – mature results of the French Phase II RTF-1 trial. *Int. J. Radiat. Oncol. Biol. Phys.*, **66**, 1152–1158.

Muto, Y., Moriwaki, H., Ninomiya, M., *et al.* (1996). Prevention of second primary tumors by an acyclic retinoid, polyprenoic acid, in patients with hepatocellular carcinoma. Hepatoma Prevention Study Group. *N. Engl. J. Med.*, **334**, 1561–1567.

Nakagohri, T., Asano, T., Kinoshita, H., *et al.* (2003). Aggressive surgical resection for hilar-invasive and peripheral intrahepatic cholangiocarcinoma. *World J. Surg.*, **27**, 289–293.

Neoptolemos, J. P., Moore, M. J., Cox, T. F., *et al.* (2012). Effect of adjuvant chemotherapy with fluorouracil plus folinic acid or gemcitabine vs observation on survival in patients with resected periampullary adenocarcinoma: the ESPAC-3 periampullary cancer randomized trial. *J. Am. Med. Ass.*, **308**, 147–156.

NICE. (2013). *Selective Internal Radiotherapy for Primary Hepatocellular Carcinoma, IPG460*. London: National Institute for Health and Care Excellence.

O'Reilly, E. M., Stuart, K. E., Sanz-Altamira, P. M., *et al.* (2001). A phase II study of irinotecan in patients with advanced hepatocellular carcinoma. *Cancer*, **91**, 101–105.

Okusaka, T., Nakachi, K., Fukutomi, A., *et al.* (2010). Gemcitabine alone or in combination with cisplatin in patients with biliary tract cancer: a comparative multicentre study in Japan. *Br. J. Cancer*, **103**, 469–474.

Oliveri, R. S., Wetterslev, J. and Gluud, C. (2011). Transarterial (chemo)embolisation for unresectable hepatocellular carcinoma. *Cochrane Database of Systematic Reviews* 2011, Issue 3. Art. No.: CD004787.

Ortner, M. E., Caca, K., Berr, F., *et al.* (2003). Successful photodynamic therapy for nonresectable cholangiocarcinoma: a randomized prospective study. *Gastroenterology*, **125**, 1355–1363.

Pereira, S., Hughes, S. K., Roughton, M., *et al.* (2010). Photostent-02; Porfimer Sodium photodynamic therapy plus stenting versus stenting alone in patients (pts) with advanced or metastatic cholangiocarcinomas and other biliary tract tumours (BTC): A multicentre, randomised phase III trial. *ESMO Congress 2010*, Abstract no: 4580.

Philip, P. A., Mahoney, M., Thomas, J., *et al.* (2004). Phase II trial of erlotinib (OSI-774) in patients with hepatocellular or biliary cancer. *Proc. Am. Soc. Clin. Oncol.*, **22** (no. 14S July 15 suppl.), 4025.

Pugh, R. N. H., Murray-Lyon, I. M., Dawson, J. L., *et al.* (1973). Transection of the oesophagus for bleeding oesophageal varices. *Br. J. Surg.*, **60**, 646–649.

Rafi, S., Piduru, S. M., El-Rayes, B., *et al.* (2011). Yttrium-90 radioembolization for unresectable standard-chemorefractory intrahepatic cholangiocarcinoma: survival, efficacy and safety study. *J. Vasc. Intervent. Radiol.*, **22** (3 Suppl), S89.

SABR UK Consortium. (2015). *Stereotactic Ablative Body Radiation Therapy (SABR): A Resource. Version 5.0. January 2015*. Available at www.actionradiotherapy.org/wp-content/uploads/2014/12/UKSABRConsortiumGuidellinesv5.pdf (accessed October 2015).

Saxena, A., Bester, L., Chua, T. C., *et al.* (2010). Yttrium-90 radiotherapy for unresectable intrahepatic cholangiocarcinoma: a preliminary assessment of this novel treatment option. *Ann. Surg. Oncol.*, **17**, 484–491.

Schwartz, J. D., Schwartz, M., Goldman, J., *et al.* (2004). Bevacizumab in hepatocellular carcinoma in patients without metastasis and without invasion of the portal vein. *Proc. Am. Soc. Clin. Oncol. (Post-Meeting edn.)*, **22** (14S July 15 suppl.), 4088.

Seong, J., Keum, K. C., Han, K. H., *et al.* (1999). Combined transcatheter arterial chemoembolization and local radiotherapy of unresectable hepatocellular carcinoma. *Int. J. Radiat. Oncol. Biol. Phys.*, **43**, 393–397.

Sharma, A., Dwary, A. D., Mohanti, B. K., *et al.* (2010). Best supportive care compared with chemotherapy for unresectable gall bladder cancer: a randomized controlled study. *J. Clin. Oncol.*, **28**, 4581–4586.

Takada, T., Amano, H., Yasuda, H., *et al.* (2002). Is postoperative adjuvant chemotherapy useful for gallbladder carcinoma? A phase III multicenter prospective randomized controlled trial in patients with resected pancreaticobiliary carcinoma. *Cancer*, **95**, 1685–1695.

UICC. (2009). *TNM Classification of Malignant Tumours*. 7th edn. Eds. L. H. Sobin, M. K. Gospodarowicz, and Ch. Wittekind. Chichester: Wiley-Blackwell.

Ursino, S., Greco, C., Cartei, F., *et al.* (2012). Radiotherapy and hepatocellular carcinoma: update and review of the literature. *Eur. Rev. Med. Pharmacol. Sci.*, **16**, 1599–1604.

Valle, J., Wasan, H., Palmer, D., *et al.* (2010). Cisplatin plus gemcitabine versus gemcitabine for biliary tract cancer. *N. Engl. J. Med.*, **362**, 1273–1281.

Verslype, C., Rosmorduc, O., Rougier, P., *et al.* (2012). Hepatocellular carcinoma: ESMO–ESDO Clinical Practice Guidelines for diagnosis, treatment and follow-up. *Ann. Oncol.*, **23**(Suppl. 7), vii41–vii48.

Weis, S., Franke, A., Mössner, J., *et al.* (2013). Radiofrequency (thermal) ablation versus no intervention or other interventions for hepatocellular carcinoma. *Cochrane Database of Systematic Reviews 2013*, Issue 12. Art. No.: CD003046.

Yang, T. S., Lin, Y. C., Chen, J. S., *et al.* (2000). Phase II study of gemcitabine in patients with advanced hepatocellular carcinoma. *Cancer*, **89**, 750–756.

Yeo, W., Mok, T. S., Zee, B., *et al.* (2005). A randomized phase III study of doxorubicin versus cisplatin/interferon alpha-2b/doxorubicin/fluorouracil (PIAF) combination chemotherapy for unresectable hepatocellular carcinoma. *J. Natl Cancer Inst.*, **97**, 1532–1538.

Yoshida, H., Tateishi, R., Arakawa, Y., *et al.* (2004). Benefits of interferon therapy in hepatocellular carinoma prevention for individual patients with chronic hepatitis C. *Gut*, **53**, 425–430.

Zoepf, T., Jakobs, R., Arnold, J. C., *et al.* (2005). Palliation of nonresectable bile duct cancer: improved survival after photodynamic therapy. *Am. J. Gastroenterol.*, **100**, 2426–2430.

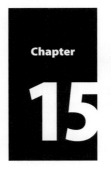

Chapter

15

Management of cancer of the exocrine pancreas

Rhian Sian Davies, Sarah Gwynne and Somnath Mukherjee

Introduction

Pancreatic cancer is the fifth commonest cause of cancer mortality in the UK. The major risk factors include smoking, diet and a history of previous total gastrectomy. There is also an association between long-standing diabetes and pancreatic cancer. Surgery is the only curative option, but fewer than 20% of patients are suitable for this. Chemotherapy is the mainstay of treatment for fit patients with advanced or metastatic cancers. Chemoradiation is an option for locally advanced inoperable (LAPC) or borderline resectable disease. Palliative care and psychosocial support are important in the management of this challenging disease.

Types of pancreatic tumour

Benign cysts can be congenital and arise from anomalous development of the pancreatic ducts. Pseudocysts are loculated collections of fluid arising from necrosis, inflammation or haemorrhage, which usually occur as a complication of acute pancreatitis. They are often solitary, can measure 5–10 cm and are often found adjacent to the pancreas in the region of the tail. Benign cystadenomas occur in elderly women and are found incidentally at autopsy or during other investigations. Microcystic and papillary–cystic are other variants found in younger women. The types of pancreatic tumour are shown in Table 15.1.

Incidence and epidemiology

There are about 8800 new cases of pancreatic cancer in the UK each year and 8700 die from the disease. The annual incidence is 9.7/100,000; peak incidence occurs for men in their eighth decade and women in their ninth decade.

Pancreatic cancer is the fifth leading cause of cancer death overall (5% of cancer mortality). The incidence is roughly equal in males and females. Most cases of the disease (80%) occur in the head of the pancreas.

Carcinoma of the exocrine pancreas

Risk factors and aetiology

Three per cent of pancreatic cancers may be inherited. Cancer family syndromes include inherited chronic pancreatitis, inherited diabetes mellitus and ataxia telangectasia syndrome.

Cigarette smoking doubles the risk. More than 1 in 4 pancreatic cancers in the UK are caused through smoking. The use of smokeless tobacco also increases the risk.

A diet rich in protein and carbohydrates and poor in fruit and fibre increases the risk of pancreatic cancer; processed meat may increase the risk.

Toxic chemicals are 2-naphthylamine, benzidine and DDT. Other risk factors are long-standing type I and type II diabetes mellitus (roughly doubles the risk), chronic pancreatitis, obesity, total gastrectomy (two to five times the risk) and pernicious anaemia.

Pathology

The pathological features of carcinoma of the pancreas are shown in Table 15.2. Pancreatic ductal adenocarcinoma is likely to arise from non-invasive precursor lesions called pancreatic intraepithelial neoplasia (PanINs) with a step-wise progression from low-grade to high-grade PanIN (carcinoma *in situ*) and thereafter to invasive adenocarcinoma.

Practical Clinical Oncology, Second Edition, ed. Louise Hanna, Tom Crosby and Fergus Macbeth. Published by Cambridge University Press. © Cambridge University Press 2015.

Table 15.1 Types of pancreatic tumour

Type	Examples
Benign tumours	Congenital cysts
	Pseudocysts
	Serous cystadenoma
	Pancreatic cysts and pseudocysts
	Papillary–cystic/microcystic
Primary tumours of exocrine pancreas	*Adenocarcinoma*
	Ductal (90% of all cases)
	Acinar
	Anaplastic
	Cystadenocarcinoma
	Adenoacanthoma
	Invasive adenocarcinoma associated with cystic mucinous neoplasm or intraductal papillary mucinous neoplasm
	Others
	Squamous cell carcinoma
	Sarcoma
	Solid and papillary neoplasms
	Borderline malignancies
	Intraductal papillary mucinous tumour with dysplasia
	Mucinous cystic tumour with dysplasia
	Pseudopapillary solid tumour
Neuroendocrine tumours of pancreas (see Chapter 39)	Islet cell tumour
	Gastrinoma
	Glucagonoma
	VIPoma
	Carcinoid
	Somatostatinoma
Metastasis	Rare (breast, lung, melanoma, non-Hodgkin lymphoma)
	More frequently metastases to retro-pancreatic lymph nodes which mimic pancreatic tumour

Table 15.2 Pathological features of pancreatic cancers

	Description
Macroscopic features	White, scirrhous, infiltrative margins
Microscopic features	Clearly recognisable glandular structures, may be mucinous, occasional adeno-squamous growth pattern
	Occasionally arise in cysts (cystadenocarcinoma) or from acinar cells (acinar cell carcinoma)

Anatomy

The pancreas is a retroperitoneal structure (peritoneum on the anterior surface only) and it lies in front of the first and second lumbar vertebrae. It has four parts: head (including uncinate process), neck, body and tail. The pancreatic duct and common bile duct pass through the head to open in the ampulla of Vater; invasion or compression of these structures leads to obstructive jaundice and pancreatic insufficiency.

Lymphatic drainage involves the pancreaticoduodenal, suprapancreatic, pyloric and pancreaticosplenic nodes which drain to the coeliac and superior mesenteric nodes.

213

The vagus and splanchnic nerves form the coeliac and superior mesenteric plexus. Posterior extension of tumour can involve the first and second coeliac ganglia, leading to back pain.

Vessels in close proximity to the pancreas include superior mesenteric vessels, portal vein, splenic vein, coeliac artery and its branches. Tumour extension to these structures is often a sign of inoperability and can lead to splenic or portal vein thrombosis.

In relation to the surrounding organs, the head of the pancreas lies within the C-loop of the duodenum and in close proximity to the stomach and jejunum. The tail abuts the hilum of the spleen and the head is close to the right kidney. The above structures along with the liver and the spinal cord are likely to be included in the radiation fields when planning radiotherapy to the pancreas.

Clinical presentation

Pain (epigastric for head lesions, left upper quadrant for tail lesions), anorexia and weight loss are common presenting symptoms. Sudden-onset painless jaundice is a typical presentation of cancer of the head of the pancreas. Back pain relieved by leaning forward is due to infiltration of the retroperitoneal structures and usually suggests inoperability. Metastatic disease (liver, peritoneum, lung, rarely bone) is common at presentation. Clinical examination should also include careful palpation for supraclavicular lymphadenopathy (Virchow's node).

Clinical features of pancreatic cancer

Symptoms/signs from primary tumour and local spread:

- gastric outlet obstruction (duodenal spread),
- obstructive jaundice,
- cholangitis,
- steatorrhoea (obstruction of bile duct by primary or malignant lymphadenopathy),
- back pain (spread to retroperitoneum and coeliac plexus),
- new-onset diabetes mellitus,
- oesophageal varices (portal vein thrombosis),
- altered bowel habits (infiltration of colon).

Symptoms and signs from metastatic disease:

- jaundice (extensive liver metastases),
- abdominal pain and ascites,
- Blumer's shelf (peritoneal metastasis in pouch of Douglas, which can be palpated rectally),

- shortness of breath (pulmonary metastasis, pleural effusion). Always exclude pulmonary embolism, which is a common association of pancreatic cancer,
- Virchow's node (malignant left supraclavicular node).

Paraneoplastic features:

- migratory thrombophlebitis (Trousseau's sign),
- Weber–Christian disease (subcutaneous fat necrosis, polyarthralgia, eosinophilia) – associated with acinar cell tumour,
- dermatomyositis/polymyositis.

Constitutional symptoms:

- fatigue,
- weight loss,
- anorexia,
- venous thrombo-embolism (incidence: 14.5% and 23% in observational arms from two studies evaluating thromboprophylaxis in pancreatic cancer) (Riess et al., 2009; Maraveyas et al., 2012).

Investigation and staging

Investigations are directed towards diagnosis and staging of the tumour.

Blood tests

- Full blood count, liver function tests, urea and electrolytes. Coagulation profile is necessary for patients presenting with obstructive jaundice.
- CA19-9: this tumour marker, detectable in blood, is raised in 70% of patients with pancreatic cancer. A low initial level and a fall in marker with therapy are associated with a better prognosis in all stages of the disease. The CA19-9 level needs to be interpreted with caution in patients with obstructive jaundice because this can cause high levels of the marker.

Imaging

A contrast-enhanced CT scan is usually used for local staging and to exclude metastatic disease. A dual-phase helical CT scan (arterial phase to show the pancreas and venous phase to look for liver metastasis) has been reported to have a 79% positive predictive value and a 96% negative predictive value in predicting tumour resectibility. 3D reconstruction may give additional information about the involvement of vascular structures. MRI has been shown to be equivalent to a

Table 15.3 TNM definitions of carcinoma of the pancreas

Stage	Description
TX	Primary tumour cannot be assessed
T0	No evidence of primary tumour
Tis	Carcinoma *in situ*
T1	Tumour limited to the pancreas, ≤ 2 cm in greatest dimension
T2	Tumour limited to the pancreas, > 2 cm in greatest dimension
T3	Tumour extends beyond the pancreas but without involvement of the coeliac axis or the superior mesenteric artery
T4	Tumour involves the coeliac axis or the superior mesenteric artery (unresectable primary tumour)
NX	Regional lymph nodes cannot be assessed
N0	No regional lymph node metastasis
N1	Regional lymph node metastasis
M0	No distant metastasis
M1	Distant metastasis

Adapted from UICC, 2009.

good-quality CT scan, but may be limited by cost and availability.

Endoscopic retrograde cholangiopancreaticogram (ERCP) is useful in patients presenting with obstructive jaundice. The 'double-duct' sign (occlusion of common bile duct and pancreatic duct) is almost diagnostic of pancreatic cancer; brushings obtained during the procedure can establish a malignant diagnosis (although the yield is low) and an endobiliary stent can be placed to relieve biliary obstruction.

Endoscopic ultrasound (EUS) can be used before surgery along with standard imaging to assess vascular involvement. It is also useful for obtaining a biopsy, especially in patients with a small tumour in whom a standard US or CT-guided biopsy may be difficult.

Further staging and diagnostic procedures

Laparoscopy and intraoperative US: for patients otherwise suitable for radical surgery, preoperative laparoscopy may find unsuspected peritoneal metastases. Positive peritoneal cytology has a positive predictive value of 94%, a specificity of 98% but a sensitivity of only 25% for determining unresectibility (Merchant *et al.*, 1999). Intraoperative US may detect small liver metastases not seen on conventional imaging.

Histology: in the past, pancreatic lesions have often been treated as 'cancers' based on a radiological diagnosis in the presence of raised tumour markers. It is essential to obtain a histological diagnosis prior to treatment, as it may be radiologically difficult to distinguish chronic pancreatitis from carcinoma, and CA19-9 may be spuriously elevated in the presence of obstructive jaundice. Histologically benign disease is found in up to 10% of radical resections. Rarer histological variants such as neuroendocrine tumours can be missed if a histological diagnosis is not established. CT, US or EUS-guided fine-needle aspiration (FNA) are safe procedures, and needle-track seeding is extremely rare. Obtaining a histological diagnosis is often difficult in LAPC, which may require treatment based on radiological diagnosis if several attempts at biopsy fail to secure a positive histology.

The role of PET-CT in the staging of pancreatic cancer remains uncertain. The PET PANC trial is now closed to recruitment, and the results of the trial are yet to be reported, but is aiming to address this question.

Staging classification

The TNM definitions and staging classification are shown in Table 15.3 and Table 15.4, respectively.

Treatment overview

Patients with localised disease should be discussed by a multidisciplinary team, including a pancreatic surgeon, radiologist, oncologist and pathologist. About 20% of patients have resectable disease at diagnosis with a median survival of about 24 months (Neoptolemos *et al.*, 2010). Patients who have advanced but localised tumours may have borderline resectable (BR) or LAPC disease depending on the degree of vascular involvement. Patients with BR disease may still be potentially curable, although this may require advanced surgical techniques including vascular reconstruction. Neoadjuvant therapy may be used to downstage BR tumours. Patients with LAPC are rarely downstaged to resectibility.

For patients who have LAPC or metastatic disease, management is palliative and the treatment goals include symptom control, optimising quality of life and improving overall survival. Palliative care should be involved early in the course of the disease for symptom control as well as for psychosocial and holistic support. Patients with pancreatic cancer are often underweight

Table 15.4 Stage groups for carcinoma of the pancreas

Stage	Description
0	Tis, N0, M0
IA	T1, N0, M0
IB	T2, N0, M0
IIA	T3, N0, M0
IIB	T1, N1, M0
	T2, N1, M0
	T3, N1, M0
III	T4, any N, M0
IV	Any T, any N, M1

Adapted from UICC, 2009.

and input from a dietician is required at every stage of the disease.

For patients with locally advanced non-metastatic cancer, both chemotherapy alone and chemoradiation are acceptable options. Chemotherapy is appropriate for patients with LAPC and metastatic disease with a WHO performance status 0–2. Nutritional support and close collaboration with the palliative care team are needed. Endobiliary stenting (for obstructive jaundice), palliative radiotherapy and coeliac plexus nerve block (for control of local pain due to retroperitoneal infiltration) are useful.

Management of pancreatic cancer

Management of resectable disease

In the UK and many parts of Europe, the standard management of resectable disease involves radical surgery followed by adjuvant chemotherapy. Postoperative chemoradiotherapy is practised in the USA, but its role is more controversial. The goal of treatment is to achieve margin-negative resection, but positive margin rates remain high despite improvements in imaging and referral of patients to high-volume specialised units for their surgery – in the ESPAC3 trial, for example, the positive margin rate was 16% (Neoptolemos et al., 2012).

Radical surgery

Pancreatico-duodenectomy (Whipple's procedure) and pylorus-preserving pancreatico-duodenectomy (PPPD) are both considered standard operations for tumours in the head/neck/uncinate process of the pancreas, whereas distal pancreatectomy is performed for tumours of body/

tail of pancreas. Total pancreatectomy may be necessary for large tumours to achieve clear margins. Whipple's procedure is associated with higher morbidity (up to 40%) and mortality (2.4% in high-volume centres) compared to distal pancreatectomy (28.1% and 1.2%, respectively) (Birkmeyer et al., 1999; Kelly et al., 2011).

Perioperative mortality and morbidity are inversely related to a surgeon's case load (Neoptolemos et al., 1997; Birkmeyer et al., 1999) and patients should be treated by a specialist surgical team (NHS Executive, 2001). The complications of surgery include delayed gastric emptying, pancreatic fistula, sepsis, haemorrhage, malabsorption and diabetes mellitus.

Adjuvant chemotherapy

Four phase III trials have tested the role of adjuvant chemotherapy. The two earlier trials, ESPAC1 and CONKO-001, tested the benefit of 5-FU and gemcitabine, respectively, against no postoperative therapy. Subsequent trials (ESPAC3 and RTOG 97-04) have randomised patients between 5-FU and gemcitabine as adjuvant treatment options.

The ESPAC1 study randomised patients to no adjuvant therapy, adjuvant chemotherapy alone (5-FU with folinic acid, days 1–5, every 4 weeks for 6 cycles), adjuvant chemoradiation or adjuvant chemoradiation followed by chemotherapy. Patients on adjuvant chemotherapy had a significantly improved survival (median survival 20.1 months compared to 15.5 months, $p = 0.0009$) and chemoradiation was found to be detrimental (median survival 15.9 months compared to 17.9 months, $p = 0.05$; Neoptolemos et al., 2004). The radiotherapy arms of the study have been criticised for using a low-dose split-course technique, the lack of a detailed protocol and inadequate quality assurance.

The CONKO-001 study randomised patients to gemcitabine or no adjuvant therapy. The median disease-free survival (13.4 versus 6.7 months, $p < 0.001$) and overall survival (22.8 months versus 20.2 months, $p = 0.01$) were significantly better in patients treated with gemcitabine, and the benefit is maintained over time in terms of 5-year OS (20.7% vs 10.4%) and 10-year OS (12.2% vs 7.7%) (Oettle et al., 2013).

ESPAC3 randomised 434 patients between 5-FU with folinic acid and gemcitabine, demonstrated a similar overall survival between the two arms (median survival 23.0 and 23.6 months, respectively), but Grade 3/4 toxicity was lower in the gemcitabine arm (Neoptolemos et al., 2012).

In the Intergroup trial RTOG 97-04, 538 patients with resected pancreatic adenocarcinoma were randomised to either gemcitabine for 3 weeks pre and 12 weeks post 5-FU-based CRT or continuous infusion 5-FU for 3 weeks pre and 12 weeks post 5-FU-based CRT regimen. There was no difference in OS between the two arms. However, there was a non-significant trend towards improved median OS and 5-year OS in favour of gemcitabine for patients with pancreatic head tumours (20.5 months, 22% vs 17.1 months, 18%, respectively; $p = 0.08$). The first site of relapse was local in 28% and distant in 73% of cases, suggesting greater need for more effective systemic therapy. (Regine *et al.*, 2011)

Based on data from these clinical trials, gemcitabine is considered standard adjuvant therapy in the UK.

Postoperative adjuvant chemoradiation

Adjuvant chemoradiation is widely practised in the USA, but not favoured in the UK and Europe. The data for adjuvant chemoradiotherapy are contentious. The potential benefit of CRT is largely based on retrospective data and one small randomised trial which included only 49 patients (Kalser and Ellenberg, 1985).

The ESPAC1 trial described above showed an overall detriment from the use of adjuvant chemoradiotherapy, but has been criticised for lack of good-quality radiotherapy. In an EORTC trial, 218 patients with pancreatic head and peri-ampullary tumours were randomised to adjuvant chemoradiotherapy (split-course) or surgery alone. There was a small improvement in survival with combined modality therapy in patients with pancreatic cancer, but this was not statistically significant (median survival 24.5 months compared to 19.0 months, 2-year survival 34% compared to 26%, $p = 0.099$). The trial was underpowered, used what would be considered a suboptimal dose and lacked quality assurance (Klinkenbijl *et al.*, 1999). A more recent trial conducted by the French group, GERCOR, randomised patients to adjuvant gemcitabine alone versus gemcitabine-based chemoradiotherapy, but failed to demonstrate benefit for addition of chemoradiotherapy with a median overall survival of 24 months in both arms (Van Laethem *et al.*, 2010).

The RTOG 0848 trial, currently open to recruitment, is randomising patients to six cycles of adjuvant gemcitabine with/without consolidation capecitabine-based CRT.

Management of borderline resectable pancreatic cancer

NCCN defines BR tumours as: unilateral or bilateral SMV or portal vein infringement, less than 50% abutment of circumference of SMA, abutment/encasement of hepatic artery or short segment occlusion of SMV. Traditionally, operating on this group of patients has been associated with a high risk of R1/R2 resection and increased risk of post-surgical morbidity/mortality. Recent specialisation of pancreatic surgery in high-volume centres and advances in perioperative care have reduced complications. A recent study from the UK retrospectively analysed the outcome of over 1500 pancreatic resections and showed no difference in complication rates between patients undergoing pancreaticoduodenectomy with vein resection (PDVR) compared to those without venous resection; although patients undergoing PDVR had more advanced tumours, median survival was comparable between these arms (18 months and 18.2 months, respectively; Ravikumar *et al.*, 2014).

The role of neoadjuvant strategies has also been investigated to downstage BR tumours prior to resection. A meta-analysis looking at prospective neoadjuvant trials in BR tumours included only 182 patients from 10 studies and showed that of the 69% of patients who went to surgery, 80% had resection and 80% of these had R0 resection (Festa *et al.*, 2013). There is only one randomised controlled trial which has compared neoadjuvant chemoradiotherapy (cisplatin/gemcitabine, 55.4 Gy) with upfront surgery. The study closed early due to poor recruitment and showed a trend towards better R0 resection rate and median survival in the neoadjuvant group (Golcher *et al.*, 2015). The ESPAC-5 trial is a randomised phase II feasibility trial which opened to recruitment in the UK in 2014, comparing immediate surgery to neoadjuvant chemotherapy (gemcitabine/capecitabine combination or FOLFIRINOX) or chemoradiotherapy in this patient group.

Currently in the UK, neoadjuvant chemotherapy or chemoradiotherapy is not routinely used outside of the context of clinical trial.

Management of locally advanced pancreatic cancer (LAPC)

Chemotherapy alone, primary chemoradiotherapy and induction chemotherapy followed by consolidation chemoradiotherapy are all considered treatment options for this patient group, but primary chemotherapy (with/without consolidation CRT) is the current treatment of choice. In LAPC, there is a high risk of micro-metastatic disease and progression occurs in 30–40% of cases within the first 3–4 months, so initiating treatment with chemotherapy is preferred over upfront chemoradiation. The role of consolidation CRT following initial 3–4 months of induction chemotherapy is currently debatable. LAP 07, a phase III trial, compared consolidation CRT with continuing chemotherapy in patients who had received 4 cycles of induction gemcitabine ± erlotinib therapy. The study showed that OS in the CRT arm was not superior to continuing chemotherapy alone. However, CRT was associated with a low rate of grade 3/4 toxicity (< 6%), a statistically significant prolongation of local control and delay in the requirement for second-line chemotherapy (Hammel *et al.*, 2013; Huguet *et al.*, 2014). Consolidation chemoradiotherapy may be considered for patients with predominant local symptoms or local-only progression following induction chemotherapy, or in patients who develop unacceptable toxicity on primary chemotherapy. As CRT may maintain local control with a low incidence of grade 3/4 toxicity, its use following induction chemotherapy may allow patients to have a period of break from chemotherapy.

Gemcitabine alone or in combination with capecitabine (GEMCAP) has been the mainstay of systemic therapy for LAPC in the UK. As discussed in the section that follows, recent trials have demonstrated an overall survival advantage with the use of FOLFIRINOX (5-FU, FA, irinotecan and oxaliplatin) and nab-paclitaxel/gemcitabine combination over gemcitabine alone; however, these trials were conducted on patients with metastatic disease. While some centres have extrapolated these results and adopted the use of these regimens for LAPC, there are no randomised trials supporting their use.

5-FU or capecitabine are traditionally used as radiosensitising drugs for the treatment of pancreatic cancer. The SCALOP trial randomised 74 patients who had received 3 cycles of induction GEMCAP chemotherapy to receive either low-dose gemcitabine (300 mg/m² weekly) or capecitabine (830 mg/m² b.d. on days of radiotherapy) in combination with radiotherapy. Although not the primary endpoint, SCALOP showed a significant OS advantage in the capecitabine arm (15.2 months versus 13.4 months, HR 0.39, $p = 0.012$) with a lower incidence of grade 3/4 haematological and non-haematological toxicity. The trial suggested that when CRT is used, a capecitabine-based regimen may

be preferable over low-dose gemcitabine (Mukherjee *et al.*, 2013).

Acceptable treatment options for LAPC are as follows.

- Chemotherapy as outlined in the metastatic section.
  - Induction chemotherapy for 3–4 cycles, followed by consolidation chemoradiotherapy (radiotherapy 50.4–54 Gy in 28–30 fractions with capeciabine 830 mg/m² p.o. b.d. on treatment days).

Management of metastatic pancreatic cancer

Since its recommendation by NICE in May 2001, single-agent gemcitabine has been the drug of choice for patients with metastatic disease and Karnofsky performance score of 50 or more. One randomised trial (Burris *et al.*, 1997) showed that it was more effective than bolus 5-FU in terms of median survival (5.6 compared to 4.4 months, $p = 0.0025$), progression-free survival (2.3 compared to 0.9 months, $p = 0.0002$) and one-year overall survival (18% compared to 2%; $p = 0.0002$). At the time of writing, gemcitabine remains the most commonly prescribed chemotherapy regimen for pancreatic cancer in the UK.

Over the last two decades, there have been nearly 50 randomised trials that have evaluated the addition of various chemotherapeutic or biological agents to gemcitabine or have tested non-gemcitabine regimens. Only three trials have been positive, and only two new drugs (erlotinib, nab-paclitaxel) have gained regulatory approval for use in pancreatic cancer since FDA approved gemcitabine in 1996.

The combination chemotherapy FOLFIRINOX has been shown to be superior to single-agent gemcitabine (11.1 months compared to 6.8 months, $p < 0.0001$) in a phase III trial ($n = 342$). However, the regimen was associated with a high incidence of grade 3/4 toxicity including neutropenia (45.7%), fatigue (23%), diarrhoea (12.7%) and neuropathy (9%) and is therefore suitable only for patients 75 years or less in age, with a performance status 0 or 1 and adequate liver and renal function (Conroy *et al.*, 2011).

The MPACT study randomised 861 patients to gemcitabine alone or in combination with albumin-bound paclitaxel (nab-paclitaxel). The overall survival was improved in the combined treatment group (8.5 months compared with 6.7 months, $p < 0.001$). Prominent grade 3/4 toxicity included neutropenia (38%), fatigue (17%) and peripheral neuropathy (17%), which was largely reversible through temporarily withholding nab-paclitaxel therapy (Von Hoff *et al.*, 2013). There has been no randomised trial of FOLFIRINOX versus gemcitabine/nab-paclitaxel.

The combination of gemcitabine with capecitabine (GEMCAP) became popular in the UK following the GEMCAP study, but this regimen is not used widely outside of the UK. The study on its own showed a trend for OS benefit when compared with gemcitabine (HR = 0.86, CI = 0.72–1.02, p = 0.08), but a meta-analysis of GEMCAP trials involving more than 900 patients, presented in the same paper, showed significant survival benefit (HR = 0.86, p = 0.02; Cunningham *et al.*, 2009). Although data are not as strong as MPACT or FOLFIRINOX, it is considered an acceptable treatment for good performance status of patients with advanced pancreatic cancer in the UK.

Treatment options

Patients with good performance status (WHO 0–1) with adequate haematological, hepatic and renal function and no contraindication to a specified chemotherapy could be offered:

- FOLFIRINOX: oxaliplatin 85 mg/m², irinotecan 180 mg/m², leucovorin 400 mg/m² and 5-FU 400 mg/m² as a bolus followed by 5-FU 2400 mg/m² as a continuous infusion for 46 hours, OR
- nab-paclitaxel 125 mg/m² 4-weekly in combination with gemcitabine 1000 mg/m² on days 1, 8 and 15. OR
- gemcitabine and capecitabine combination: gemcitabine 1000 mg/m² weekly and capecitabine 1660 mg/m² daily / 830mg/m² b.d., three weeks out of four.

Patients with borderline performance status (WHO 2) with adequate haematological, hepatic and renal function and no contraindication to gemcitabine should be offered:

- gemcitabine 1000 mg/m² days 1, 8 and 15 every 4 weeks or once weekly for weeks 1–7 then 1 week off with subsequent cycles weekly for 3 weeks out of every 4.

Patients with poor performance status (3 or 4) should not be offered chemotherapy.

Second-line chemotherapy

The CONKO study group conducted a phase III randomised trial comparing second-line oxaliplatin, folinic acid and 5-FU (OFF) to best supportive care (BSC) in patients who had progressed on first-line gemcitabine. The study closed early due to poor accrual; however, in the 46 patients randomised, median survival in the OFF group was better than the BSC group (4.82 months vs 2.30 months, p = 0.008; Pelzer *et al.*, 2011). The subsequent CONKO-003 trial randomised patients who had progressive disease on gemcitabine monotherapy to receive folinic acid and 5-FU (FF) or oxaliplatin and FF (OFF). The study demonstrated an improved median OS in the OFF group (5.9 months vs 3.3 months, p = 0.01; Oettle *et al.*, 2014).

OFF can be administered as follows:

- leucovorin (200 mg/m²) and 5-FU (2000 mg/m² as 24 hours continuous infusion) on days 1, 8, 15, 22; and oxaliplatin (85 mg/m²) on days 8 and 22; given as 6 weekly cycles.

Radiotherapy – technique, dose and fractionation

Radical radiotherapy (neoadjuvant or definitive)

As technology has moved on, intensity-modulated radiotherapy (IMRT) and 4D CT are increasingly being adopted as standard of care across the UK; they allow radiotherapy dose escalation or delivery of radical dose radiation in combination with full-dose gemcitabine, both of which are current areas of research interest. Multiple studies have now shown that compared to conventional 3D planning, IMRT delivers the radiation dose more conformally to the PTV with reduction in the mean dose to the liver, kidneys, stomach and small bowel (Milano *et al.*, 2004).

The technique for chemoradiotherapy for locally advanced disease is as follows.

- Pre-planning: it is preferable for patients to have an EDTA clearance and functioning renogram to assess total and individual renal function. GFR must be greater than 50 mL/min/1.73 m².
- Planning/localisation: CT localisation with the patient in the supine position, arms raised above the head and immobilised, ideally with the use of a chest-board and knee-fix. Intravenous contrast should be used.
- Gross tumour volume (GTV): tumour as visualised on planning scan along with lymph nodes > 1 cm diameter.

Table 15.5 Dose–volume constraints for pancreatic radiotherapy

Description	Naming convention	Variable	Optimal	Mandatory
PTV	PTV5040/5400	D99%	≥ 95%	≥ 90%
Conventional dose RT arms		D95%	≥ 97%	≥ 93%
		Dmax (0.1 cc)	≤ 105%	≤ 107%
Kidney receiving higher dose	Kidney_R or Kidney_L	V20Gy	≤ 40%	≤ 45%
Combined kidneys		V20Gy	≤ 30%	≤ 35%
Liver	Liver	V30Gy	≤ 30%	–
		Mean	≤ 28 Gy	≤ 30 Gy
Stomach	Stomach	Dmax (0.1 cc)	≤ 54 Gy	≤ 56 Gy
		V50Gy	< 5 cc	–
		V45Gy	< 75 cc	–
Small bowel	Small Bowel	Dmax (0.1 cc)	≤ 54 Gy	≤ 56 Gy
		V50Gy	< 10 cc	–
		V15Gy	< 120 cc	–
Duodenum	Duodenum	Dmax (0.1 cc)	≤ 54 Gy	≤ 56 Gy
		V50Gy	< 10 cc	–
		V15Gy	< 60 cc	–
Spinal cord PRV	SpinalCord_05	Dmax (0.1 cc)	–	≤ 45 Gy

Kidney OARs should be delineated separately and use the nomenclature specified in column 2. The reported values should be: (a) to the kidney receiving the higher dose and (b) the combined kidney dose. D95%, dose to 95% of the volume; Dmax, maximum dose to 0.1 cc; V20Gy, volume receiving 20 Gy. Adapted with permission from the SCALOP 2 radiotherapy planning and guidance document version 1.00 (4/9/2014).

- Planning target volume (PTV): where 4D CT is not available, this is defined as GTV with a 15-mm margin in the anterior–posterior direction and a 20-mm margin in the superior–inferior direction. The use of 4D CT should be encouraged. An ITV is created by combining the GTV outlines from multiple phases of respiration (at least three phases including end inspiration, end expiration and the time-weighted average or conventional 3D scan). PTV is defined as 1 cm expansion around the ITV.
- IMRT is preferred to 3D conformal radiotherapy. Where 3D conformal radiotherapy is used, common beam arrangement involves three- or four-coplanar fields – anterior–posterior beams and lateral fields angled anteriorly to reduce the dose to the kidneys.
- Dose, energy, fractionation: 50.4–54 Gy in 28–30 fractions, 1.8 Gy/fraction, using 10 MV photons, treating all fields daily, Monday to Friday. For 3D conformal radiotherapy, the maximum and minimum allowable doses within the PTV should be 107% and 95%, respectively, of the dose prescribed at ICRU 50.
- Verification: portal beam imaging taken on the first three days of treatment, weekly thereafter.
- Organs at risk and dose constraints: refer to Table 15.5.

Toxicity of chemoradiotherapy

- Gastrointestinal: anorexia, nausea and vomiting, dehydration, diarrhoea, acute gastritis; uncommon: gastrointestinal haemorrhage (may occur a few weeks after the end of chemoradiation), gastrointestinal perforation, subacute intestinal obstruction.
- Haematological: anaemia, leucopenia or thrombocytopenia (especially with gemcitabine-based chemoradiation).
- Other: fatigue, chronic renal damage, second malignancy (rare).
- General care: prophylactic anti-emetics (according to local hospital policy) and weekly clinical review.

Palliative radiotherapy

A short course of radiotherapy may be used to palliate local symptoms such as pain, bleeding or impending gastro-duodenal obstruction in patients with metastatic disease or those with locally advanced disease not suitable for chemoradiation.

The radiotherapy technique for palliative radiotherapy is as follows.

- Planning and localisation: CT localisation in a CT simulator as above.
- PTV: GTV as defined on the planning CT scan, with a 2–3 cm margin.
- Fields: anterior–posterior parallel opposed fields.
- Dose and fractionation:

  20 Gy in 5 fractions or
  30 Gy in 10 fractions.

Palliative interventions

Obstructive jaundice is a major cause of morbidity in patients with pancreatic cancer. Plastic stents are placed if surgery is planned or if the prognosis is poor. Metallic stents have a lower complication rate (infection, blockage), but cannot be replaced. Duodenal stents are used in palliative patients who develop duodenal obstruction.

Palliative surgery

In some cases of biliary and/or gastrointestinal obstruction, palliative bypass surgery is required. This entails a choledochojejunostomy and/or gastrojejunostomy.

Prognosis and prognostic factors

The overall prognosis for pancreatic cancer is poor with a 5-year survival rate of < 5%, and there has been very little improvement in survival over the past 50 years. For patients undergoing resection, the number of positive lymph nodes, the resection margin status and postoperative CA19-9 level have all been shown to be prognostic. Patients with non-metastatic LAPC have a median survival of around 10 months. Those with metastases have a median survival of around 6 months and a 1-year survival of 20% (Burris et al., 1997).

Areas of current interest

Advanced radiotherapy techniques

There has been interest in the use of stereotactic body radiotherapy (SBRT) as a means of delivering a high dose conformal radiotherapy. There are no large randomised controlled trials supporting its use at present.

Recent studies have looked at the early use of SBRT in patients with LAPC following two cycles of induction gemcitabine without the need for interruption in systemic treatment (Mahadevan et al., 2011), or concurrently with cycle 1 of gemcitabine (Gurka et al., 2013). These studies have demonstrated that the early use of SBRT may be a safe method of delivering early local therapy for those patients who have not yet developed metastatic disease; however, this will need further evaluation in larger prospective trials.

Future direction

Over decades, the quest for an effective treatment for pancreatic cancer has continued to frustrate researchers and clinicians across the globe. More recently, there has been greater understanding of the molecular aberrations that underpin the development of pancreatic cancer and its complex relationship with the tumour microenvironment. The whole exome sequencing of 99 patients with early-stage pancreatic cancer, done through collaborative effort as a part of the International Cancer Genome Consortium (ICGC), has identified over 2000 mutations and 1600 copy-number variations (Biankin et al., 2012). Sixteen significantly mutated genes were identified, including KRAS, SMAD4 (DPC4), CDKN2A (p16) and TP53, and although currently not targets for which an active treatment option exists, some of them determine prognosis and risk of metastatic disease. They may allow us to stratify patients in clinical trials and to select the most appropriate patients for locoregional therapy (surgery or radiotherapy). Known actionable targets include abnormality of the DNA repair pathway (platinum, radiotherapy), wild-type KRAS (erlotinib) and HER2 (traztuzumab), but are present in a small proportion of patients – this suggests that a potential role for personalising therapy based on whole-genome sequencing may be a way forward in this disease. A summary of current and future systemic treatment options can be found in Arslan et al. (2014).

Selection of ongoing clinical trials

Adjuvant/neoadjuvant

RTOG 0848: A phase III trial is currently looking at adjuvant treatment following resection of pancreatic head adenocarcinoma. The randomisation is between completion of six cycles of adjuvant gemcitabine alone or to proceed with adjuvant chemoradiotherapy with 5-FU or capecitabine.

APACT: A randomised phase III trial of adjuvant nab-paclitaxel plus gemcitabine versus gemcitabine alone in patients with surgically resected pancreatic adenocarcinoma.

ESPAC-4 (closed to recruitment): A randomised phase III trial comparing adjuvant combination gemcitabine–capecitabine chemotherapy with gemcitabine alone following surgical resection.

ESPAC-5 (feasibility): A randomised phase II trial comparing immediate surgery to neoadjuvant chemotherapy (gemcitabine/capecitabine combination or FOLFIRINOX) or chemoradiotherapy in patients with borderline resectable locally advanced pancreatic cancer.

Locally advanced

SCALOP II: A randomised phase II study of patients with locally advanced pancreatic cancer. Patients are treated with three cycles of induction gemcitabine and nab-paclitaxel chemotherapy, and those who have stable/responding disease will be randomised to continue same chemotherapy for a further three cycles or to receive one further cycle of gemcitabine and nab-paclitaxel followed by one of the four CRT arms: 50.4 Gy with capecitabine; 50.4 Gy with capecitabine and nelfinavir; 60 Gy with capecitabine; 60 Gy with capecitabine and nelfinavir.

RTOG 12-01: A phase II randomized trial of high versus standard intensity local or systemic therapy for unresectable pancreatic cancer.

Metastatic

SIEGE: A randomised phase II trial comparing first-line concomitant with sequential gemcitabine and nab-paclitaxel in metastatic pancreatic cancer.

References

Arslan, C. and Yalcin, S. (2014). Current and future systemic treatment options in metastatic pancreatic cancer. *J. Gastrointest. Oncol.*, **5**, 280–295.

Biankin, A. V., Waddell, N., and Kassahn, K. S. (2012). Pancreatic cancer genomes reveal aberrations in axon guidance pathway genes. *Nature*, **491**, 399–405.

Birkmeyer, J. D., Finlayson, S. R., Tosteson A. N., *et al.* (1999). Effect of hospital volume on in-hospital mortality with pancreaticoduodenectomy. *Surgery*, **125**, 250–256.

Burris, H. A. III, Moore, M. J., Anderson, J., *et al.* (1997). Improvements in survival and clinical benefit with gemcitabine as first-line therapy for patients with advanced pancreas cancer: a ramdomized trial. *J. Clin. Oncol.*, **15**, 2403–2413.

Conroy, T., Desseigne, F., Ychou, M., *et al.* (2011). FOLFIRINOX versus gemcitabine for metastatic pancreatic cancer. *N. Engl. J. Med.*, **364**, 1817–1825.

Cunningham, D., Chau, I., Stocken, D. D., *et al.* (2009). Phase III randomized comparison of gemcitabine versus gemcitabine plus capecitabine in patients with advanced pancreatic cancer. *J Clin Oncol.*, **27** (33), 5513–5518.

Festa, V., Andriulli, A., Valvano M.R., *et al.* (2013). Neoadjuvant chemo-radiotherapy for patients with borderline resectable pancreatic cancer: a meta-analytical evaluation of prospective studies. *JOP*, **14**, 618–625.

Golcher, H., Brunner, T. B., Witzigmann, H., *et al.* (2015). Neoadjuvant chemoradiation therapy with gemcitabine/cisplatin and surgery versus immediate surgery in resectable pancreatic cancer: Results of the first prospective randomized phase II trial. *Strahlenther. Onkol.*, **191**, 7–16.

Gurka, M. K., Collins, S. P., Slack, R., *et al.* (2013). Stereotactic body radiation therapy with concurrent full-dose gemcitabine for locally advanced pancreatic cancer: a pilot trial demonstrating safety. *Radiat. Oncol.*, **8**, 44.

Hammel, P., Huguet, F. and Van Laethem, J-L. (2013). Comparison of chemoradiotherapy (CRT) and chemotherapy (CT) in patients with a locally advanced pancreatic cancer (LAPC) controlled after 4 months of gemcitabine with or without erlotinib: Final results of the international phase III LAP 07 study. *J. Clin. Oncol.*, **31** (suppl; abstr LBA4003).

Huguet, F., Hammel, P., Vernerey, D., *et al.* (2014). Impact of chemoradiotherapy (CRT) on local control and time without treatment in patients with locally advanced pancreatic cancer (LAPC) included in the international phase III LAP 07 study. *J. Clin. Oncol.*, **32** (5 suppl.; abstr 4001).

Kalser, M. H. and Ellenberg, S. S. (1985). Pancreatic cancer. Adjuvant combined radiation and chemotherapy following curative resection. *Arch. Surg.*, **120**, 899–903.

Kelly, K. J., Greenblatt, D. Y., Wan, Y., *et al.* (2011). Risk stratification for distal pancreatectomy utilizing ACS-NSQIP: preoperative factors predict morbidity and mortality. *J. Gastrointest. Surg.*, **15**, 250–261.

Klinkenbijl, J.H., Jeekel, J., Sahmoud, T., *et al.* (1999). Adjuvant radiotherapy and 5-fluorouracil after curative resection of cancer of the pancreas and periampullary region: phase III trial of the EORTC gastrointestinal tract cancer cooperative group. *Ann. Surg.*, **230**, 776–782.

Mahadevan, A., Miksad, R., Goldstein, M., *et al.* (2011). Induction gemcitabine and stereotactic body radiotherapy for locally advanced nonmetastatic pancreas cancer. *Int. J. Radiat. Oncol. Biol. Phys.*, **81**, 615–622.

Maraveyas, A. Waters, J., Roy, R., *et al.* (2012). Gemcitabine versus gemcitabine plus dalteparin thromboprophylaxis in pancreatic cancer. *Eur. J. Cancer*, **48**, 1283–1292.

Merchant, N. B., Conlon, K. C., Saigo, P., *et al.* (1999). Positive peritoneal cytology predicts unresectability of pancreatic adenocarcinoma. *J. Am. Coll. Surg.*, **188**, 421–426.

Milano, M., Chmura, S. J., Garofalo, M. C., *et al.* (2004). Intensity-modulated radiotherapy in treatment of pancreatic and bile duct malignancies: toxicity and clinical outcome. *Int. J. Radiat. Oncol. Biol. Phys.*, **59**, 445–453.

Mukherjee, S., Hurt, C. N., Bridgewater, J., *et al.* (2013). Gemcitabine-based or capecitabine-based chemoradiotherapy for locally advanced pancreatic cancer (SCALOP): a multicentre, randomised, phase 2 trial. *Lancet Oncol.*, **14**, 317–326.

Neoptolemos, J. P., Russell, R. C., Bramhall, S., *et al.* (1997). Low mortality following resection for pancreatic and periampullary tumours in 1026 patients: UK survey of specialist pancreatic units. UK Pancreatic Cancer Group. *Br. J. Surg.*, **84**, 1370–1376.

Neoptolemos, J. P., Stocken, D. D., Friess, H., *et al.* (2004). A randomized trial of chemoradiotherapy and chemotherapy after resection of pancreatic cancer. *N. Engl. J. Med.*, **350**, 1200–1210.

Neoptolemos, J. P., Stocken, D. D., Bassi, C., *et al.* (2010). Adjuvant chemotherapy with fluorouracil plus folinic acid vs gemcitabine following pancreatic cancer resection: a randomized controlled trial. *J. Am. Med. Ass.*, **304**, 1073–1081.

Neoptolemos, J. P., Moore, M. J., Cox, T. F., *et al.* (2012). Effect of adjuvant chemotherapy with fluorouracil plus folinic acid or gemcitabine vs observation on survival in patients with resected periampullary adenocarcinoma: the ESPAC-3 periampullary cancer randomized trial. *J. Am. Med. Ass.*, **308**, 147–156.

NHS Executive. (2001). *Guidance on Commissioning Cancer Services- Improving Outcomes in Upper Gastro-intestinal Cancers. NHS Executive Catalogue Number 23943.* London: Department of Health.

Oettle, H., Neuhaus, P., Hochhaus, A., *et al.* (2013). Adjuvant chemotherapy with gemcitabine and long-term outcomes among patients with resected pancreatic cancer: the CONKO-001 randomized trial. *J. Am. Med. Ass.*, **310**, 1473–1481.

Oettle, H., Riess, H., Stieler, J. M., *et al.* (2014). Second-line oxaliplatin, folinic acid, and fluorouracil versus folinic acid and fluorouracil alone for gemcitabine-refractory pancreatic cancer: outcomes from the CONKO-003 trial. *J. Clin. Oncol.*, **32**, 2423–2429.

Pelzer, U., Schwaner, I., Stieler, J., *et al.* (2011). Best supportive care (BSC) versus oxaliplatin, folinic acid and 5-fluorouracil (OFF) plus BSC in patients for second-line advanced pancreatic cancer: A phase III-study from the German CONKO-study group. *Eur. J. Cancer*, **47**, 1676–1681.

Ravikumar, R., Sabin, C., Abu Hilal, M., *et al.* (2014). Portal vein resection in borderline resectable pancreatic cancer: a United Kingdom multicenter study. *J. Am. Coll. Surg.*, **218**, 401–411.

Regine, W. F., Winter, K. A., Abrams, R., *et al.* (2011). Fluorouracil-based chemoradiation with either gemcitabine or fluorouracil chemotherapy after resection of pancreatic adenocarcinoma: 5-year analysis of the U.S. Intergroup/RTOG 9704 phase III trial. *Ann. Surg. Oncol.*, **18**, 1319–1326.

Riess, U., Pelzer, G., Deutschinoff, B., *et al.* (2009). A prospective, randomized trial of chemotherapy with or without the low molecular weight heparin (LMWH) enoxaparin in patients (pts) with advanced pancreatic cancer (APC): Results of the CONKO 004 trial [abstract] *J. Clin. Oncol.*, **27** (18 Suppl. 309, abstract 4033).

UICC. (2009). *TNM Classification of Malignant Tumours*, ed. L. H. Sobin, M. K. Gospodarowicz and Ch. Wittekind, 7th edn. Chichester: Wiley-Blackwell.

Van Laethem, J. L., Hammel, P., Mornex, F., *et al.* (2010). Adjuvant gemcitabine alone versus gemcitabine-based chemoradiotherapy after curative resection for pancreatic cancer: a randomized EORTC-40013-22012/FFCD-9203/GERCOR phase II study. *J. Clin. Oncol.*, **28**, 4450–4456.

Von Hoff, D. D., Ervin, T., Arena, F. P., *et al.* (2013). Increased survival in pancreatic cancer with nab-paclitaxel plus gemcitabine. *N. Engl. J. Med.*, **369**, 1691–1703.

Chapter

16

Management of cancer of the colon and rectum

Loretta Sweeney and Richard Adams

Introduction

Colorectal cancer (CRC) is second in incidence in Europe only to lung cancer. It causes around 204,000 deaths each year. The aetiology of CRC is still unclear, but the 8- to 10-fold higher incidence in the developed world compared to that in the developing world suggests environmental causes. Around 15–20% of CRCs are of familial origin.

Screening has been adopted in the UK with faecal occult blood (FOB) testing, followed by colonoscopy if positive. Many other countries are also considering such a programme.

Surgery is the only globally accepted curative treatment. Total mesorectal excision (TME) is now well established as the most effective way of managing rectal carcinoma, although important subtleties around early T1 tumours do exist. The last 10 years have also seen a rapid increase in the use of preoperative radiotherapy, neoadjuvant and adjuvant chemotherapy and new agents for advanced disease, with small but incremental improvements in outcome.

Targeted therapies, including epithelial growth factor receptor (EGFR) inhibitors and vascular endothelial growth factor inhibitors, have been accepted into standard algorithms for the treatment of patients with advanced CRC. However, these have demonstrated no significant benefit in the adjuvant setting.

Predictive and prognostic markers have moved into routine use in this disease.

Types of colorectal tumours

The range of tumours that affect the colon and rectum is shown in Table 16.1.

Table 16.1 The range of tumours that affect the colon and rectum

Type	Examples
Non-neoplastic tumours (no malignant potential)	*Benign polyps*
	Hyperplastic polyps
	Hamartomatous polyps:
	Juvenile polyps and Peutz–Jegher polyps
	Inflammatory polyps
	Lymphoid polyps
Neoplastic epithelial tumours	*Benign polyps*
	Tubular adenoma
	Tubulo-villous adenoma
	Villous adenoma
	Malignant polyps
	Adenocarcinoma
	Carcinoid tumour
	Anal zone carcinoma
Mesenchymal tumours	*Benign*
	Leiomyoma
	Lipoma
	Neuroma
	Angioma
	Malignant
	Leiomyosarcoma
	Liposarcoma
	Malignant spindle-cell tumour
	Kaposi's sarcoma
Other	Lymphoma

Practical Clinical Oncology, Second Edition, ed. Louise Hanna, Tom Crosby and Fergus Macbeth. Published by Cambridge University Press. © Cambridge University Press 2015.

Incidence and epidemiology

The age-standardized annual incidence of CRC is 47 per 100,000 in the UK with > 41,000 new cases reported per year (CRUK; http://www.cancerresearchuk.org/cancer-info/cancerstats/types/bowel/incidence/uk-bowel-cancer-incidence-statistics, accessed July 2014.) More than 16,100 deaths (50% of rectal origin) occur per year in the UK, making CRC the second most common cause of cancer death.

There is a higher incidence of CRC in affluent Western countries and a lower incidence in Japan, Africa and South America. The peak incidence of CRC occurs at 60–70 years. The male-to-female ratios for colonic and rectal tumours are 2:3 and 2:1, respectively. In general, tumours of the colon outnumber those of the rectum by 3 to 2.

Carcinoma of the colon and rectum

Risk factors and aetiology

Family history

A family history of CRC, particularly in first-degree relatives younger than age 40, is associated with an increased risk. Genetic causes probably account for 15% of all CRCs. There are two well-recognised inherited CRC syndromes.

Lynch syndrome is an autosomal dominant condition involving defective mismatch-repair genes. It accounts for approximately 2% of CRCs. Affected gene carriers have an 80% lifetime risk of CRC. These tumours have a propensity to be right-sided, mucin-producing and less aggressive. Other associated features include an increased risk of endometrial, ovarian, gastric, pancreatic and renal malignancies.

Lynch syndrome is divided into two types.

- Lynch I describes CRC that is colon site-specific, right-sided, involves multiple tumours and is more often mucinous.
- Lynch II describes increased risk of carcinoma of both colon and endometrium, multiple tumours with an earlier age of onset.

The clinical diagnosis of Lynch syndrome is made using *Modified Amsterdam Criteria* (Vasen *et al.*, 1999). After assessment for microsatellite instability, the diagnosis is confirmed by laboratory testing for MSH1&2 and PMS1&2 mutations. Gene sequencing is performed to identify known mutations in these key mismatch-repair genes. It is notable that the majority of cancers demonstrating microsatellite instability are non-familial and are often related to epigenetic silencing of promoters by methylation.

Familial adenomatous polyposis (FAP) is an autosomal dominant condition characterised by defects in the *adenomatous polyposis coli* (APC) gene on chromosome 5. FAP accounts for fewer than 1% of all CRCs. It often manifests as a carpet of adenomatous polyps throughout the large intestine; 90% of affected individuals will have an invasive cancer by the age of 45.

There are three variants of FAP.

- Gardner's syndrome involves colorectal adenomatous polyps, osteomas and desmoid tumours.
- Turcot's syndrome involves colonic polyps associated with CNS tumours, including ependymomas and medulloblastomas.
- Attenuated FAP involves fewer adenomas and a slightly lower risk of colonic cancer.

Conditions associated with CRC

Ulcerative colitis (UC) and, to a lesser extent, Crohn's colitis are associated with CRC. The risk is greatest in patients who develop early-onset UC with a large proportion of the colon affected. These cancers are often multifocal, flat, infiltrating and poorly differentiated.

Other factors

There is a higher incidence of CRC in affluent Western countries and a lower incidence in Southeast Asia, Africa and much of South America, presumably due to dietary factors. These include a diet low in indigestible starch, high in refined carbohydrates and fat content, and a decreased intake of protective micronutrients. Increased fruit and vegetable intake results in a protective effect for colon and other cancers as suggested by case-control studies, but cohort studies in the USA provide less evidence for this finding. Other risk factors include smoking, which results in an increased risk of adenomas but with no proven increase in CRC. Low levels of physical activity and high body mass index, between 23 and 30 kg/m^2, causes a linear increase in the risk of colon cancer.

Screening and prevention

Diet

The EPIC (European Prospective Investigation into Cancer and Nutrition) study has concluded that diets deficient in fibre are associated with CRC. Recent results suggest that diets high in fish and low in red meat content may protect against CRC (Jacobs *et al.*, 1998; Key *et al.*, 2002; Bingham *et al.*, 2003).

Chemoprevention

Increasingly, evidence suggests that aspirin may have a protective effect, reducing incidence and improving survival of CRC (Chan *et al.*, 2009.) A randomised controlled trial (RCT) in patients with Lynch syndrome, CAPP2 (Burn *et al.*, 2008), has demonstrated a significant reduction in CRC incidence in those administered 600 mg aspirin per day. Interestingly no difference in polyp number formation was demonstrated in this trial.

Secondary prevention

Strategies for secondary prevention have been reviewed in an article by Agrawal and Syngal (2005). Specifically, trials are ongoing and in development to look at the impact of exercise on reducing the recurrence of CRC. These include the NCIC 'Challenge trial', which is assessing a tailored exercise intervention programme in high-risk patients post completion of adjuvant chemotherapy.

Aspirin-related secondary prevention trials include: ASCOLT (Aspirin for Dukes C and High Risk Dukes B Colorectal Cancers, NCT00565708) and 'Add-Aspirin', the UK RCT assessing the anti-cancer effects of aspirin after primary cancer therapy.

Screening strategies

Faecal occult blood (FOB)

There have been three large population-based studies (Hardcastle *et al.*, 1996). In the Nottingham trial, there was a 15% reduction in cumulative CRC mortality in the screened group; however, the false-positive rate was high, at around 90%. FOB testing is now routinely offered in the UK generally between the ages of 60 and 75. Early evidence suggests that this will result in the detection of earlier stage tumours (http://www.cancerscreening.nhs.uk/bowel/, accessed July 2014).

Sigmoidoscopy or colonoscopy

Sixty-five per cent of all CRCs are found in the rectum and sigmoid colon. Sigmoidoscopy is both sensitive and specific for these. Colonoscopy identifies more proximal tumours, but is expensive and incurs higher morbidity. These procedures have a role in malignancy prevention because premalignant polyps may be removed. When used as part of a screening programme, polypectomy has shown an approximate 60% reduction in mortality from bowel cancer. Screening programmes are now being rolled out looking at a one-off flexible sigmoidoscopy at 55 years as a strategy which may identify early neoplasm of the left colon missed by FOB testing (http://www.cancer-screening.nhs.uk/bowel/, accessed July 2014).

Strategies for patients with inflammatory bowel disease

Screening with regular colonoscopies is offered to high-risk patients and prophylactic panproctocolectomy is appropriate in selected cases.

Pathology

The adenoma–carcinoma sequence

Vogelstein described a model of transition from normal bowel, through adenomas, to carcinoma (Fearon and Vogelstein, 1990). Vogelstein's model of carcinogenesis is shown in Figure 16.1, depicting the pathway to chromosomal instability. A separate pathway characterised by microsatellite instability (MSI) occurs in hereditary non-polyposis colorectal cancer (HNPCC) along with an acquired loss of DNA mismatch repair (Rowan *et al.*, 2005).

The risk of cancer varies with the size and number of polyps:

- polyps ≤ 1 cm carry a ≤ 1% risk of invasive malignancy;
- polyps between 1 and 2 cm carry a 10% risk;
- polyps greater than 2 cm carry a 50% risk;
- 3% of CRCs are multicentric.

Features associated with an increased risk of malignant potential within colonic polyps are shown in Table 16.2.

Morphology

The morphology of colorectal adenocarcinoma is shown in Table 16.3.

Spread

Carcinoma of the colon and rectum can spread to adjacent structures such as the small or large bowel, the bladder, the uterus, and so on. Transcoelomic spread can also occur.

Regional lymph nodes are involved in 40–70% at operation; the lymph node chain usually follows

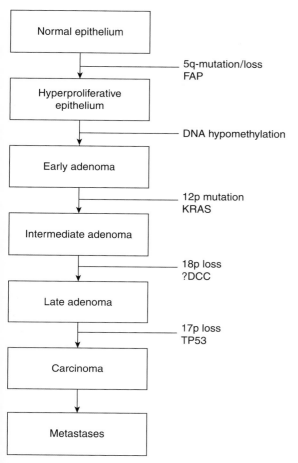

Figure 16.1 Adapted Vogelstein model of carcinogenesis for CRC. DCC, deleted in colon cancer; DNA, deoxyribonucleic acid; FAP, familial adenomatous polyposis; KRAS, Kirsten rat sarcoma viral oncogene homolog; TP53, tumour protein p53. Adapted with permission from Fearon and Vogelstein (1990).

the blood vessels. For rectal cancers these will be the pararectal lymph nodes, nodes at the bifurcation of the inferior mesenteric artery, hypogastric nodes and presacral nodes.

Haematogenous spread is most often to the liver, lungs and bone, occurring in that order of frequency. In 25–30% of patients at presentation, the tumour will be unsuitable for radical treatment.

Clinical presentation

Symptoms and signs from the primary tumour

Symptoms that occur more commonly in right-sided lesions include unexplained anaemia, ill-defined

Table 16.2 Features associated with an increased risk of malignant potential within colonic polyps

Risk category	Feature
High risk	Large size (> 1.5 cm)
	Sessile or flat
	Severe dysplasia present
	Squamous metaplasia present
	Villous architecture present
	Multiple polyps
Low risk	Small size (≤ 1 cm)
	Pedunculated
	Mild dysplasia present
	No metaplasia present
	Tubular architecture present
	Single polyp

Table 16.3 Pathological features of colorectal adenocarcinoma

Features	Description
Macroscopic	Polypoid, fungating, ulcerative or diffusely infiltrating
	Proximal tumours often grow as polypoid or fungating masses extending along one wall of the caecum or colon
	Carcinomas in the distal colon tend to be annular, stenosing tumours
Microscopic	Well-, moderately or poorly differentiated
	Spectrum from tall columnar cells akin to those found in benign polyps but with evident invasion to frankly anaplastic carcinomas
	Strong desmoplastic reactions are common, giving macroscopic firmness
	Many tumours produce mucin; rarer mucinous tumours produce sheets/pools of mucin, which carry a poor prognosis
	10% of adenocarcinomas of the colon have neuroendocrine differentiation; small-cell undifferentiated tumours are of neuroendocrine origin
	A few have signet ring appearances more commonly found in stomach or breast carcinomas
	Distal colon tumours occasionally have foci of squamous differentiation and are known as adenosquamous carcinomas

abdominal pain, an abdominal mass, weight loss and rectal bleeding.

More common in left-sided lesions are a change in bowel habit, obstruction, rectal bleeding, tenesmus and mucoid discharge.

Rectal examination can identify 75% of rectal tumours.

Criteria for referral to a specialist

Symptoms that require urgent referral to a specialist have been reviewed and are presented in NICE Clinical Guidelines (NICE, 2015a). They include:

- >40 with unexplained weight loss and abdominal pain;
- >50 with unexplained abdominal pain or weight loss;
- <60 with change in bowel habit or iron deficiency anaemia;
- >60 with anaemia even in the absence of iron deficiency;
- test shows occult blood in the faeces.

Investigation

Staging investigations

Full blood count and liver function tests should be performed; 65% of the liver can be involved before an abnormality is detected.

Carcino-embryonic antigen (CEA) is raised in 85% of patients with CRC. Higher CEA values are associated with a worse prognosis when measured preoperatively, but they do not change management.

Colonoscopy or a double-contrast barium enema is used because 5% of lesions are synchronous. Biopsy is essential.

A CT scan of the thorax abdomen and pelvis should be performed. Pelvic MRI should be performed for patients with rectal tumours, to assess the likely circumferential resection margin (CRM) and the need for preoperative therapy. Endo-anal US gives good information on size, penetration and nodal involvement of low rectal tumours and may be appropriate, especially if local excision of a rectal T1 lesion is contemplated. A PET scan is relevant only when resection of metastases is considered, to assess for occult metastatic disease. Tailored MRI of the liver to optimize assessment of patients undergoing surgical resection of liver metastases is essential (Schmoll et al., 2012).

Local staging of rectal cancer

Digital rectal examination can be accurate for T staging in up to 80% of cases. EUS is user-dependent, but it can be accurate in over 90% of cases (it can miss microscopic T3 disease). Nodal assessment is relatively poor with this modality (accurate in 50–80%).

Significant evidence now demonstrates that MRI can be used to identify the mesorectal fascia and to predict clearance at the CRM. The MERCURY study showed concordance between MRI and histological findings in the spread of tumour beyond the lamina propria (MERCURY Study Group, 2006). Updated data from the MERCURY II trial indicate that MRI staging information can offer additional benefits above and beyond post neoadjuvant therapy TNM staging, in terms of local relapse and distant relapse risk (Taylor et al., 2014).

Pathological staging of CRC

Dukes' staging has undergone various modifications and was originally used to describe rectal cancers, but it is now also accepted for colonic cancers and is shown in Table 16.4. The TNM classification is shown in Table 16.5. The data set for CRC histopathology reports has recently been updated (Loughrey et al., 2014).

Treatment for non-metastatic disease: colonic carcinoma

Surgery

Whenever possible, patients should be operated on by the specialist team. Patients presenting as an emergency should be considered for defunctioning colostomy/stenting, followed by elective definitive removal of the tumour (Athreya et al., 2006). Definitive surgery involves removing the appropriate bowel segment with its mesentery, vascular pedicle and draining lymph nodes.

Adjuvant chemotherapy for colon cancer

Adjuvant online

Data from clinical trials in colon cancer can be used to help estimate the benefit of adjuvant chemotherapy (https://www.adjuvantonline.com/colon.jsp, accessed January 2015).

T1 or T2, N0 tumours

Adjuvant chemotherapy has shown no benefit in patients with T1 or T2, N0 tumours.

Table 16.4 Dukes', TNM and AJCC/UICC staging classifications shown with approximate 5-year survival by stage

Dukes' stage (modified)	Description	Stage (AJCC/UICC)	TNM	Five-year survival (%)
	In situ	0	Tis N0 M0	100%
A	Cancer confined to submucosa or muscularis propria but not through it	I	T1 N0 M0	95%
			T2 N0 M0	90–95%
B(1)	Into but not beyond muscularis propria; no LN spread	II	T3 N0 M0	70–80%
			T4 N0 M0	
B(2)	Through the muscularis propria with no nodes involved			
C(1)	Nodes positive but not the apical node	III	Any T, N1–2, M0	40%
C(2)	Apical node positive			
D	Metastatic	IV	Any T, Any N, M1	5%

Controversially, the UK has continued to adopt AJCC version 5, although version 8 is due out in 2015.

Table 16.5 TNM classifications of CRC

Stage	Definition
T1	Tumour invades submucosa
T2	Tumour invades muscularis propria
T3	Tumour invades through muscularis propria into subserosa or into non-peritonealised pericoloic or perirectal tissue
T4	Tumour directly invades other organs/structures and/or perforates visceral peritoneum
N1	1–3 lymph nodes involved
N2	4 lymph nodes involved (12 should be examined)
M1	Presence of metastases

Adapted from the AJCC/UICC 5th edition staging of the colon and rectum, AJCC (1997).

T3 or node-positive tumours

Two meta-analyses have shown that prolonged use of a 5-FU-based regimen for longer than 3 months can improve survival in CRC. For patients with node-positive colon cancer, the benefit is about 6% at 5 years (range 2–10%; NICE, 2011). For patients with node-negative colon cancer, the increase in overall survival is 1–5% after a median follow-up of 4.2 years (Gray *et al.*, 2004), although it remains controversial whether all patients should be offered adjuvant therapy.

Current standard practice in the UK is to offer adjuvant chemotherapy to patients with Dukes' C and to selected patients with Dukes' B colon cancer. Poor-risk features identifiable in node-negative patients include serosal involvement, perforated tumours, extramural vascular invasion, less than 12 lymph nodes examined pathologically and involvement of the CRM, although these selection criteria have not yet been prospectively verified. There is now a consensus that for patients with Duke's B cancers being considered for adjuvant therapy, an assessment of MSI by genetic assessment or mismatch repair (MMR) by IHC is essential. Those with MSI-High or MMR deficiency have significantly better prognosis and thus gain minimal benefit from adjuvant chemotherapy (Sargent *et al.*, 2010). See the Appendix for a list of different adjuvant chemotherapy treatments.

Fluoropyrimidines

All adjuvant regimens are based on fluoropyrimidines. In the 1990s the following guidelines were established.

- Low-dose folinic acid (FA) is just as effective as high-dose FA (Anonymous, 2000).
- Oral fluoropyrimidines appear equally effective compared to 5-FU in the adjuvant and metastatic setting.
- When using a standard 5-FU and FA regimen, there is no advantage in extending the duration of therapy past 6 months (O'Connell *et al.*, 1998).

- All fluoropyrimidine-based regimens are associated with a risk of toxicity, notably diarrhoea, stomatitis and leucopenia. There is an increased risk of cardiac ischaemia, which can also occur in those without coronary vessel disease.
- The weekly bolus 5-FU and FA regimen is less toxic than the conventional 5-day 4-week regimen, but in a non-randomised comparison in the QUASAR trial the 5-FU/FA regimen showed no reduction in effectiveness (Kerr et al., 2000) and has become the standard bolus 5-FU regimen in the UK.
- Neutropenia is more prevalent in patients over age 70. They have a similar survival benefit from treatment (Lichtman, 2004).

Oral fluoropyrimidines

Capecitabine is as effective as and less toxic than the Mayo clinic regimen (X-ACT trial; Twelves et al., 2005) and is useful in patients with poor venous access. Capecitabine is commonly used as a single-agent adjuvant therapy in the UK. Toxicity, cost and patient preference must be taken into account when considering which therapy is most appropriate. Toxicity can specifically be increased in patients with an eGFR between 50 and 80 mL/min, so caution is advised in this group of patients (often the elderly) and those with poorly controlled, high-output ileostomy. Another oral fluoropyrimidine prodrug, tegafur-uracil, also has a role in adjuvant therapy for rectal cancers (Casado et al., 2008).

Oxaliplatin as adjuvant

Trials comparing 5-FU and FA plus oxaliplatin versus 5-FU and FA alone have both shown an improvement in disease-free survival at 3 years of about 6% (MOSAIC and NSABP C-07 trials; Andre et al., 2004; Wolmark et al., 2005), but with a greater risk of neuropathy. Oxaliplatin with a fluoropyrimidine has therefore become the standard adjuvant therapy in patients who are fit to receive it and whose risk of relapse is high. The phase III XELOXA trial (Haller et al., 2011) compared capecitabine in combination with oxaliplatin versus bolus 5-FU/FA in patients with stage III colon cancer. Its findings were in keeping with those demonstrated in the MOSAIC trial.

Irinotecan as adjuvant

Three trials have shown no benefit from adding irinotecan to adjuvant 5-FU and FA in colon cancer (Saltz et al., 2004; Ychou et al., 2005, Van Cutsem et al., 2009).

Bevacizumab and cetuximab as adjuvant therapy

Both bevacizumab and cetuximab (in KRAS wt) tumours have demonstrated no significant benefit in the adjuvant setting, as shown in the AVANT and FFCD-PETACC-8 trials (de Gramont et al., 2012; Taieb et al., 2014.)

Treatment for non-metastatic disease: rectal carcinoma

Patients whose tumours are predicted to be likely to recur after surgery alone can be selected for preoperative therapies. The risk of local recurrence following surgery is related to the CRM and nodal status. Based on the results of the MERCURY study, MRI can be used to identify three prognostic groups.

The risk categories are not universally agreed but can be considered to be:

- favourable: rT1 to rT3a (minimal extension into rectum), N0;
- unfavourable: > rT3a (significant mesorectal contamination), or N +ve *with* margin not at risk;
- advanced: T4 or CRM ≤ 1 mm.

Surgery

Surgery is technically more difficult for rectal than for colonic tumours because the pelvis is narrow, especially in the male. Very low tumours require an abdominoperineal resection (APR). For higher tumours an anterior resection is possible. Low anterior resection is associated with increased morbidity including bladder and sexual dysfunction and increased bowel frequency than for patients with higher rectal tumours.

TME is standard for rectal cancer surgery. This technique, advocated for many years by Heald, involves sharp dissection of the mesorectum. It reduces the risk of an involved resection margin (defined as ≤ 1 mm; MacFarlane et al., 1993). Patients with CRM −ve surgery had in one study a local recurrence rate of only 9% (Adam et al., 1994).

Early-stage rectal cancer

Local excision is an alternative to APR in low rectal cancers that are unlikely to have lymph node metastases. In practice this procedure is for *well-differentiated* *T1* tumours. The most common approach to local excision is trans-anal endoscopic microsurgery (TEM). In experienced surgical centres local excision can be associated with excellent results (Willett, 1999). Patients with adverse risk factors after local excision should be considered for further resection. A number of trials are currently exploring the role of external beam radiotherapy in the context of early rectal cancer. In patients for whom surgery is not considered suitable, current evidence on the efficacy and safety of low-energy contact X-ray brachytherapy for early-stage rectal cancer is adequate to support the use of this procedure. In patients for whom surgery is considered suitable, but who choose not to have an operation, the evidence on safety is adequate but the evidence on efficacy is inadequate. Therefore this procedure should only be used for these patients with special arrangements for clinical governance, consent and audit or research. (NICE, 2015b).

Adjuvant chemotherapy for rectal cancer

The clinical benefit of adjuvant chemotherapy alone for patients with rectal cancer has been difficult, as many trials have assessed the combination of chemotherapy and radiotherapy. However, the meta-analysis of trials of adjuvant chemotherapy for CRC showed a greater benefit in rectal cancer than in colon cancer (OR for mortality = 0.64; 95% CI = 0.48–0.85) and estimated the benefit to be a 9% increase in survival at 5 years (Dube *et al.*, 1997). Patients with rectal cancer currently receive the same adjuvant systemic therapy as those with colon cancer, stage for stage. Trials such as CHRONICLE in the UK (Glynne-Jones *et al.,* 2014) attempted to assess the impact of adjuvant therapy in those patients undergoing neoadjuvant chemoradiotherapy. Unfortunately, they were unable to recruit and closed early.

Radiotherapy and chemoradiotherapy in rectal cancer

There is good evidence for the use of either short-course preoperative radiotherapy (25 Gy in 5 fractions) or longer-course chemoradiotherapy (45–50.4 Gy in 25–28 fractions), both given to a planned three- or four-field volume.

The 'Sauer' study compared long-course pre- and postoperative chemoradiotherapy and showed an improvement in local control rate (13% versus 6%) in those given preoperative treatment (Sauer *et al.*, 2004). There was also more acute and late grade 3 or 4 toxicity in the postoperative group. Preoperative radiotherapy schedules have become standard practice in the UK, although there is significant variation in patients selected for neoadjuvant therapy.

Preoperative radiotherapy and chemoradiotherapy

An overview of preoperative radiotherapy trials showed a significant reduction in the odds of death or local recurrence (OR = 0.84, $p = 0.03$ and OR = 0.49, $p < 0.001$, respectively; Cammà *et al.*, 2000). A meta-analysis published in 2001 showed that local recurrence is reduced from 17% to 10%, whereas for trials in which a radiobiologically equivalent dose (RBE) of more than 30 Gy was given, recurrence was reduced from 20% to 9.8% (Colorectal Cancer Collaborative Group, 2001). For those trials that employed higher radiation doses (RBE > 30), there was a marginal survival advantage (56.5% versus 58.9%; $p = 0.04$).

Long-term follow-up (median 13 years) was provided by the Swedish Rectal Cancer Trial, which showed an 8% improvement in overall survival (38% versus 30%; $p = 0.008$) and a reduction in local recurrence from 26% to 9% ($p = 0.001$; Folkesson *et al.*, 2005). However, there was an increased risk of short-term morbidity (perineal wound infection/non-healing) and late rectal morbidity (Birgisson *et al.*, 2005).

The Dutch TME trial looked at preoperative short-course radiotherapy in more than 1800 patients. There was no survival benefit, but the local recurrence rate was significantly lower in patients who had radiotherapy (11.4% versus 5.8%; Marijnen *et al.*, 2005). The MRC CR07 trial randomised 1350 rectal cancer patients to preoperative radiotherapy (25 Gy in 5 fractions) followed by surgery, or surgery followed by selective postoperative chemoradiotherapy for CRM-positive tumours (95% had TME). This trial showed 10% CRM positivity. The local relapse rates reduced from 17% to 5% overall at 5 years in favour of preoperative radiotherapy. Node-positive patients who had CRM-negative tumours and who did not receive postoperative radiotherapy had a high local relapse rate of 17% at 5 years. Such patients should be considered for postoperative chemoradiotherapy if no neoadjuvant therapy has been given (Sebag-Montefiore *et al.*, 2009).

Follow-up from the CR07 trial assessing quality of life demonstrates a significant impact on erectile dysfunction and a trend towards greater faecal incontinence rates in those receiving preoperative short-course radiotherapy (Stephens *et al.*, 2010) compared to the postoperative chemoradiotherapy.

Oxaliplatin, irinotecan and cetuximab have all been combined with fluoropyrimidine-based

Table 16.6 Rectal cancer chemoradiotherapy trials looking at the addition of oxaliplatin

Trial	Eligibility	Fluoro-pyrimidine platform
CAO/ARO/AIO-04 $N = 637$	< 12 cm from anal verge T3/T4 cN0/N+ TRUS, CT and/or MRI	5-FU 1000 mg/m² days 1–5 + 29–33
NSABP R04 $N = 1606$	< 12 cm; resectable stage II, III TRUS or MRI–CT if T4/ N1–2	PVI 5-FU versus capecitabine
FFCD $N = 598$	Palpable; resectable; T3/4 N0–2; T2 distal anterior	Capecitabine in both arms
STAR – 01 $N = 747$	Resectable stage II, III (c stage) < 12 cm from anal verge	PVI 5FU in both arms
PETTAC 6 $N = 1090$	Stage II or III resectable or expected to become resectable < 12 cm from anal verge	Capecitabine in both arms

MRI, magnetic resonance imaging; PVI, protracted venous infusion; TRUS, transrectal ultrasound. Adapted from: Gérard *et al.*, 2010; Aschele *et al.*, 2011; Roh *et al.*, 2011; Rödel *et al.*, 2012; Schmoll *et al.*, 2014.

chemotherapy. Five phase III trials have explored the use of oxaliplatin and are shown in Table 16.6 (Gérard *et al.*, 2010; Aschele *et al.*, 2011; Roh *et al.*, 2011; Rödel *et al.*, 2012; Schmoll *et al.*, 2014). Only one has demonstrated significant benefits; however, the control arm in this trial was considered suboptimal. Irinotecan is being explored in one phase III in the UK (ARISTOTLE, Cancer Research UK; http://www.controlled-trials.com/ISRCTN09351447, accessed January 2015). Cetuximab has been explored in multiple phase II trials but has not demonstrated sufficient activity to take forward to phase III.

Postoperative radiotherapy

In the UK, postoperative radiotherapy is reserved for patients who are found to have CRM involvement at surgery and who did not receive preoperative radiotherapy. The role of postoperative radiotherapy in node-positive patients is less certain.

Practicalities of radiotherapy for rectal cancer

The UK ARISTOTLE trial (ISRCTN09351447) has defined a UK standard for outlining radiotherapy volumes. Included below are relevant edited extracts from this trial protocol for radiotherapy planning and outlining.

Patient set-up

It is recommended that appropriate immobilisation is used and that a scan/treatment position is used which the centre is familiar with. It is recognised that the supine position may be used by some centres.

A radio-opaque marker must be placed at the anal verge prior to the CT planning scan.

Patient data acquisition

The scan limits are the superior aspect of L5 superiorly to 4 cm below a radio-opaque marker indicating the anal verge or the inferior extent of tumour, whichever is more inferior. The recommended slice thickness is 3 mm.

Use of contrast

Oral contrast to show the small bowel is recommended. Gastrografin® 20 mL in 1 litre of water is taken 45–60 minutes prior to the planning scan is in routine use. The use of intravenous contrast is recommended and encouraged, but not mandated.

Definition of treatment volumes

The target volume definition process requires the delineation of gross, clinical and planning target volumes.

- **Gross tumour volume (GTV)** includes all gross sites of disease (primary, nodal and extramural vascular invasion). This information is derived from the diagnostic imaging (pelvic MRI and supplemented by pelvic CT if also available). The determination of macroscopic disease is based on a combination of clinical and radiological information.
- **Clinical target volume (CTV)** will encompass areas of microscopic spread beyond the defined GTV. The system used describes two distinct

volumes, CTVA and CTVB, which are then combined to form the Final CTV (CTVF).

- **CTVA** includes GTV + 1 cm. This defines the surrounding safety margin of potential subclinical involvement (superior, inferior, lateral, anterior and posterior).
- **CTVB** includes the mesorectum and the loco-regional nodes considered at risk of involvement.
  - This includes the nodes within the mesorectum, presacral space and the internal iliac nodes.
  - In patients with invasion of the levator muscle or sphincter complex, a 1 cm lateral and posterior margin is applied to the CTVA.
  - Uninvolved external iliac nodes are not included in CTVB.
- **Final CTV (CTVF)** is produced by combining CTVA and CTVB.
- **Planning target volume (PTV)** is defined as CTVF + 1 cm (superiorly, inferiorly, anteriorly, posteriorly and laterally). Usually, a three- or four-field plan is used with one/two posterior and two lateral fields. Typically, 45° wedges are used on the two lateral fields. Field sizes are typically 12–15 cm (S–I) × 14–17 cm for the posterior fields, and 12–15 cm (S–I) × 10–12 cm for the lateral fields.

Internationally, centres are moving to an IMRT or VMAT plan and delivery. Selected patients with significant pelvic small bowel may derive additional benefit from this. There will not be a clinical trial to evaluate this and centres must decide on the trade-off between additional time outlining and planning such cases versus the potential for increased speed of delivery per fraction.

Dose, energy and fractionation procedures are as follows.

- For preoperative short-course radiotherapy without chemotherapy, the patient receives 25 Gy in 5 fractions over 1 week, prescribed to the ICRU reference point, using 6–10 MV photons, followed by surgery at around 1 week.
- For preoperative long-course chemoradiotherapy, the patient receives 45 Gy in 25 fractions over 5 weeks (up to 50.4 Gy in 28 fractions), prescribed to the ICRU reference point, using 6–10 MV photons, followed by surgery at 6 weeks.

- The postoperative dose is 45–50 Gy in 25 fractions over 5 weeks.
- In case of residual disease in postoperative treatment, a conformal small-volume boost of 10–15 Gy can be given in 5–7 fractions.
- The total dose should be 55–60 Gy over 6.5–7 weeks to a patient with macroscopic disease.
- Inoperable or recurrent disease can be dosed with 45–50 Gy in 25 fractions; consider a boost as just mentioned to maximise local control.

Be careful if patients have adhesions, inflammatory bowel disease, diverticular disease or diabetes mellitus. The indication for treatment should be reviewed and treatment fields should be kept as small as possible to reduce toxicity.

Lasers should be used to align the patient; treat all fields isocentrically each day, set to the ICRU 50 reference point. Portal beam imaging should be taken on the first day of treatment.

Concurrent chemotherapy in combination with long-course radiotherapy often involves oral capecitabine given on *treatment days only* at 900 mg/m² p.o. b.d. Some countries continue to use 5-FU as either a continuous infusion of 5-FU at 200 mg/m² per day throughout radiotherapy treatment.

When explaining the procedure to the patient undergoing radiotherapy or chemoradiotherapy, give written information. Explain its possible side effects:

- acute: tiredness, diarrhoea, cystitis, severe and painful perineal reaction (low tumours), and cardiac toxicity. Myelosuppression is rare;
- late: menopause (in females) and infertility/sterility, impotence, bowel dysfunction and urge incontinence may occur.

The following information should be used to support the patient.

- For diarrhoea, give imodium and advise a low-residue diet with close monitoring. It is important to differentiate between tenesmus and diarrhoea and to have a good baseline history. In patients with a stoma (especially an ileostomy) assessment of diarrhoea can be very difficult. It is important to gauge hydration with simple advice around feelings of thirst and urine concentration. It is advisable to monitor these patients closely and to stop treatment/seek experienced opinion if in doubt.
- For cystitis, send MSU, treat the infection, and encourage the patient to drink fluids.

- For skin reaction, apply Epaderm® or similar emollient topically b.d., or 1% hydrocortisone cream if severe; apply Instillagel® to areas of moist desquamation (low rectal tumours).
- For anaemia, red cell transfusion can be performed (keep Hb > 100 g/L). Ensure adequate iron replacement therapy orally or intravenously if necessary.
- For neutropenia, treat the patient as per local neutropenic sepsis protocol.
- For nausea, use appropriate anti-emetics as per local protocol.

Treatment for advanced/inoperable local disease: colonic and rectal carcinoma

Inoperable primary disease

Inoperable primary disease is most common in the rectum. In some patients, clinically unresectable tumours may become operable after radiotherapy. Radiotherapy with or without chemotherapy can give useful palliation of pain and control of local disease.

In a patient with an inoperable obstructing rectal cancer, a defunctioning colostomy may provide useful palliation but will not relieve tenesmus, bleeding or mucous discharge. Trans-anal tumour ablation using laser, electrocoagulation or resectional techniques may provide better palliation and should be considered in selected cases.

Palliative radiotherapy

Patients with rectal cancer who are medically unfit for surgery, and who have symptoms of local pain, discharge, or bleeding, may be treated with palliative external beam therapy to the pelvis, either as a single fraction of 8 Gy or fractionated to 25 Gy in 5 fractions (or 20 Gy in 4 fractions) over one week. Case series have reported good tumour control with limited toxicity, which may be appropriate for patients considered surgically unfit.

Fitter patients may benefit from a higher dose of 45 Gy in 25 fractions with capecitabine chemotherapy. In the face of metastatic disease this may be preceded by systemic chemotherapy alone. Palliative radiotherapy is also beneficial for bony metastases or local bony erosion (8 Gy in a single fraction).

Patients with fixed caecal tumours may benefit from local radiotherapy (8 Gy in a single fraction), particularly if they have bleeding and recurrent anaemia.

Endoscopic therapy

Stenting of colonic and high rectal tumours is feasible and effective either for immediate relief before radical surgery or as a purely palliative procedure. Mid and low rectal tumours can be complicated by stent migration and tenesmus.

Palliative surgery

In frail patients, some surgeons will attempt to debulk rectal tumours trans-anally. UK practice at present is to leave asymptomatic primary colorectal cancers *in situ*, in the face of incurable metastatic disease, as generally complication rates are low. Even in the palliative setting, excision of a symptomatic tumour and re-anastomosis is preferable to a palliative bypass if required, as excision *may* be associated with a better survival rate and quality of life. Retrospective case series have suggested that removal of the primary tumour may improve prognosis. Currently CAIRO4 being run by the Dutch trials group is attempting to answer this question (http://clinicaltrials.gov/show/NCT01606098, accessed January 2015).

Locoregional recurrence

The 3-year survival of patients with locoregional recurrence of CRC is about 10%. Treatment with chemoradiotherapy should be considered if it has not already been given. Preoperative chemoradiation before surgical resection of recurrent disease has increased resectability rates by up to 60%. Symptom relief occurs in around 70–80% of patients treated with radiotherapy, but the median duration of relief is only 3 months.

Treatment for metastatic disease: colonic and rectal carcinoma

Surgery for isolated liver metastases

The liver and lung are the most common sites for metastatic CRC. Systemic treatment is usually the only option although, for a few patients, surgical excision of metastases or *in situ* destructive therapy may be feasible.

Around 15–20% of patients with liver metastases may benefit from primary resection. With careful patient selection, hepatectomy can achieve a 5-year survival of 20–40%. A retrospective review of 2040 patients with metachronous isolated hepatic metastases showed that those who underwent resection had a mean survival of 31 months (projected 5-year survival of 26%), whereas those patients who did not undergo resection had a mean survival of 11 months (projected 5-year survival of 2%; $p < 0.0001$; Wade *et al.*, 1996). The survival rate is worse for patients presenting with synchronous metastatic disease, those with a heavy positive lymph node burden with the primary tumour, those with a higher number of liver metastases and those with a higher CEA (Fong and Salo, 1999).

Patients should not generally be considered for surgery if there is disease outside the liver, all the hepatic veins are involved, or not enough viable liver tissue will be left after resection. Generally speaking, a minimum of 2 contiguous liver segments are required to be free of disease with > 30% normal liver to remain. Some patients with limited pulmonary metastases may also be suitable for pulmonary resection. Ongoing trials such as PulMiCC (Treasure *et al.*, 2012) are attempting to assess whether such resections of lung metastases have an impact on cure rates or on overall survival.

Neoadjuvant chemotherapy for metastatic disease

Non-randomised evidence supports the use of preoperative chemotherapy prior to resection in patients with potentially operable liver metastases (Bismuth *et al.*, 1996; Adam *et al.*, 2004). The EPOC trial (Nordlinger *et al.*, 2008) in subgroup analysis suggests that there is a small benefit from perioperative chemotherapy, but this has been variably interpreted by the international community. The *New EPOC* study (Primrose *et al.*, 2014a) evaluated the addition of cetuximab to chemotherapy and surgery for operable colorectal liver metastases in KRAS wt patients. This resulted in an unexpected finding of shorter progression-free survival with the addition of cetuximab.

In situ destructive therapies for liver metastases

Radiofrequency ablation, microwave ablation and cryotherapy

These have all been used for isolated colorectal liver metastases, but there is no RCT evidence to support their routine use. Surgery remains the standard approach for operable disease. Clinical practice in some countries has led to the use of ablative therapies as a palliative procedure in a quasi-tumour debulking scenario, but this has no supportive trial evidence.

Hepatic intra-arterial brachytherapy

Yttrium-90 labelled Sirspheres® or Theraspheres® have been approved for use as palliative therapy for patients with liver-predominant metastatic CRC after

systemic therapy has failed. There is phase II evidence to support this use (Van Hazel *et al.*, 2004). Two phase III clinical trials run in parallel SIRFLOX and FOXFIRE (ISRCTN 83867919) in Australia and the UK, respectively, are awaiting primary outcome data for analysis.

Stereotactic body radiotherapy (SBRT)

SBRT uses focused hypofractionated external beam radiotherapy utilising fiducial markers. It has been used in oligometastatic disease for CRC with limited evidence of effectiveness.

Palliative chemotherapy

A number of agents have demonstrated activity in metastatic CRC: the fluoropyrimidines including 5-FU, oral prodrugs capecitabine and combination UFT; the chemotherapy agents oxaliplatin, irinotecan, raltitrexed and mitomycin; the biological agents bevacizumab, aflibercept, cetuximab, panitumumab and regorafenib. Median overall survival has improved, from 6 to 8 months for patients managed with supportive care alone, to 10–14 months for those treated with fluoropyrimidines alone, to 22–24 months for patients receiving combination regimens including irinotecan, oxaliplatin and bevacizumab.

Palliative chemotherapy: fluoropyrimidines

A meta-analysis of five trials of palliative chemotherapy has shown improved survival with chemotherapy compared with best supportive care ($p = 0.0002$). The evidence suggests that, for patients with advanced disease, early chemotherapy before clinical deterioration improves survival by 3–6 months without any adverse impact on quality of life (NHS Executive, 1997).

Fluoropyrimidine monotherapy is used for patients who are unfit for combination chemotherapy or who have low-volume, slowly progressive metastatic disease. However, the standard therapy for fit patients is now combination chemotherapy with a fluoropyrimidine and either oxaliplatin or irinotecan (NICE, 2005). The use of single-agent capecitabine has not been compared to optimal infusional 5-FU regimens in the metastatic setting.

The optimum duration of treatment for chemotherapy is not known. A relatively standard approach in the UK is to give chemotherapy for 16 weeks followed by a break, restarting when there is evidence of progressive disease. This practice is based on evidence from the MRC COIN study (Adams *et al.*, 2011), in which patients received 3 months of chemotherapy with FOLFOX or XELOX followed by a complete break in chemotherapy or continuation until progression on treatment/excessive toxicity. Subgroup analysis, yet to be confirmed, suggest that those patients with a high baseline platelet count may have better survival if chemotherapy is maintained. The CAIRO3 Dutch trial compared 4 months of induction therapy with oxaliplatin and capecitabine followed by a complete treatment break or maintenance capecitabine and bevacizumab. This trial shows a non-statistically significant trend towards survival in the maintenance group at the expense of increased toxicity, but without significant impact on quality of life (Koopman et al., 2014).

Experience is required in deciding whether patients should be given chemotherapy. Poor performance status, low serum albumin, high alkaline phosphatase and liver involvement are independent predictors of progression; low serum albumin, high γ-glutamyl transferase and high CEA predict for poor survival.

Palliative chemotherapy: irinotecan and oxaliplatin

There is evidence to support the use of irinotecan and oxaliplatin as a first-line treatment in combination with 5-FU or capecitabine. NICE guidance 93, issued in August 2005, states that irinotecan and oxaliplatin are recommended as possible treatments for people with advanced CRC, if they are used with 5-FU. The sequencing of chemotherapy has been investigated in a number of trials, including the MRC CR08 (FOCUS) (Maughan, 2005; Tournigand et al., 2006) and CAIRO trials (Koopman et al., 2007). There is no evidence that any particular sequence is superior to another.

Novel chemotherapies

TAS-102 is a novel thymidylate synthetase inhibitor which has demonstrated efficacy when randomised against supportive care in the last-line setting and is undergoing fast-track approval in the USA.

Regional chemotherapy

Hepatic arterial infusions of chemotherapy were evaluated in the 1990s. Neither adjuvant nor palliative treatment has been shown to be effective (James et al., 2003). Novel therapies which reportedly deliver chemotherapy in higher concentration to the liver, such as in the DEBIRI trial, have demonstrated limited additional efficacy (Martin et al., 2011).

Monoclonal antibodies (MAbs) and tyrosine kinase inhibitors (TKIs)

A number of novel agents have now been licensed for mCRC.

Bevacizumab

Bevacizumab is a monoclonal antibody against the vascular endothelial growth factor (VEGF) ligand. It is licensed for first-line metastatic use. One trial randomised to first-line irinotecan and fluoropyrimidine with or without bevacizumab found that response rates increased from 34.8% to 44.8% ($p = 0.004$) and median survival increased from 15.6 to 20.3 months (HR = 0.66, $p < 0.001$) in the first-line setting (Hurwitz et al., 2004). It has also been used in combination with oxaliplatin and 5-FU or capecitabine in the first-line setting. This trial demonstrated a significant improvement in PFS with a trend towards OS benefit (Saltz et al., 2008).

Bevacizumab is licensed in the second-line setting with irinotecan, but has no head to head data to compare. Bevacizumab demonstrates no clinically significant benefit as a single agent as a maintenance therapy (Koeberle et al., 2013). Its side effects include hypertension and proteinuria, with a tendency to vascular complications events as well as a risk of bowel perforation.

Cetuximab and panitumumab

Cetuximab and panitumumab are EGFR monoclonal antibodies licensed for use in 'all RAS wild type' tumours as monotherapy in the last line or with irinotecan or oxaliplatin in first-/second-line treatment. The side-effect profile includes acneiform rash, paronychia and skin splitting in the pulps of fingers and toes. The rash is best treated aggressively with tetracycline antibiotics, moisturisers and sparing use of topical hydrocortisone. Antiseptic soaks appear to be best for paronychia. Cetuximab and panitumumab are not currently approved by NICE, although the results of the FIRE3 trial may lead to a review.

Updated data from the PRIME trial with a subgroup analysis based upon the latest validated biomarkers indicate a 5.8-month median overall survival advantage (HR = 0.78; 95% CI = 0.62–0.99; $p = 0.043$) in patients with all RAS wild-type tumours receiving FOLFOX plus panitumumab versus FOLFOX alone in the first-line setting (Douillard et al., 2013). In the updated CRYSTAL trial, analysis based upon all RAS wild-type status, patients receiving FOLFIRI plus

Appendix Colorectal chemotherapy regimens

Regimen	Mode	Doses of chemotherapy	Dose of leucovorin	Duration	Interval	Use
QUASAR	Bolus	5-FU 370 mg/m^2	20 mg/m^2	30 weeks	1 week	Adjuvant
Modified de Gramont	Bolus/ infusion	5-FU 400 mg/m^2 bolus then 2.8 g/m^2 over 46 hours	175 mg	2 days	14 days	1st line
Lokich	Continuous infusion	5-FU 300 mg/m^2 per day	–	12 weeks	–	1st line
Capecitabine	Oral	1250 mg/m^2 b.d.	–	14 days	3 weeks	1st line
Oxaliplatin modified de Gramont (FOLFOX)	Bolus/ infusion	5-FU 400 mg/m^2 bolus then 2.4 g/m^2 over 46 hours plus oxaliplatin 85 mg/m^2	175 mg	2 days	14 days	1st line with potentially resectable liver mets
Irinotecan modified de Gramont (FOLFIRI)	Bolus/ infusion	5-FU 400 mg/m^2 bolus, 2.4 g/m^2 over 46 hours plus irinotecan 180 mg/m^2	175 mg	2 days	14 days	2nd line
Irinotecan	Short infusion	350 mg/m^2	–	1 day	3 weeks	2nd line
XELOX/CAPOX (capecitabine and oxaliplatin)	Oral/ infusion	Capecitabine 1000 mg/ m^2 p.o. b.d. days 1–14 plus oxaliplatin 130 mg/m^2 over 2 hours	–	2 weeks	3 weeks	Unlicensed metastatic

cetuximab had a median overall survival advantage of 8.2 months versus those receiving FOLFIRI alone; HR = 0.69, $p = 0.0024$ (Ciardiello *et al.*, 2014).

In contrast, the MRC COIN trial randomised patients to XELOX or FOLFOX as clinician/patient choice ± cetuximab. This trial was negative when analysed based upon KRAS wild-type status (Maughan *et al.*, 2011). In the AIO FIRE3 trial of FOLFIRI + bevacizumab versus FOLFIRI + cetuximab (Heinemann *et al.*, 2013), the latter combination inferred a 3.7-month median overall survival advantage in patients harbouring a KRAS wild-type tumour. Updated analyses based upon the 'all RAS wild type' cohort of patients indicate an 8.1-month median overall survival advantage (HR = 0.70, 95% CI = 0.54–0.90, $p = 0.0059$) as per EMSO 2014 (yet to be published).

Aflibercept

Aflibercept is a monoclonal antibody VEGF trap against VEGF ligands and PGF. It is licensed in the second-line setting in combination with FOLFIRI, but is not approved by NICE. Side effects include hypertension, proteinuria and diarrhoea.

Regorafenib

Regorafenib is an oral TKI against VEGF receptor predominantly and is licensed when other available therapies have been tried or are not suitable. It is not approved by NICE.

Follow-up for colorectal carcinoma after radical therapy

There is controversy over the intensity of follow-up that should be used after resection of a primary colorectal carcinoma. This question was addressed in the UK FACS trial (Primrose *et al.*, 2014b). This trial looked at options of intensive follow-up with hospital clinical and radiological surveillance compared to GP-based follow-up. This trial controversially demonstrated no significant benefits from more aggressive follow-up. An older overview by Renehan *et al.* which included 5 trials showed a significant benefit from intensive follow-up, generally every 3 months for the first year and subsequently spreading out to every 6 months or annually (Renehan *et al.*, 2002). The evidence pointed towards a reduction in cancer-related mortality of 9–13% with an average earlier pick-up rate of metastatic disease.

Prognosis of colorectal carcinoma

The 5-year survival by stage is shown in Table 16.4.

Current clinical trials

All NCRN trials can be found at *public.ukcrn.org.uk*. A list of global trials is available at www.cancer.gov/clinicaltrials (accessed January 2015).

FOCUS4 is a multi-arm, multi-stage, phase III RCT of molecularly selected therapy in the first-line setting of metastatic CRC.

ARISTOTLE is a phase III trial of neoadjuvant chemoradiotherapy in high-risk rectal cancer randomising to standard capecitabine chemotherapy ± the addition of irinotecan as a radiosensitiser.

The CAPP3 study is a dose-finding RCT of CRC prevention using aspirin in patients with Lynch syndrome.

Genetic Factors in Colorectal Cancer studies the role of genetic factors in clinical outcome for CRC patients.

The National Study of Colorectal Cancer Genetics is an observational study. Its aim is to identify low-penetrance CRC susceptibility alleles through DNA and clinicopathological data collection.

FOXFIRE explores the use of interventional radio-embolisation in combination with FOLFOX chemotherapy in the first-line setting for liver-predominant disease.

Acknowledgements

The authors would like to acknowledge the contribution of Prof. Timothy Maughan to this chapter.

References

Adam, I. J., Mohamdee, M. O., Martin, I. G., *et al.* (1994). Role of circumferential margin involvement in the local recurrence of rectal cancer. *Lancet*, **344**, 707–711.

Adam, R., Delvart, V., Pascal, G., *et al.* (2004). Rescue surgery for unresectable colorectal liver metastases downstaged by chemotherapy: a model to predict long-term survival. *Ann. Surg*, **240**, 644–657.

Adams, R., Meade, A., Seymour, M., *et al.* on behalf of the MRC COIN Trial Investigators. (2011). Intermittent versus continuous oxaliplatin and fluoropyrimidine combination chemotherapy in the first-line treatment of patients with advanced colorectal cancer: results of the MRC COIN trial. *Lancet Oncol.*, **12**, 642–665.

Agrawal, J. and Syngal, S. (2005). Colon cancer screening strategies. *Curr. Opin. Gastroenterol.*, **21**, 59–63.

AJCC. (1997). *AJCC Cancer Staging Manual*, ed. I. D. Fleming, J. S. Cooper, D. E. Henson, *et al.*, 5th edn. Philadelphia: Lippincott-Raven.

Andre, T., Boni, C., Mounedji-Boudiaf, L., *et al.* (2004). Oxaliplatin, fluorouracil, and leucovorin as adjuvant treatment for colon cancer. *N. Engl. J. Med.*, **350**, 2343–2351.

Anonymous. (2000). Comparison of fluorouracil with additional levamisole, higher-dose folinic acid, or both, as adjuvant chemotherapy for colorectal cancer: a randomised trial. QUASAR Collaborative Group. *Lancet*, **355**, 1588–1596.

Aschele, C., Cionini, L., Lonardi, S., *et al.* (2011). Primary tumor response to preoperative chemoradiation with or without oxaliplatin in locally advanced rectal cancer: pathologic results of the STAR-01 randomized phase III trial. *J. Clin. Oncol.*, **29**, 2773–2780.

Athreya, S., Moss, J., Urquhart, G., *et al.* (2006). Colorectal stenting for colonic obstruction: the indications, complications, effectiveness and outcome – 5-year review. *Eur. J. Radiol.*, **60**, 91–94.

Bingham, S. A., Day, N. E., Luben, R., *et al.* (2003). Dietary fibre in food and protection against colorectal cancer in the European Prospective Investigation into Cancer and Nutrition (EPIC): an observational study. *Lancet*, **361**, 1496–1501; erratum in *Lancet*, 362, 1000.

Birgisson, H., Pahlman, L., Gunnarsson, U., *et al.* (2005). Adverse effects of preoperative radiation therapy for rectal cancer: long-term follow-up of the Swedish Rectal Cancer Trial. *J. Clin. Oncol.*, **23**, 8697–8705.

Bismuth, H., Adam, R., Levi, F., *et al.* (1996). Resection of nonresectable liver metastases from colorectal cancer after neoadjuvant chemotherapy. *Ann. Surg.*, **224**, 509–520.

Burn, J., Bishop, D. T., Mecklin, J. P.,*et al.* (2008). Effect of aspirin or resistant starch on colorectal neoplasia in the Lynch syndrome. *N. Engl. J. Med.*, **359**, 2567–2578.

Cammà, C., Giunta, M., Fiorica, F., *et al.* (2000). Preoperative radiotherapy for resectable rectal cancer: a meta-analysis. *J. Am. Med. Assoc.*, **284**, 1008–1015.

Casado, E., Pfeiffer, P., Feliu, J., *et al.* (2008). UFT (tegafur-uracil) in rectal cancer. *Ann. Oncol.*, **19**, 1371–1378.

Ciardiello, F., Lenz, H.J., Kohne, C. H., *et al.* (2014). Treatment outcome according to tumor *RAS* mutation status in CRYSTAL study patients with metastatic colorectal cancer (mCRC) randomized to FOLFIRI with/without cetuximab. *Ann. Oncol.*, **7**, 1346–1355.

Chan, A. T., Ogino, S. and Fuchs, C. S. (2009). Aspirin use and survival after diagnosis of colorectal cancer. *J. Am. Med. Assoc.*, **302**, 649–658.

Colorectal Cancer Collaborative Group. (2001). Adjuvant radiotherapy for rectal cancer: a systematic overview of 8507 patients from 22 randomised trials. *Lancet*, **358**, 1291–1304.

de Gramont, A., Van Cutsem, E., Schmoll, H. J., *et al.* (2012). Bevacizumab plus oxaliplatin-based chemotherapy as adjuvant treatment for colon cancer (AVANT): a phase 3 randomised controlled trial. *Lancet Oncol.*, **13**, 1225–1233.

Douillard, J. Y., Oliner, K. and Siena, S. (2013). Panitumumab-FOLFOX4 treatment and *RAS* mutations in colorectal cancer. *N. Engl. J. Med.*, **369**, 1023–1034.

Dube, S., Heyen, F. and Jenicek, M. (1997). Adjuvant chemotherapy in colorectal carcinoma: results of a meta-analysis. *Dis. Colon Rectum*, **40**, 35–41.

Fearon, E. R. and Vogelstein, B. (1990). A genetic model for colorectal tumorigenesis. *Cell*, **61**, 759–767.

Folkesson, J., Birgisson, H., Pahlman, L., *et al.* (2005). Swedish Rectal Cancer Trial: long lasting benefits from radiotherapy on survival and local recurrence rate. *J. Clin. Oncol.*, **23**, 5644–5650.

Fong, Y. and Salo, J. (1999). Surgical therapy of hepatic colorectal metastasis. *Semin. Oncol.*, **26**, 514–523.

Gérard, J., Azria, D., Gourgou-Bourgade, S., *et al.* (2010). Comparison of two neoadjuvant chemoradiotherapy regimens for locally advanced rectal cancer: results of the phase III trial ACCORD 12/0405-Prodige 2. *J. Clin. Oncol.*, **28**, 1638–1644.

Glynne-Jones, R., Counsell, N., Quirke, P., *et al.* (2014). Chronicle: results of a randomised phase III trial in locally advanced rectal cancer after neoadjuvant chemoradiation randomising postoperative adjuvant capecitabine plus oxaliplatin (XELOX) versus control. *Ann. Oncol.*, **25**, 1356–1362.

Gray, R. G., Barnwell, J., Hills, R., *et al.* (2004). QUASAR: a randomised study of adjuvant chemotherapy (CT) vs. observation including 3238 colorectal cancer patients. *J Clin Oncol, 2004 ASCO Annual Meeting Proceedings* (Post-Meeting Edition), Vol. **22**, No. 14S (July 15 Suppl.), 3501.

Haller, D. G., Tabernero, J., Maroun, J., *et al.* (2011). Capecitabine plus oxaliplatin compared with fluorouracil and folinic acid as adjuvant therapy for stage III colon cancer. *J. Clin. Oncol.*, **29**, 465–471.

Hardcastle, J. D., Chamberlain, J. O., Robinson, M. H., *et al.* (1996). Randomised controlled trial of faecal-occult-blood screening for colorectal cancer. *Lancet*, **348**, 1472–1477.

Heinemann, V., von Weikersthal, L., Decker, T., *et al.* (2013). Randomized comparison of FOLFIRI plus cetuximab versus FOLFIRI plus bevacizumab as first-line treatment of KRAS wild-type metastatic colorectal cancer: German AIO study KRK-0306 (FIRE-3). *J. Clin. Oncol.* **31**, abstr LBA3506.

Hurwitz, H., Fehrenbacher, L., Novotny, W., *et al.* (2004). Bevacizumab plus irinotecan, fluorouracil and leucovorin for metastatic colorectal cancer. *N. Engl. J. Med.*, **350**, 2335–2342.

Jacobs, D. R., Jr., Marquart, L., Slavin, J., *et al.* (1998). Whole-grain intake and cancer: an expanded review and meta-analysis. *Nutr. Cancer*, **30**, 85–96.

James, R. D., Donaldson, D., Gray, R., *et al.* (2003). Randomised clinical trial of adjuvant radiotherapy and 5-fluorouracil infusion in colorectal cancer (AXIS). *Br. J. Surg.*, **90**, 1200–1212.

Kerr, D. J., Gray, R., McConkey, C., *et al.* (2000). Adjuvant chemotherapy with 5-fluorouracil, L-folinic acid and levamisole for patients with colorectal cancer: non-randomised comparison of weekly versus four-weekly schedules – less pain, same gain. QUASAR Colorectal Cancer Study Group. *Ann. Oncol.*, **11**, 947–955.

Key, T. J., Allen, N. E., Spencer, E. A., *et al.* (2002). The effect of diet on risk of cancer. *Lancet*, **360**, 861–868.

Koeberle, D., Betticher, D. C., Von Moos, R., *et al.* (2013). Bevacizumab continuation versus no continuation after first-line chemo-bevacizumab therapy in patients with metastatic colorectal cancer: a randomized phase III noninferiority trial (SAKK 41/06). *J. Clin. Oncol.* **31** (suppl; abstr 3503).

Koopman, M., Antonini, N. F., Douma, J., *et al.* (2007). Sequential versus combination chemotherapy with capecitabine, irinotecan, and oxaliplatin in advanced colorectal cancer (CAIRO): a phase III randomised controlled trial. *Lancet*, **370**, 135–142.

Koopman, M., Simkens, L., May, A. M., *et al.* (2014). Final results and subgroup analyses of the phase 3 CAIRO3 study: maintenance treatment with capecitabine + bevacizumab versus observation after induction treatment with chemotherapy + bevacizumab in metastatic colorectal cancer (mCRC). *J. Clin. Oncol.*, **32**(5s), 3504.

Lichtman, S. M. (2004). Chemotherapy in the elderly. *Semin. Oncol.*, **31**, 160–174.

Loughrey, M., Quirke, P. and Shepherd, N. (2014). *Standards and Datasets for Reporting Cancers. Dataset for Colorectal Cancer Histopathology Reports*. Version 3. London: The Royal College of Pathologists.

MacFarlane, J. K., Ryall, R. D. and Heald, R. J. (1993). Mesorectal excision for rectal cancer. *Lancet*, **341**, 457–460.

Marijnen, C., Peeters, K., Putter, H., *et al.* (2005). Long term results, toxicity and quality of life in the TME trial. *Proc. Am. Soc. Clin. Oncol. Gastrointestinal Cancer Symposium*, Abstr. 166.

Martin, R., Joshi, J., Robbins., K., *et al.* (2011). Hepatic intra-arterial injection of drug-eluting bead, irinotecan

(DEBIRI) in unresectable colorectal liver metastases refractory to systemic chemotherapy: results of multi-institutional study. *Ann. Surg. Oncol.*, **18**, 192–198.

Maughan, T. (2005). Fluorouracil (FU), oxaliplatin, (OX), CPT-11 (irinotecan, Ir) use and sequencing in advanced colorectal cancer (ACRC): the UK MRC FOCUS (CR08) trial. *Proc. Am. Soc. Clin. Oncol. Gastrointestinal Cancers Symposium*, Abstr. 165.

Maughan, T., Adams R. A., Smith, C., *et al.* on behalf of the MRC COIN Trial Investigators. (2011). The addition of cetuximab to oxaliplatin-based first-line combination chemotherapy for advanced colorectal cancer: results of the MRC COIN trial. *Lancet*, **18**, 2103–2114.

MERCURY Study Group. (2006). Diagnostic accuracy of preoperative magnetic resonance imaging in predicting curative resection of rectal cancer: prospective observational study. *Br. Med. J.*, **333**, 779.

NHS Executive. (1997). *Cancer Guidance Sub-group of the Clinical Outcomes Group. Guidance Improving Outcomes in Colorectal Cancer: The Research Evidence.* London: Department of Health.

NICE. (2005). *Technology Appraisal 93. Colorectal Cancer (advanced) Irinotecan, Oxaliplatin and Raltitrexed (Review): Guidance.* London: NICE.

NICE. (2011). *Colorectal Cancer. The Diagnosis and Management of Colorectal Cancer. NICE Clinical Guideline CG 131.* London: NICE.

NICE. (2015a). *Suspected cancer: recognition and referral.* London. National Institute for Health and Care Excellence.

NICE. (2015b). *Low-energy contact X-ray brachytherapy (the Papillon technique) for early-stage rectal cancer. NICE interventional procedure guidance 532 London*: National Institute for Health and Care Excellence.

Nordlinger, B., Sorbye, H., Glimelius, B., *et al.* (2008). Perioperative chemotherapy with FOLFOX4 and surgery versus surgery alone for resectable liver metastases from colorectal cancer (EORTC Intergroup trial 40983): a randomised controlled trial. *Lancet*, **371**, 1007–1016.

O'Connell, M. J., Laurie, J. A., Kahn, M., *et al.* (1998). Prospectively randomised trial of postoperative adjuvant chemotherapy in patients with high-risk colon cancer. *J. Clin. Oncol.*, **16**, 295–300.

Primrose, J., Falk, S., Finch-Jones, M., *et al.* (2014a). Systemic chemotherapy with or without cetuximab in patients with resectable colorectal liver metastasis: the New EPOC randomised controlled trial. *Lancet Oncol.*, **15**, 601–611.

Primrose, J., Perera, R., Gray, A., *et al.* (2014b). Effect of 3 to 5 years of scheduled CEA and CT follow-up to detect recurrence of colorectal cancer. The FACS randomized clinical trial. *J. Am. Med. Assoc.*, **311**, 263–270.

Renehan, A. G., Egger, M., Saunders, M. P., *et al.* (2002). Impact on survival of intensive follow up after curative resection for colorectal cancer: systematic review and meta-analysis of randomised trials. *Br. Med. J.*, **324**, 813.

Rödel, C., Liersch, T., Becker, H., *et al.* (2012). Preoperative chemoradiotherapy and postoperative chemotherapy with fluorouracil and oxaliplatin versus fluorouracil alone in locally advanced rectal cancer: initial results of the German CAO/ARO/AIO-04 randomised phase 3 trial. *Lancet Oncol.*, **13**, 679–687.

Roh, M., Yothers, M., O'Connell, R., *et al.* (2011). The impact of capecitabine and oxaliplatin in the preoperative multimodality treatment in patients with carcinoma of the rectum: NSABP R-04. *J. Clin. Oncol.*, **29** (suppl; abstr 3503).

Rowan, A., Halford, S., Gaasenbeek, M., *et al.* (2005). Refining molecular analysis in the pathways of colorectal carcinogenesis. *Clin. Gastro. Hepatol.*, **3**, 1115–1123.

Saltz, L. B., Niedzwiecki, D., Hollis, D., *et al.* (2004). Irinotecan plus fluorouracil/leucovorin (IFL) versus fluorouracil/leucovorin alone (FL) in stage III colon cancer (intergroup trial CALGB C89803). *J. Clin. Oncol., 2004 ASCO Annual Meeting Proceedings* (Post-Meeting Edition), Vol. 22, No. 18S (July 15 Suppl.), 3500.

Saltz, L., Clarke, S., Diaz-Rubio, E., *et al.* (2008). Bevacizumab in combination with oxaliplatin-based chemotherapy as first-line therapy in metastatic colorectal cancer: a randomized phase III study. *J. Clin. Oncol.*, **20**, 2013–2019.

Sargent, D., Marsoni, S., Monges, G., *et al.* (2010). Defective MMR as a predictive marker for a lack of efficacy of fluorouracil-based adjuvant therapy in colon cancer. *J. Clin. Oncol.*, **28**, 3219–3226.

Sauer, R., Becker, H., Hohenberger, W., *et al.* (2004). Preoperative versus postoperative chemoradiotherapy for rectal cancer. *N. Engl. J. Med.*, **351**, 1731–1740.

Schmoll, H., Van Cutsem, E., Stein, A., *et al.* (2012). ESMO consensus guidelines for management of patients with colon and rectal cancer. A personalized approach to clinical decision making. *Ann. Oncol.*, **23**, 2479–2516.

Schmoll, H., Haustermans, K., Price, T., *et al.* (2014). Preoperative chemoradiotherapy and postoperative chemotherapy with capecitabine and oxaliplatin versus capecitabine alone in locally advanced rectal cancer: disease-free survival results at interim analysis (abstract). *J. Clin. Oncol.*, **32**(5s suppl; abstr. 3501).

Sebag-Montefiore, D., Stephens, R., Steele, R., *et al.* (2009). Preoperative radiotherapy versus selective postoperative chemoradiotherapy in patients with rectal cancer (MRC CR07 and NCIC-CTG C016): a multicentre, randomised trial. *Lancet*, **373**, 811–820.

Stephens, R., Thompson, L., Quirke, P., *et al.* (2010). Impact of short-course preoperative radiotherapy for rectal cancer on patients' quality of life: data from the Medical Research Council CR07/National Cancer Institute of Canada Clinical Trials Group C016 randomized clinical trial. *J. Clin. Oncol.*, **28**, 4233–4239.

Taieb, J., Tabernero, J., Mini, E., *et al.* (2014). Oxaliplatin, fluorouracil, and leucovorin with or without cetuximab in patients with resected stage III colon cancer (PETACC-8): an open-label, randomised phase 3 trial. *Lancet Oncol.*, **15**, 862–873.

Taylor, F. G., Quirke, P., Heald, R. J., *et al.* (2014). Preoperative magnetic resonance imaging assessment of circumferential resection margin predicts disease-free survival and local recurrence: 5-year follow-up results of the MERCURY study. *J. Clin. Oncol.*, **32**, 34–43.

Tournigand, C., Cervantes, A., Figer, A., *et al.* (2006). OPTIMOX1: a randomised study of FOLFOX4 or FOLFOX7 with oxaliplatin in a stop-and-go fashion in advanced colorectal cancer – a GERCOR study. *J. Clin. Oncol.*, **24**, 394–400.

Treasure, T., Fallowfield, L., Lees, B., *et al.* (2012). Pulonary metastasectomy in colorectal cancer: the PulMiCC trial. *Thorax*, **67**, 185–187.

Twelves, C., Wong, A., Nowacki, M. P., *et al.* (2005). Capecitabine as adjuvant treatment for stage III colon cancer. *N. Engl. J. Med.*, **352**, 2696–2704.

Van Cutsem, E., Labianca, R., Bodoky, G., *et al.* (2009). Randomized phase iii trial comparing biweekly infusional fluorouracil/leucovorin alone or with irinotecan in the adjuvant treatment of stage iii colon cancer: PETACC-3. *J. Clin. Oncol.*, **27**, 3117–3125.

Van Hazel, G., Blackwell, A., Anderson, J., *et al.* (2004). Randomised phase 2 trial of SIR-Spheres plus fluorouracil/leucovorin chemotherapy versus fluorouracil/leucovorin chemotherapy alone in advanced colorectal cancer. *J. Surg. Oncol.*, **88**, 78–85.

Vasen, H. F., Watson, P., Mecklin, J. P., *et al.* (1999). New clinical criteria for hereditary nonpolyposis colorectal cancer (HNPCC, Lynch syndrome) proposed by the International Collaborative group on HNPCC. *Gastroenterology*, **116**, 1453–1456.

Wade, T. P., Virgo, K. S., Li, M. J., *et al.* (1996). Outcomes after detection of metastatic carcinoma of the colon and rectum in a national hospital system. *J. Am. Coll. Surg.*, **182**, 353–361.

Willett, C. G. (1999). Technical advances in the treatment of patients with rectal cancer. *Int. J. Radiat. Oncol. Biol. Phys*, **45**, 1107–1108.

Wolmark, N., Wieand, H. S., Kuebler, J. P., *et al.* (2005). A phase III trial comparing FULV to FULV + oxaliplatin in stage II or III carcinoma of the colon: results of NSABP Protocol C-07. *J. Clin. Oncol. ASCO Annual Meeting Proceedings*, **23** (16 Suppl. I), 3500.

Ychou, M., Raoul, J., Douillard, J., *et al.* (2005). A phase II randomized trial of LV5FU2+CPT-11 vs. LV5FU2 alone in adjuvant high risk colon cancer (FNCLCC Accord02/FFCD9802). *J. Clin. Oncol. ASCO Annual Meeting Proceedings*, Vol. **23**, No. 16S, Part I of II (June 1 Suppl.), 3502.

Management of cancer of the anus

Richard Adams and Paul Shaw

Introduction

Anal cancer, like carcinoma of the cervix, is strongly associated with human papilloma virus (HPV) infection. In the past few decades, treatment has swung away dramatically from primary surgery to definitive chemoradiotherapy, with the evident physical and psychosocial benefits of organ preservation. Tumours of lower stage T1 or T2, N0, have an excellent outcome with chemoradiotherapy. Unfortunately, many patients present with T3, T4 or N ≥ 1 disease and they have a significant risk of both locoregional and subsequent distant failure. Half of patients still die within 5 years of treatment. Therefore, efforts are ongoing to improve outcomes via better local and systemic therapy.

Types of anal tumour

Types of anal tumour are shown in Table 17.1.

Anatomy

The anal canal extends from the rectum to the junction of the hair-bearing skin of the perianal region. It is 3–4 cm long and its walls are kept in apposition by the sphincter muscles, except during defecation. The anal margin is the perianal skin immediately adjacent to the distal limit of the anal canal. The anal verge is the lower end of the anal canal.

The tumours can be divided into three types, as follows.

1. Anal-margin tumours are usually small and well-differentiated and are more common in men.
2. Anal-canal tumours are more common than those at the anal margin. They are more common in women (male-to-female ratio ~1:2.5), are often moderately or poorly differentiated, and carry a worse prognosis.

Table 17.1 Types of anal tumour

Type	Examples
Benign	Condylomata
	Conditions that may cause swelling/ulceration
	Haemorrhoids
	Fissure
	Fistula
	Abscess
	Crohn's disease
Primary malignant	*Anal canal*
	Squamous cell carcinoma:
	Large-cell keratinising
	Large-cell non-keratinising (transitional)
	Basaloid
	Adenocarcinoma
	Small-cell carcinoma
	Malignant melanoma
	Lymphoma
	Carcinoid
	GIST
	Undifferentiated carcinoma
	Anal margin
	Squamous cell carcinoma
	Basal cell carcinoma
	Bowen's disease
	Paget's disease
Secondary malignant	Metastatic spread from other tumours: case reports only
	Direct spread from rectum, cervix, vagina, etc.

GIST, gastrointestinal stromal tumour.

Practical Clinical Oncology, Second Edition, ed. Louise Hanna, Tom Crosby and Fergus Macbeth. Published by Cambridge University Press. © Cambridge University Press 2015.

3. Dual-component tumours have both anal-margin and anal-canal components and it is not possible to define from where the tumour originated. These comprise the majority of tumours.

Incidence and epidemiology

The incidence is increasing, with 1175 new cases in the UK in 2011 (http://www.cancerresearchuk.org/cancer-info/cancerstats/, accessed December 2014), with a female to male ratio of 1.8:1. Anal cancers constitute approximately 10% of anorectal tumours; approximately 200 deaths occur per year from this cancer.

There has been a slight but steady increase in incidence in Western countries; wide geographical variation in incidence mirrors the relative risk of HPV infection (e.g. high incidence in areas of Brazil) with similar high rates of penile, vulval and cervical cancer.

The peak incidence age for anal cancer is 60–65 years, but there is a bimodal distribution that includes a younger group, ages 35–40 years.

Carcinoma of the anus

Risk factors and aetiology

Anal cancer was previously believed to be associated with chronic inflammation from haemorrhoids, fistulae and fissures, but there is no evidence to support this or an association with ulcerative colitis. A case-control study performed between 1978 and 1985 established a link between genital warts and anal cancer in women (Daling *et al.*, 1987). Men with anal cancer were more likely to be single, to have had homosexual relationships, to have practised anal-receptive intercourse or to have had sexually transmitted diseases (Daling *et al.*, 1982). The sexually transmitted agent implicated in anal cancer is HPV. The presence of the virus, especially types 16 and 18, can be found in more than 90% of cases (Tilston, 1997). It is unclear whether HPV status affects survival.

Other factors for disease include having multiple sexual partners, having other sexually transmitted viral and bacterial infections, a history of cancer or intraepithelial neoplasia of the cervix, vagina or vulva, cigarette smoking, and iatrogenic immunosuppression for organ transplant. Although anal cancer is not an AIDS-defining malignancy, an increased incidence of anal cancers is associated with HIV/AIDS.

Table 17.2 Pathological features of squamous carcinoma of the anus

Features	Description
Macroscopic	Nodular or plaque-like when small, but ulcerative and infiltrative when larger
Microscopic	Canal tumours tend to be composed of small cells with basaloid features and non-keratinisation and HPV +ve ~100%. Perianal tumours are usually large-cell, keratinising and HPV +ve in > two-thirds of cases, p16 IHC may stratify patients into prognostic groups, with p16+ patients having a better outcome

Pathology

Squamous carcinomas represent 90% of anal cancers. Cloacogenic, basaloid and transitional are all variants of squamous carcinoma, which may also be keratinising and non-keratinising. Because the natural histories and prognoses for all these subtypes are similar, they may be collectively described as epidermoid tumours. The pathological features of squamous carcinoma of the anus are shown in Table 17.2.

Anal intraepithelial neoplasia (AIN)

Anal intraepithelial neoplasia is graded from one to three as in CIN (cf. carcinoma of the cervix) and is considered precancerous (the precursor of squamous cell carcinoma of the anus). It is usually flat or raised, and ulceration is more likely to represent invasive disease.

Spread

There are abundant lymphatic channels in the anus. Overall, approximately 25% of patients have palpable inguinal nodes at presentation. However, of these, only about 50% have malignant lymphadenopathy cytologically confirmed upon fine-needle aspiration (FNA). A negative FNA does not exclude malignancy; despite this fact, excision biopsy is rarely performed in clinical practice.

Spread direct from primary

Cancer spread from the primary site is upward, submucosally to the rectum and bladder; laterally, into the ischio-rectal fossa and sphincter muscles; in women, to the vagina/urethra; and in men, to the prostate, and downward to the perianal skin in both sexes.

Lymphatic spread

Low anal tumours, anal verge tumours and anal-margin tumours spread to perirectal nodes, followed by the inguinal nodes, and then to external iliac vessels and the common iliac/para-aortic chain.

Mid and upper anal-canal tumours spread via the internal iliac nodes to the pelvis, including the hypogastric and obturator nodes and not infrequently to para-aortic/retroperitoneal nodes.

Metastatic spread

Haematogenous metastatic spread is to the liver, less frequently to the lungs and bones, and, rarely, to the brain. Fewer than 10% present with metastatic disease.

Clinical presentation

The tumour occurs as a lump or mass, either found by the patient on wiping or causing the patient discomfort. Bleeding, discharge and anal discomfort occur in about 50% of patients and about 25% are aware of a mass. The non-specific nature of the tumour can lead to a reporting delay of up to 6 months in one-third of patients. A tumour is occasionally found during an investigation of malignant inguinal lymphadenopathy. It is rare for anal cancers to present with metastases outside the pelvis.

Investigation and staging

Examination with anaesthetic may be required for formal assessment and staging of local disease. Biopsy of the primary tumour should be performed. Generally, inguinal lymph nodes are not removed, but may be subjected to FNA. Removal of inguinal nodes may lead to an increased risk of lymphoedema and wound infection with a subsequent delay or complication in the delivery of radiotherapy. FNA (for suspicious nodes) has a high false-negative rate, but detecting cancer in clinically equivocal nodes is helpful for staging and radiotherapy planning. Currently, sentinel lymph node evaluation in radiological node-negative disease is not standard but is subject to ongoing research.

A full blood count, biochemical profile and, if risk factors are present, an HIV test should be performed. A CT of the thorax abdomen and pelvis, and MRI of the pelvis should be performed. MRI is more effective at imaging the primary tumour and perirectal disease

than CT. Further investigations should be performed as clinically or biochemically indicated. PET scanning is of value in the treatment of anal cancer (Saboo et al., 2013). Many (including NCCN guidelines) now recommend PET-CT for node-positive disease; however, false-positive nodal assessment is high. PET imaging may aid in radiotherapy planning.

Stage classification

TNM classification and stage groupings

The TNM classification and stage grouping are shown in Tables 17.3 and 17.4, respectively. The staging applies to anal-canal tumours; anal-margin tumours are staged in the same way as skin tumours.

Treatment overview

Radiotherapy replaced surgery as the initial treatment in the 1980s. Evidence that concurrent chemoradiotherapy (CRT) improves local disease control compared to radiotherapy alone emerged in the 1990s. Current studies are under way to find the most effective chemoradiotherapy regimen. Abdominoperineal resection (APR) is used for patients who are unsuitable for CRT, for patients with persistent/recurrent local disease or for patients who have unmanageable late toxicity after CRT. NICE service guidance on colorectal cancer suggests that anal cancer should be managed by a network-based specialist team that includes an oncologist and a surgeon and that has established

Table 17.3 TNM classification of carcinomas of the anal canal

Stage	Definition
T1	2 cm or less
T2	Greater than 2 cm, not more than 5 cm
T3	Greater than 5 cm
T4	Of any size invading adjacent organs (e.g. vagina, urethra, bladder); involvement of sphincter muscles alone is not T4
N1	Metastasis in perirectal lymph node(s)
N2	Metastasis in unilateral internal iliac and/or unilateral inguinal lymph node(s)
N3	Metastasis in perirectal and inguinal lymph nodes and/or bilateral internal iliac and/or bilateral inguinal lymph nodes
M1	Distant metastasis present

Adapted from UICC (2009).

Table 17.4 Stage grouping for carcinomas of the anal canal

Stage	Description		
Stage 0	Tis	N0	M0
Stage I	T1	N0	M0
Stage II	T2	N0	M0
	T3	N0	M0
Stage IIIA	T1–3	N1	M0
	T4	N0	M0
Stage IIIB	T4	N1	M0
	Any T	N2	M0
	Any T	N3	M0
Stage IV	Any T	Any N	M1

Adapted from UICC (2009).

links with gynaecological and plastic surgical services. Within each radiotherapy facility, no more than two clinical oncologists should take responsibility for the care of patients with anal cancer and these should be core members of the anal cancer MDT (NICE, 2004).

If the tumour recurs locally following CRT, the only curative salvage therapy is APR.

Radical surgery for anal carcinoma

Surgery for primary tumour

Well-differentiated margin tumours less than 2 cm in diameter may be locally excised if clear surgical margins are possible. The incidence of nodal disease is less than 5%. Sentinel lymph node biopsy in this scenario may aid in treatment choices but currently remains experimental.

Abominoperineal resection is now rarely used as a primary treatment. However, if radiotherapy is contraindicated – because the patient has previously had radiotherapy to the pelvis, or there is a functioning transplanted kidney present in the pelvis – then primary surgery may be considered. It must be acknowledged, however, that this will not treat pelvic lymph nodes. Defunctioning loop colostomy or ileostomy are appropriate in the presence of bulky tumours, faecal incontinence or where there is evident fistulation, abscess or tumour invading through mucosa of adjacent organs (i.e. vagina or urethra).

The management of high-grade AINIII is uncertain. Where possible, this type of cancer should be treated by local excision, and APR should be reserved for symptomatic, uncontrolled, multifocal disease.

Adjuvant radiotherapy or CRT should be considered for patients who have undergone an excisional biopsy for an invasive tumour with positive margins, treating to a dose of at least 30 Gy (Hu et al., 1999). A selective approach may be made with respect to prophylactic inguinal nodal irradiation, with close follow-up, although the TROG Australian trial identified an unacceptable 22.5% relapse rate out of 40 patients with T1/T2 tumours treated without inguinal irradiation (Matthews et al., 2011).

Radical radiotherapy and chemoradiotherapy

Nigro et al. (1983), from the Wayne State University Cancer Center in Michigan, delivered a preoperative CRT schedule. On examination of the surgical specimen, 7 of 12 patients had no viable tumour (Nigro et al., 1974, 1983). The dose schedule was 30 Gy in 15 fractions with 2 cycles of chemotherapy (5-FU and mitomycin C (MMC), 2 cycles, 4 weeks apart). Similarly, Cummings et al. (1984) described a cohort of patients treated with CRT and compared them to a similar group of patients treated with radiation alone. The radiation given was 45–50 Gy in 25 fractions. Marked acute toxicity was seen when radiotherapy was given with 5-FU and mitomycin C (2 cycles of 5-FU, 1 g/m^2 and mitomycin C, 10 mg/m^2). A 4-week gap was therefore introduced between the two treatment phases. At 6 months, local control was achieved in 60% of the patients treated with radiotherapy alone, as opposed to 94% treated with continuous-phase chemoradiation and 93% in the split-course CRT group.

In 1996, the UKCCR published a randomised control trial of 585 patients (ACT I) that compared radiotherapy and CRT (Anal Cancer Trial Working Party, 1996). ACT I was a very successful trial, and ~30% of all patients with anal cancer in the UK took part. Local failure occurred in 39% of patients in the CRT arm versus 61% who underwent radiotherapy alone. Anal cancer deaths were reduced by 29%, but overall survival was not significantly different. Of patients who failed CRT, 50% were salvaged with surgery as opposed to 60% of patients who failed after radiotherapy alone. Chemoradiotherapy was associated with significantly greater toxicity.

The dose schedule was 45 Gy in 25 or 20 fractions with two cycles of 5-FU and mitomycin C followed by a 6-week break followed by clinical assessment. If there was less than a 50% response, patients went on to an

APR. If there was greater than a 50% response, patients received a boost, either with brachytherapy 10 Gy/day with iridium-192 (25 Gy) or EBRT 15 Gy in 6 fractions.

The radiotherapy technique was as follows: the superior border was the bottom of the S–I joints and the inferior border covered the tumour by at least 3 cm. It was recommended that the inguinal nodes were included with the use of large parallel-opposed fields, although this was not mandatory. The chemotherapy regimen was 5-FU, 1 g/m² on days 1–4 and mitomycin C, 12 mg/m² on day 1. The second cycle, given during the last week of radiotherapy, consisted of 5-FU alone. This chemotherapy regimen remains the UK standard of care, although a UK phase II trial EXTRA has indicated that 5-FU may be replaced by capecitabine on each RT treatment day in two divided doses (825 mg/m² b.d.; Glynne Jones *et al.*, 2008).

Two further trials in the USA and Europe confirmed the superiority of local control of CRT over radiotherapy alone, albeit at the expense of increased acute toxicity (Flam *et al.*, 1996; Bartelink *et al.*, 1997).

Cisplatin or MMC with radiotherapy

Three trials have explored changing the chemotherapy from MMC to cisplatin but no advantage to this approach has been demonstrated.

- The UK ACT II study (940 patients) was a 2×2 factorial design trial comparing CRT using cisplatin/5-FU versus MMC/5-FU, ± 2 cycles of adjuvant cisplatin/5-FU. There was no difference in PFS between cisplatin and MMC, and no benefit using adjuvant chemotherapy (James *et al.*, 2013).
- The US RTOG 98-11 trial (682 patients) compared 2 cycles of induction cisplatin/5-FU followed by CRT using 2 further cycles of cisplatin/5-FU versus standard CRT using MMC/5-FU. Intensification of treatment resulted in worse toxicity, tumour control, colostomy-free survival (CFS) and overall survival (Gunderson *et al.*, 2012).
- The French ACCORD-03 study (307 patients) was a 2×2 factorial design trial, comparing 2 cycles of induction cisplatin/5-FU versus no induction chemotherapy and a standard dose boost (15 Gy) versus a high dose boost (20–25 Gy) after CRT (45 Gy in 25 fractions). CFS was not improved by either induction chemotherapy or higher dose of radiotherapy (Peiffert *et al.*, 2012).

Radiotherapy technique

A temporary defunctioning colostomy should be considered if the patient has a large obstructing tumour or incontinence. Patients have traditionally been simulated and treated prone, with their hands under their head. However, with the increasing use of IMRT, institutions are moving back to a supine position to improve stability and comfort. Any such change requires close attention to the application of bolus to the primary tumour where appropriate; even small tumours may need bolus. Data have suggested that small bowel avoidance can be optimised with the patient in a prone position using a belly board and IMRT (Wiesendanger-Wittman *et al.*, 2012). A radio-opaque marker is helpful to localise the anal verge or to define the extent of tumour spread onto the perianal skin and the positioning of bolus. The bladder should be comfortably full and intravenous contrast should be administered. Small bowel contrast may be given 45–60 minutes before simulation. Bolus is often applied to the natal cleft in all anal-margin tumours and anal-canal tumours that reach a superficial level (< 2 cm).

Outlining radiotherapy

Outlining T1 N0 tumours

- GTV_A = includes the gross primary anal tumour volume;
- PTV_Anus = GTV_A with 25 mm margin.

It is at the discretion of the treating clinician whether the plan will encompass the PTV_Anus alone or if an additional PTV_Elective will be prescribed covering the pelvic and inguinal nodes at risk. This will depend on the grade and site of the tumour. It is also deemed by many that if IMRT/VMAT is used then the additional toxicity from inguinal region irradiation is more limited than when conventional radiotherapy planning is used.

Outlining T2–4 or N+ tumours

For the delineation of the elective nodal regions (CTV_E), the Australasian GastroIntestinal Tumour Group (AGITG) guidelines and atlas for IMRT in anal cancer are available for pictorial reference (Ng *et al.*, 2012). There are also detailed step-by-step directions on the website www.analimrtguidance.co.uk (accessed December 2014). Elective nodal areas should include: bilateral inguinal, femoral, external iliac, internal iliac, obturators, lower 5 cm of mesorectum (provided no mesorectal nodes are involved) and presacral lymph nodes.

Planning radiotherapy

IMRT, VMAT or equivalent are considered a standard of care for most patients receiving CRT for anal cancer. Within the UK, a consensus outlining and planning document has been developed (www.analimrtguidance.co.uk, accessed December 2014) with coordination between members of the anorectal subgroup of the National Cancer Research Institute. The volumes comprise known 'gross' disease and at-risk nodal 'elective' regions.

Dose prescription T1 N0 or T2 N0 (and T3 N0 at clinician's discretion)

- Elective – 40 Gy in 28 fractions (1.43 Gy per fraction) in 5.5 weeks.
- Gross anal disease –50.4 Gy in 28 fractions (1.8 Gy per fraction) in 5.5 weeks.

Dose prescription T4 N0 or Tany N+ (and T3 N0 at clinician's discretion)

- Elective (PTV_Elec) = 40 Gy in 28 fractions (1.43 Gy per fraction) in 5.5 weeks.
- Gross nodal disease (PTV_Nodes) = 50.4 Gy in 28 fractions (1.8 Gy per fraction) in 5.5 weeks.
- Gross anal disease (PTV_Anal) = 53.2 Gy in 28 fractions (1.9 Gy per fraction) in 5.5 weeks.

Overall treatment time

Patients with anal cancer should be treated as per Category 1 patients with avoidance of unplanned gaps in treatment where possible and compensation for gaps according to RCR guidelines (Weber *et al.* 2001; Royal College of Radiologists, 2008; Glynne-Jones *et al.*, 2011).

Chemotherapy regimen in combination with radiotherapy

The dose regimen is 5-FU 1000 mg/m^2 per day by continuous 24-hour infusion on days 1–4 and days 29–32. MMC, 12 mg/m^2, is given by i.v. bolus on day 1 (max. single dose 20 mg). 5-FU should be commenced at least 1 hour before the first fraction of radiotherapy. If GFR is 50 mL/min or less (confirmed by EDTA clearance), omit MMC. Apply caution as some patients, such as small elderly women, may have a spuriously low GFR as estimated by using the Cockcroft–Gault formula (other formulae have their own pros and cons). Weekly FBC should be obtained. If neutropenia occurs, prophylactic ciprofloxacin should be considered.

Phase II data have suggested that capecitabine may replace 5-FU in the following regimen: mitomycin 12 mg/m^2 day 1 with capecitabine 825 mg/m^2 b.d. on days of radiotherapy (Glynne-Jones *et al.*, 2008).

Implant/brachytherapy boost

Implantation alone may be suitable as a boost for T1 and T2 tumours if they:

- lie below the anal-rectal ring (proximal end of the anal canal);
- occupy less than 50% of the circumference of the canal;
- are 1 cm or less in thickness;
- have no nodal involvement.

When brachytherapy is used alone it is common to give a dose in the region of 55–60 Gy to the PTV. If used in combination with external beam radiotherapy, a dose of 45 Gy in 25 fractions to the pelvic field including inguinal lymph nodes and a brachytherapy boost of 25 Gy are used.

Brachytherapy should be performed only in specialist centres with a skilled operator. There is a high risk of dose inhomogeneity with implants in this region, which may lead to radionecrosis.

Side effects of radical radiotherapy

The side effects of radiotherapy are shown in Table 17.5. For patients with gastrointestinal symptoms following pelvic radiotherapy, an algorithm-based approach to investigation and management is advocated (Andreyev *et al.*, 2013).

Treatment for locally recurrent anal carcinoma

Formal restaging is essential; localised disease can be considered for radical resection (APR) or exenteration in selected patients. In a report from a single centre in the UK involving 254 patients treated with radiotherapy alone or with concurrent chemotherapy, there were 99 local disease failures, all but 5 being within 3 years of primary therapy (Renehan *et al.*, 2005). Age, dose and stage were significantly associated with recurrence. Of 73 patients who underwent

Table 17.5 Side effects of radiotherapy for anal cancer

Affect	Management
Acute side effects	
Lethargy	Advice re: coping with fatigue (e.g. pacing, goal-setting)
Cutaneous toxicity from dry, usually to moist, desquamation between buttocks	Expose to air; use hydrocortisone 1% cream. Occasionally, 2nd Skin® application is difficult in this area; hair dryer blowing cold can be soothing
Haematological toxicity	FBC once a week, delay if neutrophil count = 1.0×10^9/L or platelet count = 50×10^9/L
Cystitis	Alkalinisation of urine; drinking fluids; potassium citrate/cranberry juice
Diarrhoea, tenesmus	Loperamide/codeine/low-residue diet; delay RT if diarrhoea > 7 times per day and requiring parenteral support, or incontinence; postpone until under control
Crampy abdominal discomfort	Suspend treatment if guarding or significant tenderness
Late side effects	
Sterility	Consider egg harvest in consultation with local fertility clinic, although it is inadvisable to implant into a previously irradiated uterus
	Offer sperm banking to males
	DISCUSS AT CONSENT
Hormonal changes	Pre-menopausal women are highly likely to become menopausal and should be counselled re HRT as per current guidelines for HRT in early menopausal women; bone health should also be assessed
	In men hypogonadism with low testosterone is possible and in symptomatic patients should be considered for replacement
Bowel dysfunction	All patients with significant bowel dysfunction should be considered for referral to a regional gastroenterologist with an interest in radiation-related bowel damage. Screening tests for underlying aetiology should be performed and managed appropriately (Fuccio *et al.*, 2012; Andreyev *et al.*, 2013)
Anal stenosis	APR if failure to control conservatively
Faecal incontinence	APR if failure to control conservatively
Telangiectasia of the rectum/bladder leading to bleeding	Surgery if failure to control conservatively
Bowel fistula	Small bowel resection if severe, often multiple loops affected
Chronic diarrhoea	Loperamide

APR, abdominoperineal resection; FBC, full blood count; HRT, hormone replacement therapy.

surgical salvage, the 3- and 5-year survival rates were 55% and 29%, respectively.

Patients who cannot be treated with surgery and who received chemoradiotherapy 2 or more years previously may gain additional benefits in local control with further radiotherapy. New outlining and radiotherapy planning should be performed in conjunction with overlay of previous radiation fields to identify the organs at risk. Tight margins from GTV to PTV are often applied to minimise toxicity and the risk of radionecrosis. Isolated para-aortic nodes have been treated with SBRT with anecdotal success.

Isolated inguinal node recurrence in patients previously treated with CRT can be treated surgically with inguinal node block dissection if there is no disease relapse at the primary site. If the malignant lymphadenopathy is mobile/non-fixed, this treatment provides local control in about 80% of patients. The procedure is associated with a significant risk of lymphoedema, which is increased by pre- or postoperative radiation. In those patients in whom inguinal region CRT was not given (due to significant comorbidities or the presence of a small tumour), then radical CRT may be delivered, with attention to prior irradiation fields delivered to the primary tumour.

Palliative treatment for anal carcinoma

Palliative radiotherapy/chemoradiotherapy

Radiotherapy alone can be useful for patients who are unfit to receive chemotherapy. Useful palliation and even long-term disease control can be achieved with radiotherapy with a dose of 45–54 Gy in 25–30 fractions.

Fungating inguinal nodes can be treated with 30 Gy in 10 fractions, using 4–6 MV photons with bolus or, in more frail patients, 6 Gy per fraction weekly for 5–6 weeks.

Effective palliation/local control can also be achieved with a low-dose CRT regimen consisting of 30 Gy to the GTV plus a 3 cm margin with concomitant 5-FU (Charnley *et al.*, 2005).

Palliative chemotherapy

Haematogenous metastatic disease tends to occur late, but it can be rapidly progressive. Combination chemotherapy regimens are often used, such as cisplatin with 5-FU or MMC with 5-FU, giving treatment not previously used during primary CRT. Recent reports have suggested that carboplatin paclitaxel may offer a more active alternative. The International Rare Cancer Initiative has recently instigated a phase II trial (InterAACT) comparing cisplatin 5-FU with this regimen.

Follow-up after radical treatment

Clinically assess the patient at 6 weeks after the end of CRT and subsequently every 1–3 months; examination under anaesthetic (EUA) is reserved for patients who find clinical examination too uncomfortable or for those in whom local disease remains a concern. If possible, one should avoid a large biopsy in a previously irradiated area because of the risk of radionecrosis. Biopsies may result in ulceration and delayed healing, but are important to consider as currently no other modality can confirm persistent or recurrent disease over local scarring post-irradiation. It is essential to histologically confirm persistent or recurrent disease if an APR/salvage is being considered.

Special problems

Anal cancer in patients with HIV/AIDS

Patients with HIV/AIDS are at increased risk of developing anal cancer. All patients who are HIV +ve and have anal cancer (including those with CD4 count > 200 cells/mm^3) should be on highly active antiretroviral therapy (HAART). Patients treated with radiotherapy with or without chemotherapy are at increased risk of mucosal and cutaneous toxicity. Such patients should be monitored closely in collaboration with the specialist HIV team. Patients with established AIDS or a CD4 count ≤ 200 cells/mm^3 appear more likely to suffer local and haematological toxicity and it would seem appropriate to optimise retroviral therapy prior to treatment. A modified chemotherapy dose regimen, reduced PTV or a reduced radiotherapy dose should be considered for this group.

Adenocarcinoma

Although long-term stoma-free disease control has been described following radiotherapy or CRT, patients should be treated as if they have a low rectal adenocarcinoma and be offered an APR. In an attempt to reduce the involvement of the circumferential resection margin and the risk of subsequent local recurrence, pre-operative radiotherapy with or without chemotherapy is frequently given.

Prognosis

Survival

Radiotherapy and radical surgery have similar survival and local control rates, but radiotherapy has the advantage of being sphincter-sparing.

For anal-canal tumours, the 5-year survival rate with radical CRT is 65%, and the 5-year local control rate and rate of CFS is 75%. For anal-margin tumours, the rates are 80% and 85%, respectively. The average time of survival after diagnosis with metastatic disease is 8–12 months.

Prognostic factors

The principal prognostic factor of anal cancer is disease stage (i.e. TNM). Distant metastases clearly have the greatest impact on survival, whereas the T stage determines the chance of local control. Node-positive patients have a 10–20% lower 5-year survival rate than node-negative patients.

The prognosis in females is generally better than in males. HPV status, P16 immunohistochemistry, Ki-67, mitotic rate, TP53 mutation and DNA aneuploidy are also factors affecting prognosis, but it is uncertain whether these are independent of the stage of the tumour (Gilbert *et al.*, 2013).

Areas of current interest and current clinical trials

Currently, a UK phase III trial is in planning which will attempt to divide anal cancers into good and poor prognostic groups using T and N staging. T3 and T4 node-positive cancers will be randomised to dose escalation, within the same 28 fractions using a simultaneous integrated boost with IMRT or VMAT (ACT5). T1 and non-bulky T2 tumours (ACT4) will be randomised to dose de-escalation again with IMRT/VMAT as standard. Many centres have switched to an oral capecitabine with MMC schedule as indicated above.

Data collection is ongoing in relation to patient-reported outcome measures for patients receiving radical CRT for anal cancer. Regional services are being developed for patients with late toxicity from radical CRT including GI and sexual dysfunction.

An international group is reviewing the optimal staging of patients with anal cancer.

The InterAACT trial is a phase II international trial looking at identifying the optimum backbone chemotherapy for future trials in metastatic or locally incurable anal cancer. This trial is comparing cisplatin 5-FU with carboplatin paclitaxel.

No trials are planned to compare conformal CRT with IMRT/VMAT.

References

Anal Cancer Trial Working Party. (1996). Epidermoid anal cancer: results from the UKCCCR randomised trial of radiotherapy alone versus radiotherapy, 5-fluorouracil and mitomycin. *Lancet*, **348**, 1049–1054.

Andreyev, H. J., Benton, B., Lalji, A., *et al.* (2013). Algorithm-based management of patients with gastrointestinal symptoms in patients after pelvic radiation treatment (ORBIT): a randomised controlled trial. *Lancet*, **382**, 2084–2092.

Bartelink, H., Roelofsen, F., Eschwege, F., *et al.* (1997). Concomitant radiotherapy and chemotherapy is superior to radiotherapy alone in the treatment of locally advanced anal cancer: results of a phase III randomized trial of the European Organization for Research and Treatment of Cancer Radiotherapy and Gastrointestinal Cooperative Groups. *J. Clin. Oncol.*, **15**, 2040–2049.

Charnley, N., Choudhury, A., Chesser, P., *et al.* (2005). Effective treatment of anal cancer in the elderly with low-dose chemoradiotherapy. *Br. J. Cancer*, **92**, 1221–1225.

Cummings, B., Keane, T., Thomas, G., *et al.* (1984). Results and toxicity of the treatment of anal canal carcinoma by radiation therapy or radiation therapy and chemotherapy. *Cancer*, **54**, 2062–2068.

Daling, J. R., Weiss, N. S., Klopfenstein, L. L., *et al.* (1982). Correlates of homosexual behavior and the incidence of anal cancer. *J. Am. Med. Assoc.*, **247**, 1988–1990.

Daling, J. R., Weiss, N. S., Hislop, T. G., *et al.* (1987). Sexual practices, sexually transmitted diseases and the incidence of anal cancer. *N. Engl. J. Med.*, **317**, 973–977.

Flam, M., John, M., Pajak, T. F., *et al.* (1996). Role of mitomycin in combination with fluorouracil and radiotherapy, and of salvage chemoradiation in the definitive nonsurgical treatment of epidermoid carcinoma of the anal canal: results of a phase III randomized intergroup study. *J. Clin. Oncol.*, **14**, 2527–2539.

Fuccio, L., Guido, A. and Andreyev. H. J. (2012). Management of intestinal complications in patients with pelvic radiation disease. *Clin. Gastroenterol. Hepatol.*, **10**, 1326–1334.

Gilbert, D. C., Williams, A., Allan, K., *et al.* (2013). p16INK4A, p53, EGFR expression and KRAS mutation status in squamous cell cancers of the anus: correlation with outcomes following chemo-radiotherapy. *Radiother. Oncol.*, **109**, 146–151.

Glynne-Jones, R., Meadows, H., Wan, S., *et al.* (2008). EXTRA – a multicenter phase II study of chemoradiation using a 5 day per week oral regimen of capecitabine and intravenous mitomycin C in anal cancer. *Int. J. Radiat. Oncol. Biol. Phys.*, **72**, 119–126.

Glynne-Jones, R., Sebag-Montefiore, D., Adams, R., *et al.* (2011). 'Mind the gap' – the impact of variations in the duration of the treatment gap and overall treatment time in the first UK Anal Cancer Trial (ACT I). *Int. J. Radiat. Oncol. Biol. Phys.*, **81**, 1488–1494.

Gunderson, L. L. Winter, K. A., Ajani, J. A., *et al.* (2012). Long-term update of US GI Intergroup RTOG 98-11 phase III trial for anal carcinoma: survival, relapse, colostomy failure with concurrent chemoradiation involving fluorouracil/mitomycin versus fluorouracil/cisplatin. *J. Clin. Oncol.*, **30**, 4344–4351.

Hu, K., Minsky, B. D., Cohen, A. M., *et al.* (1999). 30 Gy may be an adequate dose in patients with anal cancer treated with excisional biopsy followed by combined modality therapy. *J. Surg. Oncol.*, **70**, 71–77.

James, R. D., Glynne-Jones, R., Meadows, H. M., *et al.* (2013). Mitomycin or cisplatin chemoradiation with or without maintenance chemotherapy for treatment of squamous-cell carcinoma of the anus (ACT II): a randomised, phase 3, open-label, 2 x 2 factorial trial. *Lancet Oncol.*, **14**, 516–524.

Matthews, J. H., Burmeister, B. H., Borg, M., *et al.* (2011). T1–2 anal carcinoma requires elective inguinal radiation treatment – the results of Trans Tasman Radiation Oncology Group study TROG 99.02. *Radiat. Oncol.*, **98**, 93–98.

Ng, M., Leong, T., Chander, S., *et al.* (2012). Australasian Gastrointestinal Trials Group (AGITG) contouring atlas and planning guidelines for intensity-modulated radiotherapy in anal cancer. *Int. J. Radiat. Oncol. Biol. Phys.*, **83**, 1455–1462.

NICE. (2004). *Guidance on Cancer Services. Improving Outcomes in Colorectal Cancers. Manual Update.* London: National Institute for Health and Care Excellence.

Nigro, N. D., Vaitkevicius, V. K. and Considine, B., Jr. (1974). Combined therapy for cancer of the anal canal: a preliminary report. *Dis. Colon Rectum*, **17**, 354–356.

Nigro, N. D., Seydel, H. G., Considine, B., *et al.* (1983). Combined preoperative radiation and chemotherapy for squamous cell carcinoma of the anal canal. *Cancer*, **51**, 1826–1829.

Peiffert, D., Tournier-Rangeard, L., Gérard, J. P., *et al.* (2012). Induction chemotherapy and dose intensification of the radiation boost in locally advanced anal canal carcinoma: final analysis of the randomized UNICANCER ACCORD 03 trial. *J. Clin. Oncol.*, **30**, 1941–1948.

Renehan, A. G., Saunders, M. P., Schofield, P. F., *et al.* (2005). Patterns of local disease failure and outcome after salvage surgery in patients with anal cancer. *Br. J. Surg.*, **92**, 605–614.

Royal College of Radiologists. (2008). *The Timely Delivery of Radical Radiotherapy: Standards and Guidelines for the Management of Unscheduled Treatment Interruptions, Third Edition, 2008.* London: Royal College of Radiologists.

Saboo, S. S., Zukotynski, K., Shinagare, A. B., *et al.* (2013). Anal carcinoma: FDG PET/CT in staging, response evaluation, and follow-up. *Abdom. Imaging*, **38**, 728–735.

Tilston, P. (1997). Anal human papilloma virus and anal cancer. *J. Clin. Pathol.*, **50**, 625–634.

UICC. (2009). *TNM Classification of Malignant Tumours*, ed. L. H. Sobin, M Gospodarowicz and Ch. Wittekind, 7th edn. Chichester: Wiley-Blackwell, pp. 106–109.

Weber, D. C., Kurtz, J. M. and Allal. A. S. (2001). The impact of gap duration on local control in anal canal carcionma treated by split-course radiotherapy and concomitant chemotherapy. *Int. J. Radiat. Oncol. Biol. Phys.*, **50**, 675–680.

Wiesendanger-Wittmer, E. M., Sijtsema, N. M., Muijs, C. T., *et al.* (2012). Systematic review of the role of a belly board device in radiotherapy delivery in patients with pelvic malignancies. *Radiother. Oncol.*, **102**, 325–334.

Management of gastrointestinal stromal tumours

Carys Morgan, Kate Parker and Sarah Gwynne

Introduction

Gastrointestinal stromal tumours (GISTs) are rare mesenchymal tumours that can occur anywhere in the gastrointestinal tract, although most commonly in the stomach or small intestine. GISTs have been difficult to diagnose in the past, which, along with their rarity, means their true incidence is hard to determine and probably underestimated. Until relatively recently, there were very few treatment options for patients with GIST and the prognosis for patients with advanced disease was extremely poor. However, this has changed markedly over the past decade with increases in understanding of molecular pathology. These developments have made diagnosis more accurate and have led to effective treatments with molecular-targeted therapies. As research continues, it is likely that more therapies will become available for this condition.

GISTs probably originate from the interstitial cells of Cajal (ICC) – pacemaker cells that control gut motility. The tumours are diagnosed by a combination of morphological features and immunohistochemistry staining. Oncogenesis appears to be related to dysregulation of the proto-oncogenes KIT or PDGFRA, which encode growth factor receptor tyrosine kinases. Most tumours harbour an activating mutation in KIT or less commonly PDGFRA.

Types of tumour

There are a number of gastrointestinal mesenchymal (non-epithelial) tumours which include smooth muscle tumours, schwannomas and intra-abdominal fibromatosis. GIST is the most common of the gastrointestinal soft tissue tumours.

Incidence and epidemiology

The annual incidence in the UK is between 10 and 20 per million; it is difficult to obtain an accurate count because of the cancer's rarity and because of previous difficulty in diagnosis. There are 600–1200 new cases reported per year in England and 30–60 new cases per year in Wales.

GISTs have become more reliably diagnosable since KIT expression has become detectable by immunohistochemistry, which may have changed the perceived incidence. GIST is rare before age 40; the median age at diagnosis is 60–65 years. It is rarely seen in patients < 20 years and in these cases is usually associated with a syndrome. Most studies show an equal gender distribution of the disease.

GISTs represent 1% or fewer of all primary tumours of the GI tract and 5% of soft tissue sarcomas (Duffaud and Blay, 2003).

Risk factors and aetiology

Generally GISTs are sporadic and not part of an inherited syndrome. Familial GIST, however, is associated with an inherited mutation in KIT and affected individuals have a high risk of developing GIST at a young age. This inherited disorder is associated with pigmented macules in the axilla, perineum and on the hands and face. Germline PDGFRA mutations are also seen and associated with early development of GISTs and inflammatory polyps in the stomach and small bowel.

Additionally, there are a number of rare tumour syndromes associated with GISTs.

- Carney Triad is a rare syndrome seen predominently in young females. The 'triad' of gastric GIST, paraganglioma and pulmonary chondroma is seen, but KIT and PDGFRA mutations are not seen in the GISTs associated with this.

- Carney–Stratakis syndrome is described as a germline mutation in succinate dehydrogenase; again, KIT and PDGFRA mutations are not seen.
- There is also an association with Type 1 neurofibromatosis (NF) and a subset of patients with von Recklinghausen type NF will develop multiple GISTs, usually in the small bowel.

Histogenesis and pathology

Histogenesis

GISTs are thought to originate from the precursor of the interstitial cells of Cajal (ICC). GISTs and ICC share morphological features and contain a similar form of embryonic smooth muscle myosin. They also both stain positive for CD117 (KIT). The main role of the ICC is as pacemaker cells that control gut motility.

The majority of GISTs (75–80%) have a mutation in the KIT gene, encoding a receptor tyrosine kinase. Mutations are seen most commonly in exon 11 (70% of GISTs), exon 9 (10%) and rarely in exons 13 and 17 of the KIT gene. A minority of GISTs, however, do not have a mutation in KIT but some have mutations in the gene encoding PDGFRA (platelet-derived growth factor alpha), a related receptor tyrosine kinase. In the remaining 10–15% GISTs there is no detectable mutation in either KIT or PDGFRA and these are known as wild-type tumours. These include GISTs seen as part of the rare syndromes of NF-1, Carney's triad, Carney–Stratakis syndrome and some familial GIST.

Both KIT and PDGFRA are transmembrane receptor tyrosine kinases. Ligand binding (by stem cell factor or PDGFRA, respectively) causes dimerisation of adjacent receptors, which activates the intracellular signalling cascades affecting cell proliferation, adhesion and differentiation, often via the signal transduction intermediates AKT and MAPK. Mutations often cause a change in these signals, which results in a gain of function – constitutive activation (Heinrich *et al.*, 2003).

Pathology

Macroscopic features

GISTs are located in the gastrointestinal tract, most commonly in the stomach (60–70%), small intestine (20–30%), colon, rectum and oesophagus (5–15%), and rarely do extragastrointestinal GISTs occur in other locations including the omentum, mesentery and retroperitoneum (≤ 5%).

Tumours are usually 2–30 cm in diameter at the time of diagnosis but may be 1 cm or smaller if found incidentally (known as microGIST). MicroGISTs are most common in the gastro-oesophageal area and are unlikely to be clinically significant. Most GISTs are submucosal, grow endophytically, and are often well-circumscribed with a whorled, fibroid-like appearance. Larger lesions may display cystic degeneration or necrosis.

Microscopic appearance

Microscopically, GISTs can occur as three different types:

- spindle cell (70%) – relatively uniform eosinophilic cells arranged in short fascicles or whorls;
- epithelioid (20%) – rounded cells with variably eosinophilic or clear cytoplasm;
- mixed – areas of each of the aforementioned types, either mingled together or with an abrupt transition between them.

Immunohistochemistry

Immunohistochemical testing is important in differentiating GIST from other soft tissue tumours that can appear similar on microscopy alone. The majority (95%) of GISTs stain positively with CD117 antibody that recognises an extracellular epitope of KIT (Corless *et al.*, 2004). Five per cent are CD117-negative. The vast majority are positive for DOG1 (ANO1). Table 18.1 shows the immunohistochemical features of GISTs. DOG1 is expressed ubiquitously in GISTs, irrespective of KIT and PDGFRA mutation status (Novelli *et al.*, 2010).

Metastatic deposits from other tumours can also be positive for CD117, including melanoma, angiosarcoma and seminoma.

Molecular pathology

The receptors KIT and PDGFRA are similar tyrosine kinase transmembrane receptors. Each exon encodes a different part of the receptor, for example, exon 11 in the KIT gene codes for the juxtamembrane area and exon 9 for the extracellular region involved in receptor dimerisation. The mutation type seen in KIT or PDGRFA gene can now be identified by mutational

Table 18.1 Immunohistochemical features of GIST

Immunohistochemical feature	Frequency (%)
DOG1	> 98%
CD117 (*KIT*) positive	90%
CD34 positive	60–70%
SMA positive	30–40%
S100 protein positive	5%

CD, cluster of differentiation; DOG1, ANO1; anoctamin 1, calcium-activated chloride channel; KIT, kitten; (v-kit Hardy–Zuckerman 4 feline sarcoma viral oncogene homolog); S100, S100 calcium-binding protein; SMA, smooth muscle actin. Adapted from Fletcher *et al*. (2002).

Table 18.2 The molecular classification of GISTs

Type	Description
KIT (75–80%)	Exon 11: 70% of patients
	Exon 9: 10% of patients
	Exons 13 and 17: rare (2% of patients)
PDGFRA (10%)	Exon 18: uncommon (6% of patients)
	Exons 12 and 14: rare (1.4% of patients)
Wild-type (10–15%)	Molecular aetiology unclear
Familial GIST	Germline KIT or PDGFRA mutation
Paediatric	KIT and PDGFRA mutations rare

KIT, kitten, (v-kit Hardy–Zuckerman 4 feline sarcoma viral oncogene homolog); *PDGFRA*, platelet-derived growth factor receptor, alpha polypeptide.

analysis and this forms part of the diagnostic work-up for GIST.

Mutational analysis

KIT mutations are seen in 75–80% of GISTs and the majority occur in exon 11. Point mutations, deletions, insertions and duplications are seen. Mutations are seen less commonly in exons 9, 13 and 17. Additionally, 3–5% of GISTs have an identifiable mutation in the PDGFRA gene and these are seen in exons 12, 14 and 18. KIT and PDGFRA mutations are mutually exclusive.

Around 15% have no KIT or PDGFRA mutations and these are known as wild-type GISTs and include the rare paediatric and familial syndromes. Mutations have been described in the succinate dehydrogenase complex (SDH), in BRAF, NF-1 and the RAS family (see Joensuu *et al*., 2013 for further discussion).

Mutational analysis has a number of roles. It can help to confirm the diagnosis of GIST in those where it is unclear, e.g. negative immunohistochemical staining for CD117/ DOG1. Additionally, it can provide information on the likely responsiveness to TKIs and prognosis. Some mutations confer imatinib resistance and therefore mutational testing will guide treatment options. In terms of treatment response, PDGFRA D842V-mutated GISTs are an imatinib-insensitive subgroup and should not be treated with adjuvant imatinib. This genotype is seen in approximately 10% of gastric GISTs. Additionally, exon 9 KIT mutations confer a better response to higher-dose imatinib in the metastatic setting (Gastrointestinal Stromal Tumour Meta-Analysis Group (MetaGIST), 2010) and so this treatment strategy should be considered an option in this group. Exon 9 KIT mutations are also associated with poorer prognosis than exon 11.

The molecular classification of GISTs is shown in Table 18.2.

Spread

Modes of GIST spread involve spread by the primary tumour to involve contiguous structures. Spread to lymph nodes is rare even when there is metastatic disease, but it may occur following surgery. Metastatic spread commonly includes the liver and peritoneal cavity. Lung, bone or subcutaneous sites are involved, but rarely.

Of all GISTs, there is a high rate of recurrence postoperatively between 40% and 90%, either locally or with metastatic disease.

Clinical presentation

The patient initially presents typically with an intra-abdominal tumour or as an emergency with intestinal haemorrhage or obstruction. Symptoms include gastrointestinal bleeding (50%), abdominal pain (20–50%), gastrointestinal obstruction (10–30%), tiredness and general malaise. GIST is an incidental finding and patients are asymptomatic in 20–30% of cases.

Investigation and staging

CT (or MRI) of the thorax, abdomen and pelvis should be used to look for metastases. Consider assessment of endocrine and αFP and βhCG levels to look for alternative diagnoses such as adrenal tumours and teratomas, depending on the clinical context. Percutaneous biopsy is not advised, because there is a risk of necrotic tumour leakage from the biopsy site. PET scanning and endoscopic ultrasound may add useful information for the management of some patients.

Stage classification

Malignant GIST lesions are not often classified using TNM nomenclature. GIST should be classified as localised or metastatic. Lymph node involvement is classified as metastatic, and risk stratification (described later) should be used.

Treatment

Treatment overview

It is important that these rare tumours are discussed with experts in the field including histopathologist, radiologist, surgeon and oncologist with an interest in the management of GIST. All new cases should therefore be managed by a tertiary multidisciplinary team (MDT). If the tumour is considered operable, then it should be resected following standard oncological principles; if the tumour is not operable, then a biopsy should be performed to confirm the diagnosis. Histopathological review by an experienced pathologist and MDT review should be done to confirm the diagnosis and to assess the risk of recurrence. This is based mainly on site of primary, size and mitotic rate (see discussion that follows). Additionally, mutational analysis should be carried out if further treatment is being considered.

If the tumour is fully resected, then follow-up should be done according to assessed risk (see discussion that follows) and adjuvant therapy with imatinib should be considered if there is thought to be a high risk of recurrence.

GISTs are resistant to conventional cytotoxic chemotherapy but do respond to targeted therapy as outlined in the next section (Eisenberg and Judson, 2004). If the tumour is inoperable or if residual or metastatic disease is present, then palliative imatinib therapy is the standard first-line treatment of choice.

Usually the response is assessed at 3-month intervals by CT scan. Progressive disease should be discussed at an MDT meeting with radiological review, as sometimes necrotic change with a mass can be reported as progression. In the case of stable disease or patient response, imatinib is continued until disease progression, when second-line therapy with sunitinib

is an option. Occasionally, disease can become operable, which needs to be a consideration.

Role of surgery

Surgical resection remains the best hope for a cure. It should be discussed within the relevant MDT (either the upper GI team or sarcoma team; NICE, 2006) and performed by a surgeon who is fully trained and experienced in cancer surgery in the relevant area. The primary aim is complete resection while avoiding tumour rupture. The approach depends on the presentation. Some evidence exists that preoperative imatinib may be beneficial (Eisenberg et al., 2009), but currently it should be noted that the role of imatinib in localised disease, and the role of surgery in metastatic disease, is experimental and the benefits are unclear.

Tumours larger than 2 cm

Wide local excision is required for tumours larger than 2 cm, with a margin of 1–2 cm. When adjacent organs are involved, *en bloc* dissection is necessary with the help of appropriate specialist surgeons. For tumours of the bowel, surgery will amount to a formal segmental resection with the accompanying mesentery. Because GISTs rarely metastasise to nodes, extended lymphadenectomy is not required.

Small tumours

The management of asymptomatic small (≤ 2 cm) tumours is controversial. A proportion of these have a very low risk of malignant transformation and a firm diagnosis is not always made. If these tumours are not resected, they should be re-imaged at 6 and 12 months with a CT scan or endoscopic ultrasound.

Tumours arising outside the GI tract

The tumour should be dissected from adjacent organs and then excised with a margin of normal tissue. The aim is macroscopic removal of the intact tumour mass regardless of its size.

Multiple tumours

Patients with more than one primary GIST should be referred to the cancer genetics service for advice, and each tumour should be treated as appropriate.

Role of surgery in emergency presentations

Patients may present with an obstruction and need an emergency laparotomy. If the tumour cannot be excised, a bypass procedure should be undertaken and the tumour should be biopsied. Patients then require an appropriate staging scan and an MDT discussion.

Adjuvant therapy

Adjuvant therapy with imatinib may have a role in reducing risk of recurrence in completely resected GISTs. At the time of writing, evidence was available from case reports, cohort studies and 3 RCTs. DeMatteo et al. randomised 708 patients with completely resected KIT-positive GISTs of 3 cm or more to imatinib 400 mg versus placebo for 12 months. When patients recurred, treatment was unblinded and patients were permitted to cross over to imatinib if they had previously taken placebo or increase the dose of imatinib to 800 mg/day if already taking it (DeMatteo et al., 2009). The primary endpoint was initially overall survival, but changed to recurrence-free survival (RFS). Patients assigned to the imatinib arm had a 1-year RFS of 98% versus 83% in the placebo arm ($p < 0.0001$). Grades 3 and 4 toxicities were seen in 30% of imatinib group versus 18% in the placebo arm. The study was designed prior to the development of risk stratification and patients were included irrespective of their risk of recurrence.

The Scandinavian-German study (SSGXVIII/ AIO) was published in 2012 and clearly demonstrated a marked overall survival benefit for patients offered three years of adjuvant imatinib compared with those given one year (Joensuu et al., 2012a). The study looked at patients at high risk for GIST recurrence after surgery. Patients assigned to 36 months of imatinib had a 5-year overall survival of 92.0% versus 81.7% in the 12-month arm. RFS was also longer in the 36 months group (5-year RFS 65.6% versus 47.9%).

EORTC 62024 was a randomised trial comparing adjuvant imatinib for two years with placebo in patients with localised, surgically resected, high/intermediate-risk GIST (Casali et al., 2013). Of 908 patients who were followed up for a median of 4.7 years, RFS was 84% versus 66% at 3 years, and 69% versus 63% at 5 years ($p < 0.001$); 5-year OS was 100% versus 99%. The authors concluded that adjuvant imatinib has an overt impact on short-term freedom from relapse.

Based on these data, all patients with high-risk GISTs with imatinib-sensitive mutations should be considered for 3 years of adjuvant imatinib by a specialist MDT (NICE, 2014). At present, data on treatment beyond three years in the adjuvant setting are lacking.

Systemic treatment of advanced disease

Imatinib

Indications

Indications for use of imatinib are a confirmed KIT (CD117)-positive GIST (Verweij et al., 2003b) and inoperable recurrent or metastatic disease confirmed by the MDT.

Baseline investigations

The disease should be assessed with a CT scan to allow accurate monitoring. Informed patient consent is needed (including advice to the patient on avoiding pregnancy and breast feeding). The patient's medication should be checked for drugs that interact via the p450 system. The patient's performance status and cardiac status should be assessed and baseline liver and renal function tests and FBC should be performed. The patient's weight should also be checked.

Treatment

The patient should be given imatinib 400 mg p.o. once a day continuously (van Oosterom et al., 2001; Verweij et al., 2003a), which should be taken with a large glass of water (to avoid gastric irritation). The patient should also avoid caffeine and grapefruit for 1 hour before and after receiving the dose and should avoid lying down for 1 hour afterward.

Monitoring

Two weeks after starting imatinib, check LFT and FBC, assess toxicity, measure the patient's weight (to determine fluid retention), and perform a physical and symptomatic assessment of response. Repeat this procedure at 4- to 6-week intervals. Repeat a CT or PET scan after 3 months to assess the patient's response. If there is evidence of response or stable disease then continue treatment according to toxicity parameters. Repeat the assessment with CT every 6 months or earlier if clinically indicated.

See van Oosterom et al. (2001) for more information on patient monitoring.

Toxicities

Generally imatinib is well tolerated, but toxicities include nausea and vomiting (level 1 anti-emetics are usually enough to help), diarrhoea and dyspepsia, and oedema, often periorbital or peripheral (occasionally pleural effusions, ascites). Diuretic therapy is helpful but, if oedema is severe, imatinib treatment should be stopped or the dose reduced. LFTs should be checked and treatment withheld if bilirubin levels are three times the upper limit of normal or transaminases > 5 times the upper limit. If a skin rash occurs, it is usually mild and self-limiting, but it can be severe. Occasionally neutropenia can occur often early after starting treatment (monitor FBC). Gastrointestinal bleeding also occurs, often due to response and tumour regression (van Oosterom et al., 2002).

Confirmed disease progression

NICE guidance dictates that imatinib should be discontinued when the disease progresses (NICE, 2004). Patients who remain well should be commenced on second-line therapy with sunitinib. Progression is likely to be due to development of secondary mutations which lead to resistance to imatinib.

Sunitinib

Treatment with sunitinib is standard second-line therapy following progression on imatinib (NICE, 2009). A placebo-controlled study in patients with progression or intolerance of imatinib was stopped early when an interim analysis showed increased time to tumour progression with sunitinib. Median time to tumour progression was 27.3 weeks versus. 6.4 weeks with placebo (Demetri et al., 2006).

Sunitinib is a small-molecule, multi-targeted inhibitor of all VEGFRs, PDGFRA, PDGFRB, FLT3 and KIT. It is administered orally at a dose of 50 mg daily for 4 weeks followed by a 2-week break from treatment. It is often less well-tolerated than imatinib and many patients require dose reductions (to 37.5 mg daily or further if necessary). Sometimes a lower-dose continuous treatment regimen is better tolerated, and non-randomised data suggest it is effective (The ESMO/European Sarcoma Networking Group, 2014).

Typical toxicities include fatigue, diarrhoea, nausea and skin discolouration, but can include thyroid dysfunction, hypertension, mucositis, palmar plantar erythema, hepatic toxicity and cardiac toxicities including cardiomyopathy and arrhythmias. Patients should be carefully monitored on starting therapy and in addition to usual tests should have regular blood pressure monitoring and thyroid function assessment.

Other treatment options in advanced or recurrent disease

After progression on sunitinib, there are currently no standard treatment options and entry into clinical trials should be encouraged. Sometimes nodules of resistant disease grow in previously controlled metastases. Surgery may be considered for these 'tumour-resistant clones', but treatment decisions should be individually considered because the benefit of this approach is uncertain.

Dose escalation of imatinib is controversial; occasionally, dose escalation up to 800 mg daily can lead to a further response. This is most likely to be of benefit in tumours with KIT exon 9 mutations if not previously on a higher dose. One study showed a 33% response to dose escalation, but the median duration of response was only 3 months (Zalcberg et al., 2004).

For other TKIs, see discussion of new drugs that follows.

Role of surgery in advanced or recurrent disease

Surgery may have a role in the excision of recurrent disease, debulking of advanced disease or excision of disease following response to imatinib (Bümming et al., 2003), and procedures for palliation of symptoms.

If after a good response to TKI has been achieved the possibility of achieving an R0 resection is considered likely, then surgery should be offered. If this is achieved, there is then some contention about continuation of imatinib. At least three years of adjuvant therapy would seem reasonable in the absence of data. Many would advocate continued therapy.

The survival benefit from other surgical strategies in palliative situations is currently unclear and requires further investigation. Several situations including surgical resection of a localised area of progressive disease, debulking surgery and palliation of symptomatic metastases can arise and currently each individual case should be considered on its merits, again within a specialist MDT.

A recent EORTC phase III trial (NCT00956072) evaluating the role of surgery in metastatic GIST after response to imatinib closed early after failure to accrue. This is probably due to palliative resection in this situation being carried out in many units already leading to reduced trial entry. See Meza and Wong (2011) for further discussion of surgery in advanced GIST.

Patients on imatinib can present with acute gastrointestinal haemorrhage due to tumour response. These patients should be managed intensively because the prognosis of patients on imatinib may be reasonable, with good quality of life.

Palliative radiotherapy

Historically, radiotherapy has not often played a role in the management of GIST due to large volume or widespread disease. It is, however, a radiosensitive disease and radiotherapy can be used as a palliative measure in advanced disease, for example for gastrointestinal bleeding, bone pain or mass lesions in TKI insensitive disease (Knowlton et al., 2011).

Assessing response

Contrast-enhanced CT

A response to therapy can be seen on a CT scan as early as 1 month after treatment starts. GISTs can decrease in size but may also increase in size (because of haemorrhage or myxoid degeneration). The standard RECIST criteria for assessing tumour response are therefore inadequate as the sole method to assess response (Silberman and Joensuu, 2002).

As well as changing in size, the tumour can become more homogeneous and hypoattenuated on CT, and tumour vessels and solid enhancing nodules may disappear. Therefore, it is important that the CT scans used to assess response are reported by radiologists experienced in assessing response in GIST, and that they are discussed in the MDT meeting.

Criteria to help predict response on CT, which include size and number of tumours, degree and extent of enhancement, change in Hounsfield unit, presence or absence of tumour vessels, and the presence or absence of solid nodules within the tumours, have been evaluated and were found to be better than RECIST criteria for assessing the response of GISTs to imatinib. These new criteria may make the determination of response assessment via CT more accurate.

Role of PET

Metabolic responses to imatinib can be reported as early as 24 hours after treatment and changes in FDG-PET images at 1 week have been reported compared to those seen on a CT scan at 2 months (Stroobants et al., 2003). However, FDG-PET is not routinely available for GIST in many UK centres and international response criteria for FDG-PET have not been standardised. In addition,

20% of GISTs do not take up appreciable FDG at baseline and so cannot be monitored in this way; for these tumours, CT remains the routine form of radiological assessment.

Special clinical situations

Positive surgical resection margins ('R1' resection)

Residual disease should be excised whenever possible. If not possible, patients should be started on imatinib.

Neoadjuvant imatinib

Preoperative treatment with imatinib is not standard, but can be used in some clinical scenarios. Randomised data are lacking, however. Neoadjuvant therapy may have a role in borderline resectable cases and when facilitating organ-preserving surgery in cases where primary surgery may be very extensive. It is vital to make sure that the tumour is imatinib-sensitive by mutational analysis and that an early assessment of response is carried out to avoid the potential for tumour progression. This practice is included in current ESMO clinical guidelines (The ESMO/European Sarcoma Network Working Group, 2014). PET scanning for this early assessment has been used and can be helpful.

Follow-up

Follow-up after surgery depends on the risk of recurrence. This varies greatly and is related to size and site of the tumour and mitotic rate. The most important prognostic factor is mitotic rate. Large size and non-gastric origin are also features which are associated with an increased risk of recurrence. Additionally, tumour rupture during surgery is thought to have a negative impact on outcome, but it is not incorporated into most risk stratification tables presently.

In order to quantify risk of recurrence, three commonly used patient risk stratification schemes are used, all of which have been validated: (i) the Armed Forces Institute of Pathology (AFIP) Miettinen Criteria, (ii) the Modified NIH Joensuu Criteria, and (iii) the Gold nomogram. Table 18.3 is based on the AFIP Miettinen criteria.

Follow-up imaging frequency would also depend on risk assessment. In general, all patients should have a CT scan at 3 months post-surgery.

Table 18.3 Risk of recurrence of GISTs according to the AFIP Miettinen criteria

Mitotic index	Size	Gastric	Jejunal/ileal	Duodenal	Rectal
≤ 5 per 50 high-powered fields	≤ 2 cm	None (0%)	None (0%)	None (0%)	None (0%)
	>2 cm to ≤ 5 cm	Very low (1.9%)	Low (4.3%)	Low (8.3%)	Low (8.5%)
	> 5 cm to ≤ 10 cm	Low (3.6%)	Moderate (24%)	High (34%)	High (57%)
	> 10 cm	Moderate (10%)	High (52%)	Groups combined due to low numbers	Groups combined due to low numbers
>5 per 50 high-powered fields	≤ 2 cm	Insufficient data	High (limited data)	Insufficient data	High (54%)
	> 2 cm to ≤ 5 cm	Moderate (16%)	High (73%)	High (50%)	High (52%)
	> 5 cm to ≤ 10 cm	High (55%)	High (85%)	High (86%)	High (insufficient data)
	> 10 cm	High (86%)	High (90%)	Groups combined due to low numbers	High (71%)

Adapted from Miettinen and Lasota, 2006.

Patients with very-low-risk tumours only need an annual review and no further CT scan unless clinically indicated.

For patients with low-risk tumours, repeat a CT scan at 12 months. Perform an annual review thereafter and a CT scan only if indicated clinically.

For patients with intermediate-risk tumours, repeat a CT scan at 9 months and then annually for 5 years in addition to an annual clinical review.

For patients with high-risk tumours, consider adjuvant therapy and perform a CT scan every 6 months for 3 years, then annually over the next 5 years. A clinical review should be performed every 6 months.

Prognosis

In a recent pooled analysis of operable GIST (prior to introduction of adjuvant therapy) the estimated median overall survival time was 12.4 years. Most GIST recurrences took place within the first 5 years of follow-up, and few tumours recurred after the first 10 years of follow-up. Estimated 5-year and 15-year recurrence-free survival rates after surgery were 70.5% and 59.9% (Joensuu et al., 2012b).

Prior to the use of imatinib, the prognosis for metastatic GIST was very poor (median survival 9–23 months) and this has improved significantly. Long-term results from an imatinib trial reported median survival of 57 months with 50% living over 5 years (Blanke et al.,

2008). In advanced disease the response rate to imatinib is initially between 80% and 90% (which is derived from a very small number of complete responses, around 67% partial responses and the remainder of patients with stable disease; Benjamin et al., 2003; Verweij et al., 2004; Demetri et al., 2006). The median time to progression on imatinib is around 24 months (Von Mehren et al., 2002), and the median time to achieving CR or PR is 13 weeks (Demetri et al., 2002).

Areas of current interest and clinical trials

New drugs

GIST is an area of intense research interest and there are numerous ongoing clinical trials looking at the role of other tyrosine kinase inhibitors and the use of other targeted therapies such as PI3Kinase inhibitors, MTOR antagonists and immune modulators.

Some drugs of current interest are as follows.

- Regorafenib is an oral multikinase inhibitor that demonstrated substantial activity in a phase III trial in patients after failure of imatinib and sunitinib with significant improvement in PFS compared with placebo (Demetri et al., 2013). This is considered standard third-line therapy if available.

- Masitinib is a promising multitargeted kinase inhibitor with activity against KIT, PDGFRA and FGF and is currently in phase III trials in first- and second-line scenarios.
- Dasatinib is a synthetic small-molecule inhibitor of tyrosine kinases including KIT, PDGFR, BCR-ABL and SRC. It is active when given orally, and it may have activity in imatinib-resistant patients.
- There are many other agents under investigation currently, including sorafenib, pazopanib and nilotinib.

Clinical trials

Many trials are ongoing and are needed to address the following questions and others.

- What is the optimum length of adjuvant therapy?
- What is the role of neoadjuvant imatinib?
- What is the role of debulking surgery in palliative disease?
- What is the role of other new molecular therapies?
- Which agents are active in a third-line setting?
- What is the role of targeted therapies in KIT-negative tumours?
- What is the role of new agents in resistant GIST, e.g. PGFRA Asp842Val mutations?
- What role does radiotherapy have in palliation of advanced GIST?

References

Benjamin, R. S., Ranking, C., Fletcher, C., *et al.* (2003). Phase III dose-randomized study of imatinib mesylate (STI571) for GIST: intergroup S0033 early results. *Proc. Am. Soc. Clin. Oncol.*, Abstr. 3271.

Blanke, C. D., Demetri, G. D., von Mehren, M., *et al.* (2008). Long-term results from a randomized phase II trial of standard- versus higher-dose imatinib mesylate for patients with unresectable or metastatic gastrointestinal stromal tumours expressing KIT. *J. Clin. Oncol.*, **26**, 620–625.

Bümming, P., Andersson, J., Meis-Kindblom, J. M., *et al.* (2003). Neoadjuvant, adjuvant and palliative treatment of gastrointestinal stromal tumours (GIST) with imatinib: a centre-based study of 17 patients. *Br. J. Cancer*, **89**, 460–464.

Casali, P. G., Cesne, A. L., Velasco, A. P., *et al.* (2013). Imatinib failure-free survival (IFS) in patients with localized gastrointestinal stromal tumours (GIST) treated with adjuvant imatinib (IM): the EORTC/

AGITG/FSG/GEIS/ISG randomized controlled phase 3 trial. *J. Clin. Oncol.* **31** (suppl; abstract 10500).

Corless, C. L., Fletcher, J. A. and Heinrich, M. C. (2004). Biology of gastrointestinal stromal tumors. *J. Clin. Oncol.*, **22**, 3813–3825.

DeMatteo, R. P., Ballman, K. V., Antonescu, C. R., *et al.* (2009). Adjuvant imatinib mesylate after resection of localised, primary gastrointestinal stromal tumor: a randomised, double blind, placebo-controlled trial. *Lancet*, **373**, 1097–1010.

Demetri, G. D., von Mehren, M., Blanke, C. D., *et al.* (2002). Efficacy and safety of imatinib mesylate in advanced gastrointestinal stromal tumors. *N. Engl. J. Med.*, **347**, 472–480.

Demetri, G. D., van Oosterom, A. T., Garrett, C. R., *et al.* (2006). Efficacy and safety of sunitinib in patients with advanced gastrointestinal stromal tumour after failure of imatinib: a randomised controlled trial. *Lancet*, **368**, 1329–1338.

Demetri, G. D., Reichardt, P., Kang, Y. K., *et al.* (2013). Efficacy and safety of regorafenib for advanced gastrointestinal stromal tumours after failure of imatinib and sunitinib (GRID): an international, multicentre, randomised, placebo-controlled, phase 3 trial. *Lancet*, **381**, 295–302.

Duffaud, F. and Blay, J.-Y. (2003). Gastrointestinal stromal tumors: biology and treatment. *Oncology*, **65**, 187–97.

Eisenberg, B. L. and Judson, I. (2004). Surgery and imatinib in the management of GIST: emerging approaches to adjuvant and neoadjuvant therapy. *Ann. Surg. Oncol.*, **11**, 465–475.

Eisenberg, B. L., Harris, J., Blanke, C. D., *et al.* (2009). Phase II trial of neoadjuvant/adjuvant imatinib mesylate (IM) for advanced primary and metastatic/recurrent operable gastrointestinal stromal tumor (GIST): early results of RTOG 0132/ACRIN 6665. *J. Surg. Oncol.*, **99**, 42–47.

Fletcher, C. D., Berman, J. J., Corless, C., *et al.* (2002). Diagnosis of gastrointestinal stromal tumours. A consensus approach. *Hum. Pathol.*, **33**, 459–465.

Gastrointestinal Stromal Tumour Meta-Analysis Group (MetaGIST). (2010). Comparison of two doses of imatinib for the treatment of unresectable or metastatic gastrointestinal stromal tumours: a meta-analysis of 1,640 patients. *J. Clin. Oncol.*, **28**, 1247–1253.

Heinrich, M. C., Corless, C. L., Demitri, G. D., *et al.* (2003). Kinase mutations and imatinib response in patients with metastatic gastrointestinal stromal tumor. *J. Clin. Oncol.*, **21**, 4342–4349.

Joensuu, H., Eriksson, M., Sundby Hall., K., *et al.* (2012a). One vs three years of adjuvant imatinib for operable gastrointestinal stromal tumor: a randomized trial. *J. Am. Med. Assoc.*, **307**, 1265–1272.

Joensuu, H., Vehtari, A., Riihimaki, J., et al. (2012b). Risk of recurrence of gastrointestinal stromal tumour after surgery: an analysis of pooled population-based cohorts. *Lancet Oncol.*, **13**, 265–274.

Joensuu, H., Hohenberger, P. and Corless, C. L. (2013). Gastrointestinal stromal tumour. *Lancet*, **382**, 973–983.

Knowlton, C. A., Brady, L. W. and Heintzelman, R. C. (2011). Radiotherapy in the treatment of gastrointestinal stromal tumor. *Rare Tumors*, **3**, e35.

Meza, J. M. and Wong, S. L. (2011). Surgical options in advanced/metastatic gastrointestinal stromal tumours. *Curr. Probl. Cancer*, **35**, 283–293.

Miettinen, M. and Lasota, J. (2006). Gastrointestinal stromal tumors: pathology and prognosis at different sites. *Semin. Diagn. Pathol.*, **23**, 70–83.

NICE. (2004). *Technology Appraisal 86. Imatinib for the Treatment of Unresectable and/or Metastatic Gastrointestinal Stromal Tumours*. London: NICE.

NICE. (2006). *Guidance on Cancer Services. Improving Outcomes for People with Sarcoma. The Manual*. London: NICE.

NICE. (2009). *Sunitinib for the Treatment of Gastrointestinal Stromal Tumours. NICE Technology Appraisal Guidance 179*. London: NICE.

NICE. (2014). *Imatinib for the Adjuvant Treatment of Gastrointestinal Stromal Tumours (review of NICE technology appraisal guidance 196). NICE Technology Appraisal Guidance 326*. London: NICE.

Novelli, M., Rossi, S., Rodriguez-Justo, M., et al. (2010). DOG1 and CD117 are the antibodies of choice in the diagnosis of gastrointestinal stromal tumors. *Histopathology*, **57**, 259–270.

Silberman, S. and Joensuu, H. (2002). Overview of issues related to Imatinib therapy of advanced gastrointestinal stromal tumors: a discussion amongst experts. *Eur. J. Cancer*, **38**(Suppl. 5), S66–69.

Stroobants, S., Goeminne, J., Seegers, M., et al. (2003). 18FDG-Positron Emission Tomography for the early prediction of response in advanced soft tissue sarcoma treated with imatinib mesylate. *Eur. J. Cancer*, **39**, 2012–2020.

The ESMO/European Sarcoma Network Working Group. (2014). Gastrointestinal stromal tumours: ESMO Clinical Practice Guidelines for diagnosis, treatment and follow-up. *Ann Oncol*, **25** (Suppl. 3).

van Oosterom, A. T., Judson, I., Verweij, J., et al. (2001). Safety and efficacy of Imatinib (STI571) in metastatic gastrointestinal stromal tumours: a phase I study. *Lancet*, **358**, 1421–1423.

van Oosterom, A. T., Judson, I., Verweij, J., et al. (2002). Update of phase I study of imatinib (STI571) in advanced soft tissue sarcomas and gastrointestinal stromal tumors: a report of the EORTC Soft Tissue and Bone Sarcoma Group. *Eur. J. Cancer*, **38** (Suppl. 5), S83–87.

Verweij, J., Casali, P. G., Zalcberg, J., et al. (2003a). Early efficacy comparison of two doses of Imatinib for the treatment of advanced gastrointestinal stromal tumors (GIST): interim results of a randomised phase III trial from the EORTC-STBSG, ISG and AGITG. *Proc. Am. Soc. Clin. Oncol.*, Abstr. 3272.

Verweij, J., van Oosterom, A., Blay, J. Y., etal. (2003b). Imatinib mesylate (STI-571 Glivec, Gleevec) is an active agent for gastrointestinal stromal tumours but does not yield responses in other soft tissue sarcomas that are unselected for molecular target: results form an EORTC Soft Tissue and Bone Sarcoma Group phase II study. *Eur. J. Cancer*, **39**, 2006–2011.

Verweij, J., Casali, P. G., Zalcberg, J., et al. (2004). Progression-free survival in gastrointestinal stromal tumours with high-dose imatinib: randomized trial. *Lancet*, **364**, 1127–1134.

Von Mehren, M., Blanke, C., Joensuu, H., et al. (2002). High incidence of durable responses induced by Imatinib mesylate (Gleevec) in patients with resectable and metastatic gastrointestinal stromal tumors (GISTs). *Proc. Am. Soc. Clin. Oncol.*, Abstr. 1608.

Zalcberg, J., Verweij, J., Casali, P. G., et al. (2004). Outcome of patients with advanced gastro-intestinal stromal tumours (GIST) crossing over to a daily imatinib dose of 800 mg (HD) after progression on 400 mg – an international, intergroup study of the EORTC, ISG and AGITG. *Proc. Am. Soc. Clin. Oncol.*, Abstr. 9004.

Chapter 19

Management of cancer of the breast

Delia Pudney, James Powell, Jacinta Abraham and Nayyer Iqbal

Introduction

Breast cancer accounts for 7% of all deaths from cancer and 15% of female deaths from cancer. It is the second most common cause of cancer death among women in the UK. Breast cancer most commonly presents as a lump in the breast, but the use of screening has also allowed very early cancers to be diagnosed before they can be detected clinically. The management of breast cancer has changed significantly over the past 50 years. Standard surgery used to be radical mastectomy and axillary node clearance, whereas today, patients are usually treated with breast-conserving techniques: wide local excision and sentinel lymph node biopsy followed by radiotherapy. The past few decades have also seen the development and wider use of systemic therapies: hormonal treatments, chemotherapy and targeted therapies such as trastuzumab. The mortality from breast cancer has steadily decreased over the last 20 years.

Anatomy

The female breast extends from the second to the sixth rib, and it is made up of 15–20 lobes which radiate out from the nipple. The nipple is surrounded by the areola. Each breast is divided into a central portion and four quadrants. The upper outer quadrant also contains the axillary tail. The lymphatic drainage from the breast is primarily to the axillary lymph nodes, but also to the internal mammary nodes, which lie in the thorax alongside the internal thoracic artery. A few lymphatic channels also communicate with those in the opposite breast and in the abdominal wall.

In the male and prepubertal female, the nipple and areola are small, and the breast tissue does not usually extend beyond the areola.

Types of tumour affecting the breast

Table 19.1 shows the range of tumours that can affect the breast. The most common are invasive ductal carcinoma and invasive lobular carcinoma. Invasive ductal carcinomas are positive for E-cadherin, whereas lobular carcinomas are negative for E-cadherin.

Incidence and epidemiology

Breast cancer is the most common malignancy in women in the UK and accounts for 30% of all new cancers in women. In 2011 there were 50,285 new cases of breast cancer in the UK, with 349 of these occurring in men. There is a wide geographic variation in the age-adjusted incidence of breast cancer with breast cancer occurring more commonly in Western countries (North America and Northern Europe) compared to Asian and African countries (CRUK; http://www.cancerresearchuk.org/cancer-info/cancerstats/types/breast, accessed June 2014).

Breast cancer survival has improved over the last two decades. In the UK and Ireland, the 5-year survival rate for those diagnosed up to 2007 was 79.2% compared to the European average of 81.8% (De Angelis et al., 2014). This improvement in 5-year survival is believed to be due to many factors including screening, improved treatment (improved surgical techniques, adjuvant hormone treatment and increased use of better adjuvant chemotherapy) and multidisciplinary management (Thomson et al., 2004).

Risk factors and aetiology

Breast cancer occurs predominantly in women and is rare among men. The incidence increases with age, doubling every 10 years until menopause, when the rate of increase slows. A number of risk factors for breast

Practical Clinical Oncology, Second Edition, ed. Louise Hanna, Tom Crosby and Fergus Macbeth. Published by Cambridge University Press. © Cambridge University Press 2015.

Table 19.1 Tumours that affect the breast

Type	Examples
Benign	Fibroadenoma
	Solitary cyst
	Intraduct papilloma
	Adenomas
	Duct ectasia
	Epithelial hyperplasia (without atypia)
	Sclerosing adenosis
	Radial scar
	Complex sclerosing lesion
	Atypical ductal hyperplasia
	Atypical lobular hyperplasia
Malignant primary	*Carcinoma* in situ
	Tis (ductal carcinoma *in situ*)
	Tis (lobular carcinoma *in situ*)
	Tis (Paget)
	Invasive carcinoma
	Invasive ductal carcinoma NOS or NST (75% of cases)
	Invasive lobular carcinoma (10%)
	Medullary carcinoma (5%)
	Tubular carcinoma
	Mucinous (colloid) carcinoma
	Cribriform carcinoma
	Papillary carcinoma
	Adenoid cystic carcinoma
	Apocrine carcinoma
	Secretory carcinoma
	Squamous cell carcinoma
	Inflammatory carcinoma
	Paget's carcinoma
	Metaplastic carcinoma
	Others
	Phyllodes tumour
	Sarcomas
	Vascular tumours
	Lymphoma
Malignant secondary	Melanoma
	Lung
	Ovary
	Kidney
	Stomach
	Thyroid (medullary)
	Rhabdomyosarcoma (alveolar)

NOS, not otherwise specified; NST, no special type.

cancer have been identified and include reproductive factors, a history of benign disease, previous radiation exposure, exogenous hormone therapy, dietary factors and genetic factors.

Reproductive factors

Reproductive factors include early menarche (< 12 years) and late natural menopause (the risk of cancer is halved if natural menopause occurs before age 45 years compared with 55 years). Late age at first birth (age > 40 years) and nulliparity are also associated with an increased risk of breast cancer. Women who undergo bilateral oophorectomy before the age of 35 have a reduced risk compared to women who undergo a natural menopause.

Benign breast disease

Women who have had a history of cysts, fibroadenomas or benign proliferative hyperplasia have an increased risk of breast cancer.

Exposure to radiation

Radiation exposure increases the risk of breast cancer. Women who received ionising radiation to the chest for Hodgkin's lymphoma have an increased risk of developing breast cancer, particularly if radiation was given within 6 months of menarche (Cooke *et al.*, 2013).

Exogenous hormones

The Million Women study showed that HRT users were more likely to develop breast cancer than non-users (adjusted relative risk 1.66 [95% CI 1.58–1.75]; $p < 0.0001$; Beral *et al.*, 2003). The magnitude of risk was greater for women taking oestrogen and progestin in combination than for those taking oestrogen alone ($p < 0.0001$) and the risk was higher with increasing length of HRT use.

The HABITS trial (Hormonal replacement After Breast cancer – Is It Safe?) demonstrated that the use of HRT in the early years after breast cancer diagnosis

Table 19.2 Risk categories for breast cancer

Age categories	Near population risk	Moderate risk	High risk (includes patients with BRCA1 and 2 mutations)
Lifetime risk from age 20	< 17%	> 17% but < 30%	> 30%
Risk between ages 40 and 50	< 3%	3–8%	> 8%

Adapted from NICE, 2013a.

can increase the rate of breast cancer recurrence. In this trial, 447 women were randomised to either HRT or no HRT; at a median follow-up of 4 years, 39 women randomised to receive HRT had a breast cancer recurrence compared with 17 in the no HRT arm (Holmberg *et al.*, 2008).

The data for oral contraceptives (OCs) are less consistent than those for HRT. In a large meta-analysis, there was a small increased risk of having breast cancer diagnosed in women in the 10 years after stopping combined OC. The relative risk of breast cancer in current users was 1.24 (Anonymous, 1996), but the breast cancers that developed were less likely to have spread than those in women who have never used combined OC with a relative risk of 0.88 (0.81–0.95: 2p = 0.002).

Dietary factors

Dietary factors associated with an increased risk of developing breast cancer include obesity and increased alcohol intake. Obesity increases breast cancer risk in postmenopausal women by around 50%, probably by increasing the serum concentration of oestradiol and decreasing the serum concentration of sex hormone-binding globulin, causing a substantial increase in bioavailable oestradiol. Conversely, obesity in premenopausal women reduces breast cancer risk.

Genetic factors

Breast cancer risk is doubled in women with a first-degree relative with breast cancer, with a higher risk if more than one-first degree relative is affected or has breast cancer at a young age. The recent NICE (2013a) guidance on familial breast cancer recommends the use of a carrier probability calculation method to determine which women should be referred for genetic counselling (e.g. BOADICEA and the Manchester scoring system) and defines breast cancer risk categories (see Table 19.2).

Breast cancer may result from a mutation in one or more critical genes including BRCA1, BRCA2 and TP53.

BRCA1 is located on chromosome 17q21. BRCA1 mutations account for 2% of breast cancers, increase the risk of developing breast cancer by 35–85% and are associated with early-onset breast cancer. The lifetime risk of ovarian cancer is also increased up to 60%. BRCA1 tumours tend to have more malignant pathological features and are typically ER-, PgR- and HER2-negative, often with a basal-like phenotype (Sørlie *et al.*, 2003).

The BRCA2 gene is located on a region of chromosome arm13q. The BRCA2 mutation accounts for 1% of breast cancer, and it increases the chance of breast cancer by 20–60%. The gene is also associated with a 6% lifetime risk of male breast cancer and with an increased risk of develping other cancers, such as prostate, pancreas and bladder cancer, and non-Hodgkin lymphoma. BRCA2 tumours typically express ER and PgR and tend to be of higher grade with less tubule formation.

The TP53 gene is located on chromosome 17p13. An inherited mutation in TP53 (Li–Fraumeni syndrome) is associated with a 50% lifetime risk of developing breast cancer.

Ataxia–telangiectasia (A-T) is a rare autosomal recessive disorder that renders homozygous individuals more vulnerable to cancer because of an increased risk of mutation. A-T heterozygotes are about 0.5–1% of the general population and are probably breast cancer-prone.

Cowden's syndrome (PTEN) is an autosomal dominant condition. Half of the affected females have fibrocystic disease of the breast and breast cancer, of which one-third are bilateral. Other syndromes with increased risk of breast cancer include Muir–Torre syndrome and Peutz–Jeghers syndrome.

Pathology

Almost all breast carcinomas are adenocarcinomas arising from the epithelial cells that line the terminal duct lobular.

The anatomical distribution of breast tumours includes the upper outer quadrant (50%), upper inner quadrant (10%), lower inner quadrant (10%), lower outer quadrant (10%) and central (20%). Tumours in the upper outer quadrant carry the best prognosis.

Three per cent are diffuse tumours and 5% are multicentric (i.e. in different quadrants). Multifocal means that two or more foci of disease are in the same quadrant, although the terms multicentric and multifocal are often used interchangeably.

The prognosis of breast cancer depends on clinicopathological features such as histological grade, lymph node status, tumour size and biomarkers such as expression of ER and the assessment of HER2 status.

Grade

Breast cancers are graded according to the Nottingham grading system (Elston–Ellis modification of the Scarff–Bloom–Richardson system). The grade is based on the degree of tubule formation, nuclear pleomorphism and mitotic index (Table 19.3) to give an overall grade of: grade 1 (score 3–5), grade 2 (6–7) or grade 3 (8–9).

Hormone receptor status

The ER and PgR status are established by immunohistochemistry (IHC) and a semiquantitative measure is provided by the 'H-score'. About 20% of patients are true ER-negative by these criteria (i.e. the H-score is zero). Tumours are ER-positive in more than two-thirds of postmenopausal patients, but in fewer than half of those who are premenopausal. PgRs can be identified in some breast cancers; their presence depends on an intact ER pathway. About 20% of ER-negative tumours are PgR-positive and possible reasons for their ER-negative status include a very low-level expression of ER or a false-negative result. ER-negative PgR-positive tumours account for roughly 5% of all tumours and are likely to be hormone-responsive.

HER2/neu expression

HER2 expression can be assessed by IHC with an antibody that recognises cell surface receptors (the result scored as −, 1+, 2+ or 3+), by measuring the number of gene copies with fluorescent *in situ* hybridisation (FISH) or by the level of circulating receptor protein. HER2 positivity is established by either an IHC score of 3+ or a FISH amplification of 2.1 or greater. An IHC of 2+ should be confirmed by FISH.

Table 19.3 Grading of breast cancer

Description	Categories	Score
Degree of tubule formation	> 75%	1
	10–75%	2
	< 10%	3
Nuclear pleomorphism	Mild	1
	Moderate	2
	Severe	3
Mitotic index (no. of mitoses per high-powered field)	0–9	1
	10–19	2
	> 20	3

Molecular subtyping

Microarray-based gene expression of breast cancer has demonstrated that there are multiple molecular subtypes of breast cancer (luminal A, luminal B, HER2-positive and basal-like) and these subtypes correlate with prognosis (Perou *et al.*, 2000; Sørlie *et al.*, 2001). The use of the proliferation marker Ki-67 together with ER, PgR and HER2 status may be used as 'surrogates' to define the intrinsic subtype of breast cancer (Goldhirsch *et al.*, 2013b). Ki-67 is not used routinely across the UK, however. Table 19.4 defines the agreed surrogate definitions of the intrinsic subtypes of breast cancer using the St. Gallen criteria.

Lymph nodes

Nodal staging is determined from a histopathological assessment of the excised lymph node, as only 70% of involved nodes are detectable clinically or radiologically.

Involvement of axillary nodes occurs in up to 50% of cases of symptomatic breast cancer and in 10–20% of cases of screen-detected breast cancer.

More than 90% of women with metastases to the internal mammary nodes have axillary node involvement and, in the remaining 5–10%, most have tumours involving the medial half of the breast. Internal mammary nodes have evidence of tumour in 26% of patients with inner quadrant tumours and 15% with outer quadrant tumours. In patients with axillary-node-positive breast cancer, histological sampling of the internal mammary chain reveals occult disease in 20–50% of cases; however, routine sampling of these nodes is not standard practice in the UK.

Table 19.4 Surrogate definitions of intrinsic subtypes of breast cancer

Intrinsic subtype	Clinico-pathological definition
Luminal A	**'Luminal A-like'**
	all of:
	ER and PgR positive
	HER2 negative
	Ki-67 'low'
	Recurrence risk 'low' based on multi-gene expression assay
Luminal B	**'Luminal B-like (HER2 negative)'**
	ER positive
	HER2 negative
	And *at least one of:*
	Ki-67 'high'
	PgR 'negative or low'
	Recurrence risk 'high' based on multi-gene assay
	'Luminal B-like (HER2 positive)'
	ER positive
	HER2 overexpressed or amplified
	Any Ki-67
	Any PgR
HER2 positive	**'HER2 positive (non-luminal)'**
	HER2 overexpressed or amplified
	ER and PgR absent
'Basal-like'	**'Triple negative (ductal)'**
	ER and PgR absent
	HER2 negative

Adapted from Goldhirsch *et al.* (2013b).

Spread

Routes of cancer spread include direct local spread to the chest wall, lymphatic spread and haemotogenous spread.

Lymphatic spread first involves the regional lymph nodes: the ipsilateral axillary (levels I, II and III), infra-clavicular, internal mammary and supraclavicular nodes. Any other lymph node metastasis is coded as a distant metastasis. Tumours from any site in the breast can spread to any nodal site. Internal mammary nodes are more likely to be involved in patients who also have axillary nodal disease.

Haematogenous spread moves to bone, lung, liver, brain, skin and so forth. The lobular subtype of breast cancer can spread to less-typical sites such as the gastrointestinal tract and ovary (Arpino *et al.*, 2004).

Screening and prevention

Screening

The aim of screening is to reduce mortality from breast cancer by detecting and treating it at an earlier stage. In the UK the current target screening age is 50–70 years. Women below the age of 50 are not invited for screening because the incidence of cancer is lower and the density of the breast tissue makes cancers more difficult to detect. Women over 70 years are still entitled to breast screening, although they will not be routinely invited to attend. There should be two views on the mammogram: mediolateral oblique and cranio-caudal. Taking two views rather than one increases the detection rate by 43%. The recall rate after mammography is approximately 4% across the UK with 1% going on to have a biopsy and 0.95% of the total number of women screened being diagnosed with either invasive or *in situ* cancer (NHS Cancer Screening Programmes, 2012). Mammography is less effective in women under the age of 35 because the breast is relatively radiodense. With modern screening a radiation dose of less than 1.5 mGy is standard. More information about breast cancer screening can be found at www.cancerscreening.nhs.uk (accessed December 2014).

Women with high or moderate risk of breast cancer can be offered screening with annual mammography or MRI scanning according to age and risk category (NICE, 2013a). Annual mammographic screening is offered to women aged 40–49 years at moderate and high risk of breast cancer. MRI surveillance is offered annually to women aged 30–49 with known or a > 30% risk of a BRCA1 or BRCA2 mutation and from age 20 if known or > 30% risk of TP53 mutation.

Prevention

There is no proven role for breast cancer prevention in the general population. Options for prevention in women at high risk of breast cancer include chemoprevention and prophylactic surgery.

Chemoprevention

Tamoxifen and raloxifene for 5 years are both recommended for chemoprevention in women at high risk of breast cancer, unless they are at risk or have a history of thromboembolic disease or endometrial cancer (NICE, 2013a). Neither drug has a UK licence for this indication. Anastrozole has been shown to reduce the incidence of breast cancer in women at high risk at 5 years compared with placebo from 4% to 2% (Cuzick *et al.*, 2014).

Prophylactic surgery

Women at high risk of breast cancer may choose to undergo prophylactic mastectomy which significantly reduces the risk of subsequent breast cancer. All women considering this should be given the option of reconstructive surgery (immediate or delayed).

Clinical presentation

Breast lump

A malignant breast nodule is usually solitary, unilateral, solid, hard, irregular, non-mobile and non-tender. A painful lump or lumpiness, breast distortion or pain alone should be taken seriously but are less likely to be associated with an underlying malignancy.

Skin changes

The skin may show thickening, redness, dimpling and/or inflammation. Skin dimpling or a change in contour is present in up to 25% of patients with breast cancer. A diffuse dimpling or *peau d'orange* (like orange peel) is caused by infiltration of the tumour into the subcutaneous lymphatic channels.

Nipple changes

Thickening and loss of elasticity, causing flattening or inversion of the nipple, is suspicious if it is a new finding in a breast. A persistent scaly or eczema-like lesion may be an indication of Paget's disease. Spontaneous discharge in patients older than 50 years of age is likely to be caused by carcinoma.

Regional disease

Malignant axillary lymphadenopathy is usually caused by the presence of an ipsilateral breast cancer. In the absence of evidence of another primary source of disease, patients should be managed the same as they would be for the equivalent stage of primary breast cancer where the primary has been locally resected.

Metastatic disease

Signs or symptoms of metastatic disease, most commonly affecting bone, liver, lung, brain and skin, are sometimes the presenting feature of breast cancer.

Screening

Breast cancer can present as a result of a primary screening programme in the general population, during follow-up from a previously treated breast cancer, or during screening carried out because of a strong family history. Around one-third of all breast cancers diagnosed in the UK are screen-detected.

Investigations

Triple assessment

After a complete history, triple assessment is performed including: physical examination, radiological investigation and needle biopsy. Each assessment is recorded to give a level of suspicion of malignancy from 1 (normal) to 5 (malignant) with the prefix indicating the assessment method (P = physical examination, M or R = mammogram, U = US, C = cytology and B = biopsy). Core biopsy is preferred over fine-needle aspiration as it has the advantage of providing a histological diagnosis and can differentiate between invasive and *in situ* carcinoma. The ER, PgR and HER2 status can also be tested on a biopsy specimen.

Cytology is reported as follows.

- C1 – inadequate.
- C2 – benign.
- C3 – suspicious probably benign.
- C4 – suspicious probably malignant.
- C5 – malignant epithelial cells.

Biopsy is reported as follows.

- B1 – normal breast tissue, no lesion to account for imaging findings is present (i.e. probably missed).
- B2 – benign.
- B3 – benign but may be associated with more malignant lesions nearby (i.e. diagnostic excision is necessary, e.g. atypical ductal hyperplasia or papillary lesions).
- B4 – suspicious, probably malignant, but core is crushed or there is too little tumour present (insufficient evidence for malignant diagnosis).
- B5 – malignant tumour present, either DCIS or invasive carcinoma. A provisional type and grade is usually given if possible.

Table 19.5 The T staging of breast cancer

T stage	Description
Tis	Tis (DCIS), Tis (LCIS), Tis (Paget)
T1	≤ 2 cm
T1mic	≤ 0.1 cm
T1a	> 0.1 to 0.5 cm
T1b	> 0.5 to 1 cm
T1c	> 1 to 2 cm
T2	> 2 to 5 cm
T3	> 5 cm
T4	Chest wall[a]/skin
T4a	Chest wall[a]
T4b	Skin oedema (including peau d'orange), ulceration, satellite skin nodules
T4c	Both 4a and 4b
T4d	Inflammatory carcinoma

[a] Chest wall includes ribs, intercostal muscles and serratus anterior muscle but not pectoral muscle. Dimpling of skin, nipple retraction, or other skin changes, except those in T4b and T4d, may occur in T1, T2 or T3 without affecting the classification. DCIS, ductal carcinoma *in situ*; LCIS, lobular carcinoma *in situ*. Adapted from UICC (2009).

Other tests

A full blood count, liver function tests and serum calcium level should be taken.

Patients with T1 and T2 primary breast tumours have a 2% incidence of metastatic disease, and routine staging of asymptomatic patients for metastases is not indicated. In patients with advanced (T3/T4) disease the incidence of metastatic disease is 15–20%. Staging investigations are carried out on these patients if it will affect management and include chest X-ray, liver ultrasound and bone scan. The choice of staging investigation in symptomatic patients may include CT scan (thorax/abdomen) and bone scan. MRI scanning is recommended for patients with symptoms of brachial plexopathy (Barter and Britton, 2014).

Bone marrow aspiration is performed if there is an unexplained cytopenia or a leucoerythroblastic blood smear.

Staging

The staging of breast cancer is determined by the American Joint Committee on Cancer (AJCC) and is a clinical and pathological staging system based on the

TNM classification (UICC, 2009). Table 19.5 shows the T staging for breast cancer, Table 19.6 shows the N and M staging for breast cancer and Table 19.7 shows the staging groupings for breast cancer.

Treatment: non-invasive carcinoma of the breast (Tis)

Non-invasive carcinoma of the breast comprises ductal carcinoma *in situ* (DCIS), lobular carcinoma *in situ* (LCIS) and Paget's disease of the nipple. The management of Paget's disease of the nipple is discussed later in the chapter.

Ductal carcinoma *in situ* (DCIS)

DCIS is a true premalignant condition. Between 30% and 50% of women with untreated DCIS will develop invasive breast cancer in the ipsilateral breast within 10 years of diagnosis. The most common mammographic finding in DCIS is branching microcalcification localised to a small region of breast. DCIS accounts for 20–25% of all cancer detected by screening. HER2 amplification and TP53 mutation are often found. DCIS is graded as low, intermediate and high grade, dependent on cellular features, presence of necrosis and number of mitoses. The prognosis of DCIS is associated with size, grade, distance to the resection margin and age.

Treatment options in DCIS

Surgery

Wide local excision (WLE) is the preferred treatment for localised DCIS, usually followed by adjuvant radiotherapy. If a WLE is performed, margin status can predict future recurrence. The aim is to achieve a margin status of at least 1 mm.

Mastectomy *with or without* reconstruction is recommended in patients with widespread disease (disease in two or more quadrants) or in cases in which surgical margins free of carcinoma cannot be obtained.

Axillary dissection or sampling is not recommended in cases of pure DCIS. Sentinel node biopsy is generally not needed in cases of DCIS, unless invasive cancer cannot be definitively excluded; for example, when microcalcifications are incompletely removed, or if there is extensive microcalcification or multicentric disease and a mastectomy is planned.

Table 19.6 N and M staging of breast cancer

N stage	Description	pN stage	Description
N1	Movable axillary	PN1mi	Micrometastasis > 0.2 mm ≤ 2 mm
		pN1a	1–3 axillary nodes
		pN1b	Internal mammary nodes with microscopic metastasis by sentinel node biopsy but not clinically apparent
		pN1c	1–3 axillary nodes and internal mammary nodes with microscopic metastasis by sentinel node biopsy but not clinically apparent
N2a	Axillary	pN2a	4–9 axillary nodes including at least one that is 2 mm
N2b	Internal mammary clinically detected	pN2b	Internal mammary nodes, clinically detected, without axillary nodes
N3a	Infraclavicular	pN3a	≥ 10 axillary nodes or infraclavicular node(s)
N3b	Internal mammary and axillary	pN3b	Internal mammary nodes, clinically detected, with axillary node(s) or > 3 axillary nodes and internal mammary nodes with microscopic metastasis by sentinel node biopsy but not clinically detected
N3c	Supraclavicular	pN3c	Supraclavicular
M stage description			
MX Distant metastasis cannot be assessed			
M0 No distant metastasis			
M1 Distant metastasis			

Adapted from UICC (2009).

Table 19.7 Stage groupings for breast cancer

Stage		Description	
Stage 0	Tis	N0	M0
Stage IA	T1[a]	N0	M0
Stage IB	T0	N1mi	M0
	T1	N1mi	M0
Stage IIA	T0	N1	M0
	T1[a]	N1	M0
	T2	N0	M0
Stage IIB	T2	N1	M0
	T3	N0	M0
Stage IIIA	T0	N2	M0
	T1[a]	N2	M0
	T2	N2	M0
	T3	N1, N2	M0
Stage IIIB	T4	N0, N1, N2	M0
Stage IIIC	Any T	N3	M0
Stage IV	Any T	Any N	M1

[a] T1 includes T1mic < 0.1 cm microinvasion. Adapted from UICC (2009).

Radiotherapy

Women who undergo breast-conserving surgery for DCIS should be offered adjuvant radiotherapy with an explanation of the benefits and risks. A scoring index for DCIS (Van Nuys Prognostic Index) is shown in Table 19.8, and a suggested management strategy based on the scoring system is shown in Table 19.9 (Silverstein, 2003). However, a recent systematic review has demonstrated that radiotherapy reduces local recurrence following breast-conserving surgery across all subgroups of women with DCIS (Goodwin, 2013). There is no prospective trial evidence to demonstrate whether there is a subgroup of women who do not benefit from radiotherapy for local control. Radiotherapy has no effect on survival in DCIS.

Endocrine therapy

Tamoxifen has been shown to reduce the rate of ipsilateral and contralateral DCIS; however, this benefit is small (Fisher *et al.*, 1999; Cuzick *et al.*, 2011). Tamoxifen does not affect survival and the use of tamoxifen must be balanced with its adverse effects. The IBIS II DCIS trial (closed to recruitment) is examining the use of

Table 19.8 A scoring system for DCIS

Score components	Definition
Margins[a]	
1	≥ 10 mm
2	1–9 mm
3	< 1 mm
Histological subtype	
1	Grades 1–2, no necrosis
2	Grades 1–2, necrosis present
3	Grade 3
Size	
1	≤ 1.5 cm
2	1.6–4 cm
3	> 4 cm
Age	
1	> 60 years
2	40–60 years
3	< 40 years

[a] The margin in DCIS is considered negative if it is > 10 mm; it is inadequate if it is < 1 mm. There is no uniform consensus if the margin is 1–10 mm. DCIS, ductal carcinoma *in situ*. Adapted from Silverstein (2003).

Table 19.9 Management of DCIS

Van Nuys Prognostic Index Score	Ten-year local recurrence rate (%)	Management
4–6	3	WLE
7–9	27	WLE + RT
10–12	66	Mastectomy

RT, radiotherapy; WLE, wide local excision. Adapted from Silverstein (2003).

anastrozole compared with tamoxifen following surgery for DCIS.

Lobular carcinoma *in situ* (LCIS)

LCIS is not thought to be a true premalignant condition, but rather a marker of increased risk of breast cancer. It is associated with approximately a 30% lifetime risk of developing an invasive carcinoma. The invasive cancer is usually ductal and may be present in the same or the opposite breast.

LCIS is found predominantly in premenopausal women; it is almost always multicentric in the breast and bilateral in about one-third of cases. LCIS cells are commonly ER-positive, whereas the overexpression of ERBB2 and TP53 are uncommon. LCIS is not clinically palpable or detectable by mammography, but is identified incidentally in about 1% of benign breast biopsies.

For treatment of LCIS, observation alone is the preferred option because the risk of developing invasive cancer is low (21% over 15 years). The histology of the invasive cancer tends to be favourable.

Pleomorphic LCIS is a variant of LCIS which tends to behave like DCIS. Due to the increased risk of local recurrence, there may be a role for adjuvant treatment with radiotherapy. There is no current evidence for the benefit of radiotherapy for patients with pleomorphic LCIS (Masannat *et al.*, 2013).

Bilateral mastectomy *with or without* reconstruction is preferred in special circumstances (such as a strong family history of invasive breast cancer or non-genetic predisposition) because the risk of invasive breast cancer after a diagnosis of LCIS is equal in both breasts.

Management of early breast cancer

Surgery in breast cancer

Primary disease

Modified radical mastectomy

Modified radical mastectomy involves removal of the entire breast, nipple and areola and is usually combined with an axillary node dissection (see discussion that follows).

Breast-conserving surgery

Breast conservation therapy (BCT) consists of WLE and postoperative RT. Systematic reviews have shown similar outcomes for BCT and mastectomy (Morris *et al.*, 1997; Fisher *et al.*, 2002; Veronesi *et al.*, 2002). The NSABP B-06 trial (Fisher *et al.*, 2002) randomised 1851 women with invasive breast cancer and negative margins to modified radical mastectomy, or lumpectomy plus axillary dissection and RT, or lumpectomy plus axillary dissection alone. There was no significant difference in the overall or disease-free survival at 20 years, but there was a significant difference in local recurrence (LR) at 20 years between lumpectomy plus

RT and lumpectomy alone (14.3% versus 39.2%; $p < 0.001$).

The most important surgical factor influencing LR is the completeness of excision. Current practice aims to achieve microscopically disease-free margins of at least 1 mm and it is unacceptable to have tumour cells at the surgical margin without further excision. The acceptable size of the margin is influenced by which margin is the closest and the need to minimise the degree of mutilation (e.g. the deep margin or skin margin cannot be easily increased). In cases of a positive margin, the patient should have a further excision to achieve a clear margin, but if this would lead to an unacceptable cosmetic outcome, or the patient chooses, a mastectomy should be done. It may be a reasonable option to treat selected cases with BCT using a microscopically focally positive margin in the absence of extensive intraductal tumour by RT together with a boost.

The absolute contraindications for BCT and RT include:

- previous RT to the breast or chest wall;
- RT during pregnancy;
- appearance of diffuse suspicious or malignant microcalcifications;
- widespread disease that cannot be removed by WLE through a single incision to achieve clear margins and a satisfactory cosmetic result;
- positive pathologic margin.

  Relative contraindications include:

- active connective tissue disease involving the skin (especially scleroderma and lupus);
- tumour larger than 5 cm;
- focally positive margin.

Management of the axilla

Until recently, axillary dissection (levels 1–3) was the preferred technique for all women with invasive breast cancer and at least 10 lymph nodes were needed for pathologic evaluation to accurately stage the axilla (NIH Consensus Conference, 1991).

Axillary node clearance involves clearing the axillary contents from the volume bounded by the axillary skin laterally; latissimus dorsi, teres major and subscapularis posteriorly; the lower border of the axillary vein superiorly; pectoralis muscles anteriorly; and the chest wall medially. Axillary node clearance is associated with significant morbidity including axillary pain and numbness, decreased range of arm movement, and chronic lymphoedema.

The lymph nodes of the axilla are described as levels I, II and III; these nodes are in continuity with each other, but the concept of axillary node levels is useful when discussing the extent of axillary node surgery.

Level I- lateral to the pectoralis minor

Level II- beneath pectoralis minor

Level III- superomedial to pectoralis minor

With the advent of breast screening, approximately 60–80% of women are node-negative at presentation and axillary lymph node dissection is considered overtreatment. Sentinel lymph node biopsy (SLNB) has emerged as a minimally invasive procedure that accurately assesses axillary node status (Cody *et al.*, 1999; Veronesi *et al.*, 2003; Mansel *et al.*, 2006).

The SLN (or nodes) is the first node in the regional lymphatic basin to which a tumour drains. Localisation of the SLN is possible by injecting blue dye and a radioactive colloid tracer around the tumour (peritumoural), into the dermis (subdermal) or under the nipple (subareolar), but only peritumoural injections map accurately to the internal mammary lymph nodes. The first nodal station or SLN are detectable either as visible blue nodes or as radioactive nodes detected by a hand probe. The combination of blue dye and radioisotope gives better results than either agent alone.

Localisation rates of over 95% and false-negative rates of less than 5% are possible after an initial learning curve. Compared to conventional axillary dissection, at 6 months, overall arm morbidity is less and quality of life is better. However, it is important that SLNB should meet all the following criteria.

- It should be performed by an experienced surgical team.
- The node should be clinically negative at the time of diagnosis.
- The patient should have no previous chemotherapy or hormonal therapy.

The current recommendation for women with a positive SLNB is for an axillary node clearance to be performed as a separate procedure; this invariably adds delay to any adjuvant therapy. One option to avoid a second procedure is to use intraoperative node analysis, and proceed directly to axillary node surgery if the SLN is positive. Intraoperative node analysis involves analysing a SLN at time of surgery to detect the presence of a biomarker for metastases. The two methods available are the RD-100i OSNA system and the Metasin test. The RD-100i OSNA system has been recommended by NICE as an option for detecting SLN metastases during surgery (NICE, 2013c).

Two recent studies have examined whether further axillary surgery is required in women with SLN-positive breast cancer. The Z0011 study (Giuliano *et al.*, 2011) randomised women with T1–2 breast cancer, who were clinically node-negative and were found to have 1–2 SLNs positive at the time of breast conserving surgery to either further axillary dissection or observation alone. The trial closed early because of a lower-than-expected mortality rate after 891 patients were recruited (of a planned 1900). After 6 years of follow-up there was no difference between the treatment arms in terms of overall survival or disease-free survival. The morbidity was lower in the observation arm. The Z0011 trial has led some to advocate no further surgery in women with minimal lymph node-positive disease (a significant proportion of women in both arms had micrometastases in the SLN). All patients received postoperative radiotherapy to the preserved breast and formal nodal irradiation was not allowed. There was no detailed information about the radiotherapy, and it is therefore impossible to know to what extent the lower axillary region was included in the tangential radiation fields.

The AMAROS trial randomised women with SLN-positive disease to either further surgery or axillary node irradiation (Rutgers *et al.*, 2013). The trial included 4806 women with T1–2 invasive breast cancer; all patients were randomised before axillary surgery. Seven hundred and forty-four patients in the surgical arm had a positive SLNB and 681 in the radiotherapy arm. At a median follow-up of 6 years there was no difference in overall survival or disease-free survival between the two treatment arms. There was less lymphoedema in the radiotherapy arm. The radiotherapy delivered within AMAROS was subject to rigorous quality assurance with a specified dose of 50 Gy in 25 fractions, and a target volume which included levels 1, 2 and 3 of the axilla plus the medial supraclavicular nodes.

The POSNOC trial is a non-inferiority trial randomising women with 1–2 positive SLN to no further axillary treatment or further axillary treatment (which can be with either axillary node dissection or axillary radiotherapy). Further details can be found at http://public.ukcrn.org.uk/search/StudyDetail.aspx?StudyID=16069 (accessed December 2014).

Breast reconstruction

Breast reconstruction should be offered to women with breast cancer who are undergoing mastectomy. Immediate reconstruction has economic benefits, produces better results and reduces psychosocial morbidity compared with delayed reconstruction. There is no absolute contraindication for immediate reconstruction. Relative contraindications include ischaemic heart disease, obesity, diabetes, steroid treatment, smoking and metastatic disease. Delayed reconstruction should be considered when there is a concern about tumour clearance or when postoperative RT is planned. If radiotherapy is required after reconstructive surgery there is little evidence for the safety of hypofractionated regimens.

A variety of breast reconstruction procedures are used.

- Myocutaneous flap reconstruction, using the latissimus dorsi (LD) muscle or the transverse rectus abdominus myocutaneous flap.
- An extended LD reconstruction combined with a skin-sparing mastectomy, which may or may not require an implant.
- Insertion of a breast prosthesis. A tissue expander is gradually inflated. When it is an adequate size it is removed and replaced by a permanent prosthesis which often contains silicone.
- The LD muscle and fat without overlying skin can also be used to fill defects in the breast following WLE for large tumours. The reconstruction is done as a second procedure after the histology of the WLE with a complete excision.
- Lipomodelling can be used to fill defects in the breast with the aim of restoring shape and volume to the breast.

Adjuvant radiotherapy

Role of radiotherapy following breast conserving surgery

Adjuvant whole-breast RT following breast-conserving surgery (BCS) is considered to be standard and has been shown to halve the risk of local recurrence among all subgroups of women (EBCTCG, 2011). This meta-analysis of individual data for 10,801 women in 17 trials of radiotherapy versus no radiotherapy after BCS showed that the 10-year risk of any recurrence was reduced from 35% to 19%. Radiotherapy has also been shown to reduce the risk of breast cancer death at 15 years from 20.5% to 17.2% with one cancer death avoided for every four recurrences prevented.

For women at low risk of local recurrence the absolute benefit of radiotherapy is small and a number of trials have examined whether radiotherapy can be safely omitted in older women (> 70 years) with low-risk cancers and clear margins. One study randomised 636 women aged > 70 years with clinical stage T1 N0 M0 ER-positive breast cancers treated with BCS to tamoxifen plus radiotherapy or to tamoxifen alone. At 12 years follow-up, 98% of the women who received radiotherapy were recurrence-free compared with 90% of the women who did not receive radiotherapy; there was no difference in survival (Hughes *et al.*, 2013). The PRIME 2 trial randomised 1326 women aged > 65 years with T1–2 N0 M0 ER-positive breast cancer (with clear margins) to adjuvant hormonal therapy alone or hormonal therapy plus radiotherapy. At 5 years follow-up the risk of ipsilateral tumour recurrence was 1.3% with radiotherapy and 4.1% without (Kunkler *et al.*, 2013).

RT is usually given after the patient has finished adjuvant chemotherapy. Radiation given concurrently with anthracycline-based regimens or taxanes is not recommended. Although some centres avoid the use of concurrent tamoxifen with RT because of theoretical concerns that residual tumour cells may be put into growth arrest and therefore be resistant to radiation, trials have not substantiated this concern (Ahn *et al.*, 2005; Harris *et al.*, 2005). There have been no prospective studies of concurrent hormone therapy and radiation.

The optimal timing of radiotherapy after BCS is not well defined. The effect of a delay (ranging from more than 77 days to up to 16 weeks) in starting radiotherapy has been examined in many retrospective series with the majority suggesting there is no reduction in locoregional control with delayed radiotherapy (Hershman *et al.*, 2006; Vujovic *et al.*, 2006; Livi *et al.*, 2009; Karlsson *et al.*, 2011), although it is considered good practice to start radiotherapy as soon as possible after surgery (if no chemotherapy is given).

Role of a radiation boost to the breast

A radiation boost delivered to the tumour bed has been shown to reduce the risk of local recurrence but is associated with a poorer cosmetic outcome. The EORTC boost versus no boost trials randomised 5318 patients with a microscopically complete excision (no tumour at inked margin) to an additional 16 Gy in 8 fractions or no additional RT. All patients received postoperative

RT of 50 Gy in 25 fractions. At 10 years the cumulative incidence of local recurrence was 10.2% without a boost and 6.2% with a boost ($P < 0.001$). The relative risk reduction was the same for all women regardless of age, but the absolute benefit was greatest for women aged < 40 years, with a reduction in risk from 23.99% to 13.5% (Bartelink *et al.*, 2007).

Current practice is to recommend a boost to women aged < 40 years and in women deemed at higher risk of local recurrence (e.g. positive margins, grade 3 tumours, positive lymphovascular invasion).

Role of post-mastectomy radiotherapy

Although several individual trials have shown a survival advantage for using RT after mastectomy (Overgaard *et al.*, 2004; Ragaz *et al.*, 2005), it is not considered necessary in patients who have a low risk of recurrence (node-negative, T1–2 and grade 1–2).

Women at high risk of local recurrence should be offered post-mastectomy radiotherapy routinely (T3–T4, ≥ 4 positive lymph nodes and excision margin < 1 mm).

For women with an intermediate risk of recurrence, the benefit of radiotherapy has been less certain. The SUPREMO study randomised women with 1–3 positive lymph nodes or high-risk node-negative disease (grade 3, T2 disease) to either radiotherapy or no radiotherapy. Results are awaited.

The recent EBCTCG meta-analysis has examined the effect of post-mastectomy radiotherapy in node-negative, node positive (1–3) and 4 + node-positive women. This confirms there is no additional benefit for radiotherapy in women with node-negative disease. In women with 1–3 positive lymph nodes the local recurrence rate was reduced, as was breast cancer mortality by the addition of radiotherapy (EBCTCG, 2014). In view of these findings, it would be reasonable to recommend post-mastectomy radiotherapy to women with 1–3 positive lymph nodes.

Radiotherapy to the regional lymphatics

RT to the ipsilateral SCF is associated with a reduced risk of recurrence at this site and is used in patients with the highest risk of disease such as those with more than four positive axillary lymph nodes. Axillary RT is not necessary after a complete axillary clearance. The lymph node failure rates are very low, and combined treatment to the axilla is associated with a much higher risk of lymphoedema (38.3% after axillary clearance and RT compared with 7.4% after axillary clearance alone; $p < 0.001$; Fisher *et al.*, 1980; Kissin *et al.*, 1986).

As discussed previously, radiotherapy to the axilla may be offered as an alternative to further axillary surgery in women with 1–2 positive SLNs following the AMAROS results (Rutgers *et al.*, 2013). Other indications for axillary radiotherapy include incomplete macroscopic excision and in cases where there is extensive extranodal spread.

The role of nodal irradiation in women at intermediate risk of recurrence is less certain. The MA20 trial randomised women with node-positive (1–3) or high-risk node-negative breast cancer to either whole breast RT (WBrRT) or to WBrRT + nodal irradiation. The nodal irradiation included the level 3 axillary lymph nodes, SCF nodes and internal mammary nodes. At ten years follow up there was no difference in overall survival between the two groups. There was an improvement in disease free survival of 82% in the nodal RT group and 77% in the breast RT group. This was balanced against an increased risk of pneumonitis and lymphoedema (8.4% compared with 4.5%) (Whelan *et al.*, 2015).

RT to the internal mammary nodes (IMNs) is controversial because recurrence at this site is very rare and most patients at risk receive adjuvant systemic therapy. The IMNs are difficult to treat because their exact position is often uncertain, and the RT fields that include them irradiate more normal tissue, possibly increasing the risk of cardiac complications (Arriagada *et al.*, 1988; Le *et al.*, 1990). If the internal mammary lymph nodes are known to be involved then radiotherapy can be considered.

Radiotherapy technique

Positioning

The patient is positioned supine on an angled 'breast board' with the aim of making sure the sternum is horizontal. One or both arms are abducted. For patients with very large breasts, a prone position may be used, but is not common practice in the UK. A foot rest is used to prevent the patient slipping down the breast board.

Localisation

Conventional orthogonal X-ray films or CT scanning is used. Increasingly, CT scanning is used as this allows for 3D planning. One disadvantage of CT localisation is that some patients may not fit into the bore of the CT scanner on the standard breast board. Tattoos are placed in the midline and laterally (both sides).

Target volume

- For postoperative RT to the breast, there is no GTV. The CTV is the glandular breast tissue down to the deep fascia as defined by palpation and CT scan. The PTV is the CTV with a 1 cm margin, usually allowing 5 mm skin-sparing. The PTV extends down to the deep fascia, but the treatment volume will include the ribcage and pectoral major. Following a mastectomy, the CTV includes the skin flaps, but not the muscle or the rib cage. Bolus may be used to reduce skin-sparing in women deemed at high risk of skin involvement (inflammatory tumours, positive skin margins).

- The CTV for the tumour bed boost is determined using preoperative imaging and operation notes. It is recommended that all patients have tumour bed clips placed at time of BCS to allow for better localisation of the tumour bed.

- The CTV for nodal irradiation usually includes the nodes of the SCF and level 3 axillary lymph nodes. If axillary lymph node irradiation is being used instead of axillary surgery, the target volume will include levels 1–3 of the axilla and the medial SCF nodes.

- The RTOG breast contouring atlas can be used to aid target volume definition (http://www.rtog.org/LinkClick.aspx?fileticket=vzJFhPaBipE%3d&tabid=236, accessed December 2014).

Field borders

- For conventional planning with orthogonal films, glandular breast tissue cannot be visualised, and a target volume is marked with approximate field borders as below. Tangential fields:

  - Medial – midline.
  - Lateral – mid-axillary line.
  - Superior – suprasternal notch.
  - Inferior – 1 cm below the breast tissue.
  - Deep – incorporating a maximum of 2–3 cm of lung.

- SCF and axillary field:

  - Medial – 1 cm lateral to the midline.
  - Lateral (SCF only) – the apical surgical clip defining the medial extent of axillary surgery or 1 cm lateral to the outer border of the first rib if no clips are used.
  - Lateral (SCF + axilla) – to cover axillary region laterally

- Superior – 3 cm above the clavicle; the C7/T1 junction.
- Inferior – matched to the tangential fields.
- Matching the tangential fields to a SCF field may be difficult. A skin gap is the simplest matching technique, but risks underdosing in the gap. Non-divergent beams may be created using half-beam blocking or a collimator twist.

Field arrangement (breast and chest wall)

Tangential fields are used (lateral and medial) to cover the PTV while minimising volume of lung and heart included.

Field arrangement (SCF and axilla)

For the SCF alone a single anterior field is used. When the axilla is treated, a posterior beam may be required to ensure adequate coverage of the axillary contents, particularly if the mid axillary dose is < 80% of the prescribed dose. The majority of the dose will be delivered through the anterior beam.

Dose

- 40 Gy in 15 fractions over 3 weeks has been adopted as standard practice in the UK following the publication of the START trial which showed no difference in locoregional relapse rates and less late toxicity with 40 Gy compared with 50 Gy in 25 fractions (Haviland et al., 2013).
- Alternative dose regimens include 50 Gy in 25 fractions and 45 Gy in 20 fractions.
- There is increasing interest in adjuvant breast radiotherapy with fewer, larger fractions. The FAST trial randomised 915 women (age > 50 years) with node-negative breast cancer to either 50 Gy in 25 fractions or 28.5 Gy or 30 Gy in 5 once-weekly fractions of 5.7 Gy or 6.0 Gy. At 3 years of follow-up, the 28.5 Gy arm was comparable to 50 Gy in 25 fractions in terms of cosmesis, but the 30 Gy fractionation was found to adversely affect cosmetic appearance (FAST trialists group et al., 2011).
- The FAST-Forward trial has completed recruitment of 4000 women. This trial randomised women between 40 Gy in 15 fractions compared to two other schedules, 27 Gy in 5 fractions over one week or 26 Gy in 5 fractions over one week.
- Patients who are being treated with palliative intent (fungating tumours) may be given 36 Gy in 6 fractions treating once a week with weekly review to assess skin reaction.

Planning considerations

Additional 'mini-fields' may be used to improve dose homogeneity and reduce the areas receiving > 105–107%. The use of additional fields (described as 'forward-planned IMRT' in many studies) has been shown to reduce the acute toxicity of breast radiotherapy (Pignol et al., 2008) and also leads to an improvement in late cosmesis (Donovan et al., 2007; Mukesh et al., 2013). Figure 19.1 shows a RT plan for a postoperative treatment for carcinoma of the breast.

Organs at risk

The organs at risk (OAR) include the lung and heart (left-sided treatment only). Dose constraints for the heart and lung have been defined within the START and FAST-Forward trials:

ipsilateral lung- maximum depth of 2.0 cm or V30% ≤ 17%

heart- maximum depth of 1.0 cm or V25% ≤ 5% and V5% ≤ 30%

If dose constraints cannot be met, MLC shielding may be used (ensuring adequate coverage of the tumour bed). A breath-hold technique can be used to remove the heart from the treated volume. The patient is treated during deep inspiratory breath-hold. A number of techniques have been described to achieve this.

The current UK HeartSpare (stage II) study is assessing whether voluntary deep-inspiratory breath-hold confirms effective heart-sparing in a multicentre setting (http://public.ukcrn.org.uk/search/StudyDetail .aspx?StudyID=14269, accessed December 2014).

The role of partial-breast radiotherapy

Partial-breast radiotherapy has become popular in many countries and there are a number of different techniques described, including external beam radiotherapy, single-source balloon catheter brachytherapy (MammoSite®), interstitial brachytherapy or intraoperative RT. Accelerated partial-breast irradiation (APBI) uses two fractions per day over one week, with radiation given only to the breast tissue closest to the site of the excised tumour.

The RAPID trial compared the use of ABPI radiation to the tumour bed using 3D-conformal radiotherapy with standard WBrRT and found an increased rate of poor cosmesis with ABPI (Olivotto et al., 2013). The NSABP B-39 study (which closed to recruitment

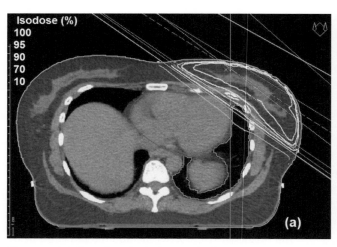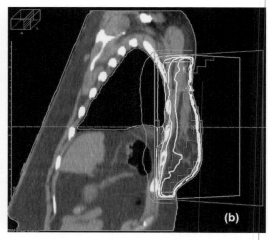

Figure 19.1 A 3D conformal radiotherapy plan for postoperative carcinoma of the breast. (a) Axial view; (b) sagittal view. In addition to the main tangential fields, small 'filler fields' have been added to improve the dose distribution and to meet the ICRU recommendations. For OARs, note how the choice of beam angles has minimised the amount of radiation received by the heart and left lung, which have been outlined to allow the dose to these organs to be calculated.

in 2013) randomised over 4000 women to either WBrRT (50 Gy in 25 fractions) or ABPI delivered by multi-catheter brachytherapy, single-entry intracavitary brachytherapy or 3D conformal radiotherapy. The UK IMPORT LOW trial has now closed; this trial compared the use of partial breast irradiation in women at low risk of recurrence (using standard fractionation to the tumour bed).

Intraoperative radiotherapy is delivered as a single dose during surgery with either electrons (6–9 MeV) or via an Intrabeam® device with 50 kV photons. The ELIOT trial compared 21 Gy intraoperative radiotherapy with electrons to standard WBrRT (50 Gy in 25 fractions with boost as needed). At 5 years the rate of ipsilateral tumour bed recurrence was higher with intraoperative radiotherapy (Veronesi *et al.*, 2013). The TARGIT-A trial used the Intrabeam® device to deliver 20 Gy to the surface of the tumour bed using 50 kV photons compared with standard WBrRT. Patients in the intraoperative arm of the trial could also receive EBRT if adverse histological features were found. The TARGIT-A trial showed non-inferiority when compared with standard WBrRT (Vaidya *et al.*, 2014).

Adjuvant systemic therapy: general

When to offer adjuvant therapy

For the adjuvant treatment in early breast cancer, international, national and local guidelines should be followed. Guidelines are widely available from national organisations such as NICE (2014) and SIGN (2013).

Breast cancer is no longer considered a single disease and classifying patients according to the molecular subtype may help direct adjuvant therapy.

Recently, multi-gene signatures have been used to distinguish between patients with high-, intermediate- or low-risk disease. The 21-gene assay (Oncotype DX®) has been shown to predict the likelihood of recurrence in women with early-stage ER+ breast cancer (up to 3 nodes positive) treated with tamoxifen. The 70-gene assay (MammaPrint®) is used to estimate the risk of distant recurrence of early breast cancer (LN up to 3+ and tumour size < 5 cm). Oncotype DX® has recently been recommended by NICE as 'an option for guiding decisions for people with ER+, lymph node negative and HER2– breast cancer' in selected cases (NICE, 2013b).

Deciding which adjuvant therapy (endocrine, chemotherapy or trastuzumab) to offer to patients has become increasingly complex and needs to take into account the risk of recurrence, the potential benefit of adjuvant therapy, comorbidities, performance status and patient preference. Table 19.10 describes the St Gallen 2013 criteria which can be helpful in selecting which adjuvant treatment to offer patients based on the molecular subtypes described in Table 19.4.

Role of adjuvant chemotherapy

The benefit of adjuvant chemotherapy in terms of overall and disease-free survival depends on the endocrine

Table 19.10 Choice of adjuvant treatment in breast cancer

Subtype	Type of therapy	Notes
'Luminal A-like'	Endocrine therapy alone in majority of cases	Chemotherapy may be considered in selected cases (high 21-gene RS, high risk on 70-gene assay or grade 3 disease)
'Luminal B-like (HER2 negative)'	Endocrine therapy for all, chemotherapy for most	
'Luminal B-like (HER2 positive)'	Chemotherapy + anti-HER2 therapy + endocrine therapy	
'HER-2 positive (non-luminal)'	Chemotherapy + anti-HER2 therapy	
'Triple negative (ductal)'	Chemotherapy	
Special histological types		
Endocrine-responsive	Endocrine therapy	Cribriform, tubular and mucinous
Endocrine-non-responsive	Chemotherapy	Apocrine, medullary, metaplastic, adenoid cystic*

*Adenoid cystic carcinoma may not require chemotherapy if node-negative. Adapted from Goldhirsch *et al.* (2013b).

responsiveness, age, the subtype of cancer and the type of chemotherapy planned. The relative and absolute benefits can be estimated using systems such as Adjuvant! Online (www.adjuvantonline.com) and should be discussed with patients thoroughly at the time of diagnosis and staging. It is important to understand that the predicted benefits of therapy are estimates and that the confidence intervals around such estimates are not usually given.

The Oncotype DX® test provides a recurrence score (RS) which stratifies patients according to risk of recurrence (low, intermediate and high) and also gives an estimate of chemotherapy benefit. Oncotype DX® has been shown to spare chemotherapy in women who were previously recommended to receive treatment based on pre-testing risk estimation (Holt *et al.*, 2013).

Adjuvant chemotherapy regimens

Adjuvant chemotherapy for breast cancer has evolved over the years. There are many possible regimens in common use and these are summarised in Table 19.11.

The first-generation chemotherapy regimens (e.g. cyclophosphamide, methotrexate and 5-FU (CMF)) did not include either anthracyclines or taxanes. The second-generation chemotherapy regimens included an anthracycline either added to CMF (such as Epi-CMF) or epirubicin or doxorubicin with 5-flurouracil and cyclophosphamide (FEC or FAC). The best results for FEC have been with doses of epirubicin of 90–100 mg/m². The addition of a taxane to an anthracycline-based regimen has shown to improve outcomes further. There are a number of taxane-based regimens including TAC (docetaxel, doxorubicin and cyclophosphamide), FEC-T (FEC followed by docetaxel) and AC-P (doxorubicin and cyclophosphamide followed by paclitaxel). 'Dose-dense' regimens usually entail two weekly treatments with G-CSF support and can be considered in patients at particularly high risk of recurrence (often node-positive, triple-negative).

The recent EBCTCG meta-analysis has compared the outcomes of different chemotherapy regimens (chemotherapy versus no chemotherapy, anthracycline versus CMF, taxanes versus anthracyclines). It showed that the higher dose anthracycline regimens and taxane-based regimens are more effective than CMF or 4AC (doxorubicin and cyclophosphamide) and reductions in risk do not appear to be affected by age (up to 70 years), nodal status, tumour size or grade, ER status or tamoxifen use. The more effective chemotherapy regimens (taxane + anthracycline or higher-dose anthracyclines) reduce breast cancer mortality by about 30%. The absolute benefits gained depend on the absolute risk of recurrence without chemotherapy (EBCTCG, 2012).

Role of adjuvant endocrine treatment

Tamoxifen is a selective ER modulator and blocks the action of oestrogen by binding to one of the activating

Table 19.11 Adjuvant chemotherapy regimens in breast cancer

Type of chemotherapy	Chemotherapy regimen	Frequency	Notes
First-generation	Cyclophosphamide 100 mg/m^2 (p.o. D1–14) Methotrexate 40 mg/m^2 (i.v. D1 and D8) 5-Flurouracil 600 mg/m^2 (i.v. D1 and D8)	Every 28 days for 6 cycles	6 cycles of standard CMF is equivalent to 4 cycles of AC (EBCTCG, 2012)
	Doxorubicin 60 mg/m^2 (i.v. D1) Cyclophosphamide 600 mg/m^2 (i.v. D1)	Every 21 days for 4 cycles	
Second-generation	5-Flurouracil 500 mg/m^2 (i.v. D1) Epirubicin 100 mg/m^2 (i.v. D1) Cyclophosphamide 500 mg/m^2 (i.v. D1)	Every 21 days for 6 cycles	(French Adjuvant Study Group, 2001). Some centres use 75 mg/m^2 of epirubicin to reduce toxicity
	Epirubicin 100 mg/m^2 (i.v. D1) Followed by: Cyclophosphamide 100 mg/m^2 (p.o. D1–14) Methotrexate 40 mg/m^2 (i.v. D1 and D8) 5-Flurouracil 600 mg/m^2 (i.v. D1 and D8)	Every 21 days for 4 cycles Every 28 days for 4 cycles	NEAT trial (Earl *et al.*, 2012)
	Docetaxel 75 mg/m^2 (i.v. D1) Cyclophosphamide 600 mg/m^2 (i.v. D1)	Every 21 days for 4 cycles	TC is superior to AC in terms of overall survival at 7 years (87% versus 82%). This regimen is of use in those for whom an antracycline is contraindicated (Jones *et al.*, 2009b)
Third-generation	Docetaxel 75 mg/m^2 (i.v. D1) Doxorubicin 50 mg/m^2 (i.v. D1) Cyclophosphamide 500 mg/m^2 (i.v. D1)	Every 21 days for 6 cycles	BCIRG 001 (Martin *et al.*, 2005). This is highly myelosuppressive and requires prophylactic G-CSF
	5-Flurouracil 500 mg/m^2 (i.v. D1) Epirubicin 100 mg/m^2 (i.v. D1) Cyclophosphamide 500 mg/m^2 (i.v. D1) Followed by: Docetaxel 100 mg/m^2 (i.v. D1)	Every 21 days for 3 cycles Every 21 days for 3 cycles	PACS 01 trial (Roché *et al.*, 2006)
	Doxorubicin 60 mg/m^2 (i.v. D1) Cyclophosphamide 600 mg/m^2 (i.v. D1) Followed by: Paclitaxel 175 mg/m^2 (i.v. D1)	Every 21 days for 4 cycles Every 21 days for 3 cycles	CALGB 9334 (Henderson *et al.*, 2003)
Dose-dense regimens	Doxorubicin 60 mg/m^2 (i.v. D1) Cyclophosphamide 600 mg/m^2 (i.v. D1) Followed by: Paclitaxel 80 mg/m^2 (i.v. D1)	Every 21 days for 4 cycles Every 7 days for 12 weeks	Weekly paclitaxel improved DFS when compared with three-weekly paclitaxel (CALGB 9334) from 76.9% (3 weekly) to 81.5% (Sparano *et al.*, 2008)
	Doxorubicin 60 mg/m^2 (i.v. D1) Cyclophosphamide 600 mg/m^2 (i.v. D1) Followed by: Paclitaxel 175 mg/m^2 (i.v. D1)	Every 14 days for 4 cycles Every 14 days for cycles	Dose-dense AC-paclitaxel was associated with an improvement in DFS from 75% to 82%. G-CSF was given routinely (Citron *et al.*, 2003)

regions of the ER. Tamoxifen is useful in the adjuvant treatment of breast cancer in both pre- and postmenopausal women with ER-positive disease. The EBCTCG has shown that tamoxifen, when given to women with ER-positive breast cancer for 5 years, reduces the annual recurrence rate by 41% and annual mortality rate by 34% (EBCTCG, 2005). The ATLAS and aTTom trials have both compared the standard 5 years with 10 years of tamoxifen and have shown a further reduction in breast cancer recurrence and mortality with 10 years of treatment (Davies et al., 2013; Gray et al., 2013).

The ER has two activation domains: AF-1 and AF-2. Tamoxifen blocks AF-2 but not AF-1 and so there remains oestrogenic activity in some tissues. Aromatase inhibitors (AIs) exert their anti-oestrogenic effects through inhibition of the aromatase enzyme, which converts circulating androgens to oestrogen. AIs are active in endocrine-responsive tumours and may be beneficial in cases of tamoxifen resistance. Anastrozole and letrozole are non-steroidal competitive inhibitors of aromatase, whereas exemestane is a steroid-irreversible AI and inhibits aromatisation *in vivo* by 98%.

Premenopausal patients

Premenopausal patients whose tumours are ER-positive should be considered for adjuvant endocrine therapy (SIGN, 2005). They should receive tamoxifen as a standard adjuvant treatment for 5 years. In the light of the ATLAS and aTTom trial results, women coming to the end of 5 years of adjuvant tamoxifen should be given the option of extending treatment to 10 years.

If chemotherapy is given, tamoxifen should be started after the chemotherapy has finished (Albain et al., 2004a). If tamoxifen is contraindicated, ovarian function suppression (OFS) with goserelin is an acceptable alternative. Tamoxifen should be avoided during pregnancy owing to its teratogenicity.

Ovarian suppression with goserelin appears to be as effective as tamoxifen and can be used in women for whom tamoxifen is contraindicated. The SOFT and TEXT trials have examined the use of ovarian suppression + tamoxifen versus ovarian suppression + exemestane, versus tamoxifen alone in pre-menopausal women with breast cancer. The results of these two trials suggest improved disease free survival in women receiving ovarian suppression + exemestane compared with either ovarian suppression + tamoxifen or tamoxifen alone. This effect appears greatest in women at

higher risk of recurrence (Francis et al., 2015; Pagani et al., 2014).

Postmenopausal patients

A number of trials have shown that AIs are more effective than tamoxifen for adjuvant treatment of post-menopausal women with ER-positive breast cancer. Tamoxifen is associated with a higher rate of gynaecological and vascular symptoms, while AIs are associated with more arthralgia and bone fractures.

Current practice is to use an aromatase inhibitor first for 5 years in post-menopausal women. Due to the risk of accelerated bone loss with AIs, the National Osteoporosis Society has produced guidance on monitoring bone health during adjuvant AI therapy (Reid et al., 2008). There is no evidence for extending adjuvant AI therapy beyond 5 years in women and decisions about extending AI therapy or switching to tamoxifen for a further 5 years should be made on an individual basis after discussion of the potential risks and benefits of extending treatment. Table 19.12 summarises the outcomes of the main trials of AIs.

Role of adjuvant trastuzumab

Trastuzumab is a chimeric antibody (95% human and 5% murine) developed against the HER2 transmembrane epidermal growth factor receptor. The use of trastuzumab in the adjuvant setting has dramatically improved the outlook of women with HER2-positive breast cancer. Table 19.13 summarises the main trials of trastuzumab in the adjuvant setting. Trastuzumab is currently given for one year and can be given as a subcutaneous injection at a fixed dose (600 mg) rather than as an intravenous infusion (Pivot et al., 2013a). The Persephone trial is comparing 6 months of trastuzumab with 12 months of trastuzumab (http://public.ukcrn.org.uk/search/StudyDetail.aspx?StudyID=4078, accessed December 2014).

The main toxicity of trastuzumab is cardiac toxicity. Patients should have left ventricular function assessed before starting trastuzumab and every 4 months during treatment. The risk of cardiac dysfunction is highest in patients receiving anthracyclines with trastuzumab, and the combination docetaxel, carboplatin and trastuzumab has a significantly lower rate of cardiac events compared with doxorubicin, cyclophosphamide and trastuzumab (Slamon et al., 2011). Guidance for the management of cardiac dysfunction in trastuzumab-treated patients has been developed (Jones et al., 2009a).

Table 19.12 Summary of the aromatase inhibitor trials

Trial (no. of patients)	Median FU (years)	Arms (duration of hormones)	DFS HR (95% CI)	OS HR (95% CI)	Reference
Upfront AI					
ATAC (9366)	10	A versus T versus T + A (5 years)	Av.T: 0.86 (0.78–0.95) Hormone receptor+	Av.T: 0.95 (0.84–1.06) Hormone receptor+	Cuzick *et al.*, 2010
BIG 1-98 (8010)	8.1	L versus T (5 years)	0.53 (0.78–0.96)	0.87 (0.77–0.99)	Regan *et al.*, 2011
TEAM (before switch) (9775)	2.75	T versus E (2.75 years)	0.89 (0.77–1.03)	NA	van de Velde *et al.*, 2011
Sequential therapy					
IES (4724)	7.5	T → E versus T → T (5 years)	0.81 (0.72–0.91)	0.53 (0.75–0.99)	Bliss *et al.*, 2012
ABCSG Trial 8 (3714)	5	T (2 years) → A (3 years) Versus T (5 years)	0.91 (0.75–1.103)	0.87 (0.64–1.16)	Dubsky *et. al.*, 2012
TEAM (9775)	5	E (5 years) versus sequential T → E	1.06 (0.91–1.24)	1.00 (0.89–1.14)	van de Velde *et al.*, 2011
Extended therapy					
MA.17 (5187)	5	L versus placebo (after 5 years of T) Results adjusted for crossover	0.52 (0.45–0.61)	0.51 (0.42–0.61)	Jin *et al.*, 2012

A, anastrozole; T, tamoxifen; L, letrozole; E, exemestane. DFS, disease-free survival; OS, overall survival; HR, hazard ratio; v. versus. Adapted from Schiavon and Smith, 2014.

Management of locally advanced breast cancer

Locally advanced breast cancer is defined as inoperable non-metastatic disease and occurs in the following stages.

- Stage IIIA (T0–3, N2, M0).
- Stage IIIB (T4, N0–2, M0).
- Stage IIIC (any T, N3).

Management

Preoperative chemotherapy, HER2-targeted therapy or endocrine therapy can be used to treat patients with large tumours not suitable for breast-conserving surgery. This treatment can be used to downstage tumours to make BCT easier and prevent mastectomy (Hanrahan *et al.*, 2005) in up to 80% of suitable patients. It should be clear at the outset whether BCT is intended, because conservation is not appropriate for patients with central tumours for whom the cosmetic outcome may be unacceptable, with multifocal tumours, or with inflammatory breast cancer. Neoadjuvant treatment also provides the opportunity to assess the sensitivity of tumours to systemic therapy by monitoring tumour response before surgery. The rate of radiological complete response (CR) is best assessed using ultrasound (± MRI) and is higher than the rate of pathological CR. In the case of radiological CR, RT may be used instead of surgery but it is associated with a higher local recurrence rate. Patients achieving pathological CR to chemotherapy have a good prognosis, and this effect on pathological CR is highest in ER-negative breast cancer patients (von Minckwitz *et al.*, 2012).

Therefore, usual treatment is neoadjuvant chemotherapy (usually anthracycline-based ± taxane) followed by BCT plus ALND plus RT with or without hormone therapy (except in women with inflammatory breast cancer), mastectomy plus ALND with or without RT, hormones or delayed breast reconstruction, or definitive RT to the breast, axilla and SCF, with or without hormones.

Table 19.13 Summary of the trastuzumab trials

Trial (no. of patients)	Median FU (years)	Arms (duration of H in weeks)	DFS HR (95% CI)	OS HR (95% CI)	Reference
NCCTG N9831 (3505)	6	AC → P AC → P → H (52) AC → PH →H (52)	[a]0.67 (0.54–0.81) [b]0.77 (0.53–1.11)	0.88 (0.67–1.15) 0.78 (0.58–1.05)	Perez *et al.*, 2011a
NSABP B-31 NCCTG N9381 joint analysis (4045)	3.9	AC → P AC → PH →H (52)	0.52 (0.45–0.60)	0.61 (0.50-0.75)	Perez *et al.*, 2011b
HERA (5102)	4	Chemo Chemo → H (52) Chemo → H (104)	0.76 (0.66–0.87) 0.99 (0.85–1.14)	0.76 (0.65–0.88) 1.05 (0.86–1.28)	Goldhirsch *et al.*, 2013a Gianni *et al.*, 2011
BCIRG 006 (3222)	5.4	AC → D AC → DH → H (52) DCarboH (52)	0.64 (0.53–0.78) 0.75 (0.63–0.90)	0.63 (0.48–0.81) 0.77 (0.60–0.99)	Slamon *et al.*, 2011
Fin Her (1010)	5.1	D/V → FEC D/V + H → FEC (9)	0.65 (0.38–1.12)	0.55 (0.27–1.11)	Joensuu *et al.*, 2009
PACS 04 (528)	4	FEC/ED FEC/ED PACS 04 H (52)	0.86 (0.61–1.22)	1.27 (0.68–2.38)	Spielmann *et al.*, 2009
PHARE (3381)	3.5	Chemo + H (26) Chemo + H (52)	1.28 (1.05–1.56)	1.47 (1.07–2.02)	Pivot *et al.*, 2013b

A, doxorubicin; C, cyclophosphamide; Carbo, carboplatin; Chemo, standard chemotherapy; D, docetaxel; E, epirubicin; F, 5-FU; H, trastuzumab; HR, hazard ratio; P, paclitaxel; V, vinorelbine.

[a]HR comparison between AC → P and AC → P → H, [b]HR comparison between and AC → P → H and AC → PH →H. (Table adapted from Pinto *et al.*, 2013.)

If there is no response to neoadjuvant chemotherapy, alternative additional chemotherapy with or without preoperative RT should be considered.

Adjuvant hormone treatment in postmenopausal women should be with an AI. Patients with HER2-positive tumours should be considered for trastuzumab.

Neoadjuvant endocrine therapy has been evaluated recently in less fit, older patients with endocrine-sensitive disease who are unlikely to tolerate chemotherapy. Letrozole is licensed for neoadjuvant therapy (followed by surgery and/or RT) in postmenopausal women with large operable or locally advanced ER-positive breast cancer. Letrozole gives a higher response rate than tamoxifen in patients with HER2-positive tumours (Bhatnagar, 2006). Letrozole or anastrozole treatment results in more patients able to undergo BCT, the complete excision rate is better, and the rates of local recurrence are low.

Management of metastatic breast cancer

The aim of treatment in metastatic breast cancer is to palliate symptoms, control disease and improve survival while keeping the toxicity of treatment to a minimum. Consideration should be given to repeating ER, PgR and HER2 assays if biopsy material is available from a metastasis, because the receptor status of the metastasis can be different from that of the primary tumour. The BRITS study showed that the switch in receptor status between primary and recurrent breast cancer tissue samples led to a change in treatment plan for 17.5% of patients (Thompson *et al.*, 2010). Median survival after diagnosis of metastatic disease can vary significantly depending on the subtype of breast cancer, with one series demonstrating a median survival of 2.2 years for the luminal A subtype compared with 0.5 years for the basal-like subtype (Kennecke *et al.*, 2010). Overall survival for patients with metastatic breast cancer, particularly for those with HER2-positive breast cancer, has improved significantly over the past three decades (Giordano *et al.*, 2004).

Hormone therapy

Hormone therapy alone is often given as first-line therapy if the patient has ER/PgR-positive metastatic disease, bone or soft tissue disease only, or is asymptomatic with minimal visceral disease. The choice of hormone therapy depends on previous treatments and menopausal status.

In postmenopausal women, AIs are more effective than tamoxifen (Mauri *et al.*, 2006). For premenopausal women who have had previous anti-oestrogen therapy and who are within one year of anti-oestrogen exposure, the preferred second-line therapy is ovarian ablation (by surgery, RT or LHRH agonists) with or without an anti-oestrogen, while for premenopausal women without previous exposure to an anti-oestrogen, initial treatment with an anti-oestrogen with or without LHRH agonists is preferred.

Second-line hormone therapy

Patients with metastatic disease often develop resistance to hormone therapy. However, for postmenopausal women who have responded to hormones, it is reasonable to offer endocrine therapies for second-line and subsequent therapy. After second-line hormonal therapy, there is little evidence to guide the choice of hormone therapy. Options include:

- non-steroidal AIs (anastrozole and letrozole);
- steroidal AI (exemestane);
- pure anti-oestrogen (e.g. fulvestrant, which lacks the oestrogen agonistic activity of tamoxifen and is given as a monthly gluteal intramuscular injection. It is at least as effective as anastrozole in patients whose disease progressed on previous endocrine therapy and has fewer side effects; Howell *et al.*, 2005);
- progestin (megestrol acetate).

Recent research has evaluated the role of the MTOR enzyme in mediating resistance to endocrine therapy in ER-positive breast cancer. ER-positive breast cancer cells that have become resistant to hormone therapy have shown activation of the PI3K/MTOR intracellular signalling pathway (Miller *et al.*, 2011). The MTOR inhibitor everolimus has been investigated in combination with exemestane and has demonstrated improved PFS in postmenopausal patients with hormone receptor-positive advanced breast cancer previously treated with non-steroidal aromatase inhibitors (Baselga *et al.*, 2012). Everolimus is licensed for use in Europe and North America for the treatment of advanced ER-positive and HER2-negative breast cancer and is not currently approved by NICE for this indication.

Premenopausal women with ER-positive disease should have ovarian ablation or suppression and then be treated as postmenopausal women. Patients who develop endocrine-resistant disease, and are suitably fit, should be considered for chemotherapy and/or trastuzumab if the disease is HER2-positive.

Chemotherapy

Chemotherapy should be considered for suitably fit patients particularly if they have ER/PgR-negative cancer, HER2-positive cancer, symptomatic visceral or hormone-refractory disease. Combination chemotherapy produces higher response rates but is associated with increased toxicity, and is more suitable for younger, fitter patients with visceral disease. In practice, sequential single-agent treatments are most often used.

An anthracycline should be the first treatment if it has not been used in the adjuvant setting. This should be followed by a taxane either as single agent or in combination, followed by oral chemotherapy (capecitabine or vinorelbine). The choice of regimen depends on patient factors such as performance status, comorbidities and acceptance of toxicity such as alopecia, tumour factors such as triple-negative cancer status, HER2 positivity and type of and response to previous chemotherapy treatment. Suitable combination regimens may include FEC (epirubicin 60 mg/m^2), EC, doxorubicin plus docetaxel/paclitaxel, CMF, docetaxel plus capecitabine, and gemcitabine plus paclitaxel (Leonard and Howell, 2000; O'Shaughnessy *et al.*, 2002).

Single-agent treatments include docetaxel, paclitaxel, albumin-bound paclitaxel, doxorubicin, epirubicin, capecitabine, vinorelbine, carboplatin and gemcitabine (Table 19.14). Some of these single-agent regimes, such as capecitabine, vinorelbine and paclitaxel, can be continued as long as there is a response.

Patients whose tumours are ER-positive may sometimes be offered endocrine maintenance treatment between courses of palliative chemotherapy unless, or until, endocrine resistance develops. However, this practice is not supported by randomised trial evidence.

Table 19.14 Single-agent chemotherapy regimens in metastatic breast cancer

Type of chemotherapy	Chemotherapy regimen	Frequency	Notes
Anthracycline	Epirubicin 50–75 mg/m² q21d or weekly 15–25 mg/m² Doxorubicin 50–75 mg/m² q21d	Every 21 days for 6 cycles	Consider cumulative lifetime anthracycline dose
Taxane	Docetaxel 75 mg/m² q21d Abraxane 260 mg/m² q21d, or 150 mg/m² d1, d8, d15 q28d Paclitaxel 70–80 mg/m² weekly	Every 21 days for 6 cycles	1st line standard in combination with trastuzumab in HER2-positive advanced disease Well tolerated
	Capecitabine 1000–1250 mg/m² d1–14 q21d		Avoids alopecia
	Vinorelbine (oral) 60–80 mg/m² d1, d8 q21d		Well tolerated in combination with trastuzumab in HER2-positive 1st line (trastuzumab and taxane naïve)
	Carboplatin AUC5-6		May be more active in triple-negative group
	Gemcitabine 1000–1250 mg/m² d1, d8 q21d		
	Eribulin		Active in heavily pretreated patients (all molecular groups)

Targeted therapy

Trastuzumab with or without chemotherapy, with or without endocrine therapy, should be considered if the tumour is HER2-positive and if there is symptomatic visceral or hormone-refractory disease (Slamon *et al.*, 2001; Cobleigh *et al.*, 1999; Albain *et al.*, 2004b; Marty *et al.*, 2005). NICE recommends the use of trastuzumab in patients with HER2-positive advanced disease in combination with taxotere after anthracycline use or as a single agent after the use of a taxane (NICE, 2002).

Single-agent trastuzumab in HER2-positive metastatic disease gives a 35% clinical response rate as a first-line treatment. There is evidence that trastuzumab plus chemotherapy produce a better PFS and response rate. Combinations are:

- trastuzumab + docetaxel;
- trastuzumab + paclitaxel;
- trastuzumab + vinorelbine;
- trastuzumab + capecitabine.

In this situation, trastuzumab is continued as a single agent after a period of combined treatment with a cytotoxic agent. Treatment with trastuzumab may be stopped in patients who develop progressive extracerebral disease, but should be continued if the site of progression

is only within the CNS. Patients on trastuzumab have a relatively high rate of isolated relapse in the CNS because trastuzumab does not effectively cross the blood–brain barrier. Such patients should be considered for radiotherapy and/or further chemotherapy. Their prognosis appears to be much better than for HER2-negative patients with CNS metastases. Lapatinib is approved for use in combination with capecitabine as second-line chemotherapy treatment in patients who progress after trastuzumab (Geyer *et al.*, 2006).

Recent advances in the management of HER2 amplified breast cancer include the development of pertuzumab, a monoclonal antibody that inhibits HER2 by binding to it and inhibiting its dimerization with HER3. Pertuzumab has been shown to improve PFS and OS in patients when used in addition to docetaxel and trastuzumab compared to docetaxel, trastuzumab and placebo (Swain *et al.*, 2013).

Managing skeletal metastases

Women with bone metastases, especially lytic, should be given a bisphosphonate, which reduces the frequency of skeletal-related events and relieves pain (Brown and Coleman, 2002). Pamidronate, clodronate, ibandronate (intravenous or oral) and zoledronic acid (intravenous) have all been shown to be effective in patients with breast cancer.

Intravenous zoledronic acid is one of the most powerful inhibitors of osteoclast activity and has been shown in the ZICE study to be preferable to oral ibandronate in preventing skeletal-related events (Barrett-Lee et al., 2014). In this study, more patients in the zoledronic acid group had renal toxic effects than in the ibandronate group (32% versus 24%), but rates of osteonecrosis of the jaw were low in both groups (1% versus < 1%).

Denosumab is a monoclonal antibody, which prevents the activation of osteoclast-mediated bone resorption by inhibiting the RANK ligand cellular membrane protein, and is given as a subcutaneous injection every 4 weeks (Baron et al., 2011). Denosumab was shown to be more effective than zoledronic acid in reducing skeletal-related events in a randomised study of more than 2000 patients with bone metastases secondary to breast cancer (Stopeck et al., 2010). Denosumab can also cause hypocalcaemia and osteonecrosis of the jaw. As with bisphosphonates, a dental assessment is recommended before treatment starts and supplementation with oral calcium and vitamin D is required throughout.

Other treatments

Patients with metastatic breast cancer develop a number of localised problems that can be treated with local RT, surgery or regional chemotherapy (e.g. intrathecal methotrexate for leptomeningeal carcinomatosis). With the improvements made in the treatment of metastatic breast cancer, cerebral metastases have become more evident particularly, as mentioned, in patients with HER2-positive disease. In patients who develop multiple brain metastases, whole-brain radiotherapy is the standard treatment, but patients who develop a solitary brain metastasis may be considered for surgical debulking or stereotactic radiotherapy using systems such as CyberKnife® or Gamma Knife®. The role of stereotactic radiotherapy is also currently being explored for 'oligometastatic' disease for sites other than the brain.

Management of recurrent disease

Half of the patients with locally recurrent disease have evidence of visceral metastasis at presentation, either clinically obvious or on restaging. Locoregional recurrence may present as chest wall, supraclavicular or axillary recurrence.

Patients with a locoregional recurrence can still be cured, but treating them may be difficult. Those with an isolated chest wall recurrence, particularly after a long disease-free interval, should be treated intensively and, although the disease-free survival at 5 years may be 25–30%, half of the patients will still be alive after 5 years. Management depends on previous treatment:

- for patients who had previous BCT, mastectomy is the usual treatment (or further WLE in highly selected cases);
- for patients who had previous mastectomy, a complete surgical resection with a clear margin should be aimed for followed by RT (chest wall and areas of lymphatic spread) if it was not given previously. Giving RT with hyperthermia is also a promising approach.

After surgery and RT, chemotherapy and endocrine treatment should be considered. Sometimes neoadjuvant chemotherapy or hormone therapy is given before surgery. Electrochemotherapy is a treatment option, approved by NICE, that can be used to palliate symptoms from a local chest wall recurrence.

Special clinical situations

Pregnancy and breast cancer

Breast cancer during pregnancy is uncommon (Eedarapalli and Jain, 2006). Patients may be diagnosed late and often have involved axillary lymph nodes, and larger tumours, which are more likely to be poorly differentiated, ER/PgR-negative and HER2-positive (slightly, 30%). Late diagnosis may be related to the endocrine effects of pregnancy or missed diagnosis caused by the tumour being difficult to detect within swollen breast tissue. It is not clear that there is any difference in prognosis, stage for stage, compared to women who are not pregnant.

Possible investigations include a mammogram, which can be safely performed with appropriate shielding of the foetus; an ultrasound scan of the breast; a chest X-ray with shielding; and an ultrasound scan of the liver.

There should be very close liaison with the obstetrician who is monitoring foetal growth and development. Management depends on the timing of the diagnosis.

During the first trimester the options are to continue pregnancy and treat with mastectomy and ALND. Adjuvant chemotherapy can begin in the second trimester. Chemotherapy cannot be given during the first trimester because of the high risk of foetal malformations (whereas the risk is only 1.3% in the second and third trimesters). Taxane, trastuzumab (risk of oligohydramnios), adjuvant RT, and adjuvant endocrine treatment can only be given postpartum. Termination, followed by standard treatment, is the other option.

During the second trimester and early third trimester, the options are mastectomy or BCT plus ALND followed by adjuvant chemotherapy. Chemotherapy should not be given later than 35 weeks to avoid haematological complications at delivery. Anthracyclines and alkylating agents can be used (e.g. in FAC chemotherapy), but methotrexate should be avoided. Adjuvant trastuzumab (risk of oligohydramnios), adjuvant RT and adjuvant endocrine treatment can only be given postpartum.

Another option is neoadjuvant chemotherapy followed by postpartum mastectomy or BCT plus ALND with or without adjuvant trastuzumab (risk of oligohydramnios), with or without adjuvant RT and adjuvant endocrine treatment.

During the late third trimester, mastectomy or BCT plus ALND can be performed followed by postpartum adjuvant chemotherapy, adjuvant trastuzumab, adjuvant RT, and adjuvant endocrine treatment as indicated.

Paget's disease

Paget's disease is a rare manifestation of breast cancer (1–4% of all breast cancers) characterised by the presence of neoplastic Paget's cells in the epidermis of the nipple areola complex (NAC). The patient presents with eczema of the areola, bleeding, ulceration and itching of the nipple. Diagnosis is often delayed. The disease is usually unilateral and occurs most frequently in the fifth or sixth decade.

Paget's disease is usually (more than 90%) associated with an underlying breast cancer, which may not be adjacent to the NAC, and about 50% of underlying tumours are palpable. For palpable tumours 90–94% are invasive cancers; if not palpable, 66–68% are DCIS.

Examination and imaging of the breast should be performed and MRI considered if no abnormality is found. Full-thickness skin biopsy of the involved NAC should be performed.

If there is only involvement of the NAC with no evidence of underlying malignancy, management options include:

- mastectomy + axillary staging;
- excision of a NAC with whole-breast RT.

If the involved NAC is associated with underlying DCIS, options include:

- mastectomy ± axillary staging;
- excision of DCIS + excision of the NAC with whole-breast RT.

If the involved NAC is associated with underlying invasive breast cancer, options include:

- mastectomy + axillary staging;
- excision of the breast tumour and excision of the NAC with whole-breast RT.

Appropriate adjuvant systemic therapy depends on the histology of the underlying breast cancer.

Male breast cancer

The median age of occurrence of breast cancer in men is in the sixth decade; it is usually ER-positive. LCIS is not found in men, and infiltrating lobular carcinoma is unusual. Local recurrence occurs in about 20% of patients.

Standard treatment involves modified radical mastectomy with or without adjuvant RT, with or without adjuvant chemotherapy, *with or without* adjuvant endocrine treatment stage for stage, similar to treatment for female breast cancer.

Bilateral breast cancer

Of patients who present with breast cancer, 1% may present with bilateral primaries in the breast. In patients with unilateral breast cancers, the annual incidence of a contralateral primary is about 0.75%.

Inflammatory breast cancer

Inflammatory breast cancer accounts for 3% of all breast cancers. It is a rare but virulent form of breast cancer with a poor prognosis. It is characterised by a rapid (less than 3 months) history of diffuse, brawny indurations of the skin with an erysipeloid edge.

The skin changes are caused by extensive involvement of dermal lymphatics. A skin biopsy usually shows dermal lymphatic invasion, but a skin biopsy is not essential to establish the diagnosis. Half the patients with inflammatory breast cancer have an underlying mass. Mammograms, ultrasound and, sometimes, MRI of the breast may be required. The aforementioned staging investigations should be carried out to look for metastases. Inflammatory breast cancers tend to be poorly differentiated, often

ER- and PgR-negative and more likely to have HER2 overexpression.

Management involves neoadjuvant chemotherapy (16% complete response, 45% partial response) followed by mastectomy and ALND plus adjuvant RT with or without adjuvant hormone, with or without adjuvant trastuzumab. In cases of complete response, radical RT may be discussed as an option. In cases of progressive disease, alternative chemotherapy, hormone therapy, and/or RT should be considered.

Prognosis

Prognostic factors

Regional lymph node status

The status of the regional lymph nodes is the most important prognostic factor and is directly related to survival and the best predictor of systemic micrometastases. Although not routinely evaluated, the presence of positive internal mammary nodes is associated with a worse prognosis.

Tumour size

The tumour size directly correlates with 10-year survival, involvement of 4 or more positive lymph nodes, and the risk of metastasis.

Tumour grade

The grade of the tumour is an important predictor of both disease-free and overall survival.

Age

Younger women (< 35 years) have a poorer prognosis than older patients with cancer of an equivalent stage. Younger women are at a higher risk of relapse with a relative risk of 1.6 for distant metastases. The rate of local recurrence after 5 years is 17% in patients under age 35 compared with 6% in those over 50.

Hormone receptor status

Patients with ER-positive tumours live longer than those with ER-negative tumours and they are more likely to respond to hormonal treatment. Patients with ER- and PgR-negative tumours have a higher complete response rate (> 30%) following neoadjuvant chemotherapy, but survival time is shorter (Colleoni et al., 2004).

Table 19.15 Five-year survival according to stage of disease

Stage	Survival at 5 years (%)
I	84
II	71
III	48
IV	18

Adapted from Miller et al. (1994).

Histological type

Histological type is one of the best predictors of long-term survival. Many of the so-called special types of invasive breast carcinoma (invasive tubular, cribriform, mucinous, papillary, microinvasive, adenoid cystic and medullary) are associated with a much better prognosis than cancer of no special type. The inflammatory type has a poor prognosis.

An extensive intraduct component (EIC) is defined as an infiltrating ductal cancer in which greater than 25% of the tumour volume is DCIS, and the DCIS extends beyond the invasive cancer into surrounding normal breast parenchyma. EIC is associated with increased local recurrence after BCT.

Lymphatic or vascular invasion

Lymphatic or vascular invasion is present in 25% of breast cancer patients and is associated with a doubling of the rate of local recurrence and high risk of short-term systemic relapse.

HER2 oncogene

Of breast cancer patients, 20% overexpress the HER2 oncogene. Gene amplification or overexpression of HER2 carries an adverse prognosis; it is also a predictive factor and patients are more likely to respond to anthracycline-based chemotherapy and to be resistant to tamoxifen.

Other markers of poor prognosis

Other indicators of poor prognosis include the following.

- High proliferation rates (measured by fraction of cells in S-phase, Ki-67 and MIB-1 monoclonal antibodies, or bromodeoxyruridine).
- Aneuploid as opposed to diploid tumours.
- TP53 accumulation, especially in the presence of abnormal expression of other markers such as p-glycoprotein, BCL2 and p21/WAF1.

Table 19.16 Ten-year survival according to the prognostic index

Prognostic group	NI scoring	Ten-year survival (%)
Excellent	≤ 2.4	94
Good	2.5 to ≤ 3.4	83
Moderate I	3.5 to ≤ 4.4	70
Moderate II	4.5 to ≤ 5.4	51
Poor	> 5.4	19

NI, Nottingham prognostic index; see Blamey (1996).

- Proteases and second-messenger systems – high concentrations of cyclic AMP, and the presence of cathepsin D, cathepsin B and matrix metalloproteinase 2.

Prognosis

The 5-year survival according to stage of the disease is shown in Table 19.15.

The Nottingham prognostic index (NI) is calculated as follows:

$$NI = (0.2 \times size) + lymph\ node\ stage + grade$$

For lymph node stage, score 1 (if N0), score 2 (if 1–3 LNs are positive), score 3 (if 4 or more LNs are positive). For grading, score 1 (for grade 1), score 2 (for grade 2) and score 3 (for grade 3).

The 10-year survival according to the Nottingham prognostic index is shown in Table 19.16.

Areas of current interest and ongoing clinical trials

Breast cancer is an extensively researched and rapidly changing area in oncology with many areas of current interest including prevention and screening, diagnosis, surgery, treatment in the neoadjuvant, adjuvant and metastatic setting, supportive care and translational research. At the time of writing there were over 150 trials listed on the website of the National Cancer Research Institute www.ncri.org.uk (accessed January 2015).

References

Ahn, P. H., Vu, H. T., Lannin, D., et al. (2005). Sequence of radiotherapy with tamoxifen in conservatively managed breast cancer does not affect local relapse rates. J. Clin. Oncol., 23, 17–23.

Albain, K., Barlow, W., O'Malley, F., et al. (2004a). Concurrent (CAFT) versus sequential (CAF-T) chemo hormonal therapy (cyclophosphamide, doxorubicin, 5-fluorouracil, tamoxifen) versus T alone for postmenopausal, node-positive, estrogen (ER) and/or progesterone (PgR) receptor-positive breast cancer: mature outcomes and new biologic correlates on phase III intergroup trial 0100 (SWOG-8814). Breast Cancer Res. Treat., 88(Suppl. 1), A-37.

Albain, K. S., Nag, S., Calderillo-Ruiz, G., et al. (2004b). Global phase III study of gemcitabine plus paclitaxel (GT) vs. paclitaxel (T) as frontline therapy for metastatic breast cancer (MBC): first report of overall survival. Proc. Am. Soc. Clin. Oncol., 23 (5), Abstr. 510.

Anonymous. (1996). Breast cancer and hormonal contraceptives: collaborative reanalysis of individual data on 53 297 women with breast cancer and 100 239 women without breast cancer from 54 epidemiological studies. Lancet, 347, 1713–1727.

Arpino, G., Bardou, V. J., Clark, G. M., et al. (2004) Infiltrating lobular carcinoma of the breast: tumor characteristics and clinical outcome. Breast Cancer Res., 6, R149–R156.

Arriagada, R., Le, M. C., Mouriesse, H., et al. (1988). Long-term effect of internal mammary chain treatment. Results of a multivariate analysis of 1195 patients with operable breast cancer and positive axillary nodes. Radiother. Oncol., 11, 213–222.

Baron, R., Ferrari, S. and Russell, R. G. 2011. Denosumab and bisphosphonates: different mechanisms of action and effects. Bone, 48, 677–692.

Barrett-Lee, P., Casbard A., Abraham, J., et al. (2014). Oral ibandronic acid versus intravenous zoledronic acid in treatment of bone metastases from breast cancer: a randomised, open label, non-inferiority phase 3 trial. Lancet Oncol., 15, 114–122.

Bartelink, H., Horiot, J.-C., Poortmans, P., et al. (2007). Impact of a higher radiation dose on local control and survival in breast-conserving therapy of early breast cancer: 10-year results of the randomised boost versus no boost EORTC 22881-10882 trial. J. Clin. Oncol., 25, 3259–3265.

Barter, S. and Britton, P., (2014). Breast cancer. In: Recommendations for Cross-Sectional Imaging in Cancer Management, second edition. ed. T. Nicholson. London: The Royal College of Radiologists.

Baselga, J., Campone, M., Piccart, M., et al. (2012). Everolimus in postmenopausal hormone-receptor-positive advanced breast cancer. N. Engl. J. Med., 366, 520–529.

Beral, V. and Million Women Study Collaborators. (2003). Breast cancer and hormone replacement therapy in the Million Women Study. Lancet, 362, 419–427.

Bhatnagar, A. S. (2006). Review of the development of letrozole and its use in advanced breast cancer and in the neoadjuvant setting. *Breast*, **15** (Suppl. 1), S3–13.

Blamey, R. W. (1996). The design and clinical use of the Nottingham Prognostic Index in breast cancer. *Breast*, **5**, 156–157.

Bliss, J. M., Kilburn, L. S., Coleman, R. E., *et al.* (2012). Disease-related outcomes with long-term follow-up: an updated analysis of the Intergroup Exemestane Study. *J. Clin. Oncol.*, **30**, 709–717.

Brown, J. E. and Coleman, R. E. (2002). The present and future role of bisphosphonates in the management of patients with breast cancer. *Breast Cancer Res.*, **4**, 24–29.

Citron, M. L., Berry, D. A., Cirrincione, C., *et al.* (2003). Randomized trial of dose-dense versus conventionally scheduled and sequential versus concurrent combination chemotherapy as postoperative adjuvant treatment of node-positive primary breast cancer: first report of Intergroup Trial C9741/Cancer and Leukemia Group B Trial 9741. *J. Clin. Oncol.*, **21**, 1431–1439.

Cobleigh, M. A.,Vogel, C. L., Tripathy, D., *et al.* (1999). Multinational study of the efficacy and safety of humanized anti-HER2 monoclonal antibody in women who have HER2-overexpressing metastatic breast cancer that has progressed after chemotherapy for metastatic disease. *J. Clin. Oncol.*, **17**, 2639–2648.

Cody, H. S. III. (1999). Sentinel lymph-node mapping in breast cancer. *Oncology (Williston Park)*, **13**, 25–34.

Colleoni, M., Viale, G., Zahrieh, D., *et al.* (2004). Chemotherapy is more effective in patients with breast cancer not expressing steroid hormone receptors: a study of preoperative treatment. *Clin. Cancer Res.*, **10**, 6622–6628.

Cooke, R., Jones, M. E., Cunningham, D., *et al.* (2013). Breast cancer risk following Hodgkin lymphoma radiotherapy in relation to menstrual and reproductive risk factors. *Br. J. Cancer*, **108**, 2399–2406.

Cuzick, J., Sestak, I., Baum, M., *et al.* (2010). Effect of anastrozole and tamoxifen as adjuvant treatment for early-stage breast cancer: 10-year analysis of the ATAC trial. *Lancet Oncol.*, **11**, 1135–1141.

Cuzick, J., Sestak, I., Pinder, S. E., *et al.* (2011). Effect of tamoxifen and radiotherapy in women with locally excised ductal carcinoma *in situ*: long-term results from the UK/ANZ DCIS trial. *Lancet*, **12**, 21–29.

Cuzick, J., Sestak, I., Forbes, J. F., *et al.* (2014). Anastrozole for prevention of breast cancer in high-risk postmenopausal (IBIS-II): an international, double-blind, randomized, placebo-controlled trial. *Lancet*, **383**: 1041–1048.

Davies, C., Pan, H., Godwin, J., *et al.* (2013). Long-term effects of continuing adjuvant tamoxifen to 10 years versus stopping at 5 years after diagnosis of oestrogen receptor-positive breast cancer: ATLAS, a randomized trial. *Lancet*, **381**, 805–816.

De Angelis, R., Sant, M., Coleman, M. P., *et al.* (2014). Cancer survival in Europe 1999–2007 by country and age: results of EUROCARE-5 – a population-based study. *Lancet Oncol.*, **15**, 23–34.

Donovan, E., Bleakley, N., Denholm, E., *et al.* (2007). Randomised trial of standard 2D radiotherapy (RT) versus intensity modulated radiotherapy (IMRT) in patients prescribed breast radiotherapy. *Radiother. Oncol.*, **82**, 254–264.

Dubsky, P. C., Jakesz, R., Milneritsch, B., *et al.* (2012). Tamoxifen and anastrozole as a sequencing strategy: a randomized controlled trial in postmenopausal patients with endocrine-responsive early breast cancer from the Austrian Breast and Colorectal Cancer Study Group. *J. Clin. Oncol.*, **30**, 722–728.

Earl, H. M., Hiller, L., Dunn, J. A., *et al.* (2012). Adjuvant epirubicin followed by cyclophosphamide, methotrexate and fluorouracil (CMF) vs CMF in early breast cancer: results with over 7 years median follow-up from the randomized NEAT/BR9601 trials. *Br. J. Cancer*, **107**, 1257–1267.

EBCTCG. (2005). Effects of chemotherapy and hormonal therapy for early breast cancer on recurrence and 15-year survival: an overview of the randomised trials. *Lancet*, **365**, 1687–1717.

EBCTCG. (2011). Effect of radiotherapy after breast-conserving surgery on 10-year recurrence and 15-year breast cancer death: meta-analysis of individual patient data for 10 801 women in 17 randomised trials. *Lancet*, **378**, 1707–1716.

EBCTCG. (2012). Comparisons between different polychemotherapy regimens for early breast cancer: meta-analyses of long-term outcome among 100 000 women in 123 randomised trials. *Lancet*, **379**, 432–444.

EBCTCG. (2014). Effect of radiotherapy after mastectomy and axillary surgery on 10-year recurrence and 20-year breast cancer mortality: meta-analysis of individual data for 8135 women in 22 randomised trials. *Lancet*, **383**, 2127–2135.

Eedarapalli, P. and Jain, S. (2006). Breast cancer in pregnancy. *J. Obstet. Gynaecol.*, **26**, 1–4.

FAST trialists group, Agrawal, R. K., Alhasso, A., *et al.* (2011). First results of the randomised UK FAST Trial of radiotherapy hypofractionation for treatment of early breast cancer (CRUKE/04/015). *Radiother. Oncol.*, **100**, 93–100.

Fisher, B., Montague, E., Redmond, C., *et al.* (1980). Findings from NSABP Protocol No. B-04-comparison of radical mastectomy with alternative treatments for primary breast cancer. I. Radiation compliance and its relation to treatment outcome. *Cancer*, **46**, 1–13.

Fisher, B., Dignam, J., Wolmark, N., *et al.* (1999). Tamoxifen in treatment of intraductal breast cancer: National Surgical Adjuvant Breast and Bowel Project B-24 randomised controlled trial. *Lancet*, **353**, 1993–2000.

Fisher, B., Anderson, S., Bryant, J., *et al.* (2002). Twenty-year follow up of a randomized trial comparing total mastectomy, lumpectomy, and lumpectomy plus irradiation for the treatment of invasive breast cancer. *N. Engl. J. Med.*, **347**, 1233–1241.

Francis, P. A., Regan, M. M., Fleming, G. F., *et al.* (2015). Adjuvant ovarian suppression in premenopausal breast cancer. *N. Eng. J. Med.*, **372**, 436–446.

French Adjuvant Study Group. (2001). Benefit of a high-dose epirubicin regimen in adjuvant chemotherapy for node positive breast cancer patients with poor prognostic factors: 5-year follow-up results of French Adjuvant Study Group 05 randomized trial. *J. Clin. Oncol.*, **19**, 602–611.

Geyer, C. E., Forster, J., Lindquist, D., *et al.* (2006). Lapatinib plus capecitabine for HER2-positive advanced breast cancer. *N. Engl. J. Med.*, **355**, 2733–2743.

Gianni, L., Dafni, U., Gelber, R. D., *et al.* (2011). Treatment with trastuzumab for 1 year after adjuvant chemotherapy in patients with HER2-positive early breast cancer: a 4-year follow-up of a randomised controlled trial. *Lancet Oncol.*, **12**, 236–244.

Giordano, S. H., Buzdar, A. U., Smith, T. L., *et al.* (2004). Is breast cancer survival improving? *Cancer*, **100**, 44–52.

Giuliano, A. E., Hunt, K. K., Ballman, K. V., *et al.* (2011). Axillary dissection vs. no axillary dissection in women with invasive breast cancer and sentinel node metastasis. *J. Am. Med. Assoc.* **305**, 569–575.

Goldhirsch, A., Gelber, R. D., Piccart-Gebhart, M. J., *et al.* (2013a). 2 versus 1 year of adjuvant trastuzumab for HER2-positive breast cancer (HERA): an open-label, randomized controlled trial. *Lancet*. **382**, 1021–1028.

Goldhirsch, A., Winer, E. P., Coates, A. S., *et al.* (2013b). Personalizing the treatment of women with early breast cancer: highlights of the St Gallen International Expert Consensus on the Primary Therapy of Early Breast Cancer 2013. *Ann. Oncol.*, **24**, 2206–2223.

Goodwin, A., Parker, S., Ghersi, D., *et al.* (2013). Post-operative radiotherapy for ductal carcinoma on situ of the breast. *Cochrane Database Syst. Rev.*, **11**. Art. No. CD000563.

Gray, R. G., Rea, D., Handley, K., *et al* (2013). aTTom: Long-term effects of continuing adjuvant tamoxifen to 10 years versus stopping at 5-years in 6,953 women with early breast cancer. *J. Clin. Oncol.*, **31**(Suppl); abstr. 5.

Hanrahan, E. O., Hennessy, B. T. and Valero, V. (2005). Neoadjuvant systemic therapy for breast cancer: an overview and review of recent clinical trials. *Exp. Opin. Pharmacother.*, **6**, 1477–1491.

Harris, E. E., Christensen, V. J., Hwang, W. T., *et al.* (2005). Impact of concurrent versus sequential tamoxifen with radiation therapy in early-stage breast cancer patients undergoing breast conservation treatment. *J. Clin. Oncol.*, **23**, 11–16.

Haviland, J. S., Owen, J. R., Dewar, J. A., *et al.* (2013). The UK standardization of breast radiotherapy (START) trials of radiotherapy hypofractionation for treatment of early breast cancer: 10-year follow-up results of two randomised controlled trials. *Lancet Oncol.*, **14**, 1086–1094.

Henderson, I. C., Berry, D. A., Demetri, G. D., *et al.* (2003). Improved outcomes from adding sequential paclitaxel but not from escalating doxorubicin dose in an adjuvant chemotherapy regimen for patients with node-positive primary breast cancer. *J. Clin. Oncol.*, **21**, 976–983.

Hershman, D. L., Wang, X., McBride, R., *et al.* (2006). Delay in initiating adjuvant radiotherapy following breast conservation surgery and its impact on survival. *Int. J. Radiat. Oncol. Biol. Phys.*, **65**, 1353–1360.

Holmberg, L., Iverson, O-E. on behalf of the HABITS Study Group. (2008). Increased risk of recurrence after hormone replacement therapy in breast cancer survivors. *J. Natl Cancer Inst.*, **100**, 475–482.

Holt, S., Bertelli, G., Humphreys, I., *et al.* (2013). A decision impact, decision conflict and economic assessment of routine Oncotype DX testing of 146 women with node-negative or pN1mi, ER-positive breast cancer in the UK. *Br. J. Cancer*, **108**, 2250–2258.

Howell, A., Pippen, J., Elledge, R. M., *et al.* (2005). Fulvestrant versus anastrozole for the treatment of advanced breast carcinoma: a prospectively planned combined survival analysis of two multicenter trials. *Cancer*, **104**, 236–239.

Hughes, K. S., Schnaper, L. A., Bellon, J. R., *et al.* (2013). Lumpectomy plus tamoxifen with or without irradiation in women 70 years of age or older with early breast cancer: long term follow-up of CALGB 9343. *J. Clin. Oncol.*, **31**, 2382–2387.

Jin, H., Tu, D., Zhao, N., *et al.* (2012). Longer-term outcomes of letrozole versus placebo after 5-years of tamoxifen in the NCIC CTG MA.17 trial: analyses adjusting for treatment crossover. *J. Clin. Oncol.*, **30**, 718–721.

Joensuu, H., Bono, P., Kataja, V., *et al.* (2009). Fluorouracil, epirubicin and cyclophosphamide with either docetaxel or vinorelbine, with or without tastuzumab, as adjuvant treatments of breast cancer: final results of the FinHer trial. *J. Clin. Oncol.*, **27**, 5685–5692.

Jones, A. L., Barlow, M. and Barrett-Lee, P. L. (2009a). Management of cardiac health in trastuzumab-treated patients with breast cancer: updated United kingdom

National Cancer Research Institute recommendations for monitoring. *Br. J. Cancer*, **100**, 684–692.

Jones, S., Homes, F. A., O'Shaughnessy, J., *et al.* (2009b). Docetaxel with cyclophosphamide is associated with an overall survival benefit compared with doxorubicin and cyclophosphamide: 7-year follow-up of US Oncology Research Trial 9735. *J. Clin. Oncol.*, **27**, 1177–1183.

Karlsson, P., Cole, B. F., Colleoni, M., *et al.* (2011). Timing of radiotherapy and outcome in patients receiving adjuvant endocrine therapy. *Int. J. Radiat. Oncol. Biol. Phys.*, **80**, 398–402.

Kennecke, H., Yerushalmi, R., Woods, R., *et al.* (2010). Metastatic behavior of breast cancer subtypes. *J. Clin. Oncol.*, **28**, 3271–3277.

Kissin, M. W., Querci della Rovere, G., Easton, D., *et al.* (1986). Risk of lymphoedema following the treatment of breast cancer. *Br. J. Surg.*, **73**, 580–584.

Kunkler, I. H., Williams, L. W., Jack, W., *et al.* (2013). The PRIME II trial: wide local excision and adjuvant hormonal therapy ± postoperative whole breast irradiation in women ≥ 65-years with early breast cancer managed by breast conservation. *San Antonio Breast Cancer Symposium*. Abstract S2-01. Presented 11 December 2013.

Le, M. G., Arriagada, R., de Vathaire, F., *et al.* (1990). Can internal mammary chain treatment decrease the risk of death for patients with medial breast cancers and positive axillary lymph nodes? *Cancer*, **66**, 2313–2318.

Leonard, R. C. and Howell, A. (2000). A systematic review of docetaxel, paclitaxel and vinorelbine in the treatment of advanced breast cancer. *Adv. Breast Cancer*, **2**, 1–3.

Livi, L., Borghesi, S., Saivea, C., *et al.* (2009). Radiotherapy timing in 4,820 patients with breast cancer: University of Florence experience. *Int. J. Radiat. Oncol. Biol. Phys.*, **73**, 365–369.

Mansel, R. E., Fallowfield, L., Kissin, M., *et al.* (2006). Randomized multicenter trial of sentinel lymph node biopsy versus standard axillary treatment in operable breast cancer: the ALMANAC trial. *J. Natl Cancer Inst.*, **98**, 599–609.

Martin, M., Pienkowski, T., Mackey, J., *et al.* (2005). Adjuvant docetaxel for node-positive breast cancer. *N. Engl. J. Med.*, **352**, 2302–2313.

Marty, M., Cognetti, F., Maraninchi, D., *et al.* (2005). Randomized phase II trial of the efficacy and safety of trastuzumab combined with docetaxel in patients with human epidermal growth factor receptor 2-positive metastatic breast cancer administered as first line treatment: the M77001 Study Group. *J. Clin. Oncol.*, **23**, 4265–4274.

Masannat, Y. A., Bains, S. K., Pinder, S. E., *et al.* (2013). Challenges in the management of pleomorphic lobular carcinoma in situ of the breast. *Breast*, **22**, 194–196.

Mauri, D., Pavlidis, N., Polyzos, N. P., *et al.* (2006). Survival with aromatase inhibitors and inactivators versus standard hormonal therapy in advanced breast cancer: a meta-analysis. *J. Natl Cancer Inst.*, **98**, 1285–1291.

Miller, T. W., Balko, J. M., Fox, E. M., *et al.* (2011). ERalpha-dependent E2F transcription can mediate resistance to estrogen deprivation in human breast cancer. *Cancer Discov.*, **1**, 338–351.

Miller, W. R., Ellis, I. O., Sainsbury, J. R. C., *et al.* (1994). ABC of breast diseases. Prognostic factors. *Br. Med. J.*, **309**, 1573–1576.

Morris, A. D., Morris, R. D., Wilson, J. F., *et al.* (1997). Breast-conserving therapy vs mastectomy in early-stage breast cancer: a meta-analysis of 10-year survival. *Cancer J. Sci. Am.*, **3**, 6–12.

Mukesh, M. B., Barnett, G. C., Wilkinson, J. S., *et al.* (2013). Randomized controlled trial of intensity-modulated radiotherapy for early breast cancer: 5-year results confirm superior overall cosmesis. *J. Clin. Oncol.*, **31**, 4488–4495.

NHS Cancer Screening Programmes. (2012). *NHS Breast Screening Programme Annual Review*. Sheffield: NHS Cancer Screening Programmes.

NICE. (2002). *Guidance on the Use of Trastuzumab for the Treatment of Advanced Breast Cancer. Technology Appraisal Guidance 34*. London: NICE.

NICE. (2013a). *Familial Breast Cancer. NICE Clinical Guideline*. http://guidance.nice.org.uk/CG164/ NICEGuidance/pdf/English. London: National Institute for Health and Clinical Excellence.

NICE. (2013b). *Gene Expression Profiling and Expanded Immunohistochemistry Tests for Guiding Adjuvant Chemotherapy Decisions in Early Breast Cancer Management: MammaPrint, Oncotype DX, IHC4 and Mammostrat. NICE Diagnostics Guidance 10*. London: National Institute for Health and Clinical Excellence.

NICE. (2013c). *Intraoperative Tests (RD-100i OSNA System and Metasin Test) for Detecting Sentinel Lymph Node Metastases in Breast Cancer. NICE Diagnostics Guidance 8*. London: National Institute for Health and Clinical Excellence.

NICE. (2014). *Early and Locally Advanced Breast Cancer. Diagnosis and Treatment. NICE Clinical Guideline 80*. London: National Institute for Health and Care Excellence.

NIH Consensus Conference. (1991). NIH consensus conference. Treatment of early-stage breast cancer. *J. Am. Med. Assoc.*, **265**, 391–395.

Olivotto, I., Whelan, T. J., Parpia, S., *et al.* (2013). Interim cosmetic and toxicity results from RAPID: a randomized trial of accelerated partial breast irradiation using three-dimensional conformal external beam radiation therapy. *J. Clin. Oncol.*, **31**, 4038–4045.

O'Shaughnessy, J., Miles, D., Vukelja, S., *et al.* (2002). Superior survival with capecitabine plus docetaxel combination chemotherapy in anthracycline-pretreated patients with advanced breast cancer: phase III trial results. *J. Clin. Oncol.*, **20**, 2812–2823.

Overgaard, M., Nielsen, H. M. and Overgaard, J. (2004). Is the benefit of post mastectomy irradiation limited to patients with 4 or more positive nodes, as recommended in international consensus reports? A subgroup analysis of the DBCG 82 b and c randomized trials. *ESTRO 2004*, Amsterdam, Abstr. 33.

Pagani, O., Regan, M. M., Walley, B. A., *et al.* (2014). Adjuvant exemestane with ovarian suppression in premenopausal breast cancer. *N. Eng. J. Med.*, **371**, 107–118.

Perou, C. M., Sørlie, T., Eisen, M. B., *et al.* (2000). Molecular portraits of human breast tumours. *Nature*, **406**, 747–752.

Perez, E. A., Surman, V. J., Davidson, N. E., *et al.* (2011a). Sequential versus concurrent trastuzumab in adjuvant chemotherapy for breast cancer. *J. Clin. Oncol.*, **29**, 4491–4497.

Perez, E. A., Romond, E. H., Suman, V. J., *et al.* (2011b). Four-year follow-up of trastuzumab plus adjuvant chemotherapy for operable human epidermal growth factor receptor 2-positive breast cancer: joint analysis of data from NCCTG N9831 and NSABP B-31. *J. Clin. Oncol.*, **29**, 3366–3373.

Pignol, J-P., Olivotto, I., Rakovitch, E., *et al.* (2008). A multicenter randomized trial of breast intensity-modulated radiation therapy to reduce acute radiation dermatitis. *J. Clin. Oncol.*, **26**, 2085–2092.

Pinto, A. C., Azambuja, E. and Piccart-Gebhart, M. (2013). How long is enough – optimal timing of anti-HER2/neu therapy in the adjuvant setting in early breast cancer. *Breast Care*, **8**, 264–269.

Pivot, X., Gligorov, J., Müller, V., *et al.* (2013a). Preference for subcutaneous or intravenous administration of trastuzumab in patients with HER2-postive early breast cancer (PrefHer): an open-label randomized study. *Lancet Oncol.*, **14**, 962–970.

Pivot, X., Romieu, G., Debled, M., *et al.* (2013b). 6 months versus 12 months of adjuvant trastuzumab for patients with HER2-positive early breast cancer (PHARE): a randomized phase 3 trial. *Lancet Oncol.*, **14**, 741–748.

Ragaz, J., Olivotto, I. A., Spinelli, J. J., *et al.* (2005). Locoregional radiation therapy in patients with high-risk breast cancer receiving adjuvant chemotherapy: 20-year results of the British Columbia randomized trial *J. Natl Cancer Inst.*, **97**, 116–126.

Regan, M. M., Neven, P., Giobbie-Hurder, A., *et al.* (2011). Assessment of letrozole and tamoxifen alone and in sequence for postmenopausal women with steroid hormone receptor-positive breast cancer: the BIG 1-98 randomised clinical trial at 8·1 years median follow-up. *Lancet Oncol.*, **12**, 1101–1108.

Reid, D. M., Doughty, J., Eastell, R., *et al.* (2008). Guidance for the management of breast cancer treatment-induced bone loss: a consensus position statement from a UK Expert Group. *Cancer Treat. Rev.*, **34**, S1–S18.

Roché, H., Fumoleau, P., Spielmann, M., *et al.* (2006). Sequential adjuvant epirubicin-based and docetaxel chemotherapy for node-positive breast cancer patients: the FNCLCC PACS 01 trial. *J. Clin. Oncol.*, **24**, 5664–5671.

Rutgers, E. J., Donker, M., Straver, M. E., *et al.* (2013). Radiotherapy or surgery of the axilla after a positive sentinel node in breast cancer patients: final analysis of the EORTC AMAROS trial (10981/22023). *J. Clin. Oncol.*, **31**(Suppl.); abstr LBA 1001.

Schiavon, G. and Smith, I. E. (2014). Status of adjuvant endocrine therapy for breast cancer. *Breast Cancer Res.*, **16**, 206–222.

SIGN. (2005). *Management of Breast Cancer in Women. A National Clinical Guideline. No. 84.* Edinburgh: Scottish Intercollegiate Guidelines Network.

SIGN. (2013). *SIGN 134. Treatment of Primary Breast Cancer. A National Clinical Guideline.* Edinburgh: Scottish Intercollegiate Guidelines Network.

Silverstein, M. J. (2003). The University of Southern California/Van Nuys prognostic index for ductal carcinoma in situ of the breast. *Am. J. Surg.*, **186**, 337–343.

Slamon, D. J., Leyland-Jones, B., Shak, S., *et al.* (2001). Use of chemotherapy plus a monoclonal antibody against HER2 for metastatic breast cancer that over expresses HER2. *N. Engl. J. Med.*, **344**, 783–792.

Slamon, D., Eiermann, W., Robert, N., *et al.* (2011). Adjuvant trastuzumab in HER2-postive breast cancer. *N. Engl. J. Med.*, **365**, 1273–1283.

Sørlie, T., Perou, C. M., Tibshirani, R., *et al.* (2001). Gene expression patterns of breast carcinomas distinguish tumour subclasses with clinical implications. *Proc. Natl Acad. Sci. USA*, **98**, 10869–10874.

Sørlie, T., Tibshirani, R., Parker, J., *et al.* (2003). Repeated observation of breast tumor subtypes in independent gene expression data sets. *Proc. Natl Acad. Sci. USA*, **100**, 8418–8423.

Sparano, J. A., Wang, M., Martino, S., *et al.* (2008). Weekly paclitaxel in the adjuvant treatment of breast cancer. *N. Engl. J. Med.*, **358**, 1663–1671.

Spielmann, M., Roché, H., Delozier, T., *et al.* (2009). Trastuzumab for patients with axillar-node-positive breast cancer: results of the FNCLCC-PACS 04 trial. *J. Clin. Oncol.*, **27**, 6129–6134.

Stopeck, A. T., Lipton, A., Body, J. J., *et al.* (2010). Denosumab compared with zoledronic acid for the treatment of bone metastases in patients with advanced breast cancer: a randomized, double-blind study. *J. Clin. Oncol.*, **28**, 5132–5139.

Swain, S. M., Kim, S. B., Cortes, J., *et al.* (2013). Pertuzumab, trastuzumab, and docetaxel for HER2-positive metastatic breast cancer (CLEOPATRA study): overall survival results from a randomised, double-blind, placebo-controlled, phase 3 study. *Lancet Oncol.*, **14**, 461–471.

Thompson, A. M., Jordan, L. B., Quinlan, P., *et al.* (2010). Prospective comparison of switches in biomarker status between primary and recurrent breast cancer: the Breast Recurrence In Tissues Study (BRITS). *Breast Cancer Res.*, **12**(6), R92.

Thomson, C. S., Brewster, D. H., Dewar, J. A., *et al.* (2004). Improvements in survival for women with breast cancer in Scotland between 1987 and 1993: impact of earlier diagnosis and changes in treatment. *Eur. J. Cancer*, **40**, 743–753.

UICC. (2009). *TNM Classification of Malignant Tumours*, 7th edn, ed. L. H. Sobin, M. Gospodarowicz and Ch. Wittekind. New York: Wiley-Liss, pp. 181–193.

Vaidya, J. S., Wenz, F., Bulsara, M., *et al.* (2014). Risk-adapted targeted intraoperative radiotherapy versus whole-breast radiotherapy for breast cancer: 5-year results for local control and overall survival from the TARGIT-A randomised trial. *Lancet*, **383**, 603–613.

van de Velde, C. J. H., Rea, D., Seynaeve, C., *et al.* (2011). Adjuvant tamoxifen and exemstane in early breast cancer (TEAM): a ransomised phase 3 trial. *Lancet*, **377**, 321–331.

Veronesi, U., Cascinelli, N., Mariani, L., *et al.* (2002). Twenty-year follow-up of a randomized study comparing breast-conserving surgery with radical mastectomy for early breast cancer. *N. Engl. J. Med.*, **347**, 1227–1232.

Veronesi, U., Orrechia, R., Maisonneuve, P., *et al.* (2013). Intraoperative radiotherapy versus external radiotherapy for early breast cancer (ELIOT): a randomized controlled equivalence trial. *Lancet Oncol.*, **14**, 1269–1277.

Veronesi, U., Paganelli, G., Viale, G., *et al.* (2003). A randomized comparison of sentinel-node biopsy with routine axillary dissection in breast cancer. *N. Engl. J. Med.*, **349**, 546–553.

von Minckwitz, G., Untch, M., Blohmer, J. U., *et al.* (2012). Definition and impact of pathologic complete response on prognosis after neoadjuvant chemotherapy in various intrinsic breast cancer subtypes. *J. Clin. Oncol.*, **30**, 1796–1804.

Vujovic, O., Yu, E., Cherian, A., *et al.* (2006). Eleven-year follow-up results in the delay of breast irradiation after conservative breast surgery in node-negative breast cancer patients. *Int. J. Radiat. Oncol. Biol. Phys.*, **64**, 760–764.

Whelan, T. J., Olivotto, I., Parulekar, W. R., *et al.* (2015). Regional nodal irradiation in early-stage breast cancer. *N. Eng. J. Med.*, **373**, 307–316.

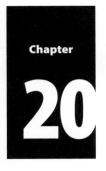

Management of cancer of the kidney

Rhian Sian Davies, Jason Lester and John Wagstaff

Introduction

Cancer of the kidney represents 4% of adult malignancies. Men are more frequently affected than women, and it commonly occurs between the ages of 50 and 70 years. More than 30% of patients present with metastatic disease. The majority of malignant tumours are adenocarcinomas, arising from the proximal renal tubular epithelium. These tumours were previously called *hypernephroma* because it was believed that they originated from adrenal rests, but they are correctly termed *renal cell carcinoma* (RCC). The main focus of this chapter is the management of RCC. Transitional cell carcinoma of the renal pelvis accounts for 5% of all renal malignancies, and is covered separately at the end of the chapter.

Types of kidney tumour

Kidney tumours can be benign, malignant primary or metastatic. Benign tumours include cysts (simple, complex, multiple), inflammatory (infection, infarction), adenoma and oncocytoma. Malignant primary tumours include RCC, lymphoma, sarcoma and renal pelvis tumours (5% of malignant renal cancers arise from the renal pelvis, and more than 90% of these are transitional cell carcinoma).

Anatomy

The kidneys are retroperitoneal structures that lie between the eleventh rib and the transverse process of the third lumbar vertebral body, each approximately 11 cm in length, the right lying slightly lower than the left. Each kidney is surrounded by perinephric fat which in turn is covered by Gerota's fascia. The right kidney abuts the liver and stomach and the left, the spleen, stomach and pancreas. The lymphatics drain along the renal vessels, on the right draining to paracaval and aortocaval nodes, and on the left to the para-aortic region.

Incidence and epidemiology

Over 10,000 new cases of kidney cancer were diagnosed in the UK in 2011 resulting in approximately 4200 deaths (Cancer Research UK website accessed July 2014). In the last 10 years kidney cancer incidence rates in the UK have increased by almost a third, and unlike in some other cancers, the death rate is still rising. Kidney cancer occurs most commonly in people 50–80 years of age. Men are more frequently affected than women; the male-to-female ratio is 5:3. It is the seventh most common cancer in men and tenth most common cancer in women in the UK.

Renal cell carcinoma

Risk factors and aetiology

Risk factors for RCC include smoking (up to one-third of cancers may be due to smoking, and there seems to be a dose–response effect), radiation, trichloroethylene, obesity, especially in women, and use of phenacetin analgesics. Possible risk factors include arsenic and cadmium. Acquired cystic kidney disease, which occurs in nearly half of patients on dialysis, is also a factor. The risk is up to 30 times greater in dialysis patients with cystic changes compared to the general population.

Occupations that may carry an increased risk of renal cell carcinoma include leather tanners, shoe workers, printing process workers and asbestos workers.

RCC risk is doubled in people with a first-degree relative with kidney cancer and quadrupled when

Practical Clinical Oncology, Second Edition, ed. Louise Hanna, Tom Crosby and Fergus Macbeth. Published by Cambridge University Press. © Cambridge University Press 2015.

the affected relative is a sibling. Genetic risk factors for RCC include Von Hippel–Lindau disease, tuberous sclerosis and adult polycystic disease. In Von Hippel–Lindau disease, the gene involved is on the short arm of chromosome 3; this disease occurs in 1 in 36,000 births and is associated with clear cell adenocarcinomas, which are often multiple and bilateral. There are two subtypes: type I, without phaeochromocytoma, and type II, with phaeochromocytoma. Tuberous sclerosis and adult polycystic disease both involve autosomal dominant inheritance; their disease incidences are 1 in 10,000 and 1 in 1000, respectively.

Pathology

Classification of renal cell tumours

The 2004 WHO classification of adult renal tumours describes categories and entities based on pathological and genetic analyses (Eble *et al.*, 2004). Table 20.1 shows the WHO classification of renal cell tumours. The pathological features of RCC are shown in Table 20.2.

Grade

The Fuhrman nuclear grading system is widely used (Fuhrman *et al.*, 1982). Several studies involving large numbers of patients have shown good correlation with survival (Murphy *et al.*, 1994). Four grades are recognised based on nuclear size, nuclear contour, and the presence of nucleoli. Mitotic activity is not considered because it varies among tumours and it does not correlate well with prognosis.

Grade I tumours demonstrate small, uniform nuclei without nucleoli. Multinucleated giant tumour cells are seen only in grade IV tumours, which occasionally may demonstrate spindling and severe nuclear anaplasia resembling a sarcoma. When tumour heterogeneity is present, the highest grade is always assigned.

Cytogenetics

Histological differentiation of benign from malignant primary renal tumours can be difficult. Cytogenetic analysis can be a useful aid. For example, clear cell carcinoma is characterised by loss of part of the short arm of chromosome 3. Regions that are frequently lost are 3p12–14, 3p21 and 3p25. Other aberrations include trisomy of chromosome 5. The WHO 2004 classification includes the rare and relatively recently described Xp11 translocation renal cell carcinoma which requires

Table 20.1 The 2004 WHO classification of renal cell tumours

Type	Examples
Benign	Papillary adenoma
	Oncocytoma
Malignant	Clear cell renal cell carcinoma (70–75% of cases)
	Multilocular clear cell renal cell carcinoma (rare)
	Papillary (formerly chromophilic) renal cell carcinoma (10–15% of cases)
	Chromophobe renal cell carcinoma (2–5% of cases)
	Collecting duct carcinoma (1% of cases)
	Renal medullary carcinoma
	Xp11 translocation carcinomas
	Carcinoma associated with neuroblastoma
	Mucinous tubular and spindle cell carcinoma
	RCC, unclassified
	Sarcomatoid change may be seen in all types of RCC and the 2004 WHO classification does not consider it a separate entity

RCC, renal cell carcinoma; WHO, World Health Organisation.

cytogenetic analysis for diagnosis. It is characterized by chromosome translocations involving the Xp11.2 breakpoint and resulting in gene fusions involving the *TFE3* transcription factor gene that maps to this locus. The genetic features of adult renal cell carcinoma are discussed in greater detail in the WHO 2004 classification (Eble *et al.*, 2004).

Clinical presentation

The tumour may remain clinically silent until metastases develop. The classic triad of pain, flank mass and haematuria occurs in only 19% of patients and predicts a poor prognosis. However, 50% of patients will have two of these symptoms.

Other symptoms include fever, sweats, weight loss, malaise and those secondary to metastatic spread, such as bone pain.

A varicocele can occur in up to 2% of males due to obstruction of the testicular vein. This will be left-sided because of the different anatomy of the left and right renal veins.

Table 20.2 Pathological features of renal cell carcinoma

Features	Description
Macroscopic	*Clear cell*: typically arises from the cortex; solid, lobulated and yellow; a pseudocapsule is often present; haemorrhage, necrosis and/or calcification are common; the tumour may contain single or multiple fluid-filled cysts *Multilocular*: cysts of variable size separated from the kidney by a fibrous capsule *Papillary*: May be bilateral or multifocal with frequent hemorrhage, necrosis and cystic degeneration *Chromophobe*: Solid and appears orange turning grey or sandy after fixation *Collecting duct*: Centrally and typically shows a firm grey–white appearance
Microscopic	*Clear cell*: clear cytoplasm, condensed hyperchromatic nuclei *Multilocular*: cysts lined by a single layer of clear to pale cells *Papillary*: centrally located small nuclei and ground-glass eosinophilic staining cytoplasm; papillary architecture; there are types I and II with different molecular defects *Chromophobe*: polygonal tumour cells with a transparent, reticulated cytoplasm; cytoplasm crowded with glycogen deposits *Collecting duct*: tubular growth pattern; basophilic cytoplasm, anaplastic nuclei

Spread

Renal cancer can spread locally, via lymphatics, and via the blood. Local spread is to the adrenal gland, renal vein, inferior vena cava, Gerota's fascia and perinephric tissue. It spreads to lymph nodes at the renal hilum, abdominal para-aortic, and paracaval regions, and via the blood to lung, bone, soft tissues, the liver, the CNS and skin.

Paraneoplastic syndromes

Paraneoplastic syndromes include hypercalcaemia (PTH-related peptide), polycythaemia (EPO-like molecule), hypertension (renin) and hepatic dysfunction (secondary to interleukin-6 production by tumour cells).

Investigation and staging

Differentiating benign from malignant tumours

There are no reliable criteria to distinguish benign renal adenomas from RCC. In 1950, a postmortem study reported that metastases were rare when renal tumours were less than 3 cm in size, and these tumours should be considered benign adenomas (Bell, 1950). With the advent of CT scans, an increasing number of small tumours that had already metastasised were reported; therefore, tumour size is no longer considered a reliable criterion to distinguish RCC (Aso and Homma, 1992). In addition, histological features of adenoma and RCC overlap, and so a biopsy may be misleading.

Abdominal ultrasound and CT detect incidental renal cysts in a significant proportion of people. Postmortem results have shown that approximately 50% of people over age 50 have one or more renal cysts, and other studies indicate that almost one-third have at least one renal cyst that is identifiable on CT (Tada *et al.*, 1983). In 1986, Bosniak created a four-part classification of cystic renal masses found on CT scans (Bosniak, 1986). The system uses Hounsfield units to categorise these lesions in order of increasing probability of malignancy. This classification system has been shown to be useful in separating tumours requiring surgery from those that can be safely followed up.

Staging investigations

Renal ultrasound can be useful in evaluating questionable cystic renal tumours if CT imaging is inconclusive. Contrast-enhanced CT scans of the thorax, abdomen and pelvis are used to look at perirenal extension, renal vein/caval involvement, lymph node enlargement and pulmonary metastases. MRI is useful for imaging the vena cava.

A bone scan, full blood count and a biochemical profile, including serum calcium, LDH and alkaline phosphatase, are also useful. A renogram (DMSA or MAG 3) should be performed if there is impaired renal function.

Table 20.3 TNM 7 staging of renal cell carcinoma

Stage	Description
Tx	Primary tumour cannot be assessed
T0	No evidence of primary tumour
T1	≤ 7 cm, confined to the kidney
T1a	≤ 4 cm
T1b	> 4 and ≤ 7 cm
T2	> 7 cm limited to the kidney
T2a	> 7 and ≤ 10 cm limited to the kidney
T2b	> 10 cm limited to the kidney
T3	Extends into major veins or perinephric tissues but not into ipsilateral adrenal gland and not beyond Gerota fascia
T3a	Grossly extends into the renal vein or its segmental (muscle-containing) branches, or invades perirenal and/or renal sinus fat but not beyond Gerota fascia
T3b	Grossly extends into vena cava below the diaphragm
T3c	Tumour grossly extends into vena cava above the diaphragm or its wall
T4	Directly invades beyond Gerota fascia including contiguous extension into the ipsilateral adrenal gland
N0	No regional nodal metastases
N1	Single regional lymph node
N2	Multiple regional lymph nodes
M0	No distant metastasis
M1	Distant metastasis

Adapted from UICC (2009).

Table 20.4 Stage grouping of renal cell cancer

Stage	Description
I	T1 N0 M0
II	T2 N0 M0
III	T3 N0 M0 or
	T1–3 N1 M0
IV	T4 N0–2 M0 or
	Any T N2 M0 or
	Any T Any N M1

Adapted from UICC (2009).

Staging classification

The regional lymph nodes are the hilar, abdominal para-aortic and paracaval nodes. Tables 20.3 and 20.4 show the TNM 7 classification and stage groupings for RCC (UICC 2009).

Treatment overview

Patients with localised or locally advanced resectable disease (stages I–III) are treated radically where possible. While the primary aim of treatment is to eliminate the cancer, it is also important to consider kidney function after surgery, particularly if patients have only one kidney or multiple tumours. For those with stage IV disease, treatment is usually palliative, although long-term survival can sometimes be achieved by resection of a single or a small number of metastases.

Treatment of localised or locally advanced resectable disease (stages I–III)

Surgery

Radical nephrectomy

Surgical resection is the treatment of choice where appropriate. This may be via an open or laparoscopic approach. Radical nephrectomy involves removal of the kidney, adrenal gland, perirenal fat and Gerota's fascia, with or without a regional lymph node dissection. Surgery can be extended to remove the tumour or tumour thrombus from the infra- and supradiaphragmatic vena cava and, rarely, the right atrium; cardiopulmonary bypass is required for the latter. In patients with bilateral stage I tumours (concurrent or subsequent), bilateral partial nephrectomy or unilateral partial nephrectomy with contralateral radical nephrectomy, when technically feasible, may be a preferred alternative to bilateral nephrectomy with dialysis or transplantation.

Laparoscopic (partial) nephrectomy

Laparoscopic nephrectomy is a less-invasive procedure. Laparoscopic surgery tends to incur less morbidity and is associated with a shorter recovery time and less blood loss. The need for pain medications is reduced, but operating room time and costs are higher. Disadvantages include concerns about spillage, limited experience and technical difficulties in defining surgical margins. A transperitoneal or retroperitoneal approach may be used. Studies of laparoscopic nephrectomy have now demonstrated clearly that the local recurrence rate (i.e. secondary to spillage) is no lower with this approach, and survival is equivalent to an open operation. Increasing evidence suggests that a partial nephrectomy is curative in selected cases (tumours < 4 cm in size).

Adjuvant treatment

Radiotherapy

Two old randomised trials showed no benefit from postoperative radiotherapy (Finney, 1973; Kjaer et al., 1987). Fatal liver damage was reported and the complication rates were high. Adjuvant radiotherapy should not be used in routine clinical practice. Studies of preoperative radiotherapy have not shown any evidence of benefit. It is not used in routine clinical practice.

Systemic therapy

An excellent overview of adjuvant trials past, present and future has recently been published (Janowitz et al., 2013).

Chemotherapy

Currently, there is no evidence supporting the use of adjuvant chemotherapy in RCC.

Immunotherapy

There is no evidence that adjuvant interferon α (IFNα) or interleukin-2 (IL-2) monotherapy improves survival following potentially curative radical nephrectomy (Clark et al., 2003; Messing et al., 2003). The EORTC 30955 trial has randomised high-risk postoperative patients (T3+ and/or N1+) to the Atzpodien regimen (see discussion later in this chapter) or to surveillance. This study is closed to recruitment and results are awaited. HYDRA is an ongoing NCRN study of similar design.

Vaccine therapy

A German trial randomised 558 radical nephrectomy patients to autologous renal tumour cell vaccine or surveillance and reported a modest improvement in progression-free but not overall survival with the vaccine (Jocham et al., 2004). This expensive treatment (18,000 Euros) is not used in routine clinical practice in the UK.

Targeted therapy

Currently, there is no evidence supporting the use of adjuvant targeted therapies in renal cell carcinoma.

Clinical trials involving all of the new targeted agents have either completed or are still recruiting, although no results are yet available (Janowitz et al., 2013).

Treatment of localised or locally advanced inoperable disease (stages I–III)

Small stage 1 cancers may be successfully treated with radiofrequency ablation (RFA) or cryotherapy when patients decline or are unfit for surgery or when a minimally invasive nephron-sparing technique is indicated. Adjuvant treatment is under investigation and should not be used routinely outside clinical trials.

Palliative treatments for localised disease include EBRT or arterial embolisation.

Treatment of stage IV or recurrent disease

The prognosis for metastatic RCC patients with stage IV or recurrent disease is relatively poor, and the vast majority are incurable. Appropriate treatment depends on many factors, including prior treatment and site of recurrence, as well as individual patient considerations. Carefully selected patients may benefit from surgical resection of localised metastatic disease, particularly if they have had a prolonged, disease-free interval since radical surgery.

Surgery

Palliative nephrectomy

Palliative nephrectomy can be performed if the burden of metastatic disease is small and the patient is fit. It may alleviate pain and bleeding and may improve paraneoplastic syndromes such as hypercalcaemia. Spontaneous regression of metastases following surgery occurs in less than 1% of cases (Montie et al., 1977). Two randomised trials have examined the role of nephrectomy in patients who were subsequently treated with interferon for metastatic disease (Flanigan et al., 2001; Mickisch et al., 2001). Both of these trials showed significantly better survival for patients undergoing nephrectomy. Nephrectomy should therefore be considered in all patients who are to undergo immunotherapy, provided their performance status is adequate.

Metastectomy

Solitary metastases can be resected, and long-term survival has been reported. As expected, patients with a long disease-free interval following surgery survive longer than those presenting with a solitary metastasis synchronous with a primary lesion (O'Dea *et al.*, 1978).

Radiotherapy

Radiotherapy to the primary tumour

Radiotherapy plays no role in the curative treatment of RCC. It can be used to control bleeding, but results are often disappointing when it is used for pain relief.

Palliative radiotherapy technique

The patient lies supine on simulator couch, knees supported by a polystyrene wedge. If using an X-ray simulator, intravenous contrast is required to define the target volume. Treatment field edges are positioned to cover part or all of the affected kidney. (Make sure you are treating the correct kidney!) Parallel-opposed anterior and posterior fields, 6–10 MV photons, on a linear accelerator are usually used. For large tumours, CT planning allows more accurate delineation of the disease and can reduce the dose to normal tissues. Doses prescribed include 20 Gy in 5 fractions over 1 week, or 6–10 Gy given as a single fraction. Side effects of radiotherapy include tiredness, nausea (give prophylactic anti-emetics) and diarrhoea.

Radiotherapy to metastases

Palliative radiotherapy can alleviate the symptoms of metastatic disease, particularly bone pain. Bone lesions from kidney cancer are lytic and can be aggressive. An 8–10 Gy single fraction or 20 Gy in 5 fractions are suitable dose fractionations. Increasingly, stereotactic body radiotherapy is being used to treat oligometastatic disease, although randomised trial evidence that this approach is beneficial is lacking.

Cytokine treatment

Interferon α

The use of cytokines in clinical practice has dropped significantly in recent years following the introduction of a variety of new and effective oral therapies for RCC, in particular the tyrosine kinase inhibitors (TKIs). An overview published in the Cochrane library (Coppin *et al.*, 2005) showed that immunotherapy (interferon and/or IL-2) produced an objective response rate (RR) of 12.9% (complete response (CR) 3.6%). This was compared with an RR of 2.5% in 10 non-immunotherapy arms and 4.3% in 2 placebo arms. The median survival was 13.3 months, which was a 3.8-month improvement compared to non-immunotherapy study arms.

In 4 studies (644 patients) the odds ratio for death at 1 year was significantly reduced by interferon therapy (OR = 0.56; 95% CI = 0.4–0.77). In this analysis the addition of anything to single-agent interferon did not significantly affect the outcome. A study of 492 patients demonstrated that interferon and/or IL-2 do not provide a survival benefit for patients with intermediate prognosis (as defined by the Groupe Francais d'Immunotherapie, Negrier *et al.*, 2005), and therefore should be considered only in patients of good prognosis (Negrier *et al.*, 2007).

No definite dose–response relationship has been proven for interferon therapy. Because tachyphylaxis usually develops, a widely used protocol is to begin with 3 million units subcutaneously 3 times weekly, escalating to 6 and then 9 million units at fortnightly intervals. Treatment should be continued until progressive disease is documented. The median time to response is 6 months.

Interleukin-2

In the Cochrane overview, IL-2 seems to incur a response rate and median survival similar to that of IFN-α (Coppin *et al.*, 2005). High-dose therapy is associated with higher complete response rates than IFN (7–8%). These responses have been shown to be very durable, with 80–85% of patients being alive after 10 years and probably cured of their disease. Side effects include flu-like symptoms, nausea, skin rashes, diarrhoea, capillary-leak syndrome, renal impairment, bone marrow suppression and, rarely, cardiac toxicity and confusion. One study (Atkins *et al.*, 2005) has shown that patients whose tumours stain positively for the expression of carbonic anhydrase IX (CAIX) have an almost 40% chance of long-term survival and possible cure. High-dose bolus IL-2 is the only therapy that has been shown to cure metastatic renal carcinoma. Selected patients who are young, have an excellent performance status, low-volume disease and whose tumours stain positively for CAIX should be considered for this therapy.

Palliative combination cytokine therapy

To date, there is no evidence that IFNα/IL-2 combinations with or without conventional chemotherapy show a survival advantage over monotherapy. High response rates have been reported with the Atzpodien regimen (IFNα, IL-2 and 5-FU), but the treatment is associated with significant toxicity and two other phase II trials failed to confirm the high response rate. A small randomised trial has shown a survival advantage of using the Atzpodien regimen compared to tamoxifen in metastatic RCC (Atzpodien et al., 2001). The RE04 trial compared IFNα with IFNα/IL-2 (Gore et al., 2010). There was no difference in either progression-free or overall survival between the two groups. Toxicity was worse in the combination arm.

Targeted treatment

Sunitinib

Sunitinib is an oral multikinase inhibitor that targets VEGFR-1, VEGFR-2, PDGFR and KIT. A phase 3 trial of 750 previously untreated patients with advanced clear cell RCC compared sunitinib with interferon-alpha (Motzer et al., 2009). Sunitinib was associated with a median progression-free survival (PFS) of 11 months compared to 5 months for interferon-alpha (HR 0.42, $p < 0.001$). There was a strong trend to improved overall survival (OS) with sunitinib (26.4 versus 21.8 months, $HR = 0.82, 95\%CI = 0.669–1.001, p = 0.051$). It is important to bear in mind that a 21.8-month median survival for interferon patients is much longer than the median survival found in the Coppin meta-analysis, suggesting that survival is likely to have been boosted by subsequent therapies in this interferon control group. A median survival of 26.4 months for sunitinib probably represents a doubling of the survival compared with interferon alone. Bevacizumab plus interferon-alpha resulted in longer PFS but not OS compared with interferon alpha alone in two similarly designed, randomised controlled trials (Escudier et al., 2007; Rini et al., 2008). Sunitinib is licensed and has NICE approval in the first-line setting for patients with advanced RCC (www.nice.org.uk/TA169, accessed November 2014).

Pazopanib

Pazopanib is an oral multikinase inhibitor that targets VEGFR-1, VEGFR-2, VEGFR-3, PDGFR, and KIT. A phase 3 trial of 435 patients with clear cell or predominantly clear-cell RCC compared pazopanib with placebo (Sternberg et al., 2010). Nearly half of the patients had previously received cytokine therapy. PFS was significantly longer in patients receiving pazopanib at 9.2 months compared with 4.2 months in patients receiving placebo ($HR = 0.46, p < 0.0001$).

Pazopanib was also compared with sunitinib in the randomised phase 3 COMPARZ trial that enrolled 1110 patients with metastatic clear-cell RCC (Motzer et al., 2013b, 2014) The primary endpoint was PFS and the trial was powered to assess the non-inferiority of pazopanib compared to sunitinib. Median PFS was 8.4 months for patients on pazopanib and 9.5 months for those on sunitinib ($HR = 1.05, 95\%CI = 0.9–1.22$). There was no difference in OS ($HR = 0.92, 95\% CI = 0.79–1.06$). Although quality of life was compared in the study, differences in the scheduled administration of the medications made this comparison difficult to interpret.

The PISCES trial was an innovative, double-blind, cross-over study in 169 patients with metastatic RCC that evaluated preference for pazopanib or sunitinib (Escudier et al., 2014). Patients with metastatic RCC were randomly assigned to pazopanib 800 mg per day for 10 weeks, a 2-week washout, and then sunitinib 50 mg per day (4 weeks on, 2 weeks off, 4 weeks on) for 10 weeks, or the reverse sequence. Of 169 randomly assigned patients, 114 met prespecified intent-to-treat criteria. Significantly, more patients preferred pazopanib (70%) over sunitinib (22%) and 8% expressed no preference ($p < 0.001$). It should be noted that 33% of the randomly assigned patients were never evaluable for the primary endpoint because of withdrawals, adverse events, lack of efficacy, deaths, and other miscellaneous reasons, limiting the prespecified analyses.

Pazopanib is licensed and NICE approved in the first-line setting for patients with advanced RCC (www.nice.org.uk/guidance/TA215, accessed November 2014).

Sorafenib

Sorafenib is an orally available multikinase inhibitor. In a phase 3 trial, 769 patients were stratified by the Memorial Sloan-Kettering Cancer Center prognostic risk category and were randomised to sorafenib or placebo. Approximately 82% of the patients had received prior IL-2 and/or interferon-alpha in both arms of the study. The median PFS for patients randomly assigned to sorafenib was 167 days compared with 84 days for patients randomly assigned to placebo ($p < 0.001$). There was no significant difference in OS.

Sorafenib is not recommended by NICE (www.nice.org.uk/guidance/TA178, accessed November 2014).

Axitinib

Axitinib has been shown to prolong progression of disease when used as second-line systemic therapy. A randomised controlled trial of 723 patients evaluated axitinib versus sorafenib in advanced RCC with a clear-cell component that had progressed during or after first-line treatment with sunitinib (54%), cytokines (35%), bevacizumab plus interferon (8%), or temsirolimus (3%) (Motzer et al., 2013a). Median PFS was 8.3 months for axitinib versus 5.7 months for sorafenib (HR = 0.656, $p < 0.0001$) The largest benefit was seen in patients who received cytokines as first-line therapy and whose median PFS was 12.2 months with axitinib compared with 8.2 months with sorafenib ($p < 0.0001$). There was no difference in OS between the two arms of the trial. Axitinib has been provisionally recommended by NICE for patients with advanced RCC after failure of treatment with a first-line kinase inhibitor or a cytokine.

Temsirolimus

Temsirolimus, an intravenously administered MTOR inhibitor, was shown to result in prolonged OS compared with interferon-alpha in a phase 3 randomised controlled trial that enrolled intermediate- and poor-risk patients (Hudes et al., 2007). The trial enrolled patients with a variety of subtypes of RCC and was not restricted to clear-cell kidney cancer. Median survival was 7.3 months in the interferon group versus 10.9 months in the temsirolimus group ($p = 0.008$), making temsirolimus the only therapy for RCC to have clearly been shown to result in longer OS than interferon-alpha using conventional statistical analysis. Temsirolimus has been licensed as an orphan drug in the European Union. It is not recommended by NICE (www.nice.org.uk/guidance/TA178, accessed November 2014).

Everolimus

Everolimus, an orally administered MTOR inhibitor, was evaluated in a double-blind, randomised placebo-controlled phase 3 trial (Motzer et al., 2008). Four hundred and ten patients with metastatic RCC with a clear-cell component that had progressed during or within 6 months of stopping treatment with sunitinib or sorafenib, or both drugs were randomly assigned in a two-to-one ratio to receive everolimus 10 mg once daily or placebo. Median PFS was 4.0 months with everolimus compared with 1.9 months with placebo. No difference in OS was reported. Everolimus is not recommended by NICE (www.nice.org.uk/guidance/TA178, accessed November 2014).

Chemotherapy

RCC is chemoresistant. Conventional chemotherapy has not been shown to give a survival advantage,

and response rates are poor (Yagoda et al., 1995). It should not be used in routine clinical practice outside a clinical trial.

Hormonal treatments

Progesterones

Progesterones were used for many years based on responses seen in animal models and a lack of any other effective systemic therapy. Response rates are 0–2%, with no proven clinical benefit (Kjaer, 1988). Patients may, however, have increased appetite and an improved feeling of well-being when on these agents. This treatment is no longer recommended.

Tamoxifen

Tamoxifen may have a low level of activity in high doses (100 mg/m^2 per day), but it is not used in routine clinical practice in the UK.

Prognosis

Survival is dependent on the stage and grade of the tumour. Following radical nephrectomy, renal vein involvement alone does not seem to adversely affect 5-year survival, but does reduce 10-year survival. In metastatic disease, increased survival is associated with good PS, absence of weight loss, presence of only pulmonary metastasis, removal of the primary tumour and a long disease-free interval between nephrectomy and the appearance of metastases.

Overall survival

Five-year survival by stage is:
- I: 60–90%;
- II: 50–70%;
- III: 20–60%;
- IV: 0–20%.

Five-year survival (M0 disease) by Furhman grade is:
- I: 90%;
- II: 90%;
- III: 55%;
- IV: 33%.

Prognostic models

Prognostic models were first developed when immunotherapy was the standard of care. The Memorial Sloan-Kettering Cancer Center (MSKCC) was the standard system and has now been validated and updated for use in the current era of targeted therapies

Table 20.5 Estimated survival for patients with kidney cancer according to number of risk factors

Number of risk factors	Risk group	Median overall survival (months)	Two-year survival (%)
0	Favourable	NR*	75
1–2	Intermediate	27	53
3–6	Poor	8.8	7

*NR, not reported. Adapted from Heng et al., 2009.

as the Heng criteria (Heng *et al.*, 2009). Patients are stratified according to the presence of six risk factors.

1. Karnofsky performance status (PS) < 80%.
2. Haemoglobin less than lower limit of normal.
3. Time from diagnosis to treatment < 1 year.
4. Corrected calcium above the upper limit of normal.
5. Platelets greater than the upper limit of normal.
6. Neutrophils greater than the upper limit of normal.

The number of risk factors present is added up and the risk is stratified as in Table 20.5.

These prognostic groupings have been used to select patients for clinical trials of targeted agents that are discussed later in this chapter.

Recently, the International Metastatic Renal Carcinoma Database Consortium performed an external validation and comparison of prognostic models in metastatic RCC (Heng *et al.*, 2013). The factors in this model were:

1. anaemia;
2. thrombocytosis;
3. neutrophilia;
4. hypercalcaemia;
5. Karnofsky performance score < 80%;
6. < 1 year from diagnosis to development of metastatic disease.

The median survivals of patients in the favourable, intermediate and poor prognostic groups were: 43.2, 22.5 and 7.8 months, respectively. It is currently unclear whether this new model will replace the MSKCC model for stratifying patients in clinical trials.

Prognostic scores have also been developed to predict the risk of relapse after radical nephrectomy. One such scoring system in use is the Leibovich score (Leibovich *et al.*, 2003). Further discussion on prognostic scores following radical surgery are beyond the scope of this chapter.

Areas of current interest and ongoing clinical trials

Immunotherapy

Kidney cancer seems to be one of the cancers most likely to respond to immunotherapy. Drugs that block PD-1 and PD-L1 are now in development and are being extensively studied in multiple tumour types. Phase 1 studies have suggested both PD-1 and PD-L1 inhibitors have some activity in advanced renal cell carcinoma and are being tested in larger clinical trials.

Ongoing clinical trials

Ongoing clinical trials open to recruitement in the UK include the following.

S-TRACT is a phase III randomised controlled trial aiming to recruit 720 patients. Patients with RCC at high risk of recurrence following radical nephrectomy are randomised to receive adjuvant sunitinib or placebo.

STAR is a phase II/III randomised controlled trial (210 patients in phase II, 1000 patients in phase III) of patients with locally advanced or metastatic RCC. Patients receiving standard first-line sunitinib or pazopaninb are randomised to either continuation of the drug or temporary cessation at the time of maximal radiological response. The outcome measures include time to strategy failure and overall survival.

SURTIME is a randomised phase III trial comparing immediate or deferred nephrectomy following 3 cycles of sunitinib in patients with synchronous metastatic RCC. The trial is aiming to recruit 458 patients, and the primary outcome measure is overall survival.

CARMENA is a randomised phase III trial aiming to recruit 1134 patients with metastatic RCC treated with sunitinib. Patients are randomised to receive sunitinib and a nephrectomy or sunitinib alone, and the primary outcome measure is overall survival.

A-PREDICT is a phase II trial aiming to recruit 99 patients with metastatic RCC unsuitable for radical nephrectomy. The patients are treated with axitinib, and the primary outcome measure is progression-free survival.

Carcinoma of the renal pelvis

Renal pelvis carcinoma is a relatively rare tumour, constituting 5% of all renal tumours; more than 90% are transitional cell carcinomas (TCCs). Squamous cell carcinoma, which is usually associated with chronic inflammation or infection of the renal pelvis, accounts for the majority of the remaining malignant tumours. Carcinoma of the renal pelvis is more common in men (male-to-female ratio of 2:1) and usually occurs between the ages of 50 and 70. The major risk factor is smoking. Other factors include phenacetin use, urban residence, work in the dye and textile industry, chronic inflammation and Balkan nephropathy. TCC is often multifocal, and up to 50% of patients with TCC may also develop bladder cancer.

The majority of patients present with frank haematuria. An intravenous urogram (IVU) will often demonstrate a filling defect in the collecting system, and CT or MRI is used to assess local extent and distant spread. Ureteroscopy allows direct visualisation and biopsy of the majority of tumours.

Localised/locally advanced disease can be treated by radical nephrectomy including total removal of the ipsilateral ureter. The role of adjuvant treatment following radical nephrectomy is under evaluation. The POUT trial is an ongoing randomised controlled trial assessing disease-free survival in patients randomised to receive adjuvant gemcitabine plus platinum-based chemotherapy versus active surveillance following a radical nephrectomy for muscle-invasive renal TCC.

Early-stage low-grade cancers are often treated with a more conservative local surgical excision. Follow-up with urine cytology and cystoureteroscopy is recommended, because up to 50% of patients will develop another renal tract cancer. The patient must be advised to stop smoking, which will greatly reduce the risk of subsequent cancers developing.

References

Aso, Y. and Homma, Y. (1992). A survey of incidental renal cell carcinoma in Japan. *J. Urol.*, **147**, 340–343.

Atkins, M., Regan, M., McDermott, D., *et al.* (2005). Carbonic anhydrase IX expression predicts outcome of interleukin 2 therapy for renal cancer. *Clin. Cancer Res.*, **11**, 3714–3721.

Atzpodien, J., Kirchner, H., Illiger, H. J., *et al.* (2001). IL-2 in combination with IFN-alpha and 5-FU versus tamoxifen in metastatic renal cell carcinoma: long-term results of a controlled randomized clinical trial. *Br. J. Cancer*, **85**, 1130–1136.

Bell, E. T. (1950). *Renal Diseases*, 2nd edn. Philadelphia, PA: Lea and Febiger.

Bosniak, M. A. (1986). The current radiological approach to renal cysts. *Radiology*, **158**, 1–10.

Clark, J., Atkins, M., Urba, W., *et al.* (2003). Adjuvant high-dose bolus interleukin-2 for patients with high-risk renal cell carcinoma: a cytokine working group randomized trial. *J. Clin. Oncol.*, **21**, 3133–3140.

Coppin, C., Porzsolt, F., Awa, A., *et al.* (2005). Immunotherapy for advanced renal cell cancer. *Cochrane Database Syst. Rev.*, **1**, CD001425.

Eble, J. N., Sauter, G., Epstein, J.I., *et al.* (2004). *Pathology and Genetics. Tumors of the Urinary System and Male Genital Organs.* Lyon: IARC Press.

Escudier, B., Pluzanska, A., Koralewski, P., *et al.* (2007). Bevacizumab plus interferon alfa-2a for treatment of metastatic renal cell carcinoma: a randomised, double-blind phase III trial. *Lancet*, **370**, 2103–2111.

Escudier, B., Porta, C., Bono, P., *et al.* (2014). Randomized, controlled, double-blind, cross-over trial assessing treatment preference for pazopanib versus sunitinib in patients with metastatic renal cell carcinoma: PISCES study. *J. Clin. Oncol.*, **32**, 1412–1418.

Finney, R. (1973). Radiotherapy in the treatment of hypernephroma: a clinical trial. *Br. J. Urol.*, **45**, 26–40.

Flanigan, R. C., Salmon, S. E., Blumenstein, B. A., *et al.* (2001). Nephrectomy followed by interferon alfa-2b compared with interferon alfa-2b alone for metastatic renal-cell cancer. *N. Engl. J. Med.*, **345**, 1655–1659.

Fuhrman, S. A., Lasky, L. C., Limas, C., *et al.* (1982). Prognostic significance of morphological parameters in renal cell carcinoma. *Am. J. Surg. Pathol.*, **6**, 655–663.

Gore, M. E., Griffin, C. L., Hancock, B., *et al.* (2010). Interferon alfa-2a versus combination therapy with interferon alfa-2a, interleukin-2, and fluorouracil in patients with untreated metastatic renal cell carcinoma (MRC RE04/EORTC GU 30012): an open-label randomised trial. *Lancet*, **375**, 641–648.

Heng, D. Y., Xie, W., Regan, M. M., *et al.* (2009). Prognostic factors for overall survival in patients with metastatic renal cell carcinoma treated with vascular endothelial growth factor-targeted agents: results from a large, multicenter study. *J. Clin. Oncol.*, **27**, 5794–5799.

Heng, D. Y., Xie, W., Regan, M. M., *et al.* (2013). External validation and comparison with other models of the

International Metastatic Renal Carcinoma Database Consortium prognostic model: a population-based study. *Lancet Oncol.*, **14**, 141–148.

Hudes, G., Carducci, M., Tomczak, P., *et al.* (2007). Temsirolimus, interferon alfa, or both for advanced renal-cell carcinoma. *N. Engl. J. Med.*, **356**, 2271–2281.

Janowitz, T., Welsh, S. J., Zaki, K., *et al.* (2013). Adjuvant therapy in renal cell carcinoma – past, present, and Future. *Semin. Oncol.*, **40**, 482–491.

Jocham, D., Richter, A., Hoffmann, L., *et al.* (2004). Adjuvant autologous renal tumour cell vaccine and risk of tumour progression in patients with renal-cell carcinoma after radical nephrectomy: phase III, randomised controlled trial. *Lancet*, **363**, 594–599.

Kjaer, M. (1988). The role of medroxyprogesterone acetate (MPA) in the treatment of renal adenocarcinoma. *Cancer Treat. Rev.*, **15**, 195–209.

Kjaer, M., Frederiksen, P. L. and Engelholm, S. A. (1987). Postoperative radiotherapy in stage II and III renal adenocarcinoma: a randomised trial by the Copenhagen Renal Cancer Study Group. *Int. J. Radiat. Oncol. Biol. Phys.*, **13**, 665–672.

Leibovich, B. C., Blute, M. L., Cheville, J. C., *et al.* (2003). Prediction of progression after radical nephrectomy for patients with clear cell renal cell carcinoma: a stratification tool for prospective clinical trials. *Cancer*, **97**, 1663.

Messing, E., Manola, J., Wilding, G., *et al.* (2003). Phase III study of interferon alfa-NL as adjuvant treatment for resectable renal cell carcinoma: an Eastern Cooperative Oncology Group/Intergroup trial. *J. Clin. Oncol.*, **21**, 1214–1222.

Mickisch, G. H., Garin, A., van Poppel, H., *et al.* (2001). Radical nephrectomy plus interferon-alfa-based immunotherapy compared with interferon-alfa alone in metastatic renal-cell carcinoma: a randomised trial. *Lancet*, **358**, 966–970.

Montie, J. E., Stewart, B. H., Straffon, R. A., *et al.* (1977). The role of adjunctive nephrectomy in patients with metastatic renal cell carcinoma. *J. Urol.*, **117**, 272–275.

Motzer, R. J., Escudier, B., Oudard, S., *et al.* (2008). Efficacy of everolimus in advanced renal cell carcinoma: a double-blind, randomised, placebo-controlled phase III trial. *Lancet*, **372**, 449–456.

Motzer, R. J., Hutson, T.E., Tomczak, P., *et al.* (2009). Overall survival and updated results for sunitinib compared with interferon alfa in patients with metastatic renal cell carcinoma. *J. Clin. Oncol.*, **27**, 3584–3590.

Motzer, R. J., Escudier, B., Tomczak, P., *et al.* (2013a). Axitinib versus sorafenib as second-line treatment for advanced renal cell carcinoma: overall survival analysis and updated results from a randomised phase 3 trial. *Lancet Oncol.*, **14**, 552–562.

Motzer, R. J., Hutson, T. E., Cella, D., *et al.* (2013b). Pazopanib versus sunitinib in metastatic renal-cell carcinoma. *N. Engl. J. Med.*, **36**, 722–731.

Motzer, R. J., Hutson, T. E., McCann, L., *et al.* (2014). Overall survival in renal-cell carcinoma with pazopanib versus sunitinib. *N. Engl. J. Med.*, **370**, 1769–1770.

Murphy, W. M., Beckwith, J. B. and Farrow, G. M. (1994). Tumors of the kidney, bladder, and related urinary structures. In: *Atlas of Tumor Pathology*, 3rd edn. Bethesda, MD: Armed Force Institute of Pathology.

Negrier, S., Gomez, F., Douillard, J. Y., *et al.* (2005). Prognostic factors of response or failure of treatment in patients with metastatic renal carcinomas treated by cytokines: a report from the Groupe Français d'Immunothérapie. *World J. Urol.*, **23**, 161–165.

Negrier, S., Perol, D., Ravaud, A., *et al.* (2007). Medroxyprogesterone, interferon alfa-2a, interleukin 2, or combination of both cytokines in patients with metastatic renal carcinoma of intermediate prognosis. *Cancer*, **110**, 2468–2477.

O'Dea, M. J., Zincke, H., Utz, D. C., *et al.* (1978). The treatment of renal cell carcinoma with solitary metastasis. *J. Urol.*, **120**, 540–542.

Rini, B.I., Halabi, S., Rosenberg, J. E., *et al.* (2008). Bevacizumab plus interferon alfa compared with interferon alfa monotherapy in patients with metastatic renal cell carcinoma: CALGB 90206. *J. Clin. Oncol.*, **26**, 5422–5428.

Sternberg, C. N., Davis, I. D., Mardiak, J., *et al.* (2010). Pazopanib in locally advanced or metastatic renal cell carcinoma: results of a randomized phase III trial. *J. Clin. Oncol.*, **28**, 1061–1068.

Tada, S., Yamagishi, J., Kobayashi, H., *et al.* (1983). The incidence of simple renal cyst by computed tomography. *Clin. Radiol.*, **34**, 437–439.

UICC. (2009). *TNM Classification of Malignant Tumours*, 7th edn, ed. L. H. Sobin, M. Gospodarowicz and Ch. Wittekind. New York: Wiley-Liss, pp. 255–257.

Yagoda, A., Abi-Rached, B., Petrylak, D., *et al.* (1995). Chemotherapy for advanced renal-cell carcinoma: 1983–1993. *Semin. Oncol.*, **22**, 42–60.

Chapter

21

Management of cancer of the bladder

Samantha Cox and Jacob Tanguay

Introduction

Bladder cancer is an important cause of morbidity and mortality and has a high incidence rate in industrialised countries. Each year in the UK, around 10,000 people develop a bladder cancer, and nearly half of those affected will die from their disease. Bladder cancers have a wide range of biological behaviours, from non-muscle-invasive cancer, which can be treated by local resection, to highly aggressive and infiltrative tumours. Radical cystectomy (RC) is the standard of care for muscle-invasive disease; however, bladder-preserving strategies may offer similar outcomes in carefully selected patients.

Types of bladder tumour

The types of bladder tumour that can occur are shown in Table 21.1.

Incidence and epidemiology

In the UK, bladder cancer is the fourth most common cancer in men and eleventh in women (CRUK; www.cancerresearchuk.org/, accessed August 2014), with 90% of cases occurring over the age of 55 and peak incidence between 65 and 73 years. The incidence rate is 11.4 per 100,000 of the population. A reduction in exposure to carcinogenic agents and a change in the cancer registry coding of carcinoma *in situ* (CIS) has decreased the incidence rate in recent years. Caucasians are affected more than other ethnicities, which may be due to genetic polymorphisms. The male to female ratio is 5:2; however, men have a survival advantage, the cause of which is unknown.

Anatomy

The bladder is a muscular sac which sits in the anterior pelvis posterior to the pubic symphysis. It changes from

Table 21.1 Types of bladder tumour

Type	Examples
Benign	Inflammatory plaques
	Transitional cell papilloma
	Inverted papilloma
	Leiomyoma
Malignant primary	*Carcinomas*
	Transitional cell carcinoma (90%)
	Squamous cell carcinoma (approx. 5%)
	Adenocarcinoma (1–2%)
	Mixed
	Small-cell carcinoma
	Others
	Sarcoma
	Lymphoma
Malignant secondary	Direct spread (e.g. from prostate, cervix, vagina)
	Distant spread from tumours at other sites

a pyramidal to an ovoid shape as it fills with urine. The normal bladder capacity is 300–400 ml and a post-void volume of greater than 50 ml is significant.

The bladder is anterior to the vagina and inferior to the uterus in women; in men it is anterior to the rectum, seminal vesicles and vasa deferentia. The apex is connected to the umbilicus by the median umbilical ligament (the embryonic remnant of the urachus), the base is supported by the pelvic floor muscles, and the prostate in men. The ureters drain obliquely into the posterolateral angles of the bladder. The trigone is the smooth triangular posterior portion which extends from the ureteric orifices to the internal urethral opening. The bladder neck is composed of organised smooth muscle

Practical Clinical Oncology, Second Edition, ed. Louise Hanna, Tom Crosby and Fergus Macbeth. Published by Cambridge University Press. © Cambridge University Press 2015.

layers forming the internal urethral sphincter, involuntary controlled by the autonomic nervous system; the skeletal muscle of the external urethral sphincter allows voluntary control of micturition.

The superior and inferior vesicular arteries (branches of the internal iliac artery) supply the majority of the bladder; a vesicular venous plexus drains to the internal iliac vein. Lymphatic drainage includes the hypogastric, obturator, internal, external and common iliac and presacral lymph nodes.

Carcinoma of the bladder

Risk factors and aetiology

The association between bladder cancer and environmental carcinogenic agents is well documented (Burger *et al.*, 2013). These agents are excreted via the urinary system resulting in direct contact with the urothelium. Tobacco smoking (2-naphthylamine, polycyclic aromatic hydrocarbons), including passive exposure, accounts for 50% of cases. Improvements in occupational health have reduced industry-related diagnoses, but these still account for around 20% of cases. Exposure to aromatic amines (benzidine, 4-aminobiphenyl), chlorinated hydrocarbons and polycyclic aromatic hydrocarbons in the manufacturing of petroleum, rubber, dye and paint was common prior to health and safety legislation. There is often a latency period of around 30 years from exposure to disease occurrence. No definitive link has been established between bladder cancer and alcohol, chlorinated water, coffee or the amount of fluid intake. Treatment for other malignancies with chemotherapy (e.g. cyclophosphamide) or pelvic ionising radiation (e.g. EBRT for prostate cancer) can also increase the incidence. Benign conditions including chronic infection (e.g. schistosomiasis due to the trematode parasite commonly seen in Africa and the Middle East causing squamous metaplasia and subsequent squamous cell carcinoma) or chronic inflammation and urinary retention are also linked to bladder cancer. Genetic polymorphisms including the glutathione *S*-transferase mu1 (GSTM1) null genotype and slow acetylation variants of N-acetyltransferase (NAT2) are associated with an increased risk (Burger *et al.*, 2013). Bladder cancer is seen in genetic conditions such as retinoblastoma (RB1) and Lynch syndrome. A positive family history in a first-degree relative doubles an individual's risk. Screening for asymptomatic haematuria with urinary tests, cytology or biomarkers is not recommended because of a lack in randomised controlled trial evidence.

Pathology

Urothelial tumours

Transitional cell (or urothelial) carcinoma (TCC) is the most common type of bladder malignancy. It is categorised according to the presence of muscle invasion and the histological grading of the tumour. The base of the bladder is most commonly affected and multiple tumours are frequent (up to 40%).

Non-muscle-invasive bladder cancer (NMIBC) accounts for 70% of TCCs and includes superficial papillary tumours restricted to the epithelium (Ta) and those involving the subepithelial connective tissue (T1). If such tumours are of low grade (G1 or G2) they are said to be of low malignant potential and are often successfully resected transurethrally. NMIBC also includes the flat, erythematous CIS which can affect any part of the urinary tract. The cells of such high-grade abnormalities are poorly differentiated, grow quickly and can progress to muscle-invasive bladder cancer (MIBC). Together, CIS and high-grade (G3) T1 lesions should be treated aggressively because they are of high malignant potential. Twenty per cent of NMIBC will become muscle-invasive and recurrence rates are as high as 50%. There is also a risk of nodal disease with high-grade T1 tumours; reportedly 10% of such patients undergoing RC and lymphadenectomy have nodal metastases (Wiesner *et al.*, 2005). Table 21.2 shows the risk stratification of NMIBC.

Other cancers

TCCs commonly contain components of squamous cell carcinoma, adenocarcinoma, small-cell or sarcomatoid elements. Such tumours are normally treated in the same way as TCCs, but it may be difficult to distinguish between a TCC with squamous differentiation and a true 'pure' squamous cell carcinoma. Pure squamous cell cancers are rare in the absence of a predisposing factor for squamous metaplasia. Small-cell carcinoma is well recognised and should be managed similarly to that of the lung, although prophylactic cranial irradiation may not be necessary due to the lower incidence of brain metastases.

Adenocarcinomas are extremely rare. They are occasionally seen in the bladder dome where they are thought to originate from a persistent urachus, but

Table 21.2 Risk stratification of non-muscle-invasive bladder cancer

NMIBC risk group	Definition	Risk of recurrence (%)	Risk of progression (%)	Mortality (%)
Low-risk tumours	Primary, solitary, Ta, low-grade/G1, <3 mm, no CIS	37	0	0
Intermediate-risk tumours	All tumours not defined in the two adjacent categories	45	1.8	0.7
High-risk tumours	Any of the following: T1 tumour High-grade/G3 tumour CIS Multiple **and** recurrent **and** large (>3 cm) Ta, G1, G2 tumours	54	15	9.5

Adapted from Babjuk *et al.* (2013) and Millán-Rodriguez *et al.* (2000).

they may also occur around the trigone (possibly originating from cystic glandularis). Definitive treatment includes partial cystectomy with resection of the bladder dome, urachal ligament and umbilicus.

Clinical presentation

Painless haematuria is the definitive symptom of bladder cancer. CIS can present like a urinary tract infection (UTI) with urgency, frequency and irritative symptoms. All microscopic and macroscopic cases of haematuria should be investigated for malignancy, even in the presence of a UTI.

Investigation

Investigations for haematuria of unknown cause

The whole of the urinary tract should be screened for tumours, stones and structural abnormalities. Urinalysis should be performed for cytology and culture, but caution is needed in attributing significant haematuria to a UTI. The specificity of urine cytology is reported to be greater than 90%, but has poor sensitivity in detecting tumours of low malignant potential. Table 21.3 summarises the classification of urine cytology results. Molecular markers are still under development. Routine bloods including FBC, U+E, LFT and bone profile should be requested.

Flexible white-light cystoscopy is generally required to diagnose bladder tumours, allowing visual and histological diagnosis of bladder abnormalities. In response to the diagnostic difficulties of NMIBC, blue-light cystoscopy (photodynamic diagnosis) has

Table 21.3 Cytological classification of urine

U1	Benign
U2	Atypical, favouring reactive
U3	Atypical, unclear if reactive or neoplastic
U4	Suspicious for malignancy
U5	Malignant

been developed as an adjunct to standard white-light cystoscopy (Mowatt *et al.*, 2011). Photosensitisation of abnormal tissue is detected with blue-light following intravesical instillation of dyes (5-aminolevulinic acid (5-ALA) or hexyl ester hexaminolevulinate (HAL)); disease appears red whereas normal tissue remains blue.

Further management if bladder tumour is confirmed

Transurethral resection of bladder tumours (TURBT) should be performed including removal of all visible tumour and taking separate biopsies from the border of the resected area and the tumour base. After a successful resection, there should be no palpable mass on EUA, but the results of bimanual examination must be considered in the context of the other staging investigations.

The histology report should include the location and grade, depth of invasion, presence or absence of CIS, lymphovascular invasion and aberrant histology. The presence or absence of necrosis may also guide therapy (see BCON study below). The presence of detrusor muscle within the specimen is important as its absence may signify an incomplete resection for which a second procedure is required. A second TURBT at 2–6 weeks is indicated for high-grade NMIBC or T1 tumours due to the risk of residual disease.

Local staging is performed with pelvic MRI or CT. CT of the chest, abdomen and pelvis and CT urography to allow assessment of the upper urinary tracts are indicated in MIBC cases being considered for radical treatment. A bone scan is not routinely indicated unless there are symptoms to suggest bony metastasis and/or in the presence of a raised serum calcium and alkaline phosphatase. PET scanning is of limited use because of interference from urinary excretion of contrast.

Staging

Tumours originate in the epithelium and infiltrate deeply into the muscle layers, penetrating through the bladder wall into perivesical fat and adjacent organs. The risk of lymph node metastases is proportional to the depth of tumour invasion (i.e. 20% for lamina propria invasion, 30% for superficial muscle invasion and 60% with full-thickness muscle invasion).

The staging system has been changed several times and care must be taken when comparing published results. The TNM staging classification is shown in Table 21.4.

Treatment of NMIBC

Following TURBT, a single dose of perioperative intravesical chemotherapy is given, reducing the rate of recurrence by 11.7% compared to TURBT alone (Sylvester *et al.*, 2004). This aims to destroy any residual unresected tumour and prevent tumour cell reimplantation from cells sloughed into the bladder during the procedure. Mitomycin C (20 mg) is the standard in the UK although epirubicin and doxorubicin may also be of benefit. A course of intravesical chemotherapy may be required (e.g. once weekly for 6 weeks) for selected at-risk individuals. Treatment is contraindicated in suspected or confirmed cases of perforation following TURBT. Toxicity related to intravesical chemotherapy includes irritative urinary symptoms and a risk of fibrosis. Patients should be monitored for myelosuppression and rash.

Intravesical immunotherapy with bacillus Calmette–Guérin (BCG) is superior to chemotherapy in reducing tumour recurrence for intermediate- and high-risk NMIBC (Shelley *et al.*, 2003); an induction course of weekly instillations for 6 weeks followed by a maintenance course (for example, weekly treatment for

Table 21.4 TNM classification for carcinoma of the bladder

Stage	Description
pTX	Primary tumour cannot be assessed
pT0	No evidence of primary tumour
Tis	Carcinoma *in situ*: 'flat tumour'
Ta	Non-invasive papillary tumour
T1	Subepithelial connective tissue
T2a	Inner half (superficial muscle)
T2b	Outer half (deep muscle)
T3a	Perivesical tissues (microscopically)
T3b	Perivesical tissues (macroscopically)
T4a	Prostatic stroma, seminal vesicles, uterus or vagina
T4b	Pelvic/abdominal wall
NX	Lymph nodes cannot be assessed
N0	Nodes free of tumour
N1	Single regional node in the true pelvis (hypogastric, obturator, external iliac or presacral)
N2	Multiple regional nodes in the true pelvis
N3	Common iliac nodal metastasis
M0	No distant metastases
M1	Distant metastases

Adapted from UICC, 2009.

3 weeks at 3, 6 and 12 months after induction) can reduce the risk of disease progression. However, it does have more side effects than chemotherapy and the optimal regimen is unknown. Immediate intravesical chemotherapy with one year BCG or chemotherapy is recommended for intermediate-risk disease, while 1–3 years of intravesical BCG is given for high-risk disease.

Absolute contraindications to BCG include instillation following difficult catheterisation or during the first 14 days after TURBT to prevent systemic absorption, symptomatic urinary tract infection and macroscopic haematuria. Relative contraindications include cases of immunosuppression or asymptomatic bacteriuria. Side effects can include flu-like and irritative urinary symptoms, to be managed conservatively with analgesics and anti-spasmodics. More serious effects include allergic reactions, granulomatous prostatitis or epididymitis and TB.

A Cochrane meta-analysis has demonstrated the efficacy of intravesical gemcitabine in certain cases of NMIBC; however, further randomised studies are required (Jones *et al.*, 2012). In low-risk patients, gemcitabine is associated with fewer adverse events than mitomycin C and there is a non-significant trend towards lower rates of recurrence and progression. Evidence suggests that recurrence rates are greater for high-risk cases treated with gemcitabine rather than intravesical BCG, but outcomes may be similar for intermediate disease. There also appears to be activity in cases of recurrent disease post-BCG.

High-risk NMIBC is an indication for RC as are recurrent disease following BCG treatment, progression to MIBC and side effects preventing completion of BCG. However, salvage BCG can be given in disease recurrence following intravesical chemotherapy or BCG for non-high-grade tumours. The MRC BS06 trial demonstrated that adjuvant radical radiotherapy following TURBT for pT1G3 bladder cancer is not associated with better survival rates compared with TURBT ± intravesical BCG (Harland *et al.*, 2007).

Follow-up should include cystoscopy and urine cytology, initially 3 months post-TURBT as this is a strong predictor for recurrence and progression. Patients should be followed up for 5 years after low-risk disease while life-long surveillance is recommended in intermediate- or high-risk disease.

Treatment of MIBC T2–T4a N0/NX M0

Patients with muscle-invasive disease are at high risk of recurrence and metastasis with TURBT alone and require further definitive treatment. RC remains the standard of care, but is a morbid procedure. It is important to first identify whether the patient is a suitable surgical candidate. Bladder cancer is strongly associated with smoking and patients often have coexistent cardiovascular and pulmonary disease. Patients may also have poor renal function due to obstructive uropathy which can be exacerbated by chemotherapy. Time should be spent assessing the patient's performance status, comorbidities and their wishes regarding available treatment options.

RC is the treatment of choice for high-risk patients (defined as cT4, CIS, multifocal tumour, incomplete TURBT and hydronephrosis) who are deemed operable. Those patients who are medically fit and of intermediate risk (cT2–3, no CIS, unifocal tumour, complete TURBT, no hydronephrosis) should have the merits of RC versus bladder preservation explained to them. Definitive chemoradiotherapy can be offered to patients who are not fit for surgery and in patients who wish for bladder preservation. There is a lack of robust

trial data to support monotherapy with chemotherapy. Radiotherapy alone is inferior to both RC and trimodality bladder preservation and should therefore be used only in patients who are unfit for these treatments.

Radical cystectomy

RC involves cystoprostatectomy for men and anterior exenteration for women, with urinary diversion using a bowel segment. Urethrectomy is indicated if the bladder neck or prostate is involved in women and men, respectively. Bilateral extended pelvic lymphadenectomy assesses nodal disease and may be associated with better 5-year progression-free survival rates than standard lymph node dissection (Gakis *et al.*, 2013). A partial cystectomy is rarely recommended. Five-year survival rates of just less than 50% have been recorded, even in multicentre studies. Positive nodal status is a poor prognostic feature. Perioperative mortality is 3% with higher morbidity rates of around 30%. Complications include bleeding, infection, thromboembolism, lymphocele formation, anastomotic leakage, bowel obstruction and sexual dysfunction.

Urostomy via an ileal conduit is the most common form of urinary diversion in which a ureteroenteric anastomosis allows free drainage of urine into an abdominal wall stoma. Other techniques include the cutaneous continent urinary diversion (formation of an abdominal pouch which is intermittently catheterised via a stoma) and the orthotopic neobladder. The latter utilises a bowel segment to form a substitute bladder which is connected to the ureters and urethral sphincter allowing micturition via contraction of the abdominal wall muscles in the majority of cases. In women, the uterus can be spared if an orthotopic neobladder is constructed. This technique is contraindicated in cases with urethral involvement.

There is no evidence that the continent urinary diversion techniques are any better than the more simple ileal conduit; however, they do require intermittent self-catheterisation and can be associated with late complications necessitating further surgical intervention. As a result, they tend to be used in patients of better performance status. Metabolic complications following urinary diversion include vitamin and bile salt malabsorption, and hyperchloraemic metabolic acidosis. Infections, skin irritation, bowel or urinary obstruction and urinary leak should be monitored for.

With outcomes and morbidity rates similar to open RC, interest in the efficacy of robotic-assisted RC and laparoscopic RC is growing; however, prospective randomised trials are needed. Although associated with longer operating times, such procedures do not require large surgical incisions and have smaller blood loss volumes. There are concerns regarding the completeness of lymph node dissection, port-site recurrence and ability to achieve negative margins. A retrospective analysis of long-term outcomes with both techniques reported similar 5-year overall survival (OS) and recurrence-free survival rates as 48% and 65%, respectively (Snow-Lisy et al., 2014).

Life-long surveillance is mandatory; however, most recurrences occur within 2 years of cystectomy. Distant recurrences frequently affect the lungs, liver and bones.

Neoadjuvant chemotherapy

The rationale for neoadjuvant chemotherapy is to improve OS rates by targeting micrometastases and downstaging the primary tumour. The ABC Meta-Analysis Collaboration established a 5% absolute survival benefit at 5 years, with OS improving from 45% to 50% (Advanced Bladder Cancer Meta-analysis Collaboration, 2003). Patients tend to tolerate chemotherapy better before surgery due to cystectomy-associated morbidity; however, neoadjuvant chemotherapy could delay potentially curative surgery. Nonetheless, neoadjuvant chemotherapy should be offered to all fit surgical candidates with adequate renal function and a complete response is associated with improved survival. Although there is a lack of randomised evidence, methotrexate, vinblastine, adriamycin and cisplatin (MVAC) and gemcitabine–cisplatin (Gem-cis) are used interchangeably; OS rates are comparable, but favour MVAC, although the non-haematological side-effect profile is better with Gem-cis (cisplatin 80 mg/m^2 day 1 and gemcitabine 1250 mg/m^2 days 1 and 8). A GFR of > 60 mL/min assessed with EDTA is necessary to avoid cisplatin-induced nephrotoxicity. Repeat cross-sectional imaging should be performed after two cycles of chemotherapy to confirm response, with a total administration of three to four cycles. There should be a gap of at least 4 weeks between the completion of neoadjuvant chemotherapy and surgery.

Adjuvant chemotherapy

A recent meta-analysis of nine RCTs has shown a survival benefit for adjuvant cisplatin-based combination chemotherapy following RC for MIBC (Leow et al., 2014). A 22% relative decrease in the risk of death and 34% relative decrease in the risk of disease recurrence

(particularly for those with high-volume nodal disease) were demonstrated. Neoadjuvant chemotherapy remains the standard of care; however, in patients who have not received this treatment and have evidence of high-volume nodal disease or extravesical spread at RC, adjuvant chemotherapy should now be considered.

Trimodality bladder-preserving strategies

In selected patients, trimodality bladder-preserving treatment with maximal TURBT followed by concurrent chemoradiotherapy (with early salvage cystectomy for recurrent disease) has similar survival rates to RC. Around 70% of patients will survive with their bladder intact, providing an attractive alternative for patients who are unfit or do not wish to undergo surgical intervention (Efstathiou et al., 2012). However, there are no prospective randomised trials directly comparing these two treatments. Important prognostic factors include patient age, tumour size, response to radiotherapy, hydronephrosis and completeness of TURBT. Acute grade ≥3 genitourinary events and gastrointestinal events are reported at 20% and 10%, respectively (James et al., 2012). Rates of late pelvic toxicity and long-term bladder function are reported to be acceptable (Efstathiou et al., 2009). Attention should be paid to symptoms or signs suggesting radiation proctitis, urinary tract strictures and haemorrhagic cystitis.

Clinicians should be aware that several RTOG studies have employed a split-course regimen. Maximal TURBT and concurrent radiotherapy to 40 Gy with cisplatin ± 5FU is given before repeat cystoscopy and biopsy; complete response to induction treatment is reported in 72% of patients who proceed to consolidation chemoradiotherapy to a total 64 Gy (Smith et al., 2013). Ten-year OS and disease-specific survival rates of 35% and 58%, respectively, are reported (Efstathiou et al., 2012).

In the UK, continuous concurrent radiotherapy and radiosensitising chemotherapy is more often used. Radiosensitisation has recently been explored in the BC2001 study in which synchronous chemoradiotherapy with 5-FU (500 mg/m^2 per day via a central venous catheter during fractions 1–5 and 16–20 of RT) and mitomycin (i.v. bolus 12 mg/m^2 on day 1 of RT) demonstrated a benefit in local control compared with standard RT alone (James et al., 2012). Locoregional disease-free survival was 67% versus 54% at 2 years. Five-year OS rates were 48% versus 35%. Acute grades 3–4 gastrointestinal side effects were more common in the chemoradiotherapy group (9.6% versus 2.7%, $p = 0.007$), but

Table 21.5 Current clinical trials in bladder cancer

EORTC 30994	Randomised phase III trial comparing immediate versus deferred chemotherapy after RC in patients with pT3–pT4 and/or N+ M0 TCC of the bladder
CALGB 90601	Randomised double-blinded phase III trial comparing gemcitabine, cisplatin and bevacizumab to gemcitabine, cisplatin and placebo in patients with locally advanced or metastatic TCC
HYMN	Phase 3 randomised multicentre study comparing hyperthermic mitomycin C and BCG for NMIBC
SUCCINT	Phase 2 study comparing standard chemotherapy with Gem-cis to Gem-cis and sunitinib for advanced TCC; recruitment is now closed and results awaited
HYBRID	Multicentre randomised phase II study of image-guided adaptive planning versus standard conformal radiotherapy using hypofractionated bladder radiotherapy (36 Gy over 6 weeks). Three conformal radiotherapy plans are generated (small, medium and large bladder) and pretreatment cone beam CT is used to select the appropriate 'plan of the day'. The primary endpoint is acute non-genitourinary toxicity in patients with pT2–T4aN0M0 unsuitable for daily radiotherapy or cystectomy

For more information, see http://www.ncri.org.uk/, accessed January 2015.

there was no significant difference for all grades 3–4 events during follow-up (8.3% versus 15.7%, $p = 0.07$). This regimen is now an attractive option, particularly for patients unsuitable for cisplatin-based treatment.

The BCON study has shown a survival benefit from hypoxic modification in addition to standard RT for stage grade 3 T1 to T4a bladder cancer. Patients were randomly assigned to RT (55 Gy in 20 fractions over 4 weeks or 64 Gy in 32 fractions over 6.5 weeks) with or without CON (inhaled carbogen before/during RT and oral nictonamide pre-RT). Three-year OS rates were 59% versus 46% ($p = 0.04$), with a significant reduction in death risk and a non-significant 11% reduction in risk of relapse. Further research is needed to both identify those with hypoxic tumours who are most likely to benefit, and for comparison with standard bladder-preserving strategies.

Life-long surveillance cystectomy is required at three-monthly intervals for the first year, six-monthly for the second year and then annually. CT imaging should be performed at 6 and 12 months, and then annually. In the event of NMIBC recurrence, patients should be managed as for a first presentation with TURBT and intravesical therapy if indicated. Any recurrent MIBC requires salvage cystectomy and is associated with poorer survival outcomes.

Planning radical radiotherapy

Set-up

Supine position on a flat couch top, arms folded across the chest and skin tattoos placed anteriorly over the pubic symphysis and laterally over the iliac crests to prevent lateral rotation. CT scanning (3-mm slices) should be used to simulate from the bottom of the ischial tuberosities to 3 cm above the dome of the bladder or the bottom of L5 (whichever is higher). The patient should have an empty rectum and empty bladder, unless partial bladder irradiation is considered.

Target volume

The CTV is the visible known tumour plus normal bladder. Information about the site and spread of the tumour should be available both from radiological investigation and cystoscopy/EUA. The PTV is 15 mm around normal bladder and 20 mm around tumour. It is standard practice in the UK to avoid nodal irradiation, despite the high risk of nodal disease, because the benefits are unclear.

Standard margins may be inadequate to allow for bladder motion in many patients. Patients particularly at risk are those with a large, dilated rectum, large tumours or tumours in the dome of the bladder (the bladder moves more superiorly). Drawing a wider margin should be considered for these patients. Trials in image-guided radiotherapy are currently recruiting (see Table 21.5).

Use of CRT/IMRT

3D planning with MLCs is strongly recommended, allowing reductions in small bowel and rectal doses. Unfortunately, dose escalation is probably not practical with the standard whole-bladder technique, because doses are limited by the tolerance of the bladder itself.

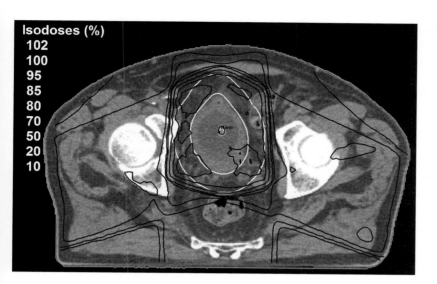

Figure 21.1 A radiotherapy plan for treating bladder cancer.

Isodoses (%)
102
100
95
85
80
70
50
20
10

A more sophisticated approach to irradiation of the bladder is needed in which a higher dose of radiation is given to the tumour with relative sparing of uninvolved areas. IMRT may be applicable, but has not yet been investigated.

Beams

One anterior and two posterior oblique wedged fields are used, depending on the bladder contour. Figure 21.1 shows a radiotherapy plan for treating bladder cancer. For the nodal irradiation technique, please refer to Chapter 22.

Doses

Single-phase treatments involve 64 Gy in 32 fractions over 6.5 weeks or 55 Gy in 20 fractions over 4 weeks.

Treatment of T4b or node-positive disease

Patients with T4b disease or nodal disease are very unlikely to be cured with radiotherapy alone. There is controversy regarding the role of surgery for patients with minimally involved lymph nodes, but some do survive with microscopic involvement of a limited number of lymph nodes. Many would consider this a systemic disease and advocate four to six cycles of systemic chemotherapy. If a good response is seen, consolidation RT to the bladder (and possibly pelvic nodes) can be considered. If nodal irradiation is considered, the patient should be planned and treated with a full bladder so that the small bowel is pushed out of the field.

Palliative chemotherapy

Bladder cancer is chemosensitive and a few patients with a relatively slow-growing TCC may achieve long remissions with combination chemotherapy. However, median survival remains disappointing at around 12 months. Although chronological age should not be used alone to define suitability for chemotherapy, many patients are elderly or in relatively poor health. Careful clinical assessment of comorbidities, fitness for cisplatin-based treatment and patient wishes is needed. The EORTC define fitness for cisplatin as GFR > 60 mL/min and PS 0–1. Ureteric stent insertion should be considered before systemic therapy if obstruction is present. Carboplatin should not be substituted for cisplatin if the patient is fit enough for the latter; response and OS rates are inferior. Non-platinum-containing regimens are also not recommended. Best supportive care is recommended for patients with PS > 2. Access to clinical trials should be considered in all cases.

In the locally advanced/metastatic setting, Gem-cis has become the standard of care (Shelley *et al.*, 2011). With similar response rates and 5-year OS rates to MVAC (13.0% versus 15.3%, $p = 0.53$), Gem-cis is associated with fewer toxicities (von der Maase *et al.*, 2005), although equivalence has not been demonstrated. The addition of paclitaxel to Gem-cis could represent an alternative first-line therapy with improved response rates and survival benefit in bladder urothelial cancer (Bellmunt *et al.*, 2012).

If patients are deemed ineligible for cisplatin, carboplatin-based regimens can be considered. The EORTC 30986 trial compared gemcitabine and carboplatin with methotrexate, carboplatin and vinblastine (M-CAVI). Both regimens demonstrated activity without significant differences in OS (9.3 versus 8.1 months, $p = 0.64$) or progression-free survival (De Santis *et al.*, 2009). Again, gemcitabine and carboplatin is preferable because of its toxicity profile.

If disease relapses within 6–12 months, a rechallenge of the first-line cisplatin-based regimen can be tried. A randomised phase III trial comparing vinflunine (a novel microtubule inhibitor) and best supportive care reported a 22% reduction in the risk of death and improved OS (6.9 versus 4.3 months) (Bellmunt *et al.*, 2013).

Palliative radiotherapy

Palliative radiotherapy may be highly effective at temporarily relieving haematuria and urinary symptoms in locally advanced and metastatic bladder cancer. It is also an option for elderly or unfit patients with clinically localised disease.

A randomised trial has shown similar palliation rates with a short, hypofractionated treatment (21 Gy in 3 fractions) compared to a higher-dose palliative treatment (35 Gy in 10 fractions; Duchesne *et al.*, 2000).

The target volume may vary widely among patients and so the technique must be determined on a case-by-case basis. Give consideration to simple AP parallel opposed fields or a four-field brick technique using virtual simulation. Treatment limited to the bladder only may improve urinary symptoms and is less toxic, particularly when delivered with a radiotherapy plan. Treatment to the whole pelvis with parallel fields permits the inclusion of pelvic lymph nodes, but can increase rectal toxicity.

A dose/fractionation schedule of 35 Gy in 10 fractions over 2 weeks or 30–36 Gy in 5–6 fractions weekly can be delivered using a CT plan, but this dose would be considered on the borderline of tolerance if parallel fields are used. If treatment to the whole pelvis is required with parallel fields, then 30 Gy in 10 fractions is better tolerated. If a smaller volume, such as the bladder only, is being treated, low-dose hypofractionated treatment is effective (e.g. 21 Gy in 3 fractions over 1 week). Even a single fraction of 8 Gy may provide relief from haematuria in a patient with poor performance status.

Clinical trials

Table 21.5 outlines some ongoing clinical trials. See http://public.ukcrn.org.uk/search/ (accessed October 2014) for more information.

Acknowledgements

The authors wish to acknowledge the contribution of Dr Stephen Williams to this chapter.

References

Advanced Bladder Cancer Meta-analysis Collaboration. (2003). Neoadjuvant chemotherapy in invasive bladder cancer: a systemic review and meta-analysis. *Lancet*, **361**, 1927–1934.

Babjuk, M., Burger, M., Zigeuner, R., *et al.* (2013). EAU guidelines on non-muscle-invasive urothelial carcinoma of the bladder: update 2013. *Eur. Urol.*, **64**, 639–653.

Bellmunt, J., von der Maase, H., Mead, G. M., *et al.* (2012). Randomized phase III study comparing paclitaxel/cisplatin/gemcitabine and gemcitabine/cisplatin in patients with locally advanced or metastatic urothelial cancer without prior systemic therapy: EORTC Intergroup Study 30987. *J. Clin. Oncol.*, **30**, 1107–1113.

Bellmunt, J., Fougeray, R., Rosenberg, J. E., *et al.* (2013). Long-term survival results of a randomized phase III trial of vinflunine plus best supportive care versus best supportive care alone in advanced urothelial carcinoma patients after failure of platinum-based chemotherapy. *Ann. Oncol.*, **24**, 1466–1472.

Burger, M., Catto, J.W., Dalbagni, G., *et al.* (2013). Epidemiology and risk factors or urothelial bladder cancer. *Eur. Urol.*, **63**, 234–241.

De Santis, M., Bellmunt, J., Mead, G., *et al.* (2009). Randomized phase II/III trial assessing gemcitabine/carboplatin and methotrexate/carboplatin/vinblastine in patients with advanced urothelial cancer 'unfit' for cisplatin-based chemotherapy: phase II – results of EORTC study 30986. *J. Clin. Oncol.*, **27**, 5634–5639.

Duchesne, G. M., Bolger, J. J., Griffiths, G. O., *et al.* (2000). A randomized trial of hypo-fractionated schedules of palliative radiotherapy in the management of bladder carcinoma: results of Medical Research Council trial BA09. *Int. J. Radiat. Oncol. Biol. Phys.*, **47**, 379–388.

Efstathiou, J. A., Bae, K., Shipley, W. U., *et al.* (2009). Late pelvic toxicity after bladder-sparing therapy in patients with invasive bladder cancer: RTOG 89–03, 95–06, 97–06, 99–06. *J. Clin. Oncol.*, **27**, 4055–4061.

Efstathiou, J. A., Spiegel, D. Y., Shipley, W. U., *et al.* (2012). Long-term outcomes of selective bladder preservation by combined-modality therapy for invasive bladder cancer: the MGH experience. *Eur. Urol.*, **61**, 705–711.

Gakis, G., Efstathiou, J., Lerner, S. P., *et al.* (2013). ICUD-EAU International Consultation on Bladder Cancer 2012: radical cystectomy and bladder preservation for muscle-invasive urothelial carcinoma of the bladder. *Eur. Urol.*, **63**, 45–57.

Harland, S. J., Kynaston, H., Grigor, K., *et al.* (2007). A randomized trial of radical radiotherapy for the management of pT1G3 NXM0 transitional cell carcinoma of the bladder. *J. Urol.*, **178**, 807–813.

James, N. D., Hussain, S. A., Hall, E., *et al.* (2012). Radiotherapy with or without chemotherapy in muscle-invasive bladder cancer. *N. Engl. J. Med.*, **366**, 1477–1488.

Jones, G., Cleves, A., Wilt, T. J., *et al.* (2012). Intravesical gemcitabine for non-muscle invasive bladder cancer. *Cochrane Database of Systematic Reviews*, Issue 1. Art. No.: CD009294.

Leow, J. J., Martin-Doyle, W., Rajagopal, P. S., *et al.* (2014). Adjuvant chemotherapy for invasive bladder cancer: a 2013 updated systematic review and meta-analysis of randomized trials. *Eur. Urol.*, **66**, 43–54.

Millán-Rodriguez, F., Chéchile-Toniolo, G., Salvador-Bayarri, J., *et al.* (2000). Primary superficial bladder cancer risk groups according to progression, mortality and recurrence. *J. Urol.*, **164**, 680–684.

Mowatt, G., N'Dow, J., Vale, L., *et al.* (2011). Photodynamic diagnosis of bladder cancer compared with white light cystoscopy: systematic review and meta-analysis. *Int. J. Technol. Assess. Health Care*, **27**, 3–10.

Shelley, M., Cleves, A., Wilt, T. J., *et al.* (2011). Gemcitabine for unresectable, locally advanced or metastatic bladder cancer. *Cochrane Database Syst Rev*, **13**(4). Art No.: CD008976.

Shelley, M. D., Court, J. B., Kynaston H., *et al.* (2003). Intravesical bacillus Calmette–Guerin versus mitomycin C for Ta and T1 bladder cancer. *Cochrane Database Syst. Rev.*, (3), CD003231.

Smith, Z.L., Christodouleas, J. P., Keefe, S. M., *et al.* (2013). Bladder preservation in the treatment of muscle-invasive bladder cancer (MIBC): a review of the literature and a practical approach to therapy. *BJU Int.*, **112**, 13–25.

Snow-Lisy, D. C., Campbell, S. C., Gill, I. S., *et al.* (2014). Robotic and laparoscopic radical cystectomy for bladder cancer: long-term oncologic outcomes. *Eur. Urol.*, **65**, 193–200.

Sylvester, R. J., Oosterlinck, W. and van der Meijden, A. P. (2004). A single immediate postoperative instillation of chemotherapy decreases the risk of recurrence in patients with stage Ta T1 bladder cancer: a meta-analysis of published results of randomized clinical trials. *J. Urol.*, **171** (6 Pt. 1), 2186–2190.

UICC. (2009). *TNM Classification of Malignant Tumours*, 7th edn, ed. L.H. Sobin, M.K. Gospodarowicz, Ch. Wittekind. Chichester: Wiley-Blackwell, pp. 262–265.

von der Maase, H., Sengelov, L., Roberts, J. T., *et al.* (2005). Long-term survival results of a randomized trial comparing gemcitabine plus cisplatin, with methotrexate, vinblastine, doxorubicin, plus cisplatin in patients with bladder cancer. *J. Clin. Oncol.*, **23**, 4602–4608.

Wiesner, C., Pfitzenmaier, J., Faldum, A., *et al.* (2005). Lymph node metastases in non-muscle invasive bladder cancer are correlated with the number of transurethral resections and tumour upstaging at radical cystectomy. *BJU Int.*, **95**, 301–305.

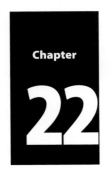

Chapter 22

Management of cancer of the prostate

Jim Barber and John Staffurth

Introduction

The biological behaviour of prostate cancer varies widely. Many tumours are found incidentally, whereas others cause signs and symptoms early on and may progress rapidly to disseminated disease. The incidence of disease is increasing, probably as a result of greater detection, yet the survival gains from earlier detection are marginal.

For men with early-stage prostate cancer, the best treatment is not known: the options are observation, surgery, external beam radiotherapy or brachytherapy. Locally advanced disease is best managed with a combination of radiotherapy and hormonal therapy. For patients with metastatic disease, the main treatment is hormonal, in the form of androgen deprivation therapy (ADT).

New technology has made a major impact on treatment techniques. Laparoscopic robot-assisted prostatectomy is superseding open prostatectomy. New techniques in radiotherapy such as intensity-modulated radiation therapy (IMRT) and image-guided radiotherapy (IGRT) offer the chance to improve the therapeutic ratio, and a range of new chemotherapeutic and hormonal agents have improved the options for men with castrate refractory prostate cancer (CRPC).

Range of tumours

Types of tumours of the prostate are shown in Table 22.1.

Incidence and epidemiology

The incidence of prostate cancer in the UK is 134 in 100,000 per year; approximately 40,000 cases occur annually, with approximately 10,000 deaths in the UK (http://www.cancerresearchuk.org/, accessed

Table 22.1 The range of tumours that occur in the prostate

Type	Examples
Benign	Benign enlargement (nodular hyperplasia)
Malignant primary	*Carcinoma*
	Adenocarcinoma (> 95%)
	Transitional carcinoma, squamous carcinoma or small-cell carcinoma (< 5%)
	Others
	Lymphoma, sarcoma, carcinosarcoma, carcinoid
Malignant secondary	Direct spread from bladder or rectum
	Metastatic spread from other primary sites is rare

January, 2015). Prostate cancer is the second most common cause of cancer death in men. Disease incidence is increasing, which is attributed primarily to increased screening. The peak incidence age is 70–75 years. The geographical distribution varies; the highest incidence occurs in Western countries and the lowest incidence is in Asia. Age-specific mortality rates have fallen slightly in both the USA and the UK, perhaps related to better treatment rather than screening, because the UK has no organised screening programme.

Anatomy

The prostate gland is in the low pelvis, behind the symphysis pubis and in front of the rectum. Laterally it is related to the anterior fibres of the levator ani muscles. It is surrounded by a pseudocapsule. It is roughly conical in shape, and its upper surface, the 'base', is in contact with the bladder. The prostate is divided into five

Practical Clinical Oncology, Second Edition, ed. Louise Hanna, Tom Crosby and Fergus Macbeth. Published by Cambridge University Press. © Cambridge University Press 2015.

Table 22.2 Pathological features of adenocarcinoma of the prostate

Features	Description
Macroscopic	Typically arise in periphery of gland posteriorly and form a firm, gritty nodule
Microscopic	Microscopic appearances are graded according to the Gleason system, which is based on degree of glandular differentiation and growth pattern within the tumour; the Gleason 'patterns' are allocated a number from 1 to 5, ranging from very well to very poorly differentiated. In the UK, guidelines restrict the use of Gleason patterns 1 and 2 to TURP chips only. For each tumour, two scores will be assigned: one for the predominant pattern and one for any secondary pattern or a small volume of a third ('tertiary') pattern if this is high grade.
	The Gleason 'grade' (or sum score) is obtained by adding the two scores, but if only one grade is seen, this is doubled (i.e. single pattern 3 would become Gleason grade $3 + 3 = 6$). For needle biopsies, the Gleason sum scores are thus Gleason 6 (3 + 3), Gleason 7 (3 + 4, 4 +3) and Gleason 8 or above (e.g. 4 + 4, 3 + 5, 4 + 5).
	For very small tumours of 1 mm or less in diameter, the diagnosis can be confirmed by immunohistochemical staining; the myoepithelial layer of cells surrounding normal glands is absent around malignant glands; this layer is difficult to see with standard haematoxylin and eosin staining, but shows clearly with high-molecular-weight cytokeratin stains.

lobes: anterior, posterior, median and two lateral; it is also divided into three zones: central, transitional and peripheral. Most prostate cancers arise in the peripheral zone. The seminal vesicles lie above and behind the prostate, between the bladder and rectum, and their ducts enter the base of the prostate.

Carcinoma of the prostate

Risk factors and aetiology

Family history is an important risk factor for disease. The relative risk doubles if one first-degree relative is diagnosed before age 70 and is four times higher if two relatives are diagnosed and if one is under age 65. Germline mutations in BRCA2 increase the risk of developing prostate cancer by up to five times. Other genetic mutations have been identified from genome-wide association studies, which lead to a small increased risk. Ethnicity is also important, with men of Afro-Caribbean descent having a higher risk of prostate cancer and an earlier disease onset than Caucasians.

Pathology

The pathological features of adenocarcinoma of the prostate are shown in Table 22.2. Important *stage information* is obtained from systematic biopsies. A high proportion of positive biopsy cores (> 50%) and the length of tumour in any individual core (e.g. > 10 mm) are highly associated with pathological T3a disease and long-term outcome after radical therapy.

Rare tumours

Transitional cell carcinomas (TCCs) may arise in the prostatic urethra or ducts and should be managed in a way similar to TCC elsewhere. Small-cell carcinomas of the prostate behave in the same way as small-cell tumours of the lung and should be treated accordingly.

Spread

Prostate carcinoma can spread locally to involve seminal vesicles and the base of the bladder. Spread to the rectum is inhibited by Denonvillier's fascia. It can also spread via lymphatics to pelvic and para-aortic lymph nodes or via the blood, most often to bone, especially spine, femur, pelvis and ribs. Spread to other organs such as liver and lung is uncommon at presentation except in very high grade cancers, but is seen in patients with castrate refractory prostate cancer (CRPC).

Screening

Serial prostate-specific antigen (PSA) testing has been used for over 30 years as a screening/diagnostic tool for early prostate cancer, but it has limitations. Many benign conditions cause rises in PSA, limiting the specificity, and some of the most aggressive cancers give only marginal elevations in PSA, limiting the sensitivity.

Many screening trials have been performed, but the results are confounded by 'out of trial' PSA testing which is routine in the USA, and have shown no reduction in prostate cancer mortality (for example the PLCO study, https://biometry.nci.nih.gov/cdas/studies/plco/). However, the European prostate cancer screening study did not suffer from this problem (http://www.erspc.org accessed January 2015) and demonstrated a significant reduction in mortality from prostate cancer in men aged 55–69 having biannual PSA tests of around 20%, now with follow-up of 13 years. To put into context, in order to save one life, 781 men are screened, and 27 cancers must be treated.

Men may have a lot to lose from overtreatment, with a significant risk of erectile dysfunction and other treatment-related morbidity. A significant proportion of men will not benefit from the treatment, and so a comprehensive screening programme could have a detrimental effect on the quality of life of a population. Because of these risks of overtreatment, there is no screening programme in the UK, but rather a 'risk management programme' which focuses on individual choice. It is relatively straightforward to recommend screening for men with a family history, BRCA2 mutations, or of Afro-Caribbean descent. However, the lack of consensus has resulted in wide variations in screening practices in primary care in the NHS, with testing primarily driven by patient demand and no clear strategy for repeating the test.

Clinical presentation

Local symptoms

Early prostate cancer rarely produces any symptoms, but many men present with lower urinary tract symptoms due to benign prostatic hypertrophy unrelated to their cancers. Similarly, erectile dysfunction is a common presentation, but thought to be coincidental in most cases. Locally advanced tumours sometimes give lower urinary tract symptoms, occasionally haematuria or haematospermia, erectile dysfunction and rarely perineal pain.

Lymph node spread or metastatic disease

Most men presenting with metastatic disease have bone metastases that cause local pain or spinal cord compression but no urinary symptoms. Some patients (< 20%) have predominantly nodal metastatic disease which can lead to lower body oedema. Lung and liver metastases are uncommon and are normally related to very high-grade disease (> Gleason 8) or CRPC. Brain metastases are virtually unknown, but extradural disease that compresses the spinal cord may occur in patients with advanced disease.

Investigation and staging

This area is currently controversial (NICE, 2014). Transrectal ultrasound (TRUS)-guided systematic sampling of the peripheral zone involving at least 10 cores covering all parts of the gland is usually performed (Prostate Cancer Risk Management Programme, 2006). Biopsies are taken from each side following a standardised protocol. Each core should be clearly labelled so that correlation can be made with a DRE and MRI scans. This technique is more likely to detect a cancer than finger- or TRUS-guided biopsy, but may not identify small tumours in large prostates or anterior tumours.

MRI clearly shows the peripheral zone of the prostate on a T2-weighted image, and tumours may be visible as a low-signal region in an area of intense high signal (on the T2-weighted image, the high-signal region is normal tissue). After a TRUS biopsy, blood may also appear as a low-signal area; because of this, some advise delaying staging scans for 4–6 weeks, but whether this improves the diagnostic power of the scan is uncertain. Comparison with T1-weighted sequences can usually distinguish between tumour and haemorrhage. Extracapsular involvement, seminal vesicle invasion and nodal disease can be identified, as well as small bone metastases that may not be seen on a bone scan.

Multi-parametric MRI (mpMRI) consists of additional MR sequences that provide functional imaging including dynamic contrast enhancement (DCE-MRI), diffusion-weighted (DW-MRI) and magnetic spectroscopy (MRS). These may add specificity and sensitivity for prostate cancer detection. In particular, it is suggested that clinically significant cancers are unlikely to give normal mpMRI results. This has led to research into alternative diagnostic pathways based on an initial mpMRI, followed by biopsy only if the mpMRI is abnormal/suspicious. In this setting it would seem sensible for the biopsy protocol to include targeting of the abnormal area on MRI. This can be achieved to some extent with a standard TRUS technique, but the alternative is a template biopsy under general anaesthetic.

CT scans give little information on the structure of the prostate, although they may be useful for nodal staging. Routine bone scans are not required

Table 22.3 TNM T-stage classification of adenocarcinoma of the prostate

TNM stage	Description
T1	No tumour palpable or visible by imaging
T1a	≤ 5% tumour in TUR chips
T1b	> 5% tumour in TUR chips
T1c	Diagnosed by TRUS biopsy
T2	Palpable tumour confined to the prostate
T2a	Tumour involves ≤ 50% of 1 lobe or less
T2b	Tumour involves >50% of 1 lobe
T2c	Tumour involves both lobes
T3	Tumour extends through prostatic capsule
T3a	Extracapsular extension
T3b	Seminal vesicle extension
T4	Tumour is fixed or invades adjacent structures such as bladder neck, rectum, pelvic wall

TRUS, transrectal ultrasound; TUR, transurethral resection.
Adapted from UICC (2009).

for low-risk patients (PSA ≤ 10 ng/mL, T ≤ 2 and Gleason score ≤ 6). Indeed, a positive bone scan is very uncommon in any patient presenting with a PSA level of 20 ng/mL or less. However, some clinicians regard a bone scan as good practice for all patients. These rules do not apply to patients who are relapsing after radical therapy or progressing on ADT; their risk of having metastatic disease should be assessed individually. Choline positron emission tomography imaging is not recommended in routine practice (NICE, 2014).

Local-stage information is provided by a combination of DRE, biopsy information, MRI scanning and pathology, especially in patients who have had radical surgery. The greater the agreement among these different methods, the more reliable the staging.

Staging classification

The 7th edition TNM T-staging classification for adenocarcinoma of the prostate is shown in Table 22.3. There is no major change from the 6th (2002) edition. Note that, in the TNM system, T1a/b tumours are rarely diagnosed today because so few trans-urethral prostatectomies (TURPs) are performed. The major clinical

distinction was between T2 and T3 disease as this identified patients who were on the borderline for surgical treatment. However, the results of trials showing the effectiveness of adjuvant post-operative radiotherapy in patients at high risk of relapse (T3a, T3b or margin positive) has led to surgery being considered for more advanced disease. Digital rectal examination (DRE) takes skill and experience and may not be highly reproducible among observers. A significant proportion of patients with early clinical T3 disease have no evidence of extensive extracapsular extension at prostatectomy.

Treatment overview

Patients with prostate cancer should be managed by a specialist MDT with equitable access to all treatment options. Patients should be allocated a named clinical nurse specialist.

Localised prostate cancer

Choices include active surveillance, radical prostatectomy, interstitial brachytherapy or external beam radiotherapy (possibly with adjuvant hormonal therapy).

Treatment results vary with known risk factors and patients should be formally allocated into a risk group (Table 22.4). Localised prostate cancer is often categorised surgically/pathologically as 'organ-confined' (pT2 or less) or 'locally advanced' (T3 or greater).

Treatment choice in localised prostate cancer

Low-risk group: untreated patients are unlikely to die from prostate cancer with mortality rates very low at 10 years. Excellent results are available with active surveillance (younger patients), watchful waiting (older patients), radiotherapy (including brachytherapy) or surgery.

Intermediate-risk group: untreated mortality is low in the first 5 years, but a small proportion will die by 10 years. Monitoring is therefore still reasonable in the elderly, but would not normally be recommended for younger patients, unless there are significant comorbidities. There is a choice of prostatectomy or radiotherapy combined with neoadjuvant hormone therapy. As an alternative to 'dose-escalated radiotherapy', high dose rate (HDR) brachytherapy can be given as a boost therapy followed by external radiation. Low dose rate (LDR) mono-brachytherapy with seeds can be performed for low volume Gleason 7 tumours, but experience is relatively limited.

Table 22.4 Risk stratification for localised prostate cancer

Risk group	Factors	Prognosis
Low	PSA < 10 ng/mL and Gleason score ≤ 6, and clinical stage T1–T2a	Excellent, 80–90% disease-free at 10 years
Intermediate	PSA 10–20 ng/mL, or Gleason score 7, or clinical stage T2b	Good, small chance of death at 10 years
High	PSA > 20 ng/mL, or Gleason score 8–10, or clinical stage ≥ T2c	Fair, significant chance of death within 10 years

High-risk group: there is a significant chance of death from prostate cancer over 10 years, and monitoring would not normally be advised, even in the elderly. Traditionally, surgery has also been avoided for these patients, as there is a high risk of positive margins; however, for early T3 tumours in selected patients, good results have been reported with radical prostatectomy when combined with postoperative radiotherapy (Bolla *et al.*, 2012). However, standard treatment for T3 disease is primary radiotherapy with neoadjuvant and/or adjuvant hormone therapy for up to 3 years. Nodal irradiation could be considered for those patients at high risk of nodal involvement.

For unfit patients, primary hormone therapy can be considered. However, the NCIC/PR07 study showed a substantial survival benefit for the addition of radiotherapy to primary hormone therapy for this group of patients (Warde *et al.*, 2011), this benefit becoming apparent at around 7 years. Primary hormone therapy is therefore used less often except in very elderly patients with high-grade tumours.

For patients with positive pelvic lymph nodes on staging, radiotherapy can be considered to prostate and pelvic lymph nodes providing there is no sign of metastatic disease elsewhere.

Observation alone (active surveillance, watchful waiting)

Observation alone can be carried out in two different ways, with different frequency of follow-up: watchful waiting and active surveillance. It is very important to agree with a patient how the monitoring will be performed, what will trigger salvage therapy, and what that treatment will be. Patient selection according to clinical risk group is important because the results of one randomised trial show a small but significant improvement in overall survival ($p = 0.04$) in patients treated immediately with prostatectomy (Bill-Axelson *et al.*, 2005).

'Watchful waiting', based on PSA monitoring, is ideal for patients who are unlikely to develop symptoms from prostate cancer during their lifetime and for whom the morbidity of treatment can therefore be avoided. This is a particularly good strategy for those men for whom hormone therapy would be considered their salvage treatment. 'Watchful waiting' is a poor description of this strategy, as follow-up is not designed to be intensive and is limited to monitoring the PSA: annual or biannual PSA monitoring would be adequate for these patients, who could be followed up in primary care.

'Active monitoring' protocols have developed greatly in the past decade and aim to detect signs of progression at an early stage and maintain the possibility of radical therapy before local progression or spread precludes it. It should be considered for men in the low-risk group.

Active monitoring protocols vary, but have become more intensive in recent years (https://www.nice.org.uk/guidance/cg175/chapter/1-recommendations, accessed January 2015). PSA monitoring and rectal examination are the backbone of monitoring and any significant changes should trigger repeat biopsy and staging investigations. Significant areas of tumour with reduced apparent diffusion coefficient (ADC) on baseline mpMRI can predict disease progression and the need for radical therapy and should be performed in all patients (van As *et al.*, 2009). Even in patients with a stable PSA, a repeat biopsy at around 1–2 years is recommended, along with a repeat mpMRI. Enlarging tumour volume on biopsy or mpMRI, or most importantly, increase in grade would be considered indications for starting treatment.

Role of surgery

Radical prostatectomy

Radical prostatectomy is a standard option for patients with T1/2 tumours, and is increasingly being offered to patients with early T3 disease in combination with an option for postoperative radiotherapy. The option to have multimodal therapy is attractive when cancer control is the highest priority.

Radical prostatectomy has some specific advantages: good published outcomes, immediate treatment, rapid access to prognostic information from pathological samples and decrease in PSA following surgery. An undetectable PSA at around 6 weeks after surgery is associated with good long-term results.

The operation is difficult because of the rich venous plexus around the prostate and the relative lack of tissue, particularly around the apex, to allow for clearance of tumour with wide margins, and should be carried out only by a specialised surgical team. The incidence of positive margins depends on the stage and risk group, and positive margin rates of around 25% are considered acceptable for early-stage disease, although higher rates would be expected in patients with early T3 disease.

The approach may be retropubic, perineal or laparoscopic and the latter may be combined with robotic assistance. Many people feel that robotic-assisted surgery has the potential to improve the results of traditional open surgery, both in terms of cancer control and reduction in complications. However, at present, clinical data to support this are limited.

The disadvantages of radical prostatectomy include high rates of erectile dysfunction (overall, at least 50%), depending on whether nerve-sparing operations can be performed, and urinary morbidity (with a small proportion of patients suffering persistent urinary incontinence).

Brachytherapy

LDR brachytherapy treatment may be performed with permanent transperineal insertion of iodine-125 seeds (with a half-life around 60 days) as sole therapy (monotherapy) as an option for patients with T2 or smaller tumours, and it is now available in some UK centres. Because the urinary toxicity can be considerable, and urinary retention can occur, it is preferable to select patients who have a good urinary flow rate (qmax 15 mL/s), relatively low International Prostate Symptoms (I-PSS) score (10 or less) and a prostate volume of 50 mL or less.

Good results, comparable to those for prostatectomy, are achieved in good-prognosis patients, but there is less experience in patients with Gleason grades of 7 and above. There is no evidence that local control is better than with external beam radiotherapy, but the treatment is attractive because very high doses of radiation (e.g. 140–145 Gy) can be given very accurately to the prostate. The procedure is an outpatient one, usually with only two visits to hospital.

Brachytherapy treatment is done under anaesthetic, and the prostate is imaged with TRUS. Intraoperative live planning is increasingly replacing the two-stage planning process. The implantation is performed through a coordinate grid mounted on the same gantry as the TRUS. Distribution of the sources is achieved by a combination of seeds and spacers introduced in each needle.

It is not practical to implant patients who have T3 disease, those who have had a previous TURP (unacceptable rates of urinary morbidity) or patients with a large (50 mL) prostate because of 'pubic arch interference'.

The acute morbidity from brachytherapy includes urinary pain, frequency and obstruction. The bowel reaction is usually not as severe as that from external beam radiotherapy, but the urinary reaction is worse.

Late morbidity includes urinary morbidity and impotence (rates similar to those with external beam radiotherapy). The urethral dose should be kept below 125 Gy if possible.

HDR afterloading brachytherapy can be performed with a Microselectron® machine using a technique very similar to that just described. Although the invasive nature of the technique limits it to one or two fractions a few hours apart, it is a practical method of delivering a radiation boost in a highly conformal fashion. HDR monotherapy for early disease using extreme hypofractionation is experimental, but is being increasingly used as a boost for locally advanced disease in combination with external beam radiotherapy (Hoskin et al., 2012).

External beam radiotherapy

Radical external beam treatment

Treatment is tailored according to clinical risk group.

For patients with low-risk disease, treatment is given to the prostate and proximal 2 cm of seminal vesicles usually without hormone therapy.

For those with intermediate-risk disease, the whole of the seminal vesicles may be included and neoadjuvant hormone therapy is standard practice, especially if patients have more than two intermediate risk factors. It may be helpful to calculate the risk of seminal vesicle invasion by the Roach equation: PSA +([Gleason – 6] × 10).

For patients with high-risk node-negative disease, prophylactic nodal irradiation should be considered along with prolonged adjuvant hormone therapy for 2–3 years. Nodal irradiation is controversial as the survival gains from whole pelvic versus prostate only RT were not statistically significant in a four-arm randomised study that also looked at neoadjuvant versus adjuvant hormone therapy (RTOG 94-13; Lawton *et al.*, 2007). However, nodal irradiation was included in the radiotherapy schedule in the majority of trials showing a survival benefit of prolonged ADT with radiotherapy (e.g. Bolla *et al.*, 2009), and new technology has rendered the treatment more acceptable. Again, it may be helpful to calculate the risk of nodal disease: 2/3 × PSA + ([Gleason – 6] × 10) using the Roach equation.

Relative contraindications to radiotherapy include a history of inflammatory bowel disease, or severe diverticulitis where perforations have been reported.

Radiotherapy planning setup

A CT planning scan is performed with the patient supine in the treatment position. One anterior and two lateral tattoos are optimal for patient set-up. If a nodal mark-up is considered, then intravenous contrast is helpful in delineating the vessels. Unwanted patient movement can be limited by using an immobilisation device (e.g. knee support). The patient is advised to hold a comfortably full bladder for treatment. Variability in rectal filling can lead to increased rectal toxicity and the risk of a geographical miss, particularly if the rectum is dilated (greater than 4 cm diameter) on the planning CT. An enema before the planning CT and each fraction of radiotherapy can prevent this problem.

Dose levels

With conventional conformal therapy and a 1 cm margin around the prostate, dose-limiting rectal toxicity occurs at around 55 Gy in 20 fractions, or 70 Gy in 35 fractions. However, boosting the dose to the prostate with a smaller margin is well tolerated and several randomised trials (e.g. UK RT01 study, http://www.ctu.mrc.ac.uk/our_research/research_areas/cancer/studies/rt01/) have shown an increase in biochemical control, but no significant survival benefit, across a variety of incremental dose comparisons. Dose-escalated radiotherapy is now standard practice.

Most departments have replaced a boost to the prostate using a two-phase approach and 'shrinking fields', a simple forward-planned 'field in field' concomitant boost or sophisticated inverse-planned IMRT. A widely used approach is to specify two dose levels: a large volume covering the prostate and seminal vesicles with a 1-cm margin (minimum coverage 76% of the dose; 56 Gy in 37 fractions), and a smaller volume with a 0.5-cm margin to cover the prostate alone (target minimum 95% of 74 Gy in 37 fractions).

With standard conformal therapy, high rectal doses can occur if the seminal vesicles curve posteriorly around the rectum. However, IMRT allows scooping out the dose around the rectum; allowing any tumour in the seminal vesicles to be included in the high-dose volume subject to rectal toxicity constraints.

For nodal irradiation, conventional wide-field pelvic radiation is associated with significantly increased gastrointestinal toxicity, and doses are limited to around 50 Gy in 37 fractions (70% of 74 Gy dose). With this technique it may not be possible to treat nodes in the posterior pelvis without incurring unacceptable rectal toxicity. Treating pelvic lymph nodes more comprehensively with higher doses and less toxicity is possible with IMRT, allowing scooping out of the dose around bladder and bowel in the central pelvis. Doses of around 54 Gy in 37 fractions (73%) can be safely delivered to the pelvic lymph nodes (Guerrero Urbano *et al.*, 2010) and a boost to any involved nodes up to 60 Gy in 37 fractions (80%) can now be considered.

Fractionation

Conventional fractionation is recommended in NICE guidelines using no more than 2 Gy per day (NICE, 2014). The total dose is 74–78 Gy over 7–8 weeks. In theory, prolonged fractionation is unlikely to improve the therapeutic ratio, taking into account that the estimated α/β ratio for prostate cancer is similar to that of the rectum. This concept is supported by the UK randomised trial of dose-escalated, forward-planned IMRT (CHHiP) which showed slightly better cancer control (statistically noninferior) with 60 Gy in 20 fractions compared to 74 Gy in 37 fractions or 57 Gy in 19 fractions and comparable late toxicity at 5 years. It is likely that many centres will adopt this approach in future. Comparison of standard fractionation with extreme hypofraction using precise image guidance and stereotactic ablative body radiotherapy (SABR) in 4–7 fractions is the subject of two forthcoming UK-based clinical trials.

Marking up guidance

The staging MRI scan and the biopsy results should be used to help define the volume, as the prostate is poorly defined on CT. The position of the prostatic apex is variable, and should be carefully defined to minimise doses to rectum and penile bulb. Any areas of extraprostatic extension should be well covered. The CTV and GTV are created using the margins described above.

If the lymph nodes are to be treated, it is recommended that CT scanning is performed with intravenous contrast. The nodal groups to be treated include the common iliac nodes from the sacral promontory, the presacral nodes, the internal iliac and obturator nodes, and the external iliac nodes down to the level of the femoral head. As pathological lymph nodes are usually closely related to the blood vessels, marking up techniques have been developed based on the expansion of a volume drawn around the vessels (e.g. http://www.rtog.org/CoreLab/ContouringAtlases/ ProstatePelvicLymphNodes.aspx, accessed January 2015). A 7-mm margin is used to generate the CTV, to which an additional 0.5 cm is added to make the PTV. Referral to the detailed guidance and atlas of pelvic nodal mark-up technique is recommended.

Optimisation of the radiotherapy plan

The DVHs for the rectum, bowel and bladder should be compared at a range of isodose levels to those of a standard optimal plan. The high-dose region should be limited to less than 25% of the rectal volume. Sparing of femoral heads and the penile bulb should also be considered.

Ensuring accurate treatment delivery: IGRT

With increasing doses and reduced margins, along with increasing evidence of prostate motion, image guidance based solely on portal imaging and bony anatomy is becoming obsolete. Most radiotherapy machines are fitted with the facility to perform cone beam CT imaging. Standard practice is to take a scan image every few days throughout the treatment, and use image matching software to compare the position to the planning scan ('off-line IGRT'). Daily 'online' cone beam CT, with scanning and adjustments made before each fraction is optimal but time consuming on the set. Alternatively, three gold seed markers inserted into the prostate before planning allows easy and reproducible set-up with each fraction. While this is probably ideal, it requires an invasive procedure to insert the seeds; it is mandatory for SABR therapy.

Postoperative adjuvant radiotherapy

It is now standard to offer patients with persistently detectable PSA levels at 6 weeks (> 0.1 ng/mL) and perhaps positive margins immediate adjuvant postoperative radiotherapy. Significantly better disease-free survival was shown in a randomised trial of radiotherapy without hormone therapy (Bolla *et al.*, 2012). The timing of radiotherapy and the optimal duration of hormone therapy are the subject of the RADICALS study (http://www.radicals-trial.org/, accessed January 2015) which should establish the optimal strategy. It may be reasonable to offer patients with Gleason 7 tumours a short course of neoadjuvant hormone therapy, and those with high-grade tumours 2–3 years of treatment. 'Super-sensitive' PSA assays may help in selecting patients for postoperative treatment.

The target volume is guided by the pathological findings and the preoperative imaging and is challenging to define reproducibly. It includes the surgical anastomosis and the prostate bed. It extends anteriorly to the pubic symphysis, posteriorly to include the rectum, laterally the neurovascular bundles and the adjacent ilio-obturator muscles. The superior margin is the bladder neck, and inferiorly, to within approximately 15 mm of the penile bulb. Seminal vesicle remnants are often present after surgery and can be included depending on the pathological findings.

Particular attention should be given to the location of any positive margins in the specimen. If there are positive nodes, then nodal irradiation can be considered as above.

The dose given is somewhat lower than for primary therapy, 60–64 Gy in 30–32 fractions or 52.5–55 Gy in 20 fractions.

Follow-up after radiotherapy

Follow-up should be designed to monitor patients for relapse, but also to address the complications of treatment. For example, radiation-induced enteropathy can benefit from specialist advice from gastroentrologists with expertise in the condition, but it is also important to exclude coincidental inflammatory bowel disease and large bowel malignancy, particularly as there is a small risk of radiation-induced malignancy in the bowel. Advice about the management of erectile dysfunction should be provided.

A risk-stratified approach to follow-up should be used, in which low-risk patients could be reasonably discharged to primary care after a couple of years, but high-risk patients kept on follow-up indefinitely.

Serial estimations of PSA every 6–12 months can establish relapse, defined as three successive increases in PSA above a nadir value, or alternatively nadir + 2 ng/mL (Buyyounouski *et al.*, 2005). DRE is not necessary as part of the follow-up provided the PSA remains at baseline levels.

In patients who have received radiotherapy alone without hormone therapy, a stable PSA 4–5 years later probably indicates a cure. Cure rates are highest in those patients with a PSA nadir of less than 0.5 ng/mL. In those patients who have received neoadjuvant hormone therapy, relapses may not become apparent until even later.

Patients who relapse following radiotherapy should have a careful assessment of the rate of disease progression. Slow rises in PSA could be observed without intervention, but patients with rapidly rising PSA levels (doubling time 6 months or less) or in those with metastatic disease should be considered for hormone therapy.

A few patients relapse with apparently localised disease after restaging with TRUS biopsy and imaging, and could be considered for a salvage prostatectomy in a specialist centre, although this is controversial and not recommended by NICE. Surgery is difficult after radiotherapy and the complication rate is quite high.

Novel approaches such as cryotherapy and high-intensity focussed ultrasound (HIFU) are also associated with significant toxicity following radiotherapy. So far there is not enough evidence of effectiveness and safety to justify their routine use outside clinical trials.

Sexual dysfunction: how to decide between surgery, radiotherapy and surveillance

For a proportion of men, preservation of sexual function is a high priority, particularly for younger men with low-risk tumours. Erectile dysfunction is common in patients treated for prostate cancer and no treatment is free from this complication. It may be caused by nerve damage following prostatectomy, radiation, or the consequence of ADT. In addition, reduced or dry ejaculation is common with both radiotherapy and surgery.

Active monitoring is a good option for younger patients who have low-risk disease and who wish to maintain their potency; unfortunately, these patients are often those most concerned about long-term cancer outcomes.

Long-term erectile function rates are similar for the different treatments, but there are significant differences in the timing. After a nerve-sparing radical prostatectomy, it may take some time for erections to recover after the trauma of the surgery, although there can be significant nerve regeneration over 6–12 months and many patients recover well. It is difficult to predict whether a satisfactory nerve-sparing procedure can be performed in advance of surgery, but a clear explanation of the expected surgical outcome is very helpful for the patient.

With external beam radiotherapy without hormone therapy, the majority of patients who are potent before treatment will remain so afterwards, but potency may decline over the subsequent years because of late radiation effects on nerves, vessels and the penile bulb. The results following brachytherapy are similar, although loss of erections may occasionally occur immediately after the implant. The addition of neoadjuvant hormone therapy will usually lead to a prolonged period of loss of libido and erectile dysfunction, although satisfactory recovery may occur.

Although PDE5 inhibitors such as sildenafil can help, they are ineffective in patients after non-nerve-sparing prostatectomy, and the majority of patients on hormonal therapy. There are effective alternatives, such as intracavernosal injections, but for most men these are not seen as an acceptable option.

In making treatment choices, it is important to establish whether or not erectile function is an important issue and clarify the issues discussed above; this may only be possible if the patient is interviewed on their own without their partner or family members.

Principles of hormonal therapy (see Chapter 3)

Prostate cancer is driven by the androgen receptor pathway, and inhibition of this can be performed in different ways.

LHRH analogues: surgical castration by subcapsular orchidectomy or medical castration with a subcutaneous depot injection of a LHRH analogue, provides the same biochemical result: a castrate level of testosterone. With LHRH analogues, patients should initially be prescribed an antiandrogen to prevent tumour flare (see Chapter 3). The majority of patients respond to these agents initially, but castration resistance can develop after one or two years.

LHRH inhibitors: results with the new inhibitor degaralix gives similar results to LHRH analogues, but without the testosterone flare. It is useful when emergency therapy is needed, but may cause skin reactions, and the depot preparation lasts only one month.

Steroidal anti-androgens: the use of drugs such as cyproterone acetate and diethylstilboestrol has declined with the availability of newer drugs. Although they can be active in selected patients, there is a risk of fluid retention and thromboembolic complications.

Non-steroidal anti-androgens: bicalutamide and flutamide are non-steroidal anti-androgens (NSAAs) that result in a normal or high testosterone level and high gonadotrophin levels. A more potent anti-androgen, enzalutamide, is now available, which has given impressive results as combined androgen blockade in castration-refractory patients. If used as monotherapy without an LHRH analogue, the high gonadotrophin levels may cause troublesome gynaecomastia.

Adrenal synthesis inhibitors have been used for many years: corticosteroids (particularly 0.5 mg of dexamethasone) and ketoconazole all have modest benefit. However, the newer agents such as abiraterone acetate inhibit the Cyp17 pathway, and have strong activity in castration-refractory patients. They must be given in combination with low-dose corticosteroids, but have few side effects apart from troublesome hypokalaemia in some patients.

Adjuvant and neoadjuvant hormonal therapy

There have been a number of trials of neoadjuvant and adjuvant therapy (see Chapter 3) using LHRH analogues. The LHRH antagonist degaralix also appears effective as a neoadjuvant therapy.

High risk

A common finding of the trials is that the greatest survival benefit from prolonged hormone therapy is seen in patients with high-grade tumours who should be offered treatment with an LHRH analogue for 3 years or longer.

Intermediate risk

For patients with Gleason grades 7, a short period of neoadjuvant hormone therapy (3–6 months) combined with radiotherapy gives a significant disease-free survival benefit, and there are also reductions in the planned target volume, which may reduce radiation toxicity. There appears to be marginal benefit from continuing hormone therapy beyond this time.

Low risk

Any potential benefit in tumour control must be offset against considerable morbidity including impotence, sweats and flushes, depression and a long-term effect on bone density. For patients in the low-risk group, neoadjuvant hormone therapy is not appropriate.

Other agents

Although morbidity may be less with bicalutamide (Wirth *et al.*, 2004), there is no apparent survival benefit from its use and it cannot currently be recommended for adjuvant therapy. Adjuvant therapy with agents such as docetaxel, abiraterone and enzalutamide is under investigation.

Palliative treatments

Treatments for metastatic disease: sequencing of therapy

A sequence of systemic therapies is now available, guided by regular clinical assessment, serial PSA and scans. These include the hormonal agents (LHRH analogues and antagonists, androgen receptor antagonists, adrenal synthesis inhitors and corticosteroids), cytotoxics, radioisotopes, bisphosphonates and immunotherapy.

Hormone therapy with LHRH analogues is the mainstay of treatment. Initial LHRH analogue therapy can give several years of response. The PSA falls to a low level (in many cases < 0.1 ng/mL) and the median duration of biochemical response is around 18 months. Clinical relapse often occurs after about 2 years, but there is wide variation. Few patients die before 2 years, but few live more than 5 years (James *et al.*, 2014).

Monotherapy with bicalutamide is an alternative to an LHRH analogue in patients who wish to maintain their sexual activity, but it has a number of drawbacks, including severe gynecomastia and poorer long-term cancer control. The gynecomastia can be reduced by prophylactic radiotherapy to the breast buds with 8 Gy orthovoltage irradiation or tamoxifen.

It is standard practice to continue the LHRH analogue even after the development of castration resistance. When the PSA starts to rise, maximal androgen blockade (MAB) with bicalutamide is often used, but the response to therapy is often short-lived. At this stage, novel hormone therapies such as abiraterone or enzalutamide or docetaxel chemotherapy are options if available. Chemotherapy can give several months of response, but when disease progression occurs, abiraterone or enzalutamide are indicated. The optimal sequencing of novel hormone therapies has not been tested in clinical trials and is not known, although abiraterone and enzalutamide have been shown to be effective when given before or after chemotherapy. Dexamethasone can be considered as a third-line treatment.

While cytotoxic chemotherapy is arduous for elderly patients or those with comorbidities, the novel hormone agents are well tolerated but not currently available in the NHS. For these patients, the best option is dexamethasone 0.5 mg, which can give excellent responses in a small proportion of patients.

Emergency hormone treatments

Patients may occasionally present as an emergency with spinal cord compression or upper urinary tract obstruction. The LHRH agonist, degaralix, gives rapid falls in testosterone and is now the treatment of choice for patients who present with these critical complications.

Palliative radiotherapy and radioisotope therapy

External beam radiotherapy is an effective treatment for bone metastases. Single-fraction treatments (e.g. 8 Gy) usually give rapid pain relief. Patients with spinal symptoms should be considered for MRI scanning of the spine, to exclude metastases threatening the spinal cord or nerve roots; suspect areas should be treated with higher doses (e.g. 30 Gy in 10 fractions). Strontium-89 therapy (e.g. 150 MBq) gives longer-lasting pain relief for multiple sites of disease, but patients who have widespread, multiple bone metastases can suffer from severe and prolonged bone marrow suppression, which can be fatal.

Because of this, radium-223 has been investigated as an alternative and has shown a survival benefit in one clinical trial (Parker et al., 2013). As it emits short-range alpha particles, the penetration into the bone marrow is less, and it is well tolerated, although it has to be given monthly. NICE guidance currently recommends its use only in patients who have chemotherapy.

Cytotoxic chemotherapy

A combination of docetaxel (75 mg/m^2 every 3 weeks) and prednisolone increases median survival by 2–3 months compared to mitoxantrone and prednisolone (Tannock et al., 2004). A maximum of 10 cycles of docetaxel is recommended by NICE guidance for fit

patients (at least KPS 60%) and is tolerated better when used early, before problems with bone marrow reserve occur. The main toxicities are fatigue and allergic reactions, which can be reduced by premedication with high-dose dexamethasone (8 mg b.d. starting 24 hours before chemotherapy). Treating patients with docetaxel again on relapse is not recommended. Cabazitaxel has been shown to be effective as a second-line therapy after docetaxel (TROPIC study; de Bono et al., 2010), but is not currently available for use in the NHS.

PSA is not a reliable marker of a response after treatment has been completed.

Docetaxel has been tested in hormone-naive patients as an 'adjuvant therapy'. For example, in a large trial of around 3000 patients with locally advanced and metastatic cancer randomised in the STAMPEDE study, there were substantial and significant survival benefits in patients with metastatic disease randomised to docetaxel at the start of hormone therapy, and this approach is likely to become standard practice. Patients with locally advanced, non metastatic cancers also benefitted to a similar degree, but statistical significance was not reached.

Bisphosphonates

The role of bisphosphonates in the prevention of skeletal-related events in prostate cancer is less clear than in breast cancer. Pathological fractures are relatively uncommon and most men with painful bone metastases respond very well to external beam radiotherapy. Extensive trials with first-generation bisphosphonates (clodronate and pamidronate) have shown little benefit. While the more potent zoledronate can reduce the incidence of skeletal complications (Saad et al., 2004), it is perhaps less widely used given the availability of other more effective treatments, and is not recommended in NICE guidance. The place of early zoledronate therapy in hormone-naive patients will be better defined by the results from the STAMPEDE trial.

Patients with advanced prostate cancer have an increased rate of osteoporosis, which may be exacerbated by the use of long-term ADT, which is associated with both a reduction in bone mineral density and an increased fracture risk. A baseline bone density scan is recommended, with annual or biannual repeats based on the results, and treatment with bisphosphonates according to local protocols if there are significant changes. Denosumab is a potent alternative for patients who are intolerant to bisphosphonates.

Areas of current interest

Role of stereotactic ablative body radiotherapy (SABR)

SABR is widely used for the radical treatment of non-small-cell lung cancer. There is great interest in hypofractionation for prostate cancer. IMRT and IGRT can reduce the volume of rectum irradiated for most patients, but is time-consuming. Initial reports of extreme hypofractionation in low-risk prostate cancer with Cyberknife® are encouraging, but SABR can also be delivered with conventional linear accelerators. The use of SABR should be considered experimental (see below).

Role of imaging-guided subvolume boosts

Some patients have intraprostatic tumour nodules that may be the site of local recurrence. These can be visualised with mpMRI and perhaps choline PET. IMRT and daily IGRT can be used to deliver boosts accurately to these small volumes, and early phase trials are on to ensure that the side effects are acceptable.

Ongoing clinical trials

The STAMPEDE trial is a trial for patients commencing on long-term hormone therapy and has studied: celecoxib, docetaxel, zoledronic acid, abiraterone, and in 2015 is currently investigating the role of local radiotherapy in metastatic disease and a combination abiraterone–enzalutamide arm.

The PACE trial is an ongoing trial of SABR versus radical prostatectomy or conventionally fractionated radiotherapy.

The RADICALS trial is an ongoing trial of immediate or delayed postoperative radiotherapy and a trial of ADT duration in combination with postoperative radiotherapy.

The CHHIP study has closed for recruitment but is yet to report tumour control outcomes (Dearnaley et al., 2012); it compared 74 Gy in 37 fractions with moderately hypofractionated treatment (57 Gy in 19 fractions and 60 Gy in 20 fractions).

The PROTECT study has closed for recruitment, but is yet to report outcomes; it randomised screen-detected prostate cancer patients to prostatectomy, radical radiotherapy or surveillance.

References

Bill-Axelson, A., Holmberg, L., Ruutu, M., et al. (2005). Radical prostatectomy versus watchful waiting in early prostate cancer. N. Engl. J. Med., **352**, 1977–1984.

Bolla, M., de Reijke, T. M., Van Tienhoven, G., et al. (2009). Duration of androgen suppression in the treatment of prostate cancer. N. Engl. J. Med., **360**, 2516–2527.

Bolla, M, van Poppel, H., Tombal, B., et al. (2012). Postoperative radiotherapy after radical prostatectomy for high-risk prostate cancer: long-term results of a randomised controlled trial (EORTC trial 22911). Lancet, **380**, 2018–2027.

Buyyounouski, M. K., Hanlon, A. L., Eisenberg, D. F., et al. (2005). Defining biochemical failure after radiotherapy with and without androgen deprivation for prostate cancer. Int. J. Radiat. Oncol. Biol. Phys., **63**, 1455–1462.

Dearnaley, D. P., Syndikus, I., Sumo, G., et al. (2012). Conventional versus hypofractionated high-dose intensity-modulated radiotherapy for prostate cancer: preliminary safety results from the CHHiP randomised controlled trial. Lancet Oncol., **13**, 43–54.

de Bono, J. S., Oudard, S., Ozguroglu, M., et al. (2010). TROPIC Investigators. Prednisone plus cabazitaxel or mitoxantrone for metastatic castration-resistant prostate cancer progressing after docetaxel treatment: a randomised open-label trial. Lancet, **376**, 1147–1154.

Guerrero Urbano, T., Khoo, V., Staffurth J., et al. (2010). Intensity-modulated radiotherapy allows escalation of the radiation dose to the pelvic lymph nodes in patients with locally advanced prostate cancer: preliminary results of a phase I dose escalation study. Clin. Oncol. (R. Coll. Radiol.), **22**, 236–244.

Hoskin, P. J., Rojas, A. M., Bownes, P. J., et al. (2012). Randomised trial of external beam radiotherapy alone or combined with high-dose-rate brachytherapy boost for localised prostate cancer. Radiother. Oncol., **103**, 217–222.

James, N. D., Spears, M. R., Clarke, N. W., et al. (2014). Survival with newly diagnosed metastatic prostate cancer in the "docetaxel era": data from 917 patients in the control arm of the STAMPEDE Trial (MRC PR08, CRUK/06/019). Eur. Oncol., [Epub ahead of print]: pii: **S0302–2838**(14)00969–5. doi: 10.1016/j.eururo.2014.09.032.

Lawton, C. A., Desilvio, M. and Roach, M. 3rd. (2007). An update of the phase III trial comparing whole pelvic to prostate only radiotherapy and neoadjuvant to total androgen suppression: updated analysis of RTOG 94–13, with emphasis on unexpected hormone/radiation interactions. Int. J. Radiat. Oncol. Biol. Phys., **69**, 646–655.

NICE. (2014). Prostate Cancer: Diagnosis and Treatment. Clinical Guideline. Commissioned by the National Institute for Health and Care Excellence. Cardiff: National Collaborating Centre for Cancer.

Parker, C., Nilsson, S., Heinrich, D., et al. (2013). Alpha emitter radium-223 and survival in metastatic prostate cancer. N. Engl. J. Med., **369**, 213–223.

Prostate Cancer Risk Management Programme. (2006). *Undertaking a Trans-rectal Ultrasound Guided Biopsy of the Prostate.* Sheffield: NHS Cancer Screening Progamme.

Saad, F., Gleason, D. M., Murray, R., *et al.* (2004). Long-term efficacy of zoledronic acid for the prevention of skeletal complications in patients with metastatic hormone-refractory prostate cancer. *J. Natl Cancer Inst.,* **96**, 879–882.

Tannock, I. F., de Wit, R., Berry, W. R., *et al.* (2004). Docetaxel plus prednisone or mitoxantrone plus prednisone for advanced prostate cancer. *N. Engl. J. Med.,* **351**, 1502–1512.

UICC. (2009). *TNM Classification of Malignant Tumours,* ed. L. H. Sobin, M. Gospodariowicz and Ch. Wittekind, 7th edn. Chichester: Wiley-Blackwell.

van As, N. J., de Souza, N. M., Riches, S. F., *et al.* (2009). A study of diffusion-weighted magnetic resonance imaging in men with untreated localised prostate cancer on active surveillance. *Eur. Urol.,* **56**, 981–987.

Warde, P., Mason, M. D., Ding, K., *et al.* (2011), Combined androgen deprivation therapy and radiation therapy for locally advanced prostate cancer: a randomised, phase 3 trial. *Lancet Oncol.,* **378**, 2104–2111.

Wirth, M. P., See, W. A., McLeod, D. G., *et al.* (2004). Bicalutamide 150 mg in addition to standard care in patients with localized or locally advanced prostate cancer: results from the second analysis of the early prostate cancer program at median followup of 5.4 years. *J. Urol.,* **172**, 1865–1870.

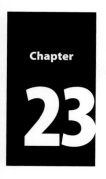

Management of cancer of the testis

Jim Barber and Satish Kumar

Introduction

The treatment of testicular cancer is a success story for oncology, with high cure rates even for patients with advanced metastatic disease. The management has changed little over the past 20 years, with refinements in some areas, and standard protocols are well developed. Nonetheless, patients with testicular cancer are best managed by specialised multidisciplinary teams.

Range of cancers

The range of testicular cancers is shown in Table 23.1.

Germ cell tumours

Incidence and epidemiology

The annual incidence of germ cell tumours in the UK is approximately 800 and incidence is increasing in virtually all European countries. The reason for the rise in incidence in the Western world is not known. A clear birth cohort effect has been identified, for example, in Scandanavian migrants, implicating pre- and postnatal environmental factors. It is speculated that environmental pollutants (for example, pesticides and numerous other candidates) could act as 'hormonal disruptors' in promoting cryptorchidism and infertility (see below).

Risk factors and aetiology

Around 2% of cases report an affected first-degree relative, and there is a 10-fold increased relative risk in a brother of an affected relative. There is wide variation in incidence between different populations which could be also accounted for by genetic factors.

A range of conditions associated with subnormal testicular development, such as testicular maldescent,

Table 23.1 Range of testicular cancers

Type	Examples
Germ cell tumours	Seminoma
	Teratoma (non-seminomatous germ cell tumour)
	Mixed tumour (seminoma and teratoma)
	Spermatocytic seminoma
Non-germ cell tumours	Sex cord/gonadal stromal tumours; Leydig cell tumours, sertoli cell tumours
	Haemopoietic tumours (lymphoma, leukaemic infiltrate)
	Metastatic tumours
	Mesenchymal tumours (embryonal rhabdomyosarcoma, leiomyosarcoma, etc.)
Benign conditions which could be confused with tumours	Epidermoid cyst

Klinefelter's syndrome, Down's syndrome and subfertility, are also associated with a higher risk of cancer.

Testicular maldescent (cryptorchidism) is associated with an approximately 10-fold increased risk of a testicular tumour. Orchidopexy, if done when the child is young enough (probably before 2 years of age), partially reduces this risk. The mechanism of carcinogenesis is unknown, but it is likely that a loss of inhibitory feedback to the pituitary gland from the abnormal germinal epithelium may predispose a person to cancer by continued hormonal stimulation of the germ cells. It is standard practice to perform orchidopexy on maldescended testes because this is thought to reduce their malignant potential.

Practical Clinical Oncology, Second Edition, ed. Louise Hanna, Tom Crosby and Fergus Macbeth. Published by Cambridge University Press. © Cambridge University Press 2015.

Table 23.2 British and American (WHO) systems of classification of teratoma/'non-semoioma'

British	American/WHO	Microscopic appearance
Teratoma differentiated	Mature teratoma; immature teratoma	Differentiated tissue only
Malignant teratoma intermediate	Teratoma with embryonal carcinoma and/or yolk sac tumour	Undifferentiated tumour and/or yolk sac tumour with differentiated tissue present
Malignant teratoma undifferentiated	Embryonal carcinoma	Undifferentiated malignant teratoma only (may include yolk sac elements)
Malignant teratoma trophoblastic	Choriocarcinoma (implies that this is the only element present, high risk for brain metastases)	Malignant trophoblast (syncytiotrophoblast plus cytotrophoblast)

Screening

There is no evidence that population screening for testicular cancer reduces mortality, which would be expected in a rare disease with effective treatment available. Despite periodic health education campaigns directed towards young males, the US Preventive Services Task Force concluded that screening was more likely to do harm than good. Testicular cancer patients should all be taught testicular self-examination, because they run a particularly high risk of second, contralateral cancers.

Pathology and classification of germ cell neoplasms

Germ cell neoplasms can be classified into the following.

- Intratubular germ cell neoplasia – abnormal germ cells within the seminiferous tubules which resemble germ cells at early stages of differentiation.
- Teratoma or 'non-seminoma' – macroscopically firm nodular tumour with areas of haemorrhage and necrosis. For microscopic features see Table 23.2.
- Seminoma, which can be *classical* or *spermatocytic*. Classical seminomas have fibrous septa, lymphocytic infiltrate, typical large round cells with distinct cell borders, clear cytoplasm and large nuclei and prominent nucleoli. They may coexist with non-seminoma (designated a mixed tumour), but 'pure seminomas' may nonetheless contain a few syncytiotrophoblastic elements. Spermatocytic seminomas have a superficial resemblance to classical seminoma, but are a distant relation. There are three types of cells

with different nuclear size: large, small and intermediate. Some nuclei may exhibit a presence of nuclear thread-like chromatin.

Table 23.2 shows the subgroups of teratoma/non-seminoma. It is important for those treating patients with testicular cancer to be aware of the differences between the WHO and British systems, which are highlighted in this table.

Pattern of spread

The 'first station' lymph nodes for tumours of the testis are the inter-aortocaval nodes for right-sided tumours (located in the midline) and the left para-aortic nodes for left-sided tumours (located near the left renal hilum).

In patients who have had ipsilateral inguino-scrotal surgery in the past (e.g. orchidopexy as a child, but probably not vasectomy), anastomotic lymphatics can develop between the testicular/spermatic cord lymphatics and local lymphatics in the groin. In these patients, the pelvic lymph nodes may be at higher risk of spread. Theoretically, this should not affect patients who had *contralateral* surgery only. This is important for planning radiotherapy, but less relevant today as early-stage seminoma is treated more with chemotherapy as an adjuvant therapy. Table 23.3 shows patterns of spread for seminoma and teratoma.

Clinical presentation

The majority of patients present with a painless testicular swelling which is sometimes discovered after trauma. On examination, the mass normally appears to be in the testis. It is useful to know that extratesticular swellings are usually benign epididymal cysts or represent epididymitis, whereas tumours in the

Table 23.3 Modes of spread for seminoma and teratoma

Mode of spread	Seminoma	Teratoma (non-seminoma)
Local (invasion of local non-testicular structures is rare)	Rete testis (signifies increased risk of nodal involvement)	Rete testis as for seminoma
Lymphatic	Highly predictable in a stepwise manner direct to para-aortic nodes and then to pelvic and mediastinal nodes	Similar to seminoma but less predictable
Blood borne (N.B., incidence is 50% in the presence of vascular invasion)	Relatively uncommon	Common in lungs; rare in liver, brain and bone but this signifies a poor prognostic group

epididymis are extremely rare. Breast enlargement is rare and usually associated with a high βhCG level.

Patients with advanced disease can present with non-specific symptoms such as fatigue and weight loss, associated with back pain. They may present with dyspnoea due to lung metastases or associated pulmonary emboli. A para-aortic mass may cause ureteric obstruction, hydronephrosis and occasionally renal failure.

Mediastinal germ cell tumours may present with classic signs and symptoms of superior vena caval obstruction.

Investigation and staging

Tumour markers

Serum tumour markers are important in staging and in monitoring therapy.

βhCG arises from syncytiotrophoblastic elements and is raised in 10–20% of patients with seminoma and around 35% of those with teratoma. Most stage 1 seminoma patients have normal markers, although marginal increases in βhCG (5–10 IU/L) are common and levels tend to fall to less than 1 IU/L after orchidectomy. Levels of βhCG much over 100 IU/L are normally associated with teratoma, but are occasionally seen in patients with seminoma containing syncytiotrophoblastic elements. Massive increases in βhCG may indicate metastatic choriocarcinoma.

αFP arises from yolk sac elements. It is raised in around 60% of patients who have teratoma, but not in patients with seminoma. Borderline elevation and/or fluctuation of αFP levels (up to around 20 ng/mL) is common, and in many patients no obvious cause can be found. Repeating the measurement of αFP levels weekly can clarify the situation rapidly because patients with active cancer generally have exponentially rising αFP levels.

LDH is required for allocation of prognostic grouping. A baseline hormone profile (testosterone, etc.) may be useful.

Mature teratoma, while not containing any frankly malignant elements, can metastasise and systemic chemotherapy is occasionally required.

Patients with pure choriocarcinoma classically present with a small 'burned out' primary and brain metastases.

Other investigations

When a patient is suspected of having a testicular cancer, initial investigation should consist of testicular ultrasound and a check for serum tumour markers. These should be measured preoperatively in all patients.

If a tumour is confirmed, most patients should undergo a high inguinal orchidectomy because a scrotal incision may result in disruption to the normal lymphatic drainage and predispose the patient to involvement of the iliac or inguinal nodes.

However, in patients with very high marker levels, or particularly in those who are unwell with severe symptoms from metastatic disease, the orchidectomy may be deferred until after chemotherapy treatment.

CT scanning of the chest, abdomen and pelvis should be performed in all patients, before surgery if possible; MRI of the brain should be considered if there is choriocarcinoma or the patient is in a poor prognostic group (particularly with a very high βhCG level).

Staging/prognostic grouping of testicular tumours

For practical purposes, most clinicians make use of the excellent Royal Marsden Hospital staging system

Table 23.4 Stage groupings for testicular tumours

Royal Marsden Hospital stage/IGCCC prognostic group	Description
0	*In situ* carcinoma
I	Tumour confined to testis, normal staging scans αFP/βhCG must fall to normal
	Can be further divided into high-risk (LVI-positive) and low-risk (LVI-negative)
IM	Persistently raised tumour markers after orchidectomy (uncommon with better quality CT scanning)
II (N.B. usually seminoma only)	Infradiaphragmatic lymph node involvement
	IIa < 2 cm
	IIb 2–5 cm
	IIc > 5 cm
III	Supradiaphragmatic lymph node involvement
	IIIa < 2 cm
	IIIb 2–5 cm
	IIIc > 5 cm
IV	Extranodal metastases
	IVa < 2 cm
	IVb 2–5 cm
	IVc > 5 cm
	Lung metastases: L1 < 3 lesions; L2 > 3 lesions; L3 > 3 lesions > 2 cm
	H+ liver; B+ brain; N+ neck node; M+ mediastinum

αFP, alpha feto-protein; βhCG, beta human chorionic gonadotrophin; CT, computed tomography; IGCCC, International Germ Cell Consensus Classification; LVI, lymphovascular invasion.

Table 23.5 Prognostic categories for testicular tumours

Prognostic group	Description
'Good-prognosis' metastatic 95% cure	All of the following: αFP < 1000 ng/mL
	βhCG < 5000 IU/L
	LDH < 1.5× normal
	Testicular primary site
'Intermediate-prognosis' metastatic 80% cure	Any of the following: αFP 1000–10,000 ng/mL
	βhCG 5000–50,000 IU/L
	LDH 1.5–10× normal
	Primary site – retroperitoneal teratoma, or any non-testicular seminoma site
'Poor-prognosis' metastatic 50% cure	Any of the following: αFP > 10,000 ng/mL
	βhCG > 50,000 IU/L
	LDH > 10× normal
	Mediastinal teratoma primary site
	Liver/brain/bone metastases ('non-pulmonary visceral metastatic disease')

αFP, alpha feto-protein; βhCG, beta human chorionic gonadotrophin; LDH, lactate dehydrogenase. Adapted from IGCCCG (1997).

The stage groupings and prognostic categories are shown in Tables 23.4 and 23.5, respectively.

Management of intratubular germ cell neoplasia

Intratubular germ cell neoplasia (IGCN) is frequently found alongside germ cell tumours and in the contralateral testis in around 5% of cases. It is the accepted precursor of testicular cancer, and some studies suggest a 50% progression rate to cancer within a few years.

The risk of contralateral IGCN is high in patients with testicular atrophy (Harland *et al.*, 1998). There is probably a weak association with testicular microlithiasis, although, more often than not, the conditions occur independently.

Some experts advocate routine biopsy of the contralateral testicle at the time of the orchidectomy, whereas others perform a biopsy only for high-risk patients (i.e. with a testicular volume < 15 mL).

for early disease (stage I teratoma and seminoma, stage II seminoma), but decision-making in stage II teratoma and all stage III cases and above is made by using prognostic groupings according to the International Germ Cell Consensus Classification (IGCCCG, 1997). Technically speaking, prognostic group allocation is determined from the nadir levels of αFP and βhCG after orchidectomy, not from the preoperative levels.

If IGCN is found, it can be eliminated by treatment with radiotherapy, for example, 20 Gy in 10 fractions; however, such treatment may cause infertility. Many IGCN patients already have borderline hypogonadism, and radiotherapy (even at 20 Gy) may further disrupt Leydig cell function. In the past, quality of life may be poor in patients who are on testosterone replacement therapy because of the lack of high-quality depot preparations, but long-acting depot injections of testosterone are now available. Side effects of testosterone replacement include acne, polycythaemia, fluid retention, sleep apnoea and testosterone-induced prostate growth.

An alternative to biopsy and radiotherapy is a combination of testicular self-examination and annual ultrasonic follow-up. Ultimately, the decision must rest with the patient.

Treatment overview: teratoma and seminoma

Stage I disease

Seminoma is exquisitely sensitive to both radiotherapy and chemotherapy, so adjuvant therapy is commonly used in stage I disease, even when the relapse risk is low. In stage I teratoma the threshold for offering adjuvant therapy is higher, because the chemotherapy regimen (BEP) is more toxic, and patients are managed solely with surveillance, although there is a trend towards the use of adjuvant BEP in high-risk patients. Because teratomas produce tumour markers more commonly than seminomas, surveillance is easier in patients with teratoma.

Metastatic disease

Patients with seminoma may be treated with radiotherapy up to stage II, but all other patients with metastatic disease should receive combination chemotherapy.

Treatment of stage I and II seminoma

Stage I seminoma

Around 15–20% of patients with stage I disease will relapse after orchidectomy, primarily and predictably within the para-aortic nodes. Tumour size and rete testis invasion are considered to be predictive of a higher rate of relapse. Tumours of 4 cm or greater have a higher relapse rate of around 25% with the group less than 4 cm having an overall relapse rate of around 13%

(SWENOTECA database, Tandstad et al., 2014); rete testis invasion is also associated with an increased risk, but is less consistently reported as an independent predictor of relapse. Lymphovascular invasion is also a high-risk factor, but may be unreliable in seminoma as it can appear as an artefact of slide preparation.

Adjuvant radiotherapy

Adjuvant radiotherapy to the para-aortic nodes has been practised for over 50 years, with a relapse rate of around 5%. Given the young age of the patients and that the majority will not relapse, the long-term consequences must be carefully considered. There is a well-documented increased risk (2–3) of second malignancies within the radiation portals (stomach, pancreas, bladder and kidney; Bokemeyer and Schmoll, 1995), and also an increased risk of cardiovascular disease, with around a doubling of risk of cardiac events reported from both M.D. Anderson Hospital, Texas and The Royal Marsden Hospital in large retrospective series.

Surveillance

Relapses are seldom detected by tumour markers or chest X-ray (CXR), so regular CT scanning is essential; it is usually done every 3–6 months in the first year, and then rapidly scaled down to annual scanning. Occasionally, relapses can occur after several years. MRI surveillance of para-aortic nodal disease, when combined with CXR and tumour markers, is an alternative using less radiation exposure: this is the subject of a recently completed UK trial (TRISST) which should also clarify the optimum surveillance follow-up schedule for these patients.

Adjuvant chemotherapy

Adjuvant chemotherapy with a single cycle of carboplatin AUC 7 gives 2-year tumour control and survival rates equivalent to adjuvant para-aortic radiotherapy (TE19, Oliver et al., 2005). In the SWENOTECA population study, the relapse rate after carboplatin was a little higher than in TE19 (Tandstad et al., 2014), but this has been attributed to enrichment of the population by patients with larger tumours. The use of two cycles of carboplatin has been suggested, but if the dosing is performed using the AUC then this is probably unnecessary. Relapse after 3 years follow-up is a very rare event (only one patient receiving carboplatin in the TE19 trial relapsed after this time) and so scanning is recommended for around 3 years.

So which option?

Given the relatively high chance of relapse with the larger tumours (4 cm), adjuvant therapy would seem advisable in these cases rather than surveillance. Many oncologists in the UK use a single cycle of carboplatin, and this practice is becoming more accepted internationally. Despite the risk of second malignancy and cardiovascular disease, radiotherapy is still widely used in the USA. The pattern of relapse with adjuvant carboplatin is quite different from that after radiotherapy; in patients having radiotherapy the relapses are mainly in the chest and pelvis, whereas in those treated with carboplatin the relapses tend to occur in the para-aortic region. This finding suggests that the treatments are to some extent complementary and gives a rationale for combining them in the treatment of stage II seminoma.

Stage II seminoma

Traditionally, patients with stage IIa/IIb seminoma are treated with 'dog-leg' radiotherapy with a boost for bulky disease. Treatment failure is considerably more likely than in stage I disease, and around 20% of patients will relapse and require chemotherapy, which seems unacceptably high. A single course of carboplatin before radiotherapy is effective in reducing the relapse rate to around 5% (Patterson et al., 2001). Single institution series (Parker et al., 2011) suggest that para-aortic strip (rather than dog-leg) nodal irradiation alone may be adequate, given the effectiveness of carboplatin in reducing relapse rates in clinically uninvolved nodal areas (see following text).

Combination chemotherapy (with EP; see the section on chemotherapy) is often used to treat patients with stage IIc (bulky) seminoma. The advantages of better cancer control rates must be offset against the greatly increased morbidity and a small chance of treatment-related death. The location of the tumour is also important in making the treatment decision. For example, even quite large, centrally sited inter-aortocaval nodes (often associated with right-sided tumours) can be treated with radiotherapy and a single cycle of carboplatin, whereas left-sided nodes may overlie the left kidney and require combination chemotherapy to avoid irradiation of a large portion of the kidney.

Technique of radiotherapy in seminoma: strips and dog-legs

For adjuvant treatment 20 Gy in 10 fractions is adequate to sterilise microscopic seminoma and a para-aortic field alone (rather than a dog-leg) is adequate (Fossa et al., 1999). The reduction in dose probably reduces the acute toxicity, and using a smaller treatment volume probably reduces the chance of second malignancies. Whereas a dose of 20 Gy is now well-accepted for stage I disease, it has not been tested in stage IIa/b disease, and 30 Gy in 15 fractions is widely used.

Treatment is planned most easily using a CT planning scan and, given the low dose, can be delivered using parallel fields. The kidneys can be outlined as organs at risk and shielded using the MLCs.

Patients with a low risk of microscopic pelvic disease: para-aortic field only

The standard target volume for stage I seminoma patients is the para-aortic nodes from around T11 to L5. Care must be taken, particularly for left-sided tumours, to ensure that the field extends to the medial border of the left kidney. The lateral borders of the target volume lie around 4–4.5 cm from the midline.

Patients with a higher risk of microscopic pelvic disease

'Dog-leg' fields have traditionally been used for stage I patients who have a history of testicular maldescent or scrotal violation, or for stage II patients. However, a single dose of carboplatin would be preferable to pelvic irradiation in controlling micrometastatic disease in the pelvis and we would recommend irradiation of the pelvic only in stage II patients with documented pelvic lymph nodes, in combination with a single cycle of carboplatin.

Pathological para-aortic nodes must be identified on the planning scan (if done without contrast enhancement then with the aid of diagnostic imaging). For left-sided nodes, there is a fine balance between allowing sufficient lateral margins and including too much of the left kidney. Most pathological nodes lie within the traditional 8–9 cm field width, but occasionally eccentrically located nodes may occur outside this range.

The dog-leg field is similar to the para-aortic field but extends inferiorly to include the ipsilateral iliac nodes to the level of the obturator foramen. The lateral border of the field normally extends to the pelvic side wall, and medially the bladder; central pelvic contents can usually be shielded. The addition of the dog-leg field increases the treatment volume considerably, and so the risk of second malignancy is likely to be much higher than with a para-aortic field alone.

Scrotal irradiation, using kilovoltage radiation and lead shielding over the contralateral testicle, is occasionally used for patients who have had an extensive tumour in the spermatic cord or had scrotal violation during surgery. However, with so much uncertainty about the site of residual disease, chemotherapy may be preferred in these patients.

Toxicity of radiotherapy

Most patients experience some nausea, but this usually can be controlled by the use of 5-HT3 antagonist drugs. Mild tiredness is common, and occasionally it can be prolonged for some months.

A dog-leg field may deliver around 40 cGy of scattered radiation to the scrotum throughout a course of treatment, depending on the field size and machine used (considerably more than with a para-aortic strip alone). Even at this dose, there is a well-documented drop in sperm counts to, in some cases, subfertile levels, and sperm banking should be considered. Patients should be also advised to avoid conception for 6–12 months to avoid the possibility of a teratogenic effect.

The risk of second cancers is as discussed earlier.

Treatment of stage I teratoma

Patients without lymphovascular invasion: low risk of relapse

Teratomas are treated in a similar fashion regardless of subtype, which has little independent significance in prognosis. The chance of relapse in patients without lymphovascular invasion is less than 20% and as many of these patients have positive tumour markers at diagnosis, they are best managed by surveillance. The risks of adjuvant chemotherapy and/or retroperitoneal surgery outweigh the benefits, and most patients who relapse can be cured with systemic chemotherapy.

Tumour markers should return to normal levels after surgery and weekly/fortnightly marker samples should be taken until this occurs. Monthly visits are recommended initially, but after the first 6–12 months the interval between visits can be extended. A typical schedule may be every 2 months in year two, every 3 months in year three, every 4–6 months in years four and five, and then annually. Tumour-marker estimations should be done at all visits and a CXR is usually taken, although this rarely identifies first relapse.

Follow-up CT scanning is done at around 3 months and at 1 year; the value of extra CT scanning is debated. The MRC trial TE08 (Mead *et al.*, 2006) showed little difference in outcomes in 400 patients randomised between 2 or 5 CT scans during the initial 2 years of follow-up, and 2 scans seems reasonable for low-risk patients, although high-risk patients were not sufficiently represented in this study to extend this policy to all patients (see below).

Patients with lymphovascular invasion: high risk of relapse

If the tumour shows lymphovascular invasion, the chances of a relapse are high even with a negative CT scan – around 45%. PET scanning is little more reliable, with a 37% relapse rate in PET-negative patients (TE22 trial; Huddart *et al.*, 2006) and cannot be recommended as a staging tool. There are three ways of managing these patients.

- *Surgical staging (with two cycles of BEP for pN+ disease).* In the USA (but not in the UK), 'staging' retroperitoneal lymph node dissections are routinely performed for stage I patients. Patients with positive para-aortic nodes at surgery (pathological stage II disease) may be cured with surgery alone, but there is a high relapse rate. Therefore, most receive adjuvant chemotherapy (two cycles of BEP), which has been shown to reduce recurrence but not improve overall survival (Williams *et al.*, 1987). There is a strong feeling outside the USA that staging surgery adds morbidity but does little to affect the long-term outcome.
- *Adjuvant chemotherapy (1–2 cycles of BEP).* Two cycles of BEP for all patients at a high risk of recurrence has been shown to reduce the rate of relapse to approximately 2% (Cullen *et al.*, 1996). Although this practice is highly effective and is standard management in many centres in the UK, adjuvant chemotherapy has a distinct morbidity and mortality risk. Robust data are available, however, to support a single cycle of BEP in high-risk patients which is more attractive as adjuvant therapy (3.4% relapse rate in the SWENOTECA study; Tandstad *et al.*, 2013) and the UK 111 study of a single cycle of BEP, recently completed, will give more data on this issue.
- *Surveillance (with 3× BEP for those who relapse).* Surveillance is a reasonable practice, provided

the patients are monitored carefully, particularly in the first 6–12 months; consideration should be given to scanning every 3 months in the initial period. Some patients are not psychologically suited to this approach and it must be explained carefully. Surveillance is a more attractive option than it was a few years ago now that salvage therapy is usually limited to 3× BEP rather than 4× BEP. For those who relapse, the majority would be in the good-prognosis metastatic group and would therefore receive 3× BEP.

Patients with borderline nodal enlargement

Sometimes, a CT scan shows para-aortic nodes that are larger than normally expected but not quite large enough to meet formal radiological size criteria for enlargement. In this situation, it can be difficult to determine whether the lymph nodes are affected by cancer. Nodes are more likely to be pathological if they are in the expected location for the side of tumour and if the patient is in the high-risk group. PET scanning is often performed but may be misleading and is not recommended. Early repeat CT scanning after approximately 6–12 weeks, combined with regular marker estimations, usually provides enough information to decide whether the nodes are pathologically involved.

Treatment of metastatic disease: BEP chemotherapy

Most patients with metastases should be cured, but the outcome depends mostly on the patient's prognostic group. Patients with good-prognosis disease (including those with stage IM disease and most of those relapsing after surveillance) are adequately treated by three cycles of BEP (bleomycin, etoposide, cisplatin), whereas four cycles would be recommended for all other patients (with the omission of bleomycin in the final cycle if the patient is at high risk for bleomycin toxicity – see below).

The BEP regimen has been extensively tested over the past 30 years and is currently the best regimen for testicular cancer. Attempts to reduce the toxicity of BEP have been unsuccessful. Bleomycin can cause potentially fatal pneumonitis, but its omission reduces cure rates by several per cent. Substituting carboplatin ('BEC') for cisplatin ('BEP') reduces the renal toxicity and makes the regimen more acceptable, but is also less effective.

There have also been several attempts to increase the effectiveness of BEP, particularly in patients with poor-prognosis disease. Several trials of intensive schedules (e.g. BOP/VIP, VIP, high-dose BEP, and most recently, high-dose chemotherapy with stem cell support) have simply resulted in more toxicity and similar overall survival rates. There is international interest in exploring the use of accelerated BEP (a two-week compressed schedule using G-CSF) which is well tolerated, quick and efficient, and does not have excessive toxicity (Grimison et al., 2014).

For patients with metastatic seminoma, there is less evidence that bleomycin is essential, and it is often left out of the regimen. The standard regimen is either 3× BEP or 4× EP. It has been shown that single-agent carboplatin (four cycles) is less effective than four cycles of EP (Horwich et al., 2000), but for elderly, unfit patients, or those in renal failure, carboplatin alone can deliver acceptable cure rates with few treatment-related deaths.

Confusion about BEP may occur because there are so many different 'recipes'. For example, the 3- and 5-day BEP schedules have been shown to give the same cure rates in good-prognosis disease (but have not been tested in the other groups), but at the price of slightly increased toxicity (gastrointestinal and tinnitus) for the 3-day version. Many centres in the UK use the 3-day BEP schedule to save on bed occupancy, but 5-day BEP can be safely given with patients as an outpatient. There is also a 'low-dose' BEP (etoposide total dose 360 mg/m² per cycle). Table 23.6 shows two versions of BEP chemotherapy.

Practical management of BEP cisplatin

Renal damage is rare if adequate hydration is given with magnesium replacement. Most patients have good renal function, but GFR should be measured by EDTA clearance before starting chemotherapy. For a patient with good renal function, a GFR estimated before each cycle using the Cockcroft–Gault formula is adequate. Severe vascular toxicity (myocardial infarction and stroke) has been reported in young men receiving BEP and has been attributed to the cisplatin component; the mechanism is unknown, but may be reversible vascular spasm. A switch to carboplatin should be considered if this occurs.

Bleomycin lung

Bleomycin may cause a potentially fatal pneumonitis, which is partially dose-related and is rarely seen

Table 23.6 Two versions of BEP chemotherapy

Regimen	Description
Standard 5-day BEP	Weekly bleomycin 30,000 IU, i.v. (D2, 8, 15) should be given regardless of blood count
	Total dose of bleomycin 270,000–360,000 IU
	Days 1–5 cisplatin 20 mg/m²
	Days 1–5 etoposide 100 mg/m²
Standard 3-day BEP	Weekly bleomycin 30,000 IU, i.v. (D2, 8, 15) should be given regardless of blood count
	Total dose of bleomycin 270,000–360,000 IU
	Days 1 and 2 cisplatin 50 mg/m²
	Days 1–3 etoposide 165 mg/m²

at cumulative doses of less than 270,000 IU. The risk increases sharply at doses above 360,000 IU. The risks of giving bleomycin should be carefully considered in those who have multiple risk factors for bleomycin toxicity: age over 40 years, those with poor renal function (GFR < 80 mL/min; O'Sullivan et al., 2003) and smokers.

A clinical respiratory assessment should be made before each treatment, especially before cycles three and four, when bleomycin toxicity is more common. A history of gradually increasing shortness of breath and a dry cough are worrying but non-specific symptoms. Monitoring lung function tests during chemotherapy is sometimes recommended, but test interpretation is difficult because lung function deteriorates in most patients during chemotherapy.

Thromboembolic disease is a very common complication in hospitalised patients with a large para-aortic mass, and thromboprophylaxis should be considered. For patients who present with significant dyspnoea or pulmonary changes, the possibility of a pulmonary embolism or bleomycin lung should be considered in addition to infection. A CT pulmonary angiogram can help to distinguish bleomycin lung (diffuse or basal patchy fibrosis/exudates) from thromboembolic disease.

Residual mass postchemotherapy: teratoma

When a teratoma metastasises, it may differentiate into mature teratoma (particularly if TD is present in the orchidectomy specimen). Following chemotherapy,

the malignant elements of the tumour may be completely cleared but residual mature teratoma may remain, because it is not sensitive to chemotherapy. It is no longer considered acceptable to observe a residual mass. Mature teratoma has the potential to grow slowly over time and may undergo subsequent malignant change, and it is likely that malignant change within mature teratoma is the major cause of late relapse following chemotherapy (after 2 years).

Residual para-aortic disease may be resected by retroperitoneal lymph node dissection (RPLND; Hendry et al., 1993). RPLND is a major operation, with a significant risk of infection and pulmonary embolus, and recovery may take several weeks. It is important to consider the timing of the operation, which can coincide with the peak of bleomycin lung toxicity if performed too soon. The operation is highly specialised and may require vascular expertise to deal with residual disease tightly adherent to major blood vessels. Potency is usually normal afterwards, but patients may experience retrograde ejaculation and lose fertility as a result.

When selecting patients for RPLND, it is useful to know that small residual lymph nodes (< 1 cm) may resolve completely over a period of several months and usually represent necrotic residues. However, any persisting masses much larger than this, or indeed persisting nodes of any size, are likely to contain mature teratoma. FDG-PET may be more accurate than CT in identifying residual malignancy, but cannot distinguish mature teratoma from fibrosis, and surgery should still be considered (De Wit et al., 2006).

A small proportion (around 10%) of resected specimens contain residual cancer (i.e. frankly malignant cells), although the pathological identification of malignant elements can be difficult. Residual viable malignancy is associated with a high incidence of relapse, and further chemotherapy (possibly second-line) should be considered.

Residual mass postchemotherapy: seminoma

Residual masses after chemotherapy for seminoma are not normally resected; they are often extremely vascular, difficult to remove and infrequently contain active cancer. Assuming the diagnosis of pure seminoma was correct, mature teratoma should not complicate the issue. There is evidence that PET scanning of seminomatous residual mass may be considerably more helpful in identifying residual cancer than in teratoma (De Wit et al., 2006). False negatives do occur, but it would be reasonable to offer radiotherapy to patients with a PET-positive residual mass. Those who are PET-negative are usually managed with observation, but those at high risk of relapse (e.g. those receiving second-line chemotherapy) might be considered for radiotherapy.

Fertility and hormonal issues

Patients should be offered the option of sperm banking before combination chemotherapy. However, for those patients who receive a single cycle of carboplatin or para-aortic radiotherapy, sperm banking may not be necessary, as studies on serial FSH levels following carboplatin have shown no significant effect.

Approximately 50% of men requiring chemotherapy for metastatic disease will have low sperm counts before chemotherapy. Of those with normal counts, about 50% will have regained normal counts 2 years after chemotherapy and 80% at 5 years (Lampe *et al.*, 1997).

There is a high incidence of hypogonadism among testicular cancer patients not only due to orchidectomy and chemotherapy, but also because of the association of testicular cancer with testicular atrophy and subfertility. A hormonal assessment should be made part of routine follow-up and testosterone replacement therapy should be considered.

Relapsed disease and the role of high-dose chemotherapy with peripheral stem cell support

If a durable remission is not obtained with 4× BEP, some patients can be cured with conventional second-line chemotherapy. This comprises cisplatin with one or two new drugs not previously used. If the patient has previously received bleomycin, it should not form part of the relapse regimen because of the toxicity risk. For patients who received BEP the first time around, suitable regimens would be VIP (VP16 [etoposide], ifosfamide, cisplatin) or TIP (paclitaxel, ifosfamide, cisplatin).

High-dose chemotherapy (HDCT) with escalation of the cisplatin dose is limited by renal toxicity, but carboplatin can be given at an AUC of up to 20 with stem cell support. There is a relatively low risk of treatment-related death of around 3% and this treatment has been in use for many years with many enthusiasts.

As previously mentioned, HDCT as first-line therapy has shown no benefit in randomised trials

and is not currently recommended. It is widely but inconsistently used after first relapse, but again randomised trials have shown disappointing results. The IT-94 study (Pico *et al.*, 2005) of a single transplant after salvage chemotherapy showed no advantage to the transplant (although there were many protocol violations), whereas a German Testicular Group trial of three high-dose treatments compared to one was stopped early due to excessive toxicity (Lorch *et al.*, 2007), without any benefit to the triple transplant.

While the issue is unresolved, an international retrospective database of roughly 1500 patients treated in first relapse (around half being treated with HDCT) has suggested a benefit for early HDCT (Lorch *et al.*, 2011) *except* for those with all the following good prognostic features:

- testicular primary,
- at least 3 months marker remission following BEP,
- αFP and βHCG in the 'good prognosis range',
- no liver, bone or brain metastases.

The result showed perhaps a greater benefit to HDCT than expected, taking into account the randomised data, with a hazard ratio of 0.44 for progression-free survival and 0.65 for overall survival. It is reasonable to select patients with multiple good prognostic features for a trial of second-line chemotherapy and reserve HDCT for second relapse, but for other patients, consideration of a transplant should be discussed at an early stage on first relapse. An international trial of two cycles of salvage chemotherapy followed by two HDCT treatments is being planned.

Patients who relapse late (arbitrarily, at more than 2 years) form a distinct subgroup, where the prognosis is worse. Histology sometimes shows an adult solid tumour (probably arising from residual mature teratoma) rather than a germ cell tumour, and may be marker-negative. Such recurrences do not respond well to standard chemotherapy regimens. Surgery should be considered initially, particularly if there is a potentially operable tumour at a single site. For patients with metastatic disease, however, there is normally little choice but to try second-line chemotherapy with consideration of HDCT and surgery afterwards depending on response to chemotherapy.

Palliative treatments

Patients who are not thought to be curable with second-line chemotherapy, or who relapse after second-line chemotherapy, may be suitable for palliative therapy in addition to best supportive care.

Germ cell cancers occasionally are slow growing and chronically recurring. Multiple remissions can be seen with repeated chemotherapy treatment. It is worthwhile considering surgical debulking of disease, and even palliative radiotherapy in selected cases and long remissions may be seen. A variety of novel agents are being tested; for example, CDK4/6 inhibitors.

Follow-up

Late recurrences are rare in patients with testicular germ cell tumours and follow-up to detect recurrence may not be needed after 5 years, except in those presenting with metastatic NSGCTs (Shahidi et al., 2002).

Special clinical situations: spermatocytic seminoma

Spermatocytic seminoma is said to account for fewer than 5% of seminomas and typically occurs in older men. It bears some histological resemblance to, and can be confused with, seminoma. Although it originates from germ cells, there is a dispute as to whether it should be classified as a germ cell tumour, because it is not descended from germ cell carcinoma in situ. It has no ovarian counterpart and is not associated with the usual risk factors for testicular cancer. Anaplastic transformation is reported, which can be confused with embryonal carcinoma, but does not appear to change the prognosis.

Spermatocytic seminoma is usually benign and slow growing, but can occasionally grow very large. Metastatic disease is virtually unknown, but there are occasional reports of sarcomatous transformation associated with the development of metastatic disease.

Sex cord stromal tumours

Sex cord stromal tumours are similar to their ovarian counterparts. The Sertoli cells provide support for spermatogenesis, and the Leydig cells secrete testosterone. They are usually classified as benign, but there are a few case reports of metastases occurring. Unfortunately, there are no well-defined pathological criteria that can predict aggressive behaviour.

Most oncologists in the UK take a conservative approach to management of these tumours. An orchidectomy and a staging CT scan should be performed. In the unlikely event of para-aortic nodal disease being found, surgery could be considered, with a node dissection if technically possible, and a cure attempted.

Close follow-up can cause much unnecessary anxiety in patients who essentially have benign tumours of little significance. It would be reasonable to monitor testosterone and gonadotrophin levels in these patients, though, because these levels have virtually never been estimated preoperatively, it is not generally known whether the tumours secrete hormones or not.

For the very occasional patient with inoperable or metastatic disease, cytotoxic chemotherapy could be considered. However, there is no established regimen with documented activity, and it should be recognised that BEP chemotherapy is unlikely to give significant responses.

References

Bokemeyer, C. and Schmoll, H. J. (1995). Treatment of testicular cancer and the development of secondary malignancies. J. Clin. Oncol., 13, 283–292.

Cullen, M. H., Stenning, S. P., Parkinson, M. C., et al. (1996). Short-course adjuvant chemotherapy in high-risk stage I nonseminomatous germ cell tumors of the testis: a Medical Research Council report. J. Clin. Oncol., 14, 1106–1113.

De Wit, M., Hartmann, M., Brenner, W., et al. (2006). [18F]-FDG-PET in germ cell tumors following chemotherapy: results of the German multicenter trial. J. Clin. Oncol., 24(18 Suppl.), 4521.

Fossa, S. D., Horwich, A., Russell, J. M., et al. (1999). Optimal planning target volume for stage I testicular seminoma: a Medical Research Council randomized trial. J. Clin. Oncol., 17, 1146.

Grimison, P. S, Stockler, M. R., Chatfield, M., et al. (2014). Accelerated BEP for metastatic germ cell tumours: a multicenter phase II trial by the Australian and New Zealand Urogenital and Prostate Cancer Trials Group (ANZUP). Ann. Oncol., 25, 143–148.

Harland, S. J., Cook, P. A., Fossa, S. D., et al. (1998). Intratubular germ cell neoplasia of the contralateral testis in testicular cancer: defining a high risk group. J. Urol., 160, 1353–1357.

Hendry, W. F., A'Hern, R. P., Hetherington, J. W., et al. (1993). Para-aortic lymphadenectomy after chemotherapy for metastatic non-seminomatous germ cell tumours: prognostic value and therapeutic benefit. Br. J. Urol., 71, 208–213.

Horwich, A., Oliver, R. T., Wilkinson, P. M., et al. (2000). A medical research council randomized trial of single agent carboplatin versus etoposide and cisplatin for advanced metastatic seminoma. Br. J. Cancer, 83, 1623–1629.

Huddart, R., O'Doherty, M., Padhani, A., *et al.* (2006). A prospective study of 18FDG PET in the prediction of relapse in patients with high risk clinical stage I (CS1) non-seminomatous germ cell cancer (NSGCT): MRC study TE22. *J. Clin. Oncol.*, **24**(18 Suppl.), 4520.

IGCCCG. (1997). International Germ Cell Consensus Classification: a prognostic factor-based staging system for metastatic germ cell cancers. *J. Clin. Oncol.*, **15**, 594–603.

Lampe, H., Horwich, A., Norman, A., *et al.* (1997). Fertility after chemotherapy for testicular germ cell cancers. *J. Clin. Oncol.*, **15**, 239–245.

Lorch, A., Kollmannsberger, C., Hartmann, J. T., *et al.* (2007). Single versus sequential high-dose chemotherapy in patients with relapsed or refractory germ cell tumors: a prospective randomized multicenter trial of the German Testicular Cancer Study Group. *J. Clin. Oncol.*, **25**, 2778–2784.

Lorch, A., Bascoul-Mollevi, C., Kramar, A., *et al.* (2011). Conventional dose versus high dose chemotherapy as first salvage treatment in male patients with metastatic germ cell tumours, an international database. *J. Clin. Oncol.*, **29**, 2178–2184.

Mead, G. M., Rustin, G. J., Stenning, S. P., *et al.* (2006). Medical Research Council trial of 2 versus 5 CT scans in the surveillance of patients with stage I non-seminomatous germ cell tumours of the testis. *J. Clin. Oncol.*, **24** (18 Suppl.), 4519.

Oliver, R. T., Mason, M., Mead, G. M., *et al.* (2005). Radiotherapy versus single-dose carboplatin in adjuvant treatment of stage I seminoma: a randomised trial. *Lancet*, **366**, 293–300.

O'Sullivan, J. M., Huddart, R. A., Norman, A. R., *et al.* (2003). Predicting the risk of bleomycin lung toxicity in patients with germ-cell tumours. *Ann. Oncol.*, **14**, 91–96.

Parker, K., Smith, C. and Barber, J. (2011). Case series of 16 patients with stage II seminoma treated with sequential carboplatin AUC7 then para-aortic radiotherapy. *Clin. Oncol. (R. Coll. Radiol.)*, **23**, 70.

Patterson, H., Norman, A. R., Mitra, S. S., *et al.* (2001). Combination carboplatin and radiotherapy in the management of stage II testicular seminoma: comparison with radiotherapy treatment alone. *Radiother. Oncol.*, **59**, 5–11.

Pico, J. L., Rosti, G., Kramar, A., *et al.* (2005). A randomised trial of high-dose chemotherapy in the salvage treatment of patients failing first-line platinum chemotherapy for advanced germ cell tumours *Ann. Oncol.*, **16**, 1152–1159.

Shahidi, M., Norman, A. R., Dearnaley, D. P., *et al.* (2002). Late recurrences in 1263 men with testicular germ cell tumors. Multivariate analysis of risk factors and implications for management. *Cancer*, **95**, 520–530.

Tandstad, T., Cavallin-Stahl, E., Dahl, O., *et al.* (2013). One course of adjuvant BEP in clinical stage I, nonseminoma: mature and expanded results from the SWENOTECA group. *J. Clin. Oncol.*, **31** (Suppl.; abstr. 4553).

Tandstad, T., Cavallin-Stahl, E., Dahl, O., *et al.* (2014). Management of clinical stage I seminomatous testicular cancer: a report from SWENOTECA. *J. Clin. Oncol.*, **32** (Suppl.; abstr. 4508).

Williams, S. D., Birch, R., Einhorn, L. H., *et al.* (1987). Treatment of disseminated germ-cell tumors with cisplatin, bleomycin, and either vinblastine or etoposide. *N. Engl. J. Med.*, **316**, 1435–1440.

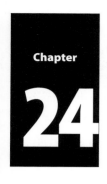

Management of cancer of the penis

Jim Barber

Range of tumours

The range of tumours affecting the penis is shown in Table 24.1.

Incidence and epidemiology

Penile cancer is relatively uncommon with around 350 cases annually in the UK, although in Asia, Africa and South America (e.g. Uganda, Brazil) the disease is more common. The peak incidence is in men over age 70, but a substantial number of cases occur in much younger men.

The national audit of penile cancer in England has shown a slow rise in the incidence of penile cancer from 1990 to 2009, although mortality has not significantly increased (http://www.ncin.org.uk/publications, accessed August 2014). A similar pattern reported in Denmark (Baldur-Felskov *et al.*, 2012) was attributed to low circumsion rates, and there is also speculation that increasing rates of HPV infection may be contributing.

Risk factors and aetiology

Penile cancer risk is increased with a history of genital warts, but is less consistently associated with HPV than is cervical carcinoma. Most studies have only identified HPV subtypes 16 and 18 in around 50% of cases of classic squamous cell tumours (Stankiewicz *et al.*, 2011), although there is a more consistent association with carcinoma *in situ* (Dillner *et al.*, 2000). Factors that affect HPV infection – including geography, number of sexual partners and circumcision – may all affect the incidence.

Circumcision at birth reduces the risk considerably, although the protective effect of circumcision is less in men without phimosis. Poor hygiene may be a

Table 24.1 Range of tumours affecting the penis

Type of tumour	Examples
Benign	Condylomata acuminata
	Bowenoid papulosis
	Leiomyoma
	Balanitis xerotica obliterans (premalignant)
	Carcinoma *in situ* (erythroplasia of Queyrat, Bowen's disease)
Malignant primary	Squamous carcinoma
	Verrucous carcinoma (very low risk of metastasis)
	Others
	Basal cell carcinoma
	Kaposi's sarcoma
	Melanoma
	Sarcoma
Malignant secondary	e.g. from bladder, prostate

factor, although smegma has now been discounted as a carcinogen.

Phimosis itself increases the risk and makes early detection more difficult; tumours are more likely to present late.

Vaccination against high-risk HPV subtypes has been proposed for boys in addition to the programme for girls and is currently under evaluation in high-risk groups (for example, men who have sex with men).

Pathology

A number of premalignant lesions are recognised. *Balanitis xerotica obliterans* is the penile equivalent of lichen planus and is associated with a small risk of invasive cancer. *Intraepithelial carcinoma* presents in a variety of shapes, from nodules to erythematous plaques. It is designated *erythroplasia of Queyrat* if it appears on the glans or prepuce, or *Bowen's disease* if it involves the skin. The risk of transformation to invasive squamous cell carcinoma (SCC) is around 30% for carcinoma *in situ* on the glans.

A range of *invasive squamous cancers* occur, rather similar to those seen in the anal or vulval region: classic, well- to poorly differentiated squamous cell cancers, a basaloid variant and a number of *verrucous tumours* (e.g. giant condylomata, Bushke Lowenstein tumour).

The classic squamous cell tumours behave in a fashion similar to that of squamous tumours elsewhere. The risk of local recurrence and metastatic spread is highly dependent on the stage and grade of the tumour, and most deaths from penile cancer result from the more aggressive G3 lesions. Penile cancer usually metastasises quite systematically through the local lymphatics, first to the inguinal nodes (bilateral disease is quite frequent) and then to the pelvic nodes. Pelvic nodal metastases have not been reported in the absence of inguinal nodes.

Verrucous tumours may exhibit features of viral change (koilocytosis). Their pattern of invasion is to advance on a broad front, in a destructive rather than invasive fashion, and they are thought to metastasise only rarely. There are case reports of anaplastic transformation, which may be spontaneous but sometimes appears to be related to radiotherapy treatment. The current literature (although sparse) would suggest that this is a relatively rare event, probably occurring in fewer than 5% of cases.

Occasionally, the penis is involved with Kaposi's sarcoma, basal cell carcinomas or melanoma. It can also be involved by metastases from other sites. Both bladder and prostate cancer can invade the penis locally, but the diagnosis rarely causes any difficulty.

Diagnosis and staging

Review by a specialist MDT is recommended at the outset. For small tumours an attempt at local excision is a reasonable first step. Larger tumours should, if possible, be biopsied and fully staged before starting the patient on definitive local therapy.

Traditional staging of penile cancer simply consists of a clinical examination of the primary and of inguinal lymph nodes. Clinically negative groins were often subjected to close clinical observation only, or in high-grade cancers staging node dissections were performed. However, staging has been improved in recent years, which avoids under- or overtreatment.

For the primary cancer, ultrasound scan (US) and MRI (with prostoglandin E1) can give information regarding corporal involvement, and MRI can differentiate between cavernosal and spongiosum involvement, which can assist with planning surgery. Both are classified as T2, but spongiosum involvement has a worse prognosis: a limitation of the current TNM system.

For patients with at least T2 tumours or any with G3 histology or vascular invasion, occult metastatic disease in the groin can be safely excluded by dynamic sentinel node biopsy using isosulphan blue and Tc-99m colloid. The technique has high sensitivity and specificity and avoids the need to perform unnecessary staging groin dissections (Tanis *et al.*, 2002; Lam *et al.*, 2013).

CT and/or MRI of the pelvis would be considered standard management for these patients. Although reactive nodes are commonly seen on CT scanning, lymph nodes with a necrotic centre or an irregular margin are highly likely to be pathological (Graafland *et al.*, 2011). There are numerous reports on further staging in these patients with PET-CT (Graafland *et al.*, 2009), but no clear evidence that it is superior in sensitivity to contrast-enhanced CT.

Clinically or radiologically suspicious nodes should be confirmed by ultrasound-guided FNA.

Although distant metastases are rare, it would be reasonable to complete staging with CT scanning of the chest and abdomen if there is clinical or radiological evidence of nodal disease in the groin.

Staging

The TNM staging classification for penile carcinoma is shown in Table 24.2.

Treatment overview

The treatment of patients with penile cancer is multi-modal and may involve a urologist, an andrologist, a plastic surgeon, an oncologist, a specialist dermatology pathologist and a specialist nurse. In the UK, NICE guidance recommendations for supraregional specialisation has led to the formation of 12

Chapter

25

Management of cancer of the ovary

Rachel Jones and Louise Hanna

Introduction

Ovarian cancer is the fifth most common cancer in women and the second most common gynaecological cancer, but the most common cause of death from gynaecological malignancy in the Western world. Epithelial ovarian cancer, fallopian tube cancer and peritoneal cancer share similar characteristics and behaviour and are treated in the same way. Ovarian cancer has been named a 'silent killer' because of its lack of symptoms during early stages. Around 90% of ovarian cancers arise from the epithelium. Two-thirds of patients present with stage III or IV disease, with increasing abdominal symptoms including ascites. Treatment typically depends on a combination of surgery and chemotherapy. In recent years there has been interest in the role of biological treatments, particularly the angiogenesis inhibitor, bevacizumab. Over the past 40 years there has been a modest increase in the survival from ovarian cancer in the UK, attributable primarily to the use of platinum-based chemotherapy, and around 40% of patients are expected to survive for 5 years or more.

Types of tumour affecting the ovary

The WHO classification of tumours of the ovary defines broad categories of ovarian tumours (WHO classification, 2003):

- surface epithelial–stromal tumours;
- sex cord–stromal tumours;
- germ cell tumours;
- tumours of the rete ovarii;
- miscellaneous tumours;
- lymphomas and haematopoietic tumours;
- secondary tumours.

Surface epithelial–stromal tumours are classified as benign, borderline or malignant. The subtypes are serous, mucinous, endometrioid, malignant mixed müllerian tumour (carcinosarcoma), clear cell, transitional cell, squamous cell, mixed and undifferentiated or unclassified.

Sex cord–stromal tumours are classified as granulosa tumours (including granulosa cell tumours and theca-fibroma tumours), sertoli cell tumours, sex-cord tumours of mixed or unclassified cell types, gynandroblastoma and steroid cell tumours.

Germ cell tumours are classified as primitive germ cell tumours (including dysgerminoma, yolk sac tumour and embryonal carcinoma), biphasic or triphasic teratomas (including immature teratoma and mature teratoma), and monodermal teratoma (composed of a single type of tissue and includes struma ovarii, which is composed of thyroid cells).

Incidence and epidemiology

The annual incidence of ovarian cancer in the UK is 17 per 100,000 women, ranging from 14 per 100,000 in Northern Ireland to 20 per 100,000 in Wales. Approximately 7000 cases are reported per year in the UK. The incidence of ovarian cancer in British women has been decreasing since the early 2000s (Cancer Research UK; www.cancerresearchuk.org, accessed December 2014). Epithelial ovarian cancer is predominantly a disease of the Western world and is commonest in older postmenopausal women with over 80% of cases in women over 50 years. Borderline tumours or hereditary cancers, particularly those associated with the BRCA1 gene, occur at a younger age.

Practical Clinical Oncology, Second Edition, ed. Louise Hanna, Tom Crosby and Fergus Macbeth. Published by Cambridge University Press. © Cambridge University Press 2015.

Epithelial–stromal cancers

Risk factors and aetiology

Risk factors and protective factors for ovarian carcinoma

Family history

- Having a first-degree relative with breast or ovarian cancer doubles the risk.
- Having a relative with cancer of the stomach, intestine or lung or lymphoma also increases the risk of ovarian cancer.
- Germline mutations in either the BRCA1 or BRCA2 genes are inherited in an autosomal dominant fashion, and they significantly increase the risk of breast and ovarian cancer in affected individuals.
- Carriers of a germline mutation in BRCA1 have an overall risk for breast cancer of 56–68% and for ovarian cancer of 16–39% (Struewing et al., 1997; Risch et al., 2001; Antoniou et al., 2003).
- Carriers of a germline mutation in BRCA2 have an overall risk for breast cancer of 45–54% and for ovarian cancer of 11–16% (Struewing et al., 1997; Antoniou et al., 2003).
- BRCA mutations also increase the risk of fallopian tube and peritoneal carcinoma. The distal fallopian tube was the dominant site of origin for early malignancies in approximately 6% of BRCA-positive women undergoing ovarian risk reduction surgery (Callahan et al., 2007).
- Women with hereditary non-polyposis colorectal cancer syndrome have a 40–60% lifetime risk for colon cancer, a 40–60% lifetime risk for endometrial cancer and a 12% lifetime risk for ovarian cancer (Lu et al., 2005).

Other risk factors and protective factors

There is increasing evidence from case-controlled and cohort studies that several factors affect the risk of ovarian cancer. These factors have been reviewed (Hanna and Adams, 2006) and are summarised in the following list. These factors are important when considering possible strategies to reduce the risk of ovarian cancer in high-risk women.

- Protective factors – pregnancy, breast feeding, use of the oral contraceptive pill, tubal ligation and hysterectomy.
- Possible protective factors – late menarche, early menopause, exercise, outdoor lifestyle (possibly linked to vitamin D), diet rich in fruit and vegetables (e.g. tomatoes and carrots, which contain carotenoids).
- Risk factors – infertility, high socioeconomic status.
- Possible risk factors – long-term HRT, obesity, occupational exposure (e.g. industrial chemicals, organic dusts, asbestos).

Aetiology

Epithelial ovarian carcinoma was traditionally thought to arise from the surface epithelium of the ovary or from entrapped epithelial cells in inclusion cysts. However none of the hypotheses completely explain all the epidemiology data and there is an emerging concept that the identified histological subtypes arise through various pathways with differences in epidemiological and genetic risk factors which lead to fundamental differences in their response to treatment and overall prognosis. This has been demonstrated with the identification of intra-epithelial precursor lesions (serous tubal intra-epithelial cancer or STIC) being detected in the fimbria of BRCA mutation carriers. This has led to the identification of the distal fallopian tube as the possible site for the development of invasive serous carcinoma (Kindelberger et al., 2007). It has also been proposed that clear cell and endometrioid carcinomas originate from ovarian endometriosis (Sato et al., 2000).

Pathology of epithelial–stromal ovarian tumours

Tumours are classified as benign, borderline or malignant (see Table 25.1).

Malignant epithelial–stromal tumours account for 90% of ovarian cancers and can be classified as type 1 or type 2 tumours. Type 1 tumours generally tend to be low grade and clinically less aggressive and include low-grade serous, low-grade endometrioid, clear cell, mucinous and transitional cell (Brenner) carcinomas. Type 1 tumours all demonstrate a distinct molecular profile and usually develop through a sequence of events similar to the adenoma-carcinoma sequence demonstrated in colonic cancer. They are most commonly associated with specific mutations including KRAS, BRAF, ERBB2, PTEN, PIK3CA (Kurman

Table 25.1 Pathological features of epithelial–stromal tumours

Type	Macroscopic features	Microscopic features
Benign	Commonly smooth walled and cystic	Regular architecture with uniform cells, rare mitoses
Borderline	Frequently cystic or solid, but without haemorrhage or necrosis	Some features of malignancy such as irregular architecture, multilayering of cells and mitotic activity, but basement membrane remains intact
Malignant	Solid and/or cystic with areas of haemorrhage and necrosis, frequently with tumour extending into the peritoneal cavity	Variable architecture from infiltrative glands to poorly defined solid areas; cells range from well-differentiated to poorly differentiated, with nuclear and cytoplasmic atypia and frequent mitoses

et al., 2010). Type 2 tumours are more common and tend to be more aggressive and genetically unstable presenting at a more advanced stage. These tumours include high-grade serous, high grade endometrioid, mixed müllerian tumour (carcinosarcoma) and undifferentiated carcinomas. These tumours are associated with a high frequency of TP53 mutations (Kurman *et al.*, 2010). There is growing recognition that the subtype of ovarian carcinoma predicts its biological behaviour and response to treatment as well as identifying targets for future treatment options. Most ovarian cancers are high-grade serous carcinomas.

Spread

The predominant modes of spread of ovarian cancer are local and peritoneal. Local spread is to the fallopian tubes, uterus, vagina, bowel, bladder and pelvic side wall. Peritoneal spread is to any peritoneal surface, particularly omentum, paracolic gutters, bowel mesentery and the undersurface of the right diaphragm. Spread to other mesothelial cavities includes pleural effusion and pericardial effusion; lymph node spread involves pelvic lymph nodes and para-aortic lymph nodes. Around 9% of patients with apparently stage I cancers have lymph node metastases (Ayhan *et al.*, 2008). Haematogenous spread occurs to the liver (rare), bone and lung (very rare).

Screening and prevention

In theory it should be possible to improve the survival of ovarian cancer patients by detecting and treating the disease at an early stage. Early treatment is hindered by lack of detailed knowledge of the natural history of ovarian cancer and the absence of a known precancerous lesion. Any screening test would require a low number of false-positive tests, because the diagnostic and therapeutic intervention is invasive (i.e. laparotomy).

Women at high risk of ovarian cancer, such as those with a strong family history or proven BRCA1 or BRCA2 mutation carriers, may be offered surveillance using transvaginal ultrasound (TVS) and serum CA125 levels. This was studied in the UKFOCSS trial and the early results confirm that screening may need to be done more frequently than annually with prompt surgical intervention to offer a better chance of early-stage detection (Rosenthal *et al.*, 2013). Further results on the more frequent screening arm from this trial are awaited.

In the general population, the UKCTOCS study has randomly assigned 200,000 postmenopausal women to no treatment, annual CA125 screening with TVS as a second-line test (multimodal screening [MMS]) or TVS alone. Results published so far have shown the sensitivity of MMS and ultrasound screening (US) is around 85–90% for all primary ovarian and tubal cancers with specificity higher in the MMS group (Menon *et al.*, 2009). However, the impact of screening on mortality is still awaited.

Strategies for the prevention of ovarian cancer for high-risk women include prophylactic salpingo-oophorectomy, which dramatically reduces the risk of ovarian cancer. Women undergoing this procedure still have a small subsequent risk of papillary serous peritoneal cancer (Meeuwissen *et al.*, 2005). Women with genetic predispositions to ovarian cancer should also be offered advice on screening and prevention for other potential tumour sites, such as the breast in BRCA-positive women and the bowel in women with HNPCC.

Recent NICE guidance recommends that BRCA testing should be offered to individuals whose chance of a mutation is 10% or more and this has led genetic departments to consider how to offer genetic testing to women with high-grade serous cancer in which the chance of a genetic mutation may be as high as 16–21% (Liu *et al.*, 2012).

Clinical presentation

Ovarian cancer is known as a 'silent killer' because symptoms may be absent or vague and non-specific in early stages. The most common symptoms include increased abdominal girth, persistent bloating, pelvic and abdominal pain, early satiety, nausea or anorexia, and increased urinary urgency or frequency.

Other symptoms include vague bowel symptoms, weight loss, back pain, shoulder tip pain, peripheral oedema, shortness of breath (pleural or pericardial effusion) or, rarely, symptoms from metastatic disease such as jaundice. Ovarian cancer only rarely causes neurological symptoms due to paraneoplastic cerebellar degeneration, neuropathy or brain metastases. Clinical signs include a pelvic mass, abdominal mass, ascites and pleural effusion.

Investigation and staging

Initial tests for patients presenting with only a pelvic mass include TVS and serum CA125, with αFP and βhCG if the patient is less than 40 years old.

For patients with a pelvic mass only, the relative malignancy index (RMI) can predict the chances of malignancy. The RMI is the product of the serum CA125 level (IU/mL), the ultrasound score (U) and menopausal status (M). The ultrasound result is scored depending on the number of the following characteristic features; multilocular cyst, solid areas, bilateral lesions, ascites and intra-abdominal metastases. If there are no characteristic features U = 0, one characteristic feature U = 1and U=3 if there are 2–5 characteristic features. Menopausal status is scored as 1 if premenopausal and 3 if postmenopausal. According to the NICE clinical guideline 122, any patient with a RMI ≥ 250 should be referred to a specialist gynae-oncology multidisciplinary team (NICE, 2011). Such patients should undergo further staging investigations with chest X-ray (CXR) and CT scan of the abdomen and pelvis.

Tests for patients with clinically advanced disease include FBC, renal, liver and bone profiles; serum CA125; CT scan of the abdomen and pelvis; CXR. In advanced disease, if patients are receiving neoadjuvant chemotherapy, a tissue diagnosis by histology,

e.g. percutaneous image-guided omental biopsy, is considered gold standard, although cytology from an ascites tap can be used if biopsy is not possible (NICE, 2011).

Staging classification

The most commonly used staging classification is that of the Fédération Internationale de Gynécologie et d'Obstétrique (FIGO). It has been updated recently and includes fallopian tube and peritoneal cancer (Prat, 2013). It is shown in Table 25.2.

Treatment overview

The standard treatment approach in the UK had initially been for a primary surgical approach to allow accurate surgical staging and attempt optimal debulking. However, in advanced-stage patients (stages III/IV) there is now the option of neoadjuvant chemotherapy and interval debulking. Following primary surgery, almost all patients receive adjuvant platinum-based chemotherapy. The exceptions are patients who have undergone optimal surgical staging and have low-risk disease when clinical surveillance is appropriate.

Conservative surgery with unilateral oophorectomy and wedge biopsy of the contralateral ovary is an option for patients wishing to retain fertility and who have good-prognosis tumours (e.g. borderline tumours, germ cell tumours and stage IA epithelial cancers).

Surgery

Surgery is used to obtain histology, accurately stage the tumour, and aims to achieve maximal cytoreduction. For patients with advanced disease, a meta-analysis confirmed that maximal cytoreduction is associated with improved overall survival, and referral to expert centres for surgery may be the best available way of improving overall survival (Bristow *et al.*, 2002). The importance of referral to specialist gynaecological oncology centres is highlighted in several national guidelines (SIGN, 2003). The current Gynecologic Oncology Group definition of optimal cytoreduction is residual disease to less than 1 cm in maximum diameter; however, there is increasing evidence that achieving no visible disease improves response rates to chemotherapy, is associated with less platinum resistance and improved survival and may become the new definition of optimal reduction (Winter *et al.*, 2008).

Table 25.2 Fédération Internationale de Gynécologie et d'Obstétrique (FIGO) staging of cancer of the ovary, fallopian tube and peritoneum

Stage	Description
I	Tumour confined to the ovaries or fallopian tubes
IA	Limited to one ovary (capsule intact) or fallopian tube, no tumour on ovarian or fallopian tube surface, no malignant cells in ascites or peritoneal washings
IB	Tumour limited to both ovaries (capsules intact) or fallopian tubes, no tumour on ovarian or fallopian tube surface, no malignant cells in ascites or peritoneal washings
IC	Tumour limited to one or both ovaries or fallopian tubes with any of the following:
	IC1 Surgical spill, capsule ruptured
	IC2 Capsule ruptured before surgery or tumour on ovarian or fallopian tube surface
	IC3 Malignant cells in ascites or peritoneal washings
II	Tumour involves one or both ovaries or fallopian tubes with pelvic extension (below pelvic brim) or primary peritoneal cancer
	IIA Extension and/or implants in uterus and/or tubes
	IIB Extension to other pelvic intraperitoneal tissues
III	Tumour involves one or both ovaries or fallopian tubes, or primary peritoneal cancer, with cytologically or histologically confirmed spread to the peritoneum outside the pelvis and/or metastasis to the retroperitoneal lymph nodes
	IIIA1 Positive retroperitoneal lymph nodes only (cytologically or histologically proven)
	IIIA1(i) Metastasis up to 10 mm in greatest dimension
	IIIA1(ii) Metastasis more than 10 mm in greatest dimension
	IIIA2 Microscopic extrapelvic (above the pelvic brim) peritoneal involvement with or without positive retroperitoneal lymph nodes
	IIIB Macroscopic peritoneal metastasis beyond pelvis up to 2 cm in greatest dimension, with or without metastasis to the retroperitoneal lymph nodes
	IIIC Macroscopic peritoneal metastasis beyond the pelvis more than 2 cm in greatest dimension, with or without metastasis to the retroperitoneal lymph nodes (includes extension of tumour to capsule of liver and spleen without parenchymal involvement of either organ)
IV	Distant metastasis excluding peritoneal metastases
	IVA Pleural effusion with positive cytology
	IVB Parenchymal metastases and metastases to extra-abdominal organs (including inguinal lymph nodes and lymph nodes outside of the abdominal cavity)

Adapted from Prat (2013).

Surgical procedure

In the recent NICE clinical guideline 122 for ovarian cancer, optimal surgical staging for ovarian cancer constitutes: midline laparotomy to allow thorough assessment of the abdomen and pelvis; a total abdominal hysterectomy, bilateral salpingo-oophorectomy and infracolic omentectomy; biopsies of any peritoneal deposits; random biopsies of the pelvic and abdominal peritoneum; and retroperitoneal lymph node assessment. Lymph node assessment involves sampling of retroperitoneal lymphatic tissue from the para-aortic and pelvic side walls if there is a palpable abnormality or random sampling if there is no palpable abnormality (NICE, 2011). Ascites or peritoneal washings are also sent for cytological analysis. There is now increased interest in the role of frozen section in early ovarian cancer to allow the necessary surgical staging to be done without the need for a second staging procedure. If it is not possible to remove the tumour fully, deposits are debulked as much as possible, including bowel resection and splenectomy if necessary and appropriate. There are differing views over the extent of random peritoneal biopsies that are required to stage the disease fully.

Fertility-sparing options

Conservative surgery is an option for patients wishing to retain fertility and who have good-prognosis tumours (e.g. borderline tumours, germ cell tumours and stage IA epithelial cancers). In these women the affected ovary alone may be removed, leaving the contralateral ovary and uterus intact. A synchronous tumour in the contralateral ovary or uterus should be excluded as far as possible with wedge resection of the ovary and endometrial curettings/hysteroscopy.

Interval debulking

Recently there has been increased use of neoadjuvant chemotherapy with interval debulking. There is currently no clear consensus for which patients this is the preferred treatment option, but it is generally used in those considered poor candidates for up-front surgery due to either location or volume of disease or medical comorbidities. The recent CHORUS trial reported that in FIGO III–IV patients neoadjuvant chemotherapy was associated with increased rates of optimal debulking, a reduction in early mortality and similar survival (Kehoe *et al.*, 2013). These results are consistent with the findings of the EORTC 55971 trial and strengthen the evidence for this approach in advanced ovarian cancer (Vergote *et al.*, 2010).

When maximum cytoreduction has been achieved during initial surgery, there is no benefit from a further laparotomy. Occasionally, second-look surgery may be appropriate if initial debulking was unsuccessful, but these decisions are individualised and should be made within the context of the specialist MDT.

Systemic anti-cancer therapy

First-line treatment

The role of postoperative chemotherapy has been the subject of randomised trials over the past two decades. The Advanced Ovarian Cancer Trialists Group found a benefit from platinum-based compared to non-platinum regimens, and that carboplatin and cisplatin were equally effective (Anonymous, 1991). There was a trend towards a benefit for platinum-containing combination chemotherapy rather than single-agent platinum; however, the subsequent ICON 2 study showed that single-agent carboplatin was as effective as

Table 25.3 Summary of paclitaxel trials

Trial	FIGO stage	Chemotherapy	OS (m)
GOG 111	III and IV	TP vs	38
(McGuire et al., 1996)		PCyclo	24
OV10	IIB–IV	TP vs	36
(Piccart et al., 2000a)		PCyclo	26
GOG132	III and IV	TP vs	26.6
(Muggia et al., 2000)		T vs	26.0
		P	30.2
ICON 3 (ICON Group, 2002)	80% III and IV	TP vs	36.1
	20% I and II	CAP or Carbo	35.4

A, doxorubicin; C, Cyclo = cyclophosphamide; Carbo, carboplatin; OS(m), overall survival in months; P, cisplatin; T, paclitaxel.

CAP (cyclophosphamide, doxorubicin and cisplatin; Anonymous, 1998).

For stage I disease, the ICON 1 and the ACTION trials (Trimbos *et al.*, 2003) showed a 7% survival benefit in patients who received platinum-based chemotherapy. Therefore, many UK oncologists would offer adjuvant chemotherapy for patients with stage I disease except for those considered low-risk. However, the classification of low-risk patients varies among professionals. Recent NICE clinical guideline 122 suggests that chemotherapy can be omitted in patients with stage IA/B grade 1/2 disease, provided adequate surgical staging has been carried out (NICE, 2011).

In advanced disease, there have been four pivotal trials studying the use of paclitaxel in addition to platinum-based chemotherapy. The GOG 111 and OV10 trials showed a highly significant benefit to adding paclitaxel, while the GOG 132 and ICON 3 trials did not. There has been much debate over why these trials have shown inconsistent results. The trials are summarised in Table 25.3. More recently, a meta-analysis demonstrated that platinum combination was better than monotherapy and that the platinum–taxane combination was better than platinum plus a non-taxane (Kyrgiou *et al.*, 2006). Several trials have compared the addition of a third chemotherapeutic agent, but none have demonstrated any significant improvement in progression-free or overall survival (Bookman *et al.*, 2009).

Due to the inconsistent trial results, the role of paclitaxel has been reviewed in NICE guidance no. 55 (NICE, 2003), which emphasises that women should be involved in making choices about their treatment. It recommends that paclitaxel in combination with platinum-based chemotherapy or platinum-based chemotherapy alone should be offered as alternatives for first-line chemotherapy in the treatment of ovarian cancer. The risks and benefits should be made available and the decision made after discussion. The NICE guidance does not specify any particular stage of disease, but emphasises that factors to be taken into account include the side-effect profile of the treatments, the stage of disease, the extent of surgical treatment and the disease-related performance status.

There have been several recent developments in the systemic management of ovarian cancer including the use of dose-dense chemotherapy regimens and incorporation of the biological agent bevacizumab into current chemotherapy regimens. A recent Japanese study compared adjuvant 3-weekly carboplatin and paclitaxel versus 3-weekly carboplatin and weekly paclitaxel for 6 cycles in stage II–IV ovarian cancer patients. It demonstrated an improvement in progression-free and overall survival with the benefit being greatest in suboptimally debulked patients (Katsumata *et al.*, 2012). There was no difference in the rates of febrile neutropenia, but a higher rate of treatment discontinuation in the weekly arm due to side effects, especially myelotoxicity. A European trial compared weekly carboplatin and paclitaxel with the 3-weekly combination in 822 patients with stage IC-IV ovarian cancer and reported no significant difference in progression free survival between the two treatment arms. However in this trial the weekly regimen was associated with a reduction in toxicity (Pignata *et al.*, 2014). The results of the recently completed ICON 8 trial are awaited; this was a 3-arm trial comparing 3-weekly carboplatin and paclitaxel, 3-weekly carboplatin and weekly paclitaxel and weekly carboplatin and paclitaxel. At present the three-weekly regimen remains standard with consideration of bevacizumab as discussed later.

Angiogenesis is now recognised as an important factor promoting ovarian cancer growth. Bevacizumab is an antibody against VEGF and has been studied extensively in ovarian cancer. Its main toxicities include hypertension, gastrointestinal disturbance, haemorrhage, proteinuria, arterial and venous thromboembolism and bowel perforation. In the first-line setting, two randomised controlled trials investigated carboplatin and paclitaxel with the addition of bevacizumab throughout chemotherapy and as maintenance. GOG 218 found a significant increase in progression-free survival from 10 to 14.1 months but no overall survival benefit when bevacizumab (15 mg/kg) was added to 6 cycles of carboplatin and paclitaxel then continued to a total of 22 cycles of bevacizumab in women with stage III/IV disease who had primary cytoreductive surgery (Burger *et al.*, 2011). ICON 7 included high-risk early-stage as well as advanced ovarian cancer patients and found no difference in overall survival when bevacizumab (7.5 mg/kg) was added to 6 cycles of carboplatin and paclitaxel and continued to 18 cycles in total of bevacizumab (Oza *et al.*, 2015). However, a in a pre-defined sub-group of high-risk patients (stage IV, suboptimally debulked IIIC) a significant survival benefit was seen with the addition of bevacizumab (restricted mean survival 34.5 versus 39.3 months with bevacizumab, log rank $p = 0.03$). Within the UK NICE subsequently reviewed bevacizumab at its licensed dose of 15 mg/kg and did not approve its use in the UK (Technology appraisal TA 284; NICE, 2013).

The challenge is therefore how to combine the potential of dose-dense chemotherapy and bevacizumab. A further US trial GOG-262 also compared carboplatin and weekly paclitaxel versus the 3 weekly combination but allowed bevacizumab at the discretion of the investigator (Chan *et al.*, 2013). The small subset of patients who received weekly paclitaxel without bevacizumab appeared to have similar progression-free survival to those receiving bevacizumab and this raises the question whether weekly paclitaxel or bevacizumab may achieve the same outcome in these high-risk patients. The UK trial ICON 8B aims to address this.

Single-agent carboplatin for ovarian cancer

- Pretreatment investigations include information from surgery, imaging, pathology, FBC, U + E, creatinine, LFT and estimate of renal function (e.g. EDTA clearance).
- The options should be discussed according to NICE guidance, and written information given about side effects and precautions (e.g. monitoring temperature).

Table 25.4 NICE descriptions of cancer types following platinum-based chemotherapy

Category	Description
Platinum-sensitive ovarian cancer	Relapse more than 12 months after response to platinum-based treatment
Partially platinum-sensitive ovarian cancer	Relapses 6–12 months after response to platinum-based treatment
Platinum-resistant ovarian cancer	Relapses less than 6 months after response to platinum-based treatment
Platinum-refractory ovarian cancer	Does not respond to platinum-based treatment

Adapted from NICE (2005).

- A chemotherapy regimen is carboplatin AUC × 5–6 i.v.i. over half an hour (AUC [area under curve] = GFR + 25), repeated every 21 days, for a total of 6 cycles.
- Anti-emetics include dexamethasone and metoclopramide.
- Side effects include nausea (treat with anti-emetics), febrile neutropenia (pretreatment education and treat with antibiotics according to local neutropenia/septic shock policy), anaemia (give red cell transfusion) and thrombocytopenia (give platelet transfusion).

Paclitaxel and carboplatin for ovarian cancer

- Pretreatment investigations include information from surgery, imaging, pathology, FBC, U + E, creatinine, LFT and estimate of renal function (e.g. EDTA clearance).
- The options should be discussed according to NICE guidance. Written information should be given, including a description of relevant side effects (e.g. monitoring temperature and the management of alopecia).
- A chemotherapy regimen is paclitaxel (175 mg/m^2 over 3 hours) and carboplatin (AUC × 5–6 over half an hour), repeated every 21 days for a total of 6 cycles.
- Patient premedication includes dexamethasone, chlorphenamine and ranitidine to reduce the risk of hypersensitivity reactions.

- Side effects, in addition to those listed for single-agent carboplatin, include alopecia (offer use of scalp-cooling, wig, head scarf), peripheral neuropathy (consider stopping paclitaxel if persistent), and muscle and joint aches (provide simple analgesics).

Recurrent disease

Despite improvements in surgical technique and adjuvant chemotherapy, unfortunately the majority of patients with advanced ovarian cancer will relapse. The decision on which chemotherapy regimen to use at relapse is influenced by many factors including previous toxicity, but predominantly the time since completing previous platinum-based chemotherapy (platinum-free interval). The NICE Technology Appraisal no. 91 (NICE, 2005) addresses the issues surrounding further chemotherapy and describes the categories as shown in Table 25.4.

Indication for treatment

Due to the high rate of relapse of ovarian cancer patients, it is important to ensure that chemotherapy is instigated at the appropriate time. Once the disease has recurred it is unlikely to be curable, and therefore the aim of treatment is to improve symptoms and quality of life. There has been much interest in CA125 and its role in follow-up and guiding initiation of treatment and this was examined in the MRC OV05 trial. This study enrolled patients with a normal CA125 following platinum-based chemotherapy. If the CA125 levels rose to more than twice the upper limit of normal, they were randomised to immediate or delayed chemotherapy. Although patients in the immediate chemotherapy arm started chemotherapy 4.8 months earlier on average, there was no associated survival benefit compared to those starting treatment when symptomatic. In addition, the immediate chemotherapy arm reported a worse quality of life (Rustin et al., 2010). These results have influenced local follow-up and demonstrated that it is safe to delay starting further chemotherapy with a rising CA125 if the patient is asymptomatic with only small volume relapse.

Chemotherapy for platinum-sensitive relapse

The majority of patients with recurrent disease will have previously received platinum-based chemotherapy, either alone or in combination with paclitaxel. In patients with platinum-sensitive or

Table 25.5 Response rates to single-agent chemotherapy in platinum-sensitive and platinum-resistant disease

Chemotherapy regimen	Platinum-sensitive disease (RR)	Platinum-resistant/-refractory disease (RR)
Paclitaxel 3 weekly (Peripheral neuropathy, myalgia, arthralgia, myelosuppression)	13–50% (ten Bokkel Huinink *et al.*, 2004; Piccart *et al.*, 2000b; Cantu *et al.*, 2002)	22–33% (Trimble *et al.*, 1993; Thigpen *et al.*, 1994)
Paclitaxel weekly		21–56% (Markman *et al.*, 2006; Kaern *et al.*, 2002)
PLDH (Cardiac toxicity, skin rash, palmar-plantar erythrodysaesthesia)	28% (Muggia and Hamilton, 2001)	20% (Gordon *et al.*, 2004)
Topotecan (Myelosuppression)	19–33% (Herzog, 2002)	5–18% (Herzog, 2002)
Gemcitabine (Myelosuppression, flu-like symtoms)	29% (Ferrandina *et al.*, 2008)	9% (Mutch *et al.*, 2007)
Etoposide (Myelosuppression, GI disturbance)	34% (Rose *et al.*, 1998)	27% (Rose *et al.*, 1998)

PLDH, pegylated liposomal doxorubicin hydrochloride; RR, response rate.

partially platinum-sensitive ovarian cancer, further platinum-based therapy is recommended except in women with an allergy to platinum-based compounds. In these patients there is evidence that if they are able to tolerate combination therapy, this is associated with an improved response rate and survival.

The parallel ICON 4/AGO-OVAR 2.2. trials randomised women with platinum-sensitive relapse to paclitaxel plus platinum-based chemotherapy or conventional platinum-based chemotherapy. Overall, there was a 7% improvement in survival at 2 years in women receiving paclitaxel and platinum, including those women who had already received paclitaxel (Parmar *et al.*, 2003). The subsequent CALYPSO trial demonstrated that the combination carboplatin and PLDH (pegylated liposomal doxorubicin hydrochloride) was 'non-inferior' to the carboplatin-paclitaxel combination. This study demonstrated an improvement in progression-free survival in favour of carboplatin and PLDH but no significant difference in overall survival (Wagner *et al.*, 2012). The side-effect profile of the PLDH–carboplatin combination was also favourable because it was associated with less alopecia and no neuropathy, which was important in patients who may have had residual toxicity from their initial chemotherapy.

The combination gemcitabine and carboplatin is commonly used in the US following the GCIG study which compared the combination with single-agent carboplatin and demonstrated an improved response rate and improvement in progression-free survival, although no overall survival benefit in favour of the combination (Pfisterer *et al.*, 2006).

Overall, the choice of the second agent in platinum doublet chemotherapy is often determined by the individual patient factors, such as the toxicity of the treatment and the convenience of administration.

Other non-platinum-containing regimens are also being investigated. Trabectedin improved the response rate and reduced the risk of progression when added to PLDH in the OVA-301 study. The greatest benefit was in the partially platinum-senstive subgroup and this is being investigated further in the INOVATYON trial comparing trabectedin and PLDH against carboplatin and PLDH (Poveda *et al.*, 2011). There is also interest in whether the use of a non-platinum agent is able to prolong the platinum-free interval and increase the response to further carboplatin.

The addition of bevacizumab to gemcitabine and carboplatin gave an improved response rate and median progression-free survival but not overall survival in the OCEANS study when bevacizumab was continued as maintenance until disease progression (Aghajanian *et al.*, 2012).

In patients with platinum-sensitive relapse, although combination regimens are recommended, not all patients are able to tolerate them either due to platinum sensitivity, toxicities from previous chemotherapy or associated comorbidities. In these patients, single-agent treatments may be considered. Response rates to single-agent drugs are reviewed in Table 25.5.

In patients with known BRCA-mutated (germline and/or somatic) ovarian cancer there is now a maintenance treatment available following complete or partial response to second-line platinum based chemotherapy. Olaparib, a poly ADP-ribose (PARP) inhibitor is licensed following results of a phase 2 study which demonstrated improved progression-free survival compared with placebo (median PFS 11.2 versus 4.3 months, p < 0.0001) (Ledermann *et al.*, 2014).

Chemotherapy for platinum-refractory/-resistant relapse

There are several chemotherapy drugs available in patients relapsing on or within 6 months of platinum-based chemotherapy (Table 25.5). There is no clear evidence of benefit from a combination regimen, and single-agent regimens are usually adopted. There is some guidance on sequencing in the NICE Technology Appraisal 91, which recommends paclitaxel and PLDH as options for second-line or subsequent treatment in this group of patients, but advises that topotecan is used only as a second-line treatment for women with platinum-resistant and platinum-refractory ovarian cancer for whom paclitaxel and PLDH are considered inappropriate (NICE, 2005). It should be noted that this guidance is currently under review and may subsequently change.

There is also interest in the use of bevacizumab in the platinum-resistant setting. The AURELIA study investigated single-agent paclitaxel, topotecan or PLDH with or without bevacizumab (15 mg/kg). Crossover to single agent bevacizumab was permitted after progression with chemotherapy alone. Median progression-free survival was 3.4 months with chemotherapy alone compared with 6.7 months with addition of bevacizumab. Overall response rate was also increased from 11.8% to 27.3% (p = 0.001). The overall survival trend was not significant (Pujade-Lauraine

et al., 2014). Four patients developed GI perforation (2.2%) and other toxicity included hypertension and proteinuria.

Allergy to platinum chemotherapy

Patients may develop an allergy to carboplatin and experience anaphylaxis during the infusion. Prompt treatment with chlorphenamine, hydrocortisone, with or without adrenaline, is required. In grade 1 or 2 hypersensitivity reactions, rechallenge with increased prophylaxis can be considered but after grade 3 or 4 reactions carboplatin should not be readministered and the regimen should be changed. Patients may then tolerate cisplatin chemotherapy, which is usually given with extra steroid cover as a precaution. Rarely desensitisation schedules can be considered.

Other treatments for palliation

Patients with ovarian cancer may experience symptoms of recurrent ascites, pleural effusion or bowel obstruction, particularly when their disease becomes chemotherapy-resistant.

Ascites

Patients present with symptoms of abdominal distension and discomfort, shortness of breath and poor appetite. Paracentesis under ultrasound guidance can be done as a day case procedure. An indwelling peritoneal catheter allows regular drainage in the community for patients with intractable ascites.

Pleural effusion

Patients present with shortness of breath and/or chest discomfort. Pleural aspiration (removal of approximately 1.5 L of fluid) provides rapid relief and may be done as a day case. Recurrence may be prevented by pleurodesis, which requires a chest drain to allow drainage of fluid to 'dryness'.

Bowel obstruction

Bowel obstruction may be acute or subacute. Patients present with colicky abdominal pain, constipation and vomiting. The characteristic X-ray changes may not be apparent in the early stages. These symptoms are usually managed conservatively at first, but early surgical intervention should be considered when appropriate e.g. if there is a single site of obstruction in a patient who is likely to respond to further chemotherapy. Vomiting caused by bowel obstruction may respond to resting the bowel and nasogastric tube placement for drainage. Symptoms may respond to hyoscine butyl-bromide, cyclizine, or octreotide. There is limited evidence that chemotherapy is helpful in this setting.

Pelvic pain or PV bleeding

Patients with local pelvic symptoms may benefit from palliative radiotherapy to the whole pelvis (e.g. 20–30 Gy in 5–10 fractions over 1–2 weeks). This treatment is usually limited to patients whose disease is confined to the pelvis and in whom chemotherapy is not appropriate.

Hormones

The response rate to tamoxifen is low, at approximately 10%, but it may be beneficial in patients whose disease has a long natural history. Newer agents including letrozole may also be considered and present an attractive option for some patients due to the low toxicity profile.

Prognosis

Survival for ovarian cancer has improved with the 5-year survival rate increasing from 21% to 46% over the last 30 years.

There is also an improved trend for relative survival by age and FIGO stage with patients aged 15–39 having a 5-year survival of 87% compared with 17% for patients aged over 80 years. The 5-year survival for patients with stage 1 disease is 90% compared to 3% in those with stage IV disease (Cancer Research UK, http://www.cancerresearchuk.org/cancer-info/cancerstats/, accessed December 2013).

Areas of current interest

Areas of current interest in ovarian cancer include the following.

- Ovarian cancer screening.
- The role of cytoreduction in relapsed epithelial ovarian cancer – DESKTOP III is a RCT comparing the efficacy of additional tumour debulking surgery versus chemotherapy alone for recurrent platinum-sensitive ovarian cancer.
- Use of non-platinum drugs to artificially prolong the platinum-free interval.
- Intraperitoneal chemotherapy, which has received much interest since the publication of the GOG 158 and GOG 172 studies, which showed a benefit in optimally debulked patients who receive intraperitoneal chemotherapy (Runowicz, 2006). PETROC/OV21 is a current trial assessing the feasibility of delivering IP chemotherapy in the UK.
- HIPEC – heated intraperitoneal chemotherapy in optimally debulked patients
- The role of other new systemic agents, e.g.:
  o farletuzumab, a humanised monoclonal Ab to folate receptor α;
  o PARP inhibitors, e.g. olaparib both in known BRCA mutation patients and sporadic ovarian cancer patients displaying BRCAness;
  o pazopanib, an oral tyrosine kinase inhibitor against VEGF, PDGF and KIT receptors;
  o cediranib, an oral inhibitor of VEGFR 1, 2 and 3 - results from ICON 6 showed a survival benefit when given with chemotherapy and as maintenance in platinum sensitive relapsed disease but with increased toxicity so a further trial is awaited.

At the time of writing there were over 50 trials for ovarian and fallopian tube cancer open to recruitment and registered with the National Cancer Research Clinical Studies Group – Gynaecological (http://csg.ncri.org.uk/, accessed January 2015). The full list is available on the website and includes trials in primary treatment, recurrent disease, prevention, diagnosis supportive care and observational/translational studies.

Borderline ovarian tumours

Borderline ovarian tumours are epithelial tumours of low malignant potential characterised by a lack of stromal invasion in the ovary. Typically, they affect women at a younger age than does invasive cancer. Most borderline tumours are either serous or mucinous; approximately half of all cases are serous and one-third are mucinous. Most patients with borderline tumours present with early-stage disease; however, stage III disease can occur. The mainstay of treatment is surgery, with maximal cytoreduction, but there is a role for conservative surgery in young women with early or localised disease who wish to retain their fertility. Women treated conservatively require close follow-up because the contralateral ovary may become affected. The role of adjuvant chemotherapy remains to be defined, with no proven benefit shown. Recurrent disease, however, may respond to platinum-based chemotherapy. The prognosis is significantly better than for invasive cancer; the 5-year survivals for stage I and stage III disease are up to 99% and 55–75%, respectively (WHO classification, 2003). For patients with stage III disease, the prognosis is worse if the peritoneal implants are invasive rather than growing on the surface of the peritoneum (Longacre et al., 2005).

Pseudomyxoma peritonei

Pseudomyxoma peritonei refers to the condition involving abundant mucinous ascites in the pelvis and abdominal cavity, surrounded by fibrous tissue. The associated tumour cells may be benign, borderline or malignant. The finding of associated mucinous ovarian tumours usually indicates metastatic disease from the appendix or elsewhere in the GI tract rather than primary ovarian disease. The optimal management consists of removal of the tumour and complex peritonectomy, which is frequently combined with intraperitoneal chemotherapy (Moran and Cecil, 2003). The long-term prognosis is poor.

Granulosa cell tumour of the ovary

Granulosa cell tumours account for less than 5% of all ovarian tumours. There are two distinct histological types. The first is the juvenile granulosa cell tumour, which accounts for 5% of granulosa cell tumours, occurs up to the age of 30, and nearly always presents in stage I. The second type is adult granulosa cell, which occurs from middle to old age and accounts for around 95% of cases.

Presentation may be with non-specific abdominal or pelvic symptoms, vaginal bleeding (due to endometrial hyperplasia or adenocarcinoma, and associated with excess endogenous oestrogen produced by tumour cells), or acute tumour rupture and haemoperitoneum (due to the vascular nature of the tumour).

Most patients present with stage I disease, and the treatment for young women is conservative fertility-sparing surgery (unilateral salpingo-oophorectomy). Older women are treated with total abdominal hysterectomy, bilateral salpingo-oophorectomy and infracolic omentectomy.

The role of adjuvant treatment has yet to be defined, and randomised trials are lacking for this uncommon disease. Many oncologists reserve further treatment until relapse, although adjuvant treatment with BEP chemotherapy has been advocated by some for stage IC disease with a high mitotic index or stage II–IV, based on the results of non-randomised studies.

For patients with residual or recurrent disease, responses to platinum-based chemotherapy regimens have been reported, including combinations of platinum, etoposide and bleomycin, or platinum, vinblastine and bleomycin, or platinum and paclitaxel. Adult granulosa cell tumours are typically slow growing, and debulking surgical resections can be used to control disease. Radiotherapy may also have a role in delaying the progression of inoperable disease. There have also been responses reported to hormonal therapy, such as progestagens or gonadorelin analogues.

The most important prognostic factor is stage of disease; age, tumour rupture and amount of residual disease have also been reported as significant. The survival for stage I disease is reported to be around 90% at 5 years, whereas for those with advanced-stage disease it is around 30%. Relapses have been reported 20 years after the original presentation and, for this reason, prolonged follow-up is recommended.

Ovarian germ cell tumours

Ovarian germ cell tumours are a diverse group of tumours. The majority are mature teratomas (most commonly benign cystic tumours, also known as dermoid cysts), which have a peak incidence around the age of 30 years. Germ cell tumours are classified as follows.

- Primitive germ cell tumours, including dysgerminoma and yolk sac tumour (also called endodermal sinus tumour); yolk sac tumour is characteristically positive for αFP.
- Biphasic or triphasic tumours, including immature teratoma and mature teratoma. Immature teratoma is graded (1–3) according to the amount of immature neuroepithelial tissue present.
- Monodermal teratoma including struma ovarii, a benign mature teratoma composed of thyroid tissue.

Malignant germ cell tumours

The malignant germ cell tumours account for less than 5% of all ovarian cancers and are most common in women under the age of 20, the peak age being around 18. The majority of malignant tumours are unilateral, and patients typically present with pain and a pelvic mass. Investigations should include αFP and βhCG.

Surgical management involves unilateral oophorectomy only, in the majority of cases. More radical surgery should be avoided because fertility can usually be preserved without compromising the chance of a cure. Many would advise a programme of postoperative surveillance for patients with stage IA dysgerminoma or grade 1 stage I immature teratoma, with regular and frequent clinical, biochemical and radiological assessment. For others and those who relapse on surveillance, chemotherapy with bleomycin, etoposide and cisplatin (BEP) is frequently curative. The overall rate of survival for patients with malignant germ cell tumours is around 90%. A series involving 59 patients with metastatic ovarian germ cell tumours treated with chemotherapy had a 3-year survival of 87.8%, with no relapses occurring more than 3 years after treatment (Bower et al., 1996).

References

Aghajanian, C., Blank, S., Goff, B., et al. (2012). OCEANS: a randomized, double-blind, placebo-controlled Phase III trial of chemotherapy with or without bevacizumab in patients with platinum-sensitive recurrent epithelial ovarian, primary peritoneal or fallopian tube cancer. J. Clin. Oncol., 30, 2039–2045.

Anonymous. (1991). Chemotherapy in advanced ovarian cancer: an overview of randomised clinical trials. Br. Med. J., 303, 884–893.

Anonymous. (1998). ICON2: randomised trial of single-agent carboplatin against three-drug combination of CAP (cyclophosphamide, doxorubicin and cisplatin) in women with ovarian cancer. Lancet, 352, 1571–1576.

Antoniou, A., Pharoah, P. D., Narod, S., et al. (2003). Average risks of breast and ovarian cancer associated with BRCA1 or BRCA2 mutations detected in case series unselected for family history: a combined analysis of 22 studies. Am. J. Hum. Genet., 72, 1117–1130.

Ayhan, A., Gultekin, M., Dursun, P., et al. (2008). Metastatic lymph node number in epithelial ovarian carcinoma: does it have any clinical significance? Gynecol. Oncol., 108, 428–432.

Bookman, M., Brady, M., McGuire, W., et al. (2009). Evaluation of new-platinum-based treatment regimens in advanced-stage ovarian cancer: a phase III trial of the Gynecologic Cancer Intergroup. J. Clin. Oncol., 27, 1419–1425.

Bower, M., Fife, K., Holden, L., et al. (1996). Chemotherapy for ovarian germ cell tumours. Eur. J. Cancer, 32A, 593–597.

Bristow, R. E., Tomacruz, R. S., Armstrong, D. K., et al. (2002). Survival effect of maximal cytoreductive surgery for advanced ovarian carcinoma during the platinum era: a meta-analysis. J. Clin. Oncol., 20, 1248–1259.

Burger, R., Brady, M., Brookman, M., et al. (2011). Incorporation of bevacizumab in the primary treatment of ovarian cancer. New Engl. J. Med., 365, 2473–2483.

Callahan, M. J., Crum, C. P., Medeiros, F., et al. (2007). Primary fallopian tube malignancies in BRCA-positive women undergoing surgery for ovarian cancer risk reduction. J. Clin. Oncol., 25, 3985–3990.

Cantu, M., Buda, A., Parma, G., et al. (2002). Randomized controlled trial of single-agent paclitaxel versus cyclophosphamide, doxorubicin and cisplatin in patients with recurrent ovarian cancer who responded to first-line platinum-based regimens. J. Clin. Oncol., 20, 1232–1237.

Chan, J., Brady, M., Penson, R., et al. (2013). Phase III trial of every-3-weeks paclitaxel versus dose dense weekly paclitaxel with carboplatin +/- bevacizumab in epithelial ovarian, peritoneal, fallopian tube cancer: GOG 262 (NCT0116712). Int. J. Gynecol. Cancer, 23 (8 suppl 1), 9–10.

Ferrandina, G., Ludovisi, M., Lorusso, D., et al. (2008). Phase III trial of gemcitabine compared with pegylated liposomal doxorubicin in progressive or recurrent ovarian cancer. J. Clin. Oncol., 26, 890–896.

Gordon, A. N., Tonda, M., Sun, S., et al. (2004). Long-term survival advantage for women treated with pegylated liposomal doxorubicin compared with topotecan in a phase 3 randomized study of recurrent and refractory epithelial ovarian cancer. Gynecol. Oncol., 95, 1–8.

Hanna, L. and Adams, M. (2006). Prevention of ovarian cancer. Best Pract. Res. Clin. Obstet. Gynaecol., 20, 339–362.

Herzog, T. J. (2002). Update on the role of topotecan in the treatment of recurrent ovarian cancer. Oncologist, 7(Suppl. 5), 3–10.

ICON Group. (2002). Paclitaxel plus carboplatin versus standard chemotherapy with either single-agent carboplatin or cyclophosphamide, doxorubicin, and cisplatin in women with ovarian cancer: the ICON 3 randomised trial. Lancet, 360, 505–515.

Kaern, J., Baekelandt, M. and Trope, C. (2002). A phase II study of weekly paclitaxel in platinum and paclitaxel-resistant ovarian cancer patients. Eur. J. Gynaecol. Oncol., 23, 383–389.

Katsumata, N., Yasuda, M., Isonishi, S., et al. (2012). Long-term follow-up of a randomized trial comparing conventional paclitaxel and carboplatin with dose-dense weekly paclitaxel and carboplatin in women with advanced epithelial ovarian, fallopian rube or primary peritoneal cancer: JGOG 3016 trial. *J. Clin. Oncol.*, **15** (Suppl.), abstract 5003.

Kehoe, S., Hook, J., Nankivell, N., *et al.* (2013). Chemotherapy or upfront surgery for newly diagnosed advanced ovarian cancer: results from the MRC CHORUS trial. *J. Clin Oncol.*, **31**(Suppl.), abstract 5500.

Kindelberger, D., Lee, Y., Miron, A., *et al.* (2007). Intraepithelial carcinoma of the fimbria and pelvic serous carcinoma: evidence for a causal relationship. *Am. J. Surg. Pathol.*, **32**, 161–169.

Kurman, R. and Shih, leM. (2010). The origin and pathogenesis of epithelial ovarian cancer: a proposed unifying theory. *Am. J. Surg. Pathol.*, **34**, 433–443.

Kyrgiou, M., Salanti, G., Pavlidis, N., *et al.* (2006). Survival benefits with diverse chemotherapy regimens for ovarian cancer: meta-analysis of multiple treatments. *J. Natl Cancer Inst.*, **98**, 1655–1663.

Ledermann, J., Harter, P., Gourley, G., *et al.* (2014). Olaparib maintenance therapy in patients with platinum-sensitive relapsed ovarian cancer: a preplanned retrospective analysis of outcomes by BRCA status in a randomised phase 2 trial. *Lancet Oncol.*, **15**, 852–861.

Liu, G., Yang, D., Sun, Y., *et al.* (2012). Differing clinical impact of BRCA1 and BRCA2 mutations in serous ovarian cancer. *Pharmacogenomics*, **13**, 1523–1535.

Longacre, T. A., McKenney, J. K., Tazelaar, H. D., *et al.* (2005). Ovarian serous tumors of low malignant potential (borderline tumors): outcome-based study of 276 patients with long-term (> or = 5-year) follow-up. *Am. J. Surg. Pathol.*, **29**, 707–723.

Lu, K. H., Dinh, M., Kohlmann, W., *et al.* (2005). Gynecologic cancer as a 'sentinel cancer' for women with hereditary nonpolyposis colorectal cancer syndrome. *Obstet. Gynecol.*, **105**, 569–574.

Markman, M., Blessing, J., Rubin, S., *et al.* (2006). Phase II trial of weekly paclitaxel (80mg/m2) in platinum and paclitaxel-resistant ovarian and primary peritoneal cancers: a Gynecologic Oncology Group study. *Gynecol. Oncol.*, **101**, 436–440.

McGuire, W. P., Hoskins, W. J., Brady, M. F., *et al.* (1996). Cyclophosphamide and cisplatin compared with paclitaxel and cisplatin in patients with stage III and stage IV ovarian cancer. *N. Engl. J. Med.*, **334**, 1–6.

Meeuwissen, P. A., Seynaeve, C., Brekelmans, C. T., *et al.* (2005). Outcome of surveillance and prophylactic salpingooophorectomy in asymptomatic women at high risk for ovarian cancer. *Gynecol. Oncol.*, **97**, 476–482.

Menon, U., Gentry-Maharaj, A., Hallett, R., *et al.* (2009). Sensitivity and specificity of multimodal and ultrasound screening for ovarian cancer, and stage distribution of detected cancers: results of the prevalence screen of the UK Collaborative Trial of Ovarian Cancer Screening (UKCTOCS). *Lancet Oncol.*, **10**, 327–340.

Moran, B. J. and Cecil, T. D. (2003). The etiology, clinical presentation, and management of pseudomyxoma peritonei. *Surg. Oncol. Clin. N. Am.*, **12**, 585–603.

Muggia, F. and Hamilton, A. (2001). Phase II data on Caelyx® in ovarian cancer. *Eur. J. Cancer*, **37** (Suppl. 9), S15–18.

Muggia, F. M., Braly, P. S., Brady, M. F., *et al.* (2000). Phase III randomized study of cisplatin versus paclitaxel versus cisplatin and paclitaxel in patients with suboptimal stage III or IV ovarian cancer: a Gynecologic Oncology Group study. *J. Clin. Oncol.*, **18**, 106–115.

Mutch, D., Orlando, M., Goss, T., *et al.* (2007). Randomized phase III trial of Gemcitabine compared with pegylated liposomal doxorubicin in patients with platinum-resistant ovarian cancer. *J. Clin. Oncol.*, **25**, 2811–2818.

NICE. (2003). *Technology Appraisal Guidance – No. 55. Guidance of the Use of Paclitaxel in the Treatment of Ovarian Cancer*. London: National Institute for Clinical Excellence.

NICE. (2005). *Technology Appraisal Guidance – No. 91. Paclitaxel, Pegylated Liposomal Doxorubicin Hydrochloride and Topotecan for Second-line or Subsequent Treatment of Advanced Ovarian Cancer. Review of Technology Appraisal Guidance 28, 45 and 55*. London: National Institute for Clinical Excellence.

NICE. (2011). *Clinical Guideline 122; Ovarian Cancer – The Recognition and Initial Management of Ovarian Cancer*. London: National Institute for Clinical Excellence.

NICE. (2013). *Technology Appraisal Guidance – TA 284. Bevacizumab in Combination with Paclitaxel and Carboplatin for First-line Treatment of Advanced Ovarian Cancer*. London: National Institute for Clinical Excellence.

Oza, A. M., Cook, A. D., Pfisterer, J., *et al.*, (2015). Standard chemothrapy with or without bevacizumab for women with newly diagnosed ovarian cancer (ICON7): overall survival results of a phase 3 randomised trial. *Lancet Oncol.*, **16**, 928–936.

Parmar, M. K., Ledermann, J. A., Colombo, N., *et al.* (2003). Paclitaxel plus platinum-based chemotherapy versus conventional platinum-based chemotherapy in women with relapsed ovarian cancer: the ICON4/AGO-OVAR-2.2 trial. *Lancet*, **361**, 2099–2106.

Pfisterer, J., Plante, M., Vergote, I., *et al.* (2006). Gemcitabine and carboplatin compared with carboplatin in patients with platinum-sensitive recurrent ovarian cancer: an intergroup trial of the AGO-OVAR, the NCIC CTG and the EORTC GCG. *J. Clin. Oncol.*, **24**, 4699–4707.

Piccart, M. J., Bertelsen, K., James, K., *et al.* (2000a). Randomized intergroup trial of cisplatin-paclitaxel versus cisplatin-cyclophosphamide in women with advanced epithelial ovarian cancer: three-year results. *J. Natl Cancer Inst.*, **92**, 699–708.

Piccart, M. J., Green, J., Lacave, L., *et al.* (2000b). Oxaliplatin or paclitaxel in patients with platinum-pretreated advanced ovarian cancer: a randomized phase II study of the European Organization for Research and Treatment of Cancer gynecology group. *J. Clin. Oncol.*, **18**, 1193–1202.

Pignata, S., Scambia, G., Katsaros, D., *et al.* (2014). Carboplatin plus paclitaxel once a week versus every 3 weeks in patients with advanced ovarian cancer (MITO): a randomized, multicentre, open-label phase 3 trial. *Lancet Oncol.*, **15**, 396–405.

Poveda, A., Vergote, I., Tjulandin, S., *et al.* (2011). Trabectedin plus pegylated liposomal doxorubicin in relapsed ovarian cancer in the partially-platinum sensitive sub-population of OVA-301 phase III randomised trial. *Ann. Oncol.*, **22**, 39–48.

Prat, J. (2013). Staging classification for cancer of the ovary, fallopian tube, and peritoneum. *Int. J. Gynecol. Obstet.* http://dx.doi.org/10.1016/j.ijgo.2013.10.001

Pujade-Lauraine, E., Hilpert, F., Weber, B., *et al.* (2014). Bevacizumab combined with chemotherapy for platinum-resistant recurrent ovarian cancer: the AURELIA open-label randomized phase III trial. *J. Clin. Oncol.*, **32**, 1302–1308.

Risch, H. A., McLaughlin, J. R., Cole, D. E., *et al.* (2001). Prevalence and penetrance of germline *BRCA1* and *BRCA2* mutations in a population series of 649 women with ovarian cancer. *Am. J. Hum. Genet.*, **68**, 700–710.

Rose, P., Blessing, J., Mayer, A., *et al.* (1998). Prolonged oral etoposide as second-line therapy for platinum-resistant and platinum-sensitive ovarian carcinoma: a Gynecologic Oncology Group Study. *J. Clin. Oncol.*, **16**, 405–410.

Rosenthal, A., Fraser, L., Manchanda, R., *et al.* (2013). Results of annual screening in phase I of the United Kingdom Familial Ovarian Cancer Screening study highlight the need for strict adherence to screening schedule. *J. Clin.Oncol.*, **31**, 49–57.

Runowicz, C. (2006). Should patients with ovarian cancer receive intraperitoneal chemotherapy following initial cytoreductive surgery? *Nat. Clin. Pract. Oncol.*, **3**, 416–417.

Rustin, G., van der Burg, M., Griffin, C., *et al.* (2010). Early versus delayed treatment of relapsed ovarian cancer (MRC 0V05/EORTC 55955): a randomised trial. *Lancet*, **376**, 1155–1163.

Sato, N.,Tsunoda, H., Nishida, M., *et al.* (2000). Loss of heterozygosity on 10q23.3 and mutation of the tumor suppressor gene PTEN in benign endometrial cyst of the ovary: possible sequence progression from benign endometrial cyst to endometrioid carcinoma and clear cell carcinoma of the ovary. *Cancer Res.*, **60**, 7052–7056.

SIGN. (2003). *Guideline 75. Epithelial Ovarian Cancer*. Edinburgh: Scottish Intercollegiate Guidelines Network.

Struewing, J. P., Hartge, P., Wacholder, S., *et al.* (1997). The risk of cancer associated with specific mutations of *BRCA1* and *BRCA2* among Ashkenazi Jews. *N. Engl. J. Med.*, **336**, 1401–1408.

ten Bokkel Huinink, W., Lane, S. and Ross, G. (2004). Long-term survival in a phase III randomised study of topotecan versus paclitaxel in advanced epithelial ovarian carcinoma. *Ann. Oncol.*, **15**, 100–103.

Thigpen, J., Blessing, J., Ball, H., *et al.* (1994). Phase II trial of paclitaxel in patients with progressive ovarian carcinoma after platinum-based chemotherapy: a Gynecologic Oncology group study. *J. Clin. Oncol.* **12**, 1748–1753.

Trimble, E., Adams, J., Vena, D., *et al.* (1993). Paclitaxel for platinum-refractory ovarian cancer: results from the first 1000 patients registered to National Cancer Institute Treatment Referral Center. *J. Clin.Oncol.*, **11**, 2405–2410.

Trimbos, J. B., Parmar, M., Vergote, I., *et al.* (2003). International Collaborative Ovarian Neoplasm trial 1 and Adjuvant ChemoTherapy In Ovarian Neoplasm trial: two parallel randomized phase III trials of adjuvant chemotherapy in patients with early-stage ovarian carcinoma. *J. Natl Cancer. Inst.*, **95**, 105–112.

Vergote, I., Tropé, C. G., Amant, F., *et al.* (2010). Neoadjuvant chemotherapy or primary surgery in stage IIIC or IV ovarian cancer. *N. Engl. J. Med.*, **363**, 943–953.

Wagner, U., Marth, C., Largillier, R., *et al.* (2012). Final overall survival results of phase III GCIG CALYPSO trial of pegylated liposomal doxorubicin and carboplatin vs paclitaxel and carboplatin in platinum-sensitive ovarian cancer patients. *Br. J. Cancer*, **107**, 588–591.

Winter, E., Maxwell, L., Tian, C., *et al.* (2008). Tumor residual after surgical cytoreduction in prediction of clinical outcome in stage IV epithelial ovarian cancer: a Gynecologic Oncology Group study. *J. Clin. Oncol.*, **26**, 83–89.

WHO Classification. (2003). In *World Health Organization Classification of Tumours: Pathology and Genetics of Tumours of the Breast and Female Genital Organs*, ed. A. Tavassoli and P. Devilee. Lyon: IARC Press, Chapter 4.

Chapter

26

Management of cancer of the body of the uterus

Catherine Pembroke, Emma Hudson and Louise Hanna

Introduction

The most common tumour affecting the body of the uterus is endometrial adenocarcinoma. The major risk factor for disease is unopposed oestrogen stimulation of the endometrium, which is associated with obesity; because of this, endometrial cancer is more common among women in developed countries. Most patients present with stage I disease and have a good prognosis when treated with a combination of surgery and selective postoperative radiotherapy. Other tumours affecting the body of the uterus include the uterine sarcomas, a group of tumours that may arise from the endometrium or the myometrium. These can be aggressive tumours, but treatment may be curative for early-stage disease.

Gestational trophoblastic tumours are discussed in Chapter 30.

Types of tumour affecting the uterus

Approximately 90% of endometrial cancers are carcinomas, and approximately 90% of these are adenocarcinomas. Types of uterine tumour are shown in Table 26.1.

Incidence and epidemiology

The annual incidence of uterine cancer has risen by around 50% in the past 20 years and is currently 26 in 100,000 (CRUK National Statistics; see info.cancerresearchuk.org, accessed November 2014). In 2011 there were 8475 new cases of uterine cancer diagnosed in the UK. Uterine cancer accounts for 5% of all female malignancies and is the fourth most common cancer among women in the UK. The disease is more common in the Western world than in developing countries and more common in women with high socioeconomic status and nulliparity. The high incidence has been

Table 26.1 Types of uterine tumour

Type of tumour	Examples
Benign	Endometrial polyp
	Leiomyoma (fibroid)
Malignant primary	Endometrial carcinoma (90% of cancers)
	Uterine sarcomas
	Mixed müllerian tumour (carcinosarcoma)
	Endometrial stromal sarcoma
	Leiomyosarcoma
	Others
	Lymphoma
	Gestational trophoblastic diseases
Malignant secondary	Direct spread from:
	Ovary
	Rectum
	Bladder
	Cervix
	Vagina
	Metastatic spread (e.g. from breast)

linked with increasing levels of obesity and physical inactivity (Schouten *et al.*, 2004). Endometrial carcinoma occurs typically in the postmenopausal age group, and the median age is 60 years.

Endometrial carcinoma

Risk factors and aetiology

Approximately 80% of endometrial carcinomas are of the endometrioid type and they arise against a

Practical Clinical Oncology, Second Edition, ed. Louise Hanna, Tom Crosby and Fergus Macbeth. Published by Cambridge University Press. © Cambridge University Press 2015.

background of unopposed oestrogen stimulation, which may be endogenous or exogenous.

Factors increasing risk

Factors that increase the risk of endometrial carcinoma include increasing age, obesity, long-term exposure to unopposed oestrogens, genetic factors and atypical endometrial hyperplasia (reviewed by Amant *et al.*, 2005b).

Obesity, sometimes in association with diabetes and hypertension, causes high levels of unopposed endogenous oestrogen via conversion of androstenedione to oestrone in peripheral fat.

Exogenous oestrogens include oestrogen-only hormone replacement therapy, which should not be prescribed in women with a native uterus, or hormone-replacement therapy with fewer than 12–14 days of progestagens. Long-term tamoxifen, which is used in the treatment and prevention of breast cancer, has a weak oestrogenic effect on the uterus. Endogenous oestrogens include those secreted by granulosa cell tumours. Polycystic ovary syndrome, increasing years of menstruation, nulliparity and infertility are also associated with endometrial cancer.

Genetic factors for endometrial carcinoma include a positive family history of endometrial, breast or colorectal cancer in a first-degree relative. An uncommon autosomal dominant genetic cause is hereditary non-polyposis colorectal cancer (HNPCC, Lynch type II), which is associated with colorectal, pancreatic, endometrial, breast and ovarian cancer.

Atypical endometrial hyperplasia appears to be a premalignant phase for endometrioid adenocarcinoma (Kurman *et al.*, 1985).

Factors decreasing risk

Factors that decrease the risk of endometrial cancer include grand multiparity, oral contraceptive pill use, physical activity and a diet including some phyto-oestrogens.

Pathology

Endometrial carcinomas are classified as follows (WHO classification, 2003).

- Endometrial adenocarcinoma (including the variants with squamous differentiation, villoglandular, secretory and ciliated-cell).
- Mucinous carcinoma.
- Serous carcinoma.
- Clear cell carcinoma.
- Mixed cell adenocarcinoma.
- Squamous cell carcinoma.
- Transitional cell carcinoma.
- Small cell carcinoma.
- Undifferentiated carcinoma.
- Others.

Endometrial carcinomas can be divided into type I and type II (Bokhman, 1983). Type I cancers comprise endometrioid and mucinous types, which are oestrogen-dependent tumours and frequently associated with atypical endometrial hyperplasia. Type II cancers lack an association with oestrogen stimulation and are characterised by aggressive behaviour. The two main type II carcinomas are serous and clear cell. Typical pathological features of endometrial carcinoma are shown in Table 26.2.

Many endometrial carcinomas, particularly endometrioid carcinomas, express oestrogen and progesterone receptors. Other molecular characteristics include loss of function in tumour-suppressor pathways, in particular the PTEN pathway in type I cancers and the TP53 pathway in type II cancers.

Spread

The regional lymph nodes are the pelvic and the para-aortic nodes. The main routes of lymphatic spread in the pelvis are to the utero-ovarian, parametrial, presacral, hypogastric, external iliac and common iliac nodes (Benedet *et al.*, 2000).

Endometrial cancer can spread locally through the myometrium and to the serosal surface of the uterus, to the cervix, the parametria, the fallopian tubes, the vagina, the bladder and the rectum. It can spread to lymph nodes, particularly pelvic nodes, para-aortic nodes and mediastinal nodes. Blood-borne cancer spread occurs to the lung, bone and liver, and peritoneal spread to peritoneal surfaces can occur.

Clinical presentation

The usual presenting symptom is postmenopausal bleeding. This early sign allows prompt investigation and it means that most endometrial carcinomas are curable. Any woman with postmenopausal bleeding should be investigated because there is a 15% risk of endometrial carcinoma or hyperplasia (Gredmark *et al.*, 1995).

Most patients with endometrial adenocarcinoma present with stage I disease. A population-based study

Table 26.2 Pathological features of endometrial carcinoma

	Description
Macroscopic features	Often form a friable papillary or polypoid mass protruding into the uterine cavity
Microscopic features	Endometrioid-type tumours, which account for about 80% of endometrial carcinomas, may be graded 1–3 on the basis of glandular formation, non-squamous solid areas and nuclear atypia (WHO classification, 2003); grade 1 represents well-formed glands with no more than 5% solid non-squamous areas and no striking cytological atypia; mucinous tumours are nearly all grade 1
	Type II tumours
	Serous carcinoma has papillae, covered with highly pleomorphic tumour cells, frequent mitoses and necrosis; the probable precursor lesion is endometrial intraepithelial carcinoma (Ambros *et al.*, 1995)
	Clear cell carcinoma has clear, glycogen-filled cells and hobnail cells with highly pleomorphic nuclei, which project into lumens and papillary spaces

in Norway found 81% stage I, 11% stage II, 6% stage III and 2% stage IV disease (Abeler and Kjorstad, 1991).

About 8% of endometrial carcinomas are associated with a simultaneous ovarian carcinoma of the same histology. These tumours are generally regarded as independent tumours (Eifel *et al.*, 1982).

Clinical features of the primary tumour are postmenopausal bleeding (usual presentation), vaginal discharge, other abnormal bleeding (intermenstrual, menorrhagia, postcoital) and a pelvic mass.

Clinical features of local spread of the primary or lymphadenopathy are pelvic pain, rarely renal failure (ureteric obstruction), haematuria, bowel symptoms (e.g. constipation, rectal bleeding), and back pain (from para-aortic nodes).

Metastatic disease is sometimes detected incidentally on a chest X-ray, or causes shortness of breath, bone pain and, rarely, cachexia and jaundice.

Screening

There is no screening in use for the general population. Screening has a possible role in high-risk groups, such as women taking tamoxifen or those with HNPCC. Screening involves a combination of ultrasound, endometrial biopsy and serum CA125. There is no evidence of a clinical benefit.

Investigation and staging

Any woman presenting with unexplained postmenopausal bleeding, intermenstrual bleeding or postcoital bleeding should have a pelvic examination in primary care including a speculum examination and be referred to a rapid-access gynaecology clinic within 2 weeks.

For premenopausal women where the only abnormal bleeding is heavy menstrual bleeding, NICE guidance recommends that any accompanying pain or pressure symptoms warrant pelvic examination and further investigation (NICE, 2007).

New NICE guidance on referral for suspected endometrial cancer (NICE, 2015) recommends:

For women over 55:

- Referral via a suspected cancer pathway (2 weeks) for women with postmenopausal bleeding
- Direct access ultrasound for women with
  - unexplained symptoms of vaginal discharge who
    - are presenting for the first time or
    - have thrombocytosis or
    - report haematuria
  - visible haematuria and
    - low haemoglobin or
    - thrombocytosis or
    - high blood glucose

For women less than 55:

- Consideration of suspected cancer pathway referral for women with postmenopausal bleeding

Diagnostic investigations

Transvaginal ultrasound can detect a thickened endometrium; the endometrium is abnormal if it is greater than 4–5 mm in postmenopausal women who do not take hormone replacement therapy (Gupta *et al.*, 2002).

A hysteroscopy may be performed as an outpatient procedure under local anaesthesia and allows inspection of the uterine cavity.

Pipelle biopsy, an outpatient procedure, involves taking samples of endometrium through a long plastic tube.

Examination under anaesthetic and curettage are indicated if the patient is unable to tolerate an outpatient procedure.

- Anaesthetic assessment is important (especially for patients who are obese, hypertensive, diabetic or have heart disease).
- Inspection of vulva, vagina, cervix, bimanual palpation.
- Dilatation of the cervix, with or without hysteroscopy.
- Curettings from endocervical canal and uterine body.
- Cystoscopy or sigmoidoscopy if extension to bladder or rectum is suspected.
- Pregnancy status should be checked before the procedure in premenopausal women.

Staging investigations

Although endometrial cancer is staged surgically, it is essential to gain as much information about the extent of disease as possible.

- Imaging of the pelvis and abdomen is used to look at the depth of myometrial invasion, involvement of the cervix and possible lymph node enlargement. MRI scanning is superior to transvaginal ultrasound or CT scanning in detecting the depth of myometrial invasion (Kim *et al.*, 1995).
- Chest X-ray.
- Full blood count.
- Biochemical profile.
- Serum CA125 may be useful for follow-up.
- Bone scan is undertaken if clinically or biochemically indicated.

Staging

The most commonly used staging system is that described by the Fédération Internationale de Gynécologie et d'Obstétrique (FIGO). It is shown in Table 26.3.

Treatment overview

Stage I

Standard primary treatment is total abdominal hysterectomy (TAH), bilateral salpingo-oophorectomy

Table 26.3 Fédération Internationale de Gynécologie et d'Obstétrique (FIGO) staging of endometrial cancer

FIGO stage	Description
I	Tumour confined to the corpus uteri
IA	Invades up to less than half of myometrium
IB	Invades to equal to or more than one-half of myometrium
II	Tumour invades cervical stroma, but does not extend beyond the uterus
III	Local and/or regional spread of the tumour
IIIA	Tumour involves serosa of the corpus uteri and/or adnexae
IIIB	Vaginal and /or parametrial involvement
IIIC	Metastasis to pelvic and/or para-aortic lymph nodes
IIIC1	Positive pelvic nodes
IIIC2	Positive para-aortic nodes with or without pelvic lymph nodes
IV	Tumour invades bladder and/or bowel mucosa and/or distant metastases
IVA	Tumour invasion of bladder and/or bowel mucosa
IVB	Distant metastasis (excluding metastasis to vagina, pelvic serosa or adnexa), including metastasis to intra-abdominal metastases and/or inguinal nodes

Adapted from Pecorelli *et al.* (2009). Note that endocervical glandular involvement only should be considered as stage I and no longer as stage II. Positive cytology should be reported separately without changing the stage.

(BSO) and peritoneal washings, followed by selective radiotherapy for high-risk cases.

Laparoscopic or vaginal hysterectomy is an option for very obese patients who are unable to undergo an abdominal procedure. Patients who are medically unfit for hysterectomy also have the option of primary radiotherapy.

Patients with grade 1, stage I tumours, who are unfit for surgery or radiotherapy, may respond to intrauterine progesterone, although there are conflicting reports of the usefulness of this approach (Montz *et al.*, 2002; Dhar *et al.*, 2005).

Fertility-sparing options are considered later in the chapter.

Stage II

Patients with stage II disease are at a greater risk of occult lymph node involvement. If cervical involvement is identified preoperatively, many centres advocate a radical hysterectomy followed by postoperative radiotherapy.

Stages III–IVA

Patients with cancer at stages III–IVA may be unsuitable for surgery because the disease extends outside the uterus; in this situation, radical radiotherapy is given whenever possible. If disease extent or comorbidity prevents radical treatment, palliative radiotherapy, chemotherapy or hormonal treatment may be indicated.

Stage IVB

Patients with metastatic disease require palliative treatments, which are aimed at improving the quality of life. A symptomatic benefit may be achieved with treatments such as radiotherapy, chemotherapy or hormonal treatments. Occasionally, long-term disease control can be achieved with hormonal treatments for metastatic low-grade endometrioid cancers.

Surgical treatments

Total abdominal hysterectomy and bilateral salpingo-oophorectomy

TAH, BSO and peritoneal washings make up the standard treatment for patients with stage I endometrial cancer. A midline laparotomy incision is performed and peritoneal washings are taken. The peritoneal surfaces are inspected carefully. The uterus, fallopian tubes and ovaries are removed, the latter to exclude an ovarian metastasis or a synchronous ovarian cancer.

Laparoscopic hysterectomy

The laparoscopic hysterectomy technique results in quicker recovery, shorter hospital stays and fewer wound complications than with an open operation. A Cochrane meta-analysis of three randomised trials showed no difference in risk of death or recurrence when laparoscopy was compared with laparotomy in early endometrial cancer (Galaal et al., 2012). NICE currently supports the use of laparoscopic hysterectomy in early endometrial cancer in suitably trained centres (NICE, http://www.nice.org.uk/guidance/ipg356, accessed November 2014).

The role of lymphadenectomy in stage I cancer

Lymphadenectomy has the potential to remove occult metastases and provide further staging information to direct adjuvant treatment. Adding lymphadenectomy to standard surgery in stage I endometrial cancer did not improve overall survival (Kitchener et al., 2009). These results have supported the argument against routine lymphadenectomy in apparent stage I cancers, but there remains interest in its use in patients with high-risk features such as grade 3 or stage IB disease.

Radical hysterectomy and lymphadenectomy

For women who are known to have stage II disease prior to surgery, radical (Wertheim-type) hysterectomy is often used. The uterus, cervix, upper vagina and parametria are removed and pelvic lymphadenectomy is undertaken. In endometrial cancer, bilateral oophorectomy is also indicated because of the risk of spread to the ovary or a synchronous ovarian cancer.

Radiotherapy

Definitive radical radiotherapy

Radical radiotherapy is a standard treatment for patients with stage III endometrial cancer which is inoperable due to disease extent and when the patient is able to tolerate the procedure. Radical radiotherapy is also given as a primary treatment for patients with stage I or II disease who are medically unfit or decline surgery. Treatment involves external beam pelvic radiotherapy followed by brachytherapy. In selected patients with no adverse prognostic features, brachytherapy alone may be considered; however, the techniques may carry some uncertainty as to whether the uterine cavity is fully treated.

External beam technique:

- The patient lies supine on the couch with arms on chest, knees supported by a polystyrene wedge, and without further immobilisation. The bladder should be comfortably full. Intravenous contrast aids delineation of the nodal volumes.
- CT planning is recommended to ensure the uterus is included in the target volume. The use of orthogonal films to define fields by conventional bony landmarks carries a risk of a geographical miss. The clinical target volume includes the primary tumour, the uterus, cervix, upper vagina, parametria and adnexae. The regional lymph nodes include the internal and external iliac, obturator, presacral and common iliac nodes.

The upper border of the lymph node volume may be individualised up or down depending on the perceived risk of lymph node spread and the level of the highest involved node that is known to be involved. A PTV is grown around the CTV. It is important to remember that internal organ movement varies considerably among the structures in the pelvis, and larger CTV–PTV margins are usually required for midline structures such as the uterus, cervix and upper vagina than for the lymph nodes that are near the pelvic side wall.

- If CT planning is not available or if treatment needs to be started as an emergency, the following field borders may be marked on orthogonal X-ray images:

  - superior border – between L5 and S1 vertebrae;
  - inferior border – 2 cm below the inferior extent of the tumour (no higher than the lower border of the obturator foramina);
  - lateral borders – 1.5–2 cm outside the bony pelvic side wall;
  - posterior border – lower margin of the S2 vertebral body, approximately 2 cm in front of the sacral hollow or 2 cm behind the tumour on the staging scan;
  - anterior border – through the symphysis pubis or 2 cm in front of the tumour on the staging scan.

- A four-field conformal plan adequately covers the volume with an anterior, a posterior and two lateral fields, with roughly equal weighting from each beam.

- With regard to dose energy and fractionation, the dose is prescribed to the ICRU reference point (intersection of beams), using 6–10 MV photons. Each field is treated daily, 5 days a week. The dose schedule is 40–50.4 Gy in 1.8–2 Gy per fraction prescribed to the ICRU reference point. Typical fractionation regimens include:

  - 45 Gy in 25 fractions over 5 weeks;
  - 50.4 Gy in 28 fractions over 5.5 weeks.

- Verification is performed via portal beam or cone beam imaging taken on the first 3 days of treatment and weekly thereafter.

- If IMRT is used, the considerable internal movement of the midline pelvic structures must be accounted for when determining the CTV-PTV margin.

Brachytherapy

- Typically, a general anaesthetic is required for brachytherapy (or appropriate local or regional anaesthesia). A thorough anaesthetic assessment is required because many women in this group will have been turned down for definitive surgery because of comorbidity.

- A variety of techniques has been described, including a single-line source, an intrauterine source in combination with vaginal ovoids and packing methods such as Heyman's capsules. The uterine cavity is frequently longer than in patients with cervical cancer. There is no consensus over which dose specification points should be used. CT or MRI scanning with the applicators and the use of a computerised planning system can optimise the dose distribution. For a comprehensive review of brachytherapy in endometrial cancer, see ESTRO (2002).

- For a single uterine tube with vaginal ovoids, 'body loading' refers to a variation of the classic Manchester isodose distribution, but with greater weighting in the uterine fundus to widen the isodoses at this level.

- The dose varies depending on the relative contributions from external beam and brachytherapy, and a detailed discussion is beyond the scope of this book. Some centres advocate the use of a central shield to reduce the external beam dose to the primary tumour, thus allowing a greater contribution from brachytherapy. Examples of brachytherapy doses include the following.

(1) Following 45 Gy external beam radiotherapy, without a central shield:
  – for an intrauterine tube with two vaginal ovoids:
    - low-dose-rate dose – 25–30 Gy to point A in a single fraction with body loading;
    - high-dose-rate dose – 21–24 Gy to point A in 3–4 fractions with body loading.
  – for Heyman's capsule technique:
    - low-dose-rate dose – 35 Gy in a single fraction;
    - high-dose-rate dose – 30 Gy in 6 fractions.

Table 26.4 Toxicity from pelvic radiotherapy for endometrial cancer.

Effect	Management
Acute effects	
Tiredness	Advice (e.g. goal-setting, prioritising activity, self-pacing, treat associated anxiety/depression)
Anaemia	Red cell transfusion
Diarrhoea	Loperamide, low-residue diet
Proctitis	Rectal steroids or sucralfate
Cystitis	Exclude infection, maintain fluid intake
Skin reaction	Epaderm® or 1% hydrocortisone cream if severe
Nausea	Anti-emetics (e.g. phenothiazines, metoclopramide, steroids, 5-HT3 antagonists, benzodiazepines)
Late effects	
Gastrointestinal	Algorithm-based approach, as in Andreyev *et al.*, 2013
Haemorrhagic cystitis	Urine microscopy, renal function, cystoscopy, site-specific treatment for bleeding
Reduced bladder capacity, detrusor instability	Pelvic floor exercises, antimuscarinics, augmentation cystoplasty
Vaginal shortening and narrowing	Lubricants, vaginal dilators

(2) For brachytherapy alone, without external beam:
 – low-dose-rate dose – 50 Gy in one fraction or 75 Gy in two fractions; mean dose 2 cm from the intrauterine tube (Jones and Stout, 1986).
 – high-dose-rate dose – 34–40 Gy in 4–7 fractions 2 cm from the mid point along the uterine applicator (Nag *et al.*, 2000).

Explanation to patient

Explain the procedure to the patient, including possible side effects. Give written information and allow the patient sufficient time to make a decision. Obtain informed consent, refer to a specialist nurse counsellor.

Toxicity of radiotherapy

Some of the toxicities from pelvic radiotherapy are shown in Table 26.4. Although premature menopause and infertility are also side effects of pelvic radiotherapy, most patients undergoing this treatment are already postmenopausal.

Postoperative radiotherapy

The role of postoperative radiotherapy is the subject of much debate, although an established concept is to tailor the treatment based on the individual risk of locoregional recurrence. Risk factors include increasing depth of myometrial invasion, increasing grade, lymphovascular space invasion, clear cell or serous histology and increasing age.

Postoperative external beam radiotherapy reduces the risk of pelvic and vaginal recurrences but gives no benefit in overall survival (Aalders *et al.*, 1980; Creutzberg *et al.*, 2000; Keys *et al.*, 2004; Blake *et al.*, 2009). In the absence of a survival benefit the morbidity associated with external beam radiotherapy (EBRT) is a real concern. The PORTEC-1 trial reported rates of 26% grade 1–2 gastrointestinal toxicity. As a result, postoperative radiotherapy in the low-risk group (stage I, well-differentiated, minimally invasive) is unjustified.

The PORTEC study group defined 'high intermediate risk' (HIR) of pelvic recurrence as any two out of grade 3 tumour, deep myometrial invasion and age greater than 60 years. This group had a reduction in 10-year pelvic recurrence from 23% to 5% with the use of postoperative radiotherapy in the PORTEC-1 study (Creutzberg *et al.*, 2011). Both GOG-99 and PORTEC-1 showed that 75% of these local recurrences occurred in the vagina. As a result, PORTEC-2 trial compared the use of EBRT with vaginal vault brachytherapy in HIR patients. They demonstrated equivalent 5-year vaginal recurrence rates, disease-free and overall survival while gastrointestinal toxicity and quality of life were improved with brachytherapy (Nout *et al.*, 2010). Subsequently, vaginal brachytherapy has become a recommended adjuvant treatment for HIR disease.

For high-risk stage I disease and more advanced stages, EBRT ± vaginal vault brachytherapy is still the standard of care. These patients have the greatest risk of local recurrence without treatment and although there is no evidence of a survival advantage, a recent meta-analysis showed the published studies to be underpowered to demonstrate one (Kong *et al.*, 2012).

The definition of high-risk stage I disease in the recent PORTEC-3 study is as follows.

- Stage IA with myometrial invasion, grade 3 with documented lymphovascular space invasion (LVSI).
- Stage IB grade 3.
- Stage IA with myometrial invasion with serous or clear cell histology.

External beam technique: postoperative radiotherapy

- The patient lies supine on the couch with arms on chest, knees supported by a polystyrene wedge and without further immobilisation. The bladder should be comfortably full and a radio-opaque marker placed at the introitus. Intravenous contrast aids delineation of the nodal volumes. A CT scan is taken from L3 to 3 cm below the introitus in 3 mm slices.
- Traditional simulator or 3D conformal radiotherapy techniques treat the pelvis with a 'four-field box' technique. Equally weighted anterior, posterior and two lateral field borders are defined by the bony pelvic anatomy.
- There is an increasing trend to adopt intensity modulated radiotherapy (IMRT) enabling us to shape the dose around target volumes and to minimise dose to the organs at risk (small bowel, rectum, bladder). IMRT improves toxicity when compared with historical controls. It has been adopted in some centres in the UK.
- International consensus guidelines (Small *et al.*, 2008) have defined the postoperative CTV for IMRT. They state that the CTV should include common, external and internal iliac lymph node regions, the upper 3.0 cm of vagina and paravaginal soft tissue lateral to the vagina. If cervical stromal invasion is identified, the CTV should include the presacral lymph node region.
  - Superior CTV (above the bifurcation of the common iliac vessels)
    - border: 7 mm below the L4–L5 interspace; common iliac vessels should be outlined on axial CT slice and expanded by 7 mm in all directions. The CTV should be modified to exclude the vertebral body, psoas muscle and bowel and include lymphoceles, suspicious lymph nodes and prominent surgical clips.
  - Middle CTV (from the bifurcation to the vaginal cuff):

- presacral lymph nodes (if cervical stromal involvement) extends from sacral promentary to inferior border of S2 and should not include foramina;
- expansion of 7 mm in all directions around internal and external iliac vessels excluding the vertebral body, muscle and bowel and including lymphoceles, suspicious lymph nodes and prominent surgical clips.
- Inferior CTV (below and including the vaginal cuff):
  - lower border – 3.0 cm below the upper extent of the vagina (defined by the vaginal marker) or to 1.0 cm above the inferior extent of the obturator foramen, whichever is lowest;
  - 'nodal' volumes, internal iliac vessels are poorly visualised at this level, but volumes should be bounded posteriorly by the piriformis muscle, even if the CTV extends more than 7 mm beyond visible vasculature. At the superior border of the femoral heads, the nodal volume should be discontinued. The rectum, bladder, bone, and muscle should be excluded from the CTV;
  - vaginal and para-vaginal tissues with a 0.5 cm margin which may extend into the perivesicular or perirectal fat. Bladder and rectum should be excluded, but a minimum 1.5 cm distance between the anterior and posterior borders of the CTV are required at the midline.
- The PTV comprises the internal margin, accounting for organ motion, and the set-up margin accounting for uncertainties in its delivery. For IMRT to be of benefit, a knowledge of pelvic organ motion and image guided strategies is required to allow accurate treatment delivery avoiding geographical miss of the target and unnecessary OAR inclusion. CTV–PTV margins vary according to local guidelines and are usually greater for the vaginal tissues than for nodal regions because of the greater internal movement seen in centrally placed structures.
- If CT planning is not available, field borders are defined as for definitive radiotherapy.
- Dose-fractionation guidelines have been published by the Royal College of Radiologists

(Board of the Faculty of Clinical Oncology, The Royal College of Radiologists, 2006). Acceptable treatment regimens are as follows.

- 45–46 Gy in 1.8–2 Gy per fraction over 4.5–5 weeks.
- 40–46 Gy in 20–25 daily fractions over 4–5 weeks.
- Energy – 6–10 MV photons.
- Portal beam imaging or cone beam imaging is taken for verification on the first 3 days of treatment and weekly thereafter.

Brachytherapy technique

- No anaesthetic is required. The procedure is carried out with a vaginal cylinder (obturator or 'Dobbie') and prior examination of the patient to determine which diameter tube should be used (typically 2–3 cm). Alternatively a pair of vaginal ovoids is used.
- Doses vary among centres and depend on the amount of external beam radiotherapy given. The local protocol should always be followed. Acceptable doses after external beam therapy include:
  - high-dose rate – 15 Gy in 5 daily fractions over 5 days to the top 3–5 cm, 0.5 cm from the surface of the obturator, or 8 Gy in 2 fractions, 3–5 days apart
  - low-dose rate: 15 Gy at 0.5 cm from the obturator surface as a single fraction.
- Acceptable doses for brachytherapy alone (no EBRT) include:
  - high-dose rate: 22–25 Gy at 0.5 cm from the surface of the obturator in 4–5 fractions
  - low-dose rate: 30 Gy at 0.5 cm from the surface of the obturator as a single fraction.
- See earlier text for an explanation of side effects and toxicity discussion.

Chemotherapy

Adjuvant chemotherapy

Recent studies suggest a benefit from adjuvant chemotherapy for high-risk early-stage and locally advanced disease. When comparing adjuvant chemotherapy and radiotherapy, equivalent 5-year overall and progression-free survivals are found, suggesting they have complementary effects. Chemotherapy appeared to delay the presence of distant relapse and radiotherapy, local relapse (Maggi et al., 2006). A Cochrane systematic review (Johnson et al., 2011) showed that adjuvant chemotherapy reduced the risk of developing first relapse outside the pelvis by 5%.

There is current interest in the role of combining chemotherapy and radiotherapy in the adjuvant setting. A meta-analysis showed that adding chemotherapy in combination with postoperative radiotherapy in high risk patients gave a significant survival advantage for those with advanced disease (Park et al., 2013b). The NSGO9501/EORTC 55991 trial reported a 7% increase in progression-free survival and a trend towards increased overall survival when EBRT was preceded or followed by cisplatin-based chemotherapy (Hogberg, 2008). PORTEC-3 is a randomised trial that has completed recruitment of patients with high-risk stage I disease, stage II, stage IIIA/C or stage IIIB if myometrial invasion. Patients were randomised to either adjuvant radiotherapy or adjuvant radiotherapy plus concurrent cisplatin plus adjuvant carboplatin and paclitaxel for 4 cycles. The results are awaited.

The European Society of Medical Oncology currently recommends adjuvant chemotherapy in patients with stage III or IV cancers, and that chemotherapy should be considered in patients with intermediate or high risk stage I disease and negative prognostic factors (Colombo et al., 2013).

Chemotherapy in advanced disease

Chemotherapy may provide palliation in advanced disease. Single-agent carboplatin is well tolerated and has a response rate of around 30%, which is comparable with more toxic combinations such as cisplatin and doxorubicin. There is current interest in the combination of carboplatin and paclitaxel, which has been reported to have response rates of 63 to 87% (Akram et al., 2005; Michener et al., 2005). Response rates to second-line chemotherapy are disappointing. Options include pegylated liposomal doxorubicin and topotecan with response rates of around 10%. There is interest in a weekly paclitaxel schedule as an alternative option.

Hormonal therapy

In the adjuvant setting, a meta-analysis has shown that hormonal treatments do not improve overall survival and are associated with unacceptable cardiac morbidity and mortality (Martin-Hirsch et al., 1996).

There is current interest in the use of progestagens alone in grade 1 endometrial carcinoma as a fertility-sparing treatment. A recent review of 48 patients reported a complete response rate of 77.1% after a median treatment duration of 10 months on oral medroxyprogesterone acetate. Recurrence rates ranged from 23.1% in stage IA, G2–3 without myometrial invasion to 71.4% in patients with stage IA, G2–3 with myometrial invasion. Nine patients became pregnant after completing treatment and gave birth to 10 healthy newborns (Park *et al.*, 2013a).

For patients with advanced, metastatic or recurrent endometrial cancer not amenable to surgery, hormonal treatment may provide useful palliation. Treatments with progestins, selective oestrogen modulators and aromatase inhibitors have been evaluated and shown response rates of 9–55% with a median PFS of 4 months and a median OS of 10 months (Tsoref and Oza, 2011). Response rates of around 15–25% are achieved with medroxyprogesterone acetate. Responses are most likely to occur in patients with grade 1 tumours and in patients with a long history (Kieser and Oza, 2005). The addition of tamoxifen to progestin gives response rates of 33% for alternating schedules and 27% for combination therapy in phase II studies (Fiorica *et al.*, 2004; Whitney *et al.*, 2004). Aromatase inhibitors, such as anastrozole, show response rates of 9%. Despite these observations, a recent Cochrane review failed to demonstrate that these response rates correlated with improvements in overall survival, but did suggest that insufficient numbers may explain why no differences were seen (Kokka *et al.*, 2010).

Recurrent and metastatic disease

Selected patients with local recurrence may still be suitable for radical treatments, either radiotherapy (if not already given) or surgery (e.g. pelvic exenteration). The use of PET-CT scanning can help select patients suitable for exenteration. One study randomised high-risk stage I patients to surgery with or without radiotherapy. In the no radiotherapy group, 15% developed a locoregional relapse and most of these underwent radical radiotherapy, achieving a 5-year survival of 65% (Creutzberg *et al.*, 2003). Para-aortic nodal disease may cause severe back pain and can be palliated with an additional para-aortic radiotherapy field. Metastatic disease may respond to hormones or chemotherapy as mentioned earlier.

Prognosis

Prognostic factors

Adverse prognostic factors include increasing depth of myometrial invasion, grade 3 disease, non-endometrioid histological subtype, particularly clear cell, serous and adenosquamous and lymph node metastases.

Prognosis

Type 1 tumours represent 65% of endometrial carcinomas and the 5-year survival is 85.6%. Type 2 tumours tend to be poorly differentiated, with deep invasion of the myometrium. The 5-year survival is 58.8% (Bokhman, 1983). Serous carcinoma and clear cell carcinoma are associated with a poor prognosis because 40% of tumours are metastatic at presentation. The overall 5-year survival percentage figures are as follows (Lewin *et al.*, 2010):

- Stage IA – 89.6%,
- Stage IB – 77.6%,
- Stage II – 73.5%,
- Stage IIIA – 56.3%,
- Stage IIIB – 36.2%,
- Stage IIIC1 – 57%,
- Stage IIIC2 – 49.4%,
- Stage IVA – 22%,
- Stage IVB – 21.1%.

Areas of current interest

Molecular pathways

New avenues for treatment may be found by exploring the precise molecular pathways involved in tumour growth, such as oestrogen- and progesterone-related pathways and the molecular differences between type I and type II tumours. Upregulation of the PI3K/AKT/MTOR pathway due to loss of the tumour suppressor gene PTEN appears to be important in the pathogenesis of endometrial cancer. Some phase II studies have demonstrated responses through the inhibition of MTOR. The MTOR inhibitor temsirolimus resulted in partial responses or stable disease in 83% of chemotherapy naïve and 52% of chemotherapy treated patients (Oza *et al.*, 2011).

Ongoing clinical trials

At the time of writing, the following were open clinical trials for endometrial cancer registered with the

National Cancer Research Network (www.ncri.org.uk, accessed January 2015).

ENGOT-EN2-DGCG-EORTC-55102: a phase III trial of postoperative chemotherapy or no further treatment for patients with node-negative stage I–II intermediate- or high-risk endometrial cancer.

NCRN-2597: a randomised controlled study comparing AEZS-108 with doxorubicin as second-line therapy for locally advanced, recurrent or metastatic endometrial cancer.

PARAGON: a phase II study of aromatase inhibitors in women with potentially hormone-responsive recurrent/metastatic gynaecological neoplasms.

Uterine sarcomas

Introduction

Uterine sarcomas are uncommon tumours, which account for fewer than 5% of malignant uterine tumours, although their incidence has apparently increased in recent years, possibly because of increased detection. The age range of women affected spans from early adulthood to the postmenopausal age. Presenting symptoms include vaginal bleeding, pelvic pain, pelvic mass or an incidental finding at hysterectomy. Uterine sarcomas are defined as homologous if the sarcomatous element is derived from elements found normally in the uterus, and heterologous if the sarcomatous element is derived from elements not normally found in the uterus. Uterine sarcomas can be described according to nuclear and cytoplasmic appearances and the mitotic index (number of mitoses per 10 high-power fields). The mode of spread is local to the surrounding pelvic organs, lymphatic to lymph nodes, through the peritoneum to peritoneal surfaces, or via the blood to lung or bone. There are three main types of sarcoma of the uterus:

- leiomyosarcoma (approximately 50% of uterine sarcomas);
- carcinosarcoma (mixed müllerian tumour) (approximately 30% of uterine sarcomas);
- endometrial stromal sarcoma (approximately 20% of uterine sarcomas).

Adenosarcoma is a rare mixed tumour where the glandular component appears benign. Carcinosarcomas are staged in the same way as endometrial carcinomas, whereas leiomyosarcoma and endometrial stromal sarcoma are staged differently (see Table 26.5). The prognosis for uterine sarcoma is unfavourable, with a 30% overall 5-year survival (Livi et al., 2004).

Table 26.5 Staging of leiomyosarcoma, endometrial stromal sarcomas and adenosarcoma

Leiomyosarcoma	
Stage	Definition
I	Limited to the uterus (IA < 5 cm; IB > 5 cm)
II	Extends beyond pelvis (IIA adnexal involvement; IIB extrauterine pelvic tissue)
III	Invades abdominal tissues (IIIA one site; IIIB >1 site; IIIC metastasis to pelvic and/or para-aortic lymph nodes)
IVA	Invades bladder and/or rectum
IVB	Distant metastasis
Endometrial stromal sarcoma and adenosarcoma	
I	Limited to the uterus (IA imited to endometrium/endocervix with no myometrial invasion; IB ≤ half-myometrial invasion; > half-myometrial invasion)
II	Extends to pelvis (IIA adnexal involvement; IIB extrauterine pelvic tissue)
III	Invades abdominal tissues (IIIA one site; IIIB > 1 site; IIIC metastasis to pelvic and/or para-aortic lymph nodes)
IVA	Invades bladder and/or rectum
IVB	Distant metastasis

Adapted from FIGO, 2009.

Types of uterine sarcoma

Leiomyosarcoma

The mean age of patients with leiomyosarcoma is 55.3 years (Nordal et al., 1993). Its benign counterpart is the leiomyoma or fibroid, but malignant change in a fibroid is very rare and only about 5–10% of leiomyosarcomas arise in a pre-existing fibroid. Leiomyosarcoma is a highly malignant tumour and typically relapses distantly to liver and lung. Overall survival rates range from 15% to 25%; patients with stage I and II tumours have a 5-year survival of 40–70% (WHO classification, 2003).

Carcinosarcoma

The median age of patients with carcinosarcoma is 65 years (WHO classification, 2003). The tumour is composed of malignant epithelial cells and malignant stromal cells. Occasionally the epithelial component is benign, which is called adenosarcoma. It is accepted that mixed müllerian tumours have an epithelial origin and represent metaplastic carcinomas (WHO classification, 2003). However, the pattern of spread and prognosis are different from high-grade endometrial carcinoma; mixed müllerian tumours are more likely to spread to lymph nodes and have a poorer prognosis (Amant *et al.*, 2005a). The 3-year survival is poor at 22% (Livi *et al.*, 2004).

Endometrial stromal sarcoma

The mean age of patients is 55.3 years (Nordal *et al.*, 1993). Endometrial stromal sarcoma is classified as either low-grade or high-grade; the latter is also known as undifferentiated endometrial or uterine sarcoma (WHO classification, 2003). Low-grade tumours frequently express oestrogen receptors and progesterone receptors, whereas undifferentiated endometrial sarcomas do not. One series reported 54% of endometrial stromal sarcomas to be of low-grade type at the time of diagnosis. The overall 5-year survival was 67%, but the 5-year survival of patients with grade 3 or 4 disease was only 33% (Nordal *et al.*, 1993).

Treatment of uterine sarcomas

The main treatment of uterine sarcomas is surgery and, due to the increased risk of lymph node metastases, pelvic and para-aortic node dissection should be considered. Postoperative radiotherapy in carcinosarcomas reduces the risk of local recurrence but not progression-free or overall survival. Given the high risk of extrapelvic disease, chemotherapy can be considered, but its use is controversial because of a lack of evidence from randomised trials. In patients with leiomyosarcoma, there is no advantage from adjuvant radiotherapy (Reed *et al.*, 2008) and no evidence to suggest a benefit to adjuvant chemotherapy.

Patients with advanced or metastatic disease may respond to palliative treatments. For example, patients with metastatic endometrial stromal sarcomas may benefit from progestagens. Modest responses may be seen with palliative chemotherapy (Kanjeekal *et al.*, 2005). Response rates are typically in the order of 15–30% for regimens based on doxorubicin or ifosfamide. Gemcitabine and docetaxel have a response rate of 53% in unresectable leiomyosarcoma (Hensley *et al.*, 2002). Patients with a carcinosarcoma may respond to platinum-based chemotherapy with response rates reported between 19% and 43% (Reed, 2008).

References

Aalders, J., Abeler, V., Kolstad, P., *et al.* (1980). Postoperative external irradiation and prognostic parameters in stage I endometrial carcinoma: clinical and histopathological study of 540 patients. *Obstet. Gynecol.*, **56**, 419–427.

Abeler, V. M. and Kjorstad, K. E. (1991). Endometrial adenocarcinoma in Norway. A study of a total population. *Cancer*, **67**, 3093–3103.

Akram, T., Maseelall, P. and Fanning, J. (2005). Carboplatin and paclitaxel for the treatment of advanced or recurrent endometrial cancer. *Am. J. Obstet. Gynecol.*, **192**, 1365–1367.

Amant, F., Cadron, I., Fuso, L., *et al.* (2005a). Endometrial carcinosarcomas have a different prognosis and pattern of spread compared to high-risk epithelial endometrial cancer. *Gynecol. Oncol.*, **98**, 274–280.

Amant, F., Moerman, P., Neven, P., *et al.* (2005b). Endometrial cancer. *Lancet*, **366**, 491–505.

Ambros, R. A., Sherman, M. E., Zahn, C. M., *et al.* (1995). Endometrial intraepithelial carcinoma: a distinctive lesion specifically associated with tumours displaying serous differentiation. *Hum. Pathol.*, **26**, 1260–1267.

Andreyev, H. J., Benton, B., Lalji, A., *et al.* (2013). Algorithm-based management of patients with gastrointestinal symptoms in patients after pelvic radiation treatment (ORBIT): a randomised controlled trial. *Lancet*, **382**, 2084–2092.

Benedet, J. L., Bender, H., Jones, H. 3rd, *et al.* (2000). FIGO staging classifications and clinical practice guidelines in the management of gynecologic cancers. *Int. J. Gynecol. Obstet.*, **70**, 209–262.

Blake P., Swart A., Orton J., *et al.* (2009). Adjuvant external beam radiotherapy in the treatment of endometrial cancer (MRC ASTEC and NCIC CTG EN.5 randomised trials): pooled trial results, systematic review,and meta-analysis. *Lancet*; **373**, 137–146.

Board of the Faculty of Clinical Oncology, The Royal College of Radiologists. (2006). *Radiotherapy Dose-Fractionation*. London: Royal College of Radiologists, p. 36.

Bokhman, J. V. (1983). Two pathogenetic types of endometrial carcinoma. *Gynecol. Oncol.*, **15**, 10–17.

Colombo, N., Preti, E., Landoni, F., *et al.* (2013). Endometrial cancer: ESMO clinical practice guidelines. *Ann. Oncol.*, **24**, vi33–vi38.

Creutzberg, C. L., van Putten, W. L., Koper, P. C., *et al.* (2000). Surgery and postoperative radiotherapy versus surgery alone for patients with stage-1 endometrial carcinoma: multicentre randomised trial. *Lancet*, **355**, 1404–1411.

Creutzberg, C. L., van Putten, W. L., Koper, P. C., *et al.* (2003). Survival after relapse in patients with endometrial cancer: results from a randomized trial. *Gynecol. Oncol.*, **89**, 201–209.

Creutzberg, C. L., Nout, R. A., Lybeert, M. L., *et al.* (2011). Fifteen year radiotherapy outcomes of the randomized PORTEC-1 trial for endometrial carcinoma. *Int. J. Radiat. Oncol. Biol. Phys.*, **81**, e631–638.

Dhar, K. K., NeedhiRajan, T., Koslowski, M., *et al.* (2005). Is levonorgestrel intrauterine system effective for treatment of early endometrial cancer? Report of four cases and review of the literature. *Gynecol. Oncol.*, **97**, 924–927.

Eifel, P., Hendrickson, M., Ross, J., *et al.* (1982). Simultaneous presentation of carcinoma involving the ovary and the uterine corpus. *Cancer*, **50**, 163–170.

ESTRO. (2002). *The GEC ESTRO Handbook of Brachytherapy*, ed. A. Gerbaulet, R. Potter, J.-J. Mazeron, *et al.* Brussels: ESTRO, Chapter 15, pp. 365–401.

FIGO. (2009). FIGO staging for uterine sarcomas. *Int. J. Gynecol. Obstet.*, **104**, 179.

Fiorica, J. V., Brunetto, V. L., Hanjani, P., *et al.* (2004). Phase II trial of alternating courses of megestrol acetate and tamoxifen in advanced endometrial carcinoma: a Gynecologic Oncology Group study. *Gynecol, Oncol.*, **92**, 10–14.

Galaal, K., Bryant, A., Fisher, A., *et al.* (2012). Laparoscopy versus laparotomy for the management of early stage endometrial cancer. *Cochrane Database Syst Rev.* 2012 Sep 12;9:CD006655.

Gredmark, T., Kvint, S., Havel, G., *et al.* (1995). Histopathological findings in women with postmenopausal bleeding. *Br. J. Obstet. Gynaecol.*, **102**, 133–136.

Gupta, J. K., Chien, P. F., Voit, D., *et al.* (2002). Ultrasonographic endometrial thickness for diagnosing endometrial pathology in women with postmenopausal bleeding: a meta-analysis. *Acta Obstet. Gynecol. Scand.*, **81**, 799–816.

Hensley, M. L., Maki, R., Venkatraman, E., *et al.* (2002). Gemcitabine and docetaxel in patients with unresectable leiomyosarcoma: results of a phase II trial. *J. Clin. Oncol.*, **20**, 2824–2831.

Hogberg, T. (2008). Adjuvant chemotherapy in endometrial carcinoma: overview of randomised trials. *Clin. Oncol. (R. Coll. Radiol.)*, **20**, 463–469.

Jones, D. A. and Stout, R. (1986). Results of intracavitary radium treatment for adenocarcinoma of the body of the uterus. *Clin. Radiol.*, **37**, 169–171.

Johnson, N., Bryant, M., Miles, T., *et al.* (2011). Adjuvant chemotherapy for endometrial cancer after hysterectomy. *Cochrane Database Syst. Rev.* doi: 10.1002/14651858.CD003175.pub2

Kanjeekal, S., Chambers, A., Fung, M. F., *et al.* (2005). Systemic therapy for advanced uterine sarcomas: a systematic review of the literature. *Gynecol. Oncol.*, **97**, 624–637.

Keys, H. M., Roberts, J. A., Brunetto, V. L., *et al.* (2004). A phase III trial of surgery with or without adjunctive external pelvic radiation therapy in intermediate risk endometrial adenocarcinoma: a Gynecologic Oncology Group study. *Gynecol. Oncol.*, **92**, 744–751.

Kieser, K. and Oza, A. M. (2005). What's new in systemic therapy for endometrial cancer. *Curr. Opin. Oncol.*, **17**, 500–504.

Kim, S. H., Kim, H. D., Song, Y. S., *et al.* (1995). Detection of deep myometrial invasion in endometrial carcinoma: comparison of transvaginal ultrasound, CT and MRI. *J. Comput. Assist. Tomogr.*, **19**, 766–772.

Kitchener, H., Blake, P., Sanderock J., Parmer M., ASTEC Study Group. (2009). Efficacy of systematic pelvic lymphadenectomy in endometrial cancer (MRC ASTEC trial): a randomised study, *Lancet*; **373**, 125–136.

Kokka, F., Brockbank, E., Oram, D., *et al.* (2010). Hormonal therapy in advanced or recurrent endometrial cancer. *Cochrane Database Syst. Rev.*, **12**, CD007926.

Kong, A., Johnson, N., Kitchener, H. C., *et al.* (2012). Adjuvant radiotherapy for stage I endometrial cancer: an updated Cochrane systematic review and meta-analysis. *J. Natl Cancer Inst.*, **104**, 1625–1634.

Kurman, R. J., Kaminski, P. F. and Norris H. J. (1985). The behaviour of endometrial hyperplasia. A long-term study of 'untreated' hyperplasia in 170 patients. *Cancer*, **56**, 403–412.

Lai, C. H. and Huang, H. J. (2006). The role of hormones for the treatment of endometrial hyperplasia and endometrial cancer. *Curr. Opin. Obstet. Gynecol.*, **18**, 29–34.

Lewin, S., Herzog, T., Medel, N., *et al.* (2010). Comparative performance of the 2009 International Federation of Gynecology and Obstetrics' staging system for uterine corpus cancer. *Obstet. Gynecol.*, **116**, 1141–1149.

Livi, L., Andreopoulou, E., Shah, N., *et al.* (2004). Treatment of uterine sarcoma at the Royal Marsden Hospital from 1974 to 1988. *Clin. Oncol. (R. Coll. Radiol.)*, **16**, 261–268.

Maggi, R., Lissoni, A., Spina, M., *et al.* (2006). Adjuvant chemotherapy vs radiotherapy in high-risk endometrial carcinoma: results of a randomised trial. *Br. J. Cancer*, **95**, 266–271.

Martin-Hirsch, P. L., Lilford, R. J. and Jarvis, G. J. (1996). Adjuvant progestagen therapy for the treatment of endometrial cancer: review and meta-analysis of published randomised controlled trials. *Eur. J. Obstet. Gynecol. Reprod. Biol.*, **65**, 201–207.

Michener, C. M., Peterson, G., Kulp, B., *et al.* (2005). Carboplatin plus paclitaxel in the treatment of advanced or recurrent endometrial carcinoma. *J. Cancer Res. Clin. Oncol.*, **131**, 581–584.

Montz, F. J., Bristow, R. E., Bovicelli, A., *et al.* (2002). Intrauterine progesterone treatment of early endometrial cancer. *Am. J. Obstet. Gynecol.*, **186**, 651–657.

Nag, S., Erickson, B., Parikh, S., *et al.* (2000). The American Brachytherapy Society recommendations for high-dose-rate brachytherapy for carcinoma of the endometrium. *Int. J. Radiat. Oncol. Biol. Phys.*, **48**, 779–790.

NICE. (2007). *Heavy Menstrual Bleeding NICE Clinical Guideline 44.* London: National Institute for Health and Care Excellence.

NICE. (2015). *Suspected cancer: recognition and referral. NICE guideline.* London: National Institute for Health and Care Excellence.

Niwa, K., Tagami, K., Lian, Z., *et al.* (2005). Outcome of fertility-preserving treatment in young women with endometrial carcinomas. *Br. J. Obstet. Gynecol.*, **112**, 317–320.

Nordal, R. N., Kjørstad, K. E., Stenwigh, A. E., *et al.* (1993). Leiomyosarcoma (LMS) and endometrial stromal sarcoma (ESS) of the uterus. A survey of patients treated in the Norwegian Radium Hospital 1976–1985. *Int. J. Gynecol. Cancer*, **3**, 110–115.

Nout, R. A., Smit, V. T., Putter, H., *et al.* (2010). Vaginal brachytherapy versus pelvic external beam radiotherapy for patients with endometrial cancer of high-intermediate risk (PORTEC-2): an open-label, non-inferiority, randomised trial. *Lancet*, **375**, 816–823.

Oza. A. M., Elit, L. and Tsao, M. (2011). Phase II study of temsirolimus in women with recurrent or metastatic endometrial cancer: a trial of the NCIC clinical trials group. *J.Clin. Oncol.*, **29**, 3278–3285.

Park., J. Y., Kim, D. Y., Kim, T. J., *et al.* (2013a). Hormonal therapy for women with stage IA endometrial cancer of all grades. *Obstet. Gynecol.*, **122**, 7–14.

Park, H., Nam, E., Sunghoon, K., *et al.* (2013b). The benefit of adjuvant chemotherapy combined with postoperative radiotherapy for endometrial cancer: a meta-analysis. *Eur. J. Obstet. Gynecol. Reprod. Biol.*, **170**, 39–44.

Pecorelli, S., *et al.,* FIGO Committee on Gynecologic Oncology. (2009). Revised FIGO staging for carcinoma of the vulva, cervix, and endometrium. *Int. J. Gynecol. Obstet.*, **105**, 103–104.

Reed, N. S. (2008). The management of uterine sarcomas. *Clin. Oncol. (R Coll Radiol.)*, **20**, 470–478.

Reed, N.S., Mangioni, C., Malmström H., *et al.* (2008). Phase III randomised study to evaluate the role of adjuvant pelvic radiotherapy in the treatment of uterine sarcomas stages I and II: a European Organisation for Research and Treatment of Cancer Gynaecological Cancer Group Study (protocol 55874). *Eur. J. Cancer*, **44**, 808–818.

Schouten, L. J., Goldbohm, R. A. and van den Brandt, P. A. (2004). Anthropometry, physical activity, and endometrial cancer risk: results from the Netherlands Cohort Study. *J. Natl Cancer Inst.*, **96**, 1635–1638.

Small, W., Mell, L., Anderson P., *et al.* (2008). Consensus guidelines for the delineation of the clinical target volume for intensity modulated pelvic radiotherapy in the postoperative treatment of endometrial and cervical cancer. *Int. J. Radiat. Oncol. Biol. Phys.*, **71**, 428–434.

Tsoref, D. and Oza A. (2011). Recent advances in systemic therapy for advanced endometrial cancer. *Curr. Opin. Oncol.*, **23**, 494–500.

Whitney, C. W., Brunetto, M. F., Homesley, H. D., *et al.* (2004). Phase II study of medroxy-progesterone acetate plus tamoxifen in advanced endometrial carcinoma: a Gynecologic Oncology Group study. *Gynecol. Oncol.*, **92**, 4–9.

WHO classification. (2003). In *World Health Organization Classification of Tumours: Pathology and genetics of tumours of the breast and female genital organs*, ed. A. Tavassoli and P. Devilee. Lyon: IARC Press, Chapter 4.

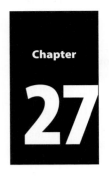

Chapter

27

Management of cancer of the cervix

Samantha Cox, Kate Parker and Louise Hanna

Introduction

Cervical cancer is the most common cause of death from female malignancy worldwide. Overall it causes more than 273,000 deaths per year, accounting for 9% of all female cancer deaths. The major risk factor is persistent human papilloma virus (HPV) infection, particularly types 16 and 18. In the UK, the incidence of invasive disease has fallen with cervical screening, and mortality rates are 60% lower than 30 years ago. The introduction of the national HPV vaccination programme should further contribute to cervical cancer prevention.

Surgery is the mainstay of treatment for early-stage cancers (stages IA1 to IB1 and small volume stage IIA). For later-stage disease, the standard is concurrent radiotherapy with cisplatin-based chemotherapy followed by brachytherapy. Prognosis is strongly related to the stage of disease at presentation. Recent improvements in the planning and delivery of radiotherapy are likely to result in better local disease control rates. In the future, recurrence in the metastatic setting will require better systemic treatment options.

Types of cervical tumour

Cervical tumours can be benign, malignant primary or malignant secondary. The range of tumours is shown in Table 27.1.

Anatomy

The cervix is an approximately 2.5 cm long, hollow structure which projects superiorly towards the body of the uterus and inferiorly into the vagina. The bladder lies anteriorly and the pouch of Douglas (which may contain small bowel) and the rectum, posteriorly. The parametria lie laterally within the broad ligaments and contain the ureters (1–2 cm from the cervix) and uterine arteries.

Table 27.1 The range of cervical tumours

Type	Examples
Benign	Endocervical polyp
Malignant primary	*Carcinomas*
	Squamous carcinoma (60–70%)
	Adenocarcinoma (15%)
	Adenosquamous carcinoma
	Undifferentiated carcinoma
	Clear cell (DES exposure)
	Small cell
	Transitional cell
	Others
	Carcinoid
	Lymphoma
	Melanoma
	Sarcoma
	Rhabdomyosarcoma (esp. paediatric)
Malignant secondary	*Direct spread from*
	Endometrium
	Bladder
	Ovary
	Vagina
	Peritoneum
	Metastatic spread from other tumours
	Breast, rarely thyroid

Incidence and epidemiology

The annual incidence of cervical cancer in the UK is approximately 9 in 100,000 cases (Cancer Research UK; http.//info.cancerresearchuk.org, accessed January 2015). It is the twelfth most common

Practical Clinical Oncology, Second Edition, ed. Louise Hanna, Tom Crosby and Fergus Macbeth. Published by Cambridge University Press. © Cambridge University Press 2015.

cancer in females, representing 2% of all cancers. Approximately 3000 new cases of cervical cancer are diagnosed annually in the UK, causing approximately 900 deaths. Overall, incidence and mortality rates have fallen since the introduction of screening. However, in the last decade there has been a 60% increase in the incidence rate for women aged 25–34 years. This is thought to be related to the younger onset of sexual activity in females and subsequent HPV infection, causing the first peak in incidence at 30–34 years; the second peak is at 80–84 years. There is a large worldwide geographical variation in disease occurrence, with the highest rates in developing countries (Ferlay *et al.*, 2004).

Carcinoma of the cervix

Risk factors and aetiology

The major risk factor for carcinoma of the cervix is HPV infection (Helmerhorst and Meijer, 2002). Although most women are exposed to HPV, it is persistent infection that leads to malignant change; types 16 and 18 confer the highest risk.

The viral proteins E6 and E7 are responsible for malignant transformation, and herpes simplex virus type 2 may act as a co-factor (Smith *et al.*, 2002). Some of the other risk factors may reflect exposure to HPV:

- early onset of sexual activity;
- early age at first pregnancy;
- multiparity;
- multiple sexual partners;
- partner who has had multiple sexual partners;
- use of an oral contraceptive pill (Moreno *et al.*, 2002);
- cigarette smoking;
- low social class;
- immunocompromise (AIDS-defining illness);
- diethylstilboestrol exposure *in utero* (clear cell carcinoma, as in vagina).

Cervical screening and prevention

Screening

Cervical screening detects abnormal cells at the dyskaryotic or precancerous stage (i.e. cervical intraepithelial neoplasia (CIN)). In 1988 the Department of Health set up the NHS Cervical Screening Programme, which has resulted in a continued reduction in the annual death rate. Women aged 25–64 years are called every 3–5 years for assessment. The proportion of eligible women being regularly screened remains stable at approximately 80%. It is worrying, however, that screening coverage in women aged 25–29 years has continued to fall since 1995 to around 59% and is associated with a significant increase in incidence rates in this age group (Trent Cancer Registry, 2011). The protective effect for adenocarcinoma appears to be less than that of squamous cell carcinoma (Boon *et al.*, 1987).

Liquid-based cytology has replaced the traditional Papanicolau smear as the standard screening technique in England and Wales (NICE, 2003). It is up to 12% more sensitive, and allows a faster turnaround time for results with fewer inadequate samples. A brush obtains cervical cells and is rinsed or broken off into a vial of preservative fluid. In the laboratory, cellular debris is removed and a thin layer of cervical cells is deposited onto a microscope slide. The results are classified by the British Society for Clinical Cytology (BSCC) as 'negative, borderline, mild, moderate, severe [dyskaryosis], ?glandular neoplasia, ?invasive, or inadequate.' In 2008, the BSCC recommended that mild dyskaryosis should be renamed low-grade dyskaryosis, and moderate and severe dyskaryosis should be categorised singularly as high-grade dyskaryosis (Denton *et al.*, 2008); however, the use of the previous classifications persists.

Table 27.2 shows the management for different cervical smear results. Colposcopy involves examination of the cervix with a low-power microscope. Acetic acid or iodine is used to stain areas of dyskaryosis white or yellow, respectively. Abnormal areas are removed using LLETZ (large loop excision of the transformation zone), LEEP (loop electro-excision procedure) or, when microinvasion is suspected, knife cone biopsy. Follow-up is essential because up to 5% of cases require further excision.

HPV testing is being introduced to the screening programme in England to triage women with borderline results or low-grade dyskaryosis. Approximately 30% of such cases test negative and can therefore avoid colposcopy and return immediately to routine recall (Kelly *et al.*, 2011); HPV-positive cases are referred for immediate colposcopy which can result in earlier detection of CIN2 or 3. Primary HPV testing of all cervical smears is currently being piloted.

Table 27.2 Management of cervical screening results

Result	Action
Normal	Repeat in 3–5 years
Inadequate	Repeat; refer for colposcopy after 3 inadequate
Borderline glandular change (nuclear change in endocervical cells)	Refer for colposcopy within 4 weeks
Borderline nuclear change in squamous cells	Repeat; refer for colposcopy after three consecutive tests
Mild (CIN 1)	Refer for colposcopy
Moderate (CIN 2)	Refer for colposcopy within 4 weeks
Severe (CIN 3)	Refer for colposcopy within 4 weeks
Possible invasion	Refer for colposcopy urgently within 2 weeks
Glandular neoplasia	Refer for colposcopy urgently within 2 weeks
Abnormal cervix or symptoms of cervical cancer	Refer to gynaecologist within 2 weeks

Management of cervical screening results, adapted from NHS Cancer Screening Programme (2010).

Table 27.3 Pathological features of invasive cervical carcinoma

Features	Description
Macroscopic	Microinvasive cancer is usually clinically undetectable; clinically detectable cancers are typically fungating, producing an obvious mass, but may be ulcerating or infiltrative
Microscopic	Keratinising (identified by presence of keratin pearls) or non-keratinising; graded according to degree of pleomorphism and mitoses; in microinvasive cancer, small finger-like processes penetrate the basement membrane
Immunocytochemistry	Cytokeratin – epithelial Mucin – adenocarcinoma

Prevention

A national HPV vaccination programme started in the UK in 2008 for girls aged 12–13 years. The quadrivalent vaccine, Gardasil®, has activity against HPV 6, 11, 16 and 18 and confers protection against genital warts and CIN 3 (in females not previously exposed to these virus types), with over 90% efficacy (Lehtinen and Dillner, 2013). Vaccination does not obviate the need for screening as there are other virus types that cause cervical cancer. The use of vaccines in cancer is discussed in Chapter 2.

Pathology

Typically, carcinoma of the cervix originates at the squamous–columnar junction. The premalignant phase of squamous cervical cancer is CIN, which is graded by cellular and nuclear atypia and mitoses. Mild, moderate and severe dyskaryosis are equivalent to CIN 1, 2 and 3, respectively; CIN 3 is carcinoma *in situ*. Invasion of the basement membrane indicates progression to true cervical cancer. In general, progression from CIN to invasive cancer takes 10–12 years. About 30% of women with CIN 3 develop invasive cancer. The pathological features of cervical cancer are shown in Table 27.3.

Immunohistochemical stains can be useful; reactivity to anti-cytokeratin antibodies suggests an epithelial origin, and reactivity to antibodies against mucin suggests adenocarcinoma. In distinguishing between endocervical and endometrial adenocarcinoma, endocervical tumours are often CEA+, p16+ and HPV+, whereas endometrial tumours are more commonly vimentin+, ER+ and PgR+.

Spread

Cervical carcinoma can spread locally (to the parametrium, vagina, ureters, bladder, rectum or peritoneum); via lymphatics to pelvic, para-aortic and mediastinal lymph nodes; or via the blood to lungs, bone and liver.

Clinical presentation

All women who present with abnormal vaginal bleeding (e.g. postcoital, intermenstrual and postmenopausal bleeding, and heavy menstrual bleeding with pain and/or pressure symptoms), vaginal discharge or dyspareunia should have a full pelvic examination in primary care including speculum examination. Any suspicion of cervical cancer should prompt an urgent referral. NICE guidance recommends referral via a suspected cancer pathway (2 weeks) for women if, on examination, the appearance of their cervix is consistent with cervical cancer (NICE, 2015).

Examination may reveal a cervix that is enlarged or ulcerated and sometimes fixed (immobile).

Clinical features of local spread or involved pelvic lymph nodes include renal failure (ureteric obstruction), frequency and dysuria, pelvic pain, bladder outflow obstruction, a change in bowel habit, rectal bleeding, haematuria, urine incontinence (vesico-vaginal fistula), faecal incontinence (recto-vaginal fistula), deep pelvic pain or lymphoedema of the legs.

Clinical features of metastatic spread include bone pain, weight loss, anorexia or cachexia, and rarely jaundice or dyspnoea.

Investigation and staging

Examination under anaesthetic and biopsy give diagnostic and staging information. Following inspection of the vulva, vagina and cervix, the cervix is palpated bimanually to estimate size, position and mobility. Parametrial invasion is best assessed via rectal examination. A cervical biopsy is taken and cystoscopy, urine cytology and sigmoidoscopy are performed.

MRI is standard to assess the primary tumour and CT or MRI of the abdomen and pelvis to assess the primary tumour and for lymph node involvement. The chest is staged using chest X-ray (CXR) or CT. PET-CT is indicated for locally advanced cervical cancer amenable to radical chemoradiotherapy (RCP and RCR, 2013).

Other investigations include FBC and a biochemical profile. EDTA clearance or estimation of creatinine clearance should be checked pre-chemoradiotherapy. Pregnancy status should be checked in premenopausal women.

Staging classification

The staging classification of cervical cancer is shown in Table 27.4. The sentinel lymph node can be within any of the pelvic groups including the pre-sacral and para-aortics; however, the external iliac, obturator, parametrial and common iliac groups are affected more often (Bader et al., 2007).

Table 27.4 Fédération Internationale de Gynécologie et d'Obstétrique (FIGO) staging of cervical cancer

FIGO stage	Description
0	Carcinoma *in situ*
I	Confined to cervix
IA	Diagnosed only by microscopy
IA1	Depth ≤ 3 mm, horizontal spread ≤ 7 mm
IA2	Depth > 3–5 mm, horizontal spread ≤ 7 mm
IB	Clinically visible or microscopic lesion greater than 1A2
IB1	≤ 4 cm in greatest dimension
IB2	> 4 cm in greatest dimension
II	Invades beyond uterus but not pelvic wall or lower third of vagina
IIA	Without parametrial invasion
IIB	With parametrial invasion
III	Extends to pelvic wall and/or lower third of vagina and/or hydronephrosis or non-functioning kidney
IIIA	Lower third of vagina only
IIIB	Pelvic wall and/or causes hydronephrosis or non-functioning kidney
IVA	Invades mucosa of bladder or rectum and/or extends beyond true pelvis
IVB	Distant metastasis

Adapted from Pecorelli (2009).

Treatment overview

Stage IA1

Stage IA1 represents microinvasive disease. The risk of lymph node metastases is so low that a simple hysterectomy is adequate (Sevin et al., 1992); postmenopausal women should undergo bilateral salpingo-oophorectomy. Knife cone biopsy alone may be sufficient in selected patients who wish to retain fertility.

Stage IA2

The risk of lymph node metastasis has been reported as 7.4% (Buckley et al., 1996) and a modified radical hysterectomy with lymph node dissection is typically carried out. Radical trachelectomy is an option for patients who wish to preserve fertility, but is limited to patients with tumours up to 2 cm with no adverse prognostic factors (such as lymphovascular space involvement). Radical radiotherapy is needed for patients who are medically unfit or decline surgery.

Stage IB1 and small-volume stage IIA

Patients with low-risk stage IB tumours (less than 4 cm) and small-volume stage IIA tumours may be treated with surgery or radical radiotherapy. The radical Wertheim hysterectomy involves removal of the uterus, upper third of the vagina and entire parametrium) and bilateral lymphadenectomy with preservation of the ovaries (if premenopausal).

Radical vaginal trachelectomy and laparoscopic lymphadenectomy is again an option for patients who wish to maintain fertility (see previously). Adjuvant radiotherapy for stage IB disease decreases the risk of progression at 5 years but not overall survival and is not used routinely (Rogers *et al.*, 2012). Postoperative cisplatin-based chemoradiotherapy is given in high-risk cases (e.g. those with positive lymph nodes, involved resection margins or parametrial involvement; Peters *et al.*, 2000).

Stage IB2 to IVA

The standard radical treatment is EBRT with concurrent cisplatin-based chemotherapy followed by brachytherapy. Radical radiotherapy alone is reserved for medically unfit patients.

In 1999, five randomised clinical trials of concurrent platinum-based chemoradiotherapy showed an overall survival benefit in patients with stages IB2 to IVA disease (Keys *et al.*, 1999; Morris *et al.*, 1999; Rose *et al.*, 1999, Whitney *et al.*, 1999; Peters *et al.*, 2000); the effect was confirmed by meta-analyses (Green *et al.*, 2001). A further systematic review and meta-analysis of 8 randomised trials demonstrated that the relative risk of death (RR) for the whole group was 0.74 (95% CI 0.64–0.86) in favour of concurrent cisplatin-based chemoradiotherapy (Lukka *et al.*, 2002). For patients with locally advanced disease, the RR was 0.78 (95% CI 0.67–0.9) and a greater benefit was apparent in high-risk early-stage disease (RR = 0.56; 95% CI 0.41–0.77).

Stage IVB

Para-aortic lymph node metastases are regarded as stage IVB disease and affected patients are often treated with radical chemoradiotherapy. Other patients with metastatic disease require palliative treatment aimed at improving quality of life. Options include chemotherapy, radiotherapy and surgery (stoma formation to relieve symptomatic fistulae).

Recurrent disease

Central pelvic recurrence following radical chemoradiotherapy requires restaging with MRI and PET-CT. Surgery can occasionally be curative provided that the disease is sufficiently clear of critical structures at the pelvic side wall and involves pelvic exenteration (anterior, posterior or total) with stoma formation (ileal conduit/colostomy). Patient selection is important because the procedure is both physically and psychologically demanding. Occasionally patients with isolated metastases such as regional lymph node recurrences may achieve complete responses to targeted treatments such as stereotactic ablative body radiotherapy.

Radical chemoradiotherapy

Radical chemoradiotherapy typically involves a two-phase technique: external beam radiotherapy to the primary plus lymph nodes together with concurrent cisplatin-based chemotherapy followed by intracavitary brachytherapy. External beam radiotherapy has traditionally been planned using orthogonal X-ray films, but use of CT planning reduces the chances of a geographical miss. A 3D conformal plan is frequently used. Use of IMRT requires an in-depth knowledge of the considerable organ movements that can occur (Jadon *et al.*, 2014).

Brachytherapy has traditionally been planned on plain radiographs to a fixed point (prescribed to point A, planned at time of brachytherapy) following clinical examination and review of diagnostic cross-sectional imaging. However, assessing adequate CTV coverage and delineation of organs at risk (OAR) are limited with such methods. In 2005 the Gynaecological (GYN) GEC-ESTRO Working Group set about implementing 3D image-based treatment planning, enabling volume-based dosimetry, optimisation of tumour dose (including dose escalation) and OAR dose (Haie-Meder *et al.*, 2005); image-guided brachytherapy (IGBT) is now accepted as the international standard. MRI assessment of GTV and CTV at both diagnosis and time of each brachytherapy application session is recommended because of its superiority in

Table 27.5 Definition of planning terminology for image-based 3D treatment planning for cervical cancer

Volume	Definition	Comments
GTV at diagnosis (GTV$_D$)	Clinical examination findings and MRI T2 weighted images	
GTV at brachytherapy (GTV$_{B1, B2, B3…}$)	Clinical examination findings and MRI T2 weighted images at *each* brachytherapy session	
High risk CTV for brachytherapy (HR-CTV$_{B1,B2,B3…}$)	All residual macroscopic tumour GTV$_B$, whole cervix and presumed extracervical tumour (grey zones on MRI)	The minimum equivalent dose in 2 Gy per fraction (EQD2) should be 75–80 Gy (a/β 10 Gy); D90 and V100 should be reported OAR minimum EQD2 dose to the most irradiated tissue 2 cm³ volume adjacent to the applicator (D2cc): Rectum: 70–75 Gy (a/β 3 Gy) Sigmoid/bowel: 70–75 Gy (a/β 3 Gy) Bladder: 90–95 Gy (a/β 3 Gy)
Intermediate risk CTV for brachytherapy (IR-CTV$_{B1,B2,B3…}$)	Areas of initial macroscopic disease but now likely to cover residual/significant microscopic tumour HR-CTV + 5–15 mm safety margin (based on GTV$_D$ and response to EBRT assessed on MRI)	
Low-risk CTV for brachytherapy (LR-CTV$_B$)	Potential microscopic disease	Volume treated by surgery or EBRT and not routinely delineated
PTV$_B$	Identical to CTV	Protocol assumes no extra margins required

CTV, clinical target volume; EBRT, external beam radiotherapy; EQD2, equivalent dose at 2 Gy; GTV, gross tumour volume; HR-CTV, high-risk CTV; IR-CTV, intermediate-risk CTV; LR-CTV, low-risk CTV; MRI, magnetic resonance imaging; OAR, organs at risk; PTV, planning target volume. Adapted from Haie-Meder *et al.*, 2005 and Pötter *et al.*, 2006.

tumour delineation and to verify applicator position; target volumes can be adapted according to response to preceding EBRT. A protocol for target volume delineation has been developed and a common planning terminology defined as shown in Table 27.5.

A single-centre study has reported excellent 3-year local control rates at 98% and 92% for tumours 2–5 cm and 5 cm in diameter, respectively; grade 3–4 late gastrointestinal and urinary morbidity was approximately 5% (Pötter *et al.*, 2011). A relative reduction in pelvic recurrence by 65–70% is also reported. MRI-based planning can also improve local control rates by dose escalation; as much as a 138% increase in the dose received by 95% of the target volume without compromising the OAR has been reported (Wachter-Gerstner *et al.*, 2003). The EMBRACE multi-centre trial will report on the local control rates

and morbidity, with survival outcomes as secondary endpoints (Pötter *et al.*, 2008).

The Royal College of Radiologists (RCR) has defined four levels of image-guided brachytherapy (RCR, 2009):

- verification of applicator position,
- accurate definition of OAR doses,
- conformation of dose distribution,
- dose escalation.

The RCR is currently facilitating the implementation of MRI-based IGBT as the future UK standard. In the interim, CT-guided planning and 3D-image verification of applicator placement is recommended; one centre has reported a 20% improvement in 3-year disease control rates with this technique (Tan *et al.*, 2009). However, CT-planning can overestimate the HR-CTV subsequently affecting D90, and is therefore recommended only for smaller tumours (< 5 cm) (Nesvacil et al., 2012).

The following discussion outlines the salient points of radical chemoradiotherapy treatment based on current UK practice.

Radiation dose and dose rate

Early data on outcomes for cervical cancer came from series incorporating low-dose-rate (LDR) brachytherapy (with caesium-137). ICRU 38 specifies the 60 Gy envelope for treatments using LDR brachytherapy and other reference points (e.g. bladder and rectum; ICRU, 1985). Use of HDR brachytherapy (with cobalt-60 or iridium-192) has increased for reasons including patient convenience (day case procedure), reduced treatment time (minutes rather than days), radiation protection and machine availability. HDR brachytherapy is deemed to be safe and efficacious with no significant difference in overall survival compared to either LDR or MDR brachytherapy (NICE, 2006); grade 3 or 4 toxicity rates are between 2% and 6%.

The relative prescribed doses of EBRT and brachytherapy depend on the initial volume of disease, the ability to displace the bladder and rectum, the degree of tumour regression during pelvic irradiation, and institutional preference (Nag et al., 2000). Doses vary, both in the UK and internationally.

Current typical dose ranges for EBRT in the UK are:

- 45 Gy in 25 fractions over 5 weeks, or
- 50.4 Gy in 28 fractions over 5.5 weeks.

The dose is prescribed to the 100% isodose using 6–10 MV photons. Each field is treated daily, 5 days a week. Carcinoma of the cervix is placed in category 1, meaning any unscheduled breaks in treatment should be corrected for (RCR, 2008).

A typical HDR brachytherapy dose is 21 Gy given in 3 fractions; alternatives include 14 Gy in 2 fractions to 24 Gy in 4 fractions. LDR and MDR dose ranges are 22.5–30 Gy and 20–22 Gy, respectively, in one or two insertions. The American Brachytherapy Society recommend treating point A to at least a total LDR equivalent of 80–85 Gy for early-stage disease and 85–90 Gy for advanced-stage disease (bearing in mind that, as the dose rate increases, it is necessary to reduce the total radiation dose and fractionate to avoid unacceptable late tissue complications) (Nag

et al., 2000). Doses used in the UK are traditionally lower at EQD2 to point A and/or D90 of 75–80 Gy (RCR, 2009). The OAR dose constraints are shown in Table 27.5.

EBRT technique

Clinical examination is performed prior to radiotherapy planning to aid the oncologist in marking the clinical target volume. The patient lies supine on a couch, head on a low headrest, with arms on chest and knees supported by a polystyrene wedge. The bladder should be comfortably full and intravenous contrast is administered. Localising tattoos are placed anteriorly and laterally. Conformal planning with a CT simulation scan and localisation markers is recommended.

The CTV includes the primary tumour, cervix, uterus, upper vagina, parametrium and regional lymph nodes. The uterosacral ligament is included if involved. Some protocols also include the ovaries, but these are not a typical site of spread. The lymph nodes typically comprise the internal and external iliac, obturator, presacral and distal common iliac nodes with extension to the proximal common iliac nodes or para-aortic nodes as required. If treating the para-aortic nodes, the doses to kidneys need to be calculated and kept within tolerance. A PTV is grown around the CTV to allow the creation of a conformal four-field plan (anterior, posterior and two lateral fields).

Traditional field borders may be marked as follows: if treatment needs to start as an emergency or where conformal planning is unavailable, the following borders are used, but adapted to ensure adequate coverage of disease:

- superior border – sacral promontory or between L4 and L5 vertebrae;
- inferior border – 2 cm below the lower extent of the clinical tumour or the inferior edge of obturator foramina;
- lateral borders – 1.5–2 cm outside the bony pelvic side wall;
- posterior border – lower border of S2 vertebra, 2 cm anterior to the sacral hollow or 2 cm behind the tumour on a CT planning scan;
- anterior border – through the symphysis pubis or 2 cm in front of the tumour.

Portal beam or cone beam imaging is taken for verification on the first 3 days of treatment and weekly thereafter.

The midline pelvic structures can move considerably. The prospect of IMRT has highlighted the need for individualised, adaptive strategies to account for daily changes in the size, shape and position of the CTV (Jadon *et al.*, 2014).

Concurrent chemotherapy

Cisplatin (40 mg/m^2) is given weekly during EBRT, with pre- and post-hydration. Chemotherapy is given approximately 1 hour before radiotherapy, but should not be given to patients with poor renal function or performance status.

Brachytherapy

Either a general anaesthetic or appropriate regional or local anaesthesia is required. A prior anaesthetic assessment reduces the risk of cancellation. Treatment is given in a specialised brachytherapy suite, allowing remote patient monitoring.

With the patient in the lithotomy position a urinary catheter is inserted. Examination under anaesthetic is performed to assess the tumour. Ultrasound guidance can be used to place a uterine sound. This enables the measurement of the uterine cavity length before dilating the cervix and inserting the intrauterine tube; either two ovoids are placed in the lateral vaginal fornices or an MRI-compatible tandem-ring is inserted. Additional interstitial brachytherapy can improve tumour coverage for bulky tumours. Vaginal packing and a rectal shield are placed and the applicators are secured in place. 3D imaging (CT, MRI or US) is recommended to verify that the interuterine tube is within the uterine canal.

The classic Manchester system of dosimetry specifies a line source inserted into the uterus with two ovoids placed in the lateral vaginal fornices. This procedure creates a pear-shaped volume around the cervix, uterus, upper vagina and immediate parametria. The dose is prescribed to Manchester point A, defined as 2 cm above the lateral vaginal fornices and 2 cm lateral to the central uterine tube. Point B is 5 cm lateral to the midline. The ICRU 38 bladder point is the posterior surface of the bladder balloon, and the rectal point is 5 mm behind the posterior vaginal wall at the level of the lower end of the intrauterine source, as shown in Figure 27.1. More recently, cross-sectional imaging has allowed the brachytherapy target volume to be individually defined and planned. Figure 27.2 shows MRI and CT

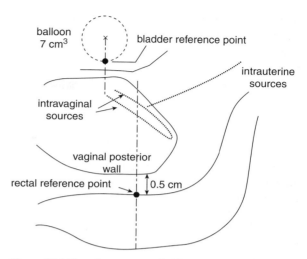

Figure 27.1 The reference points for bladder and rectum during gynaecological brachytherapy. Redrawn with permission of the ICRU, 1985: ICRU Report 38. *Dose and Volume Specification for Reporting Intracavitary Therapy in Gynaecology,* Bethesda, Maryland: International Commission on Radiation Units and Measurements; http:ICRU.org, accessed January 2015.

images of an intracavitary brachytherapy treatment for cervical cancer.

Toxicity of chemoradiotherapy

Important toxicities resulting from chemoradiotherapy for cervical carcinoma are shown in Table 27.6. The national audit of the management and outcome of carcinoma of the cervix treated with radiotherapy in 1993 found the crude rate of late severe complications to be 6.1% at 5 years (Denton *et al.*, 2000). It is well documented that late effects are under-reported by patients. Improvements in managing late effects have been made, so identification is important. The hope is that late effects will be reduced in the advent of more conformal radiotherapy planning techniques.

Postoperative radiotherapy and chemoradiotherapy

Postoperative patients found to have high-risk factors (involved lymph nodes or parametrium, positive resection margins) are treated with adjuvant chemoradiotherapy (or radiotherapy alone if medically unfit) and brachytherapy via a 2–3 cm diameter vaginal obturator.

Patient set-up and EBRT doses are the same as for definitive radiotherapy. Consensus guidelines for CTV

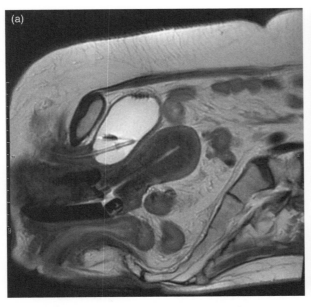
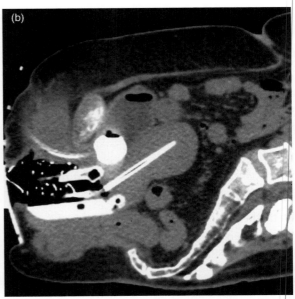

Figure 27.2 Sagittal views of an intracavitary brachytherapy treatment for carcinoma of the cervix. (a) T2-weighted MRI scan. (b) CT scan. Note the intrauterine tube, the ring applicator just below the cervix, the rectal retractor, the balloon of the urinary catheter and the vaginal packing. Note how the anatomical detail is seen most clearly on the MRI scan while the applicators are seen more easily on the CT scan.

Table 27.6 Toxicities from chemoradiotherapy for cervical carcinoma

Effect	Management
Acute effects	
Tiredness	Advice about fatigue, goal-setting; treat anxiety and depression; appropriate rest; moderate exercise if able
Anaemia	Red cell transfusion to keep Hb ≥ 120 g/L
Myelosuppression/neutropenic sepsis	Patient education, weekly review and FBC, prompt assessment and treatment of fever
Diarrhoea	Loperamide, low-residue diet
Proctitis	Rectal steroids or sucralfate
Cystitis	Exclude infection, maintain fluid intake, potassium citrate mixture 10 mL three times daily
Skin reaction	Epaderm® or 1% hydrocortisone cream if severe
Nausea	Anti-emetics, e.g. phenothiazines, metoclopramide, steroids, 5-HT3 antagonists, benzodiazepines
Peripheral neuropathy/renal impairment	Clinical monitoring; modify cisplatin dose as necessary
Late effects	
Gastrointestinal symptoms	Algorithm-based approach as in Andreyev *et al.*, 2013
Haemorrhagic cystitis	Urine microscopy, renal function, cystoscopy, site specific treatment for bleeding
Reduced bladder capacity, detrusor instability	Pelvic floor exercises, anti-muscarinics, augmentation cystoplasty
Vaginal shortening and narrowing	Lubricants, vaginal dilators
Menopause	Hormone replacement therapy
Infertility	Adoption, surrogacy

5-HT3, 5 hydroxy-tryptamine 3; Hb, haemoglobin.

delineation using IMRT are available (Small *et al.*, 2008); the external and internal iliac, obturator, presacral and common iliac nodes are included, as are the upper vagina and parametrium. The regional lymph node CTV can be created by adding a 7-mm margin to the pelvic vessels, excluding normal tissues on each slice (bladder, bowel, muscle and bone) connecting the external and internal iliac regions to cover the obturator nodes and adding a presacral nodal region. Anisotropic margins are recommended for PTV expansion, as the internal movement is much greater for the vagina than for the nodal regions.

HDR prescriptions at 0.5-cm depth include 11 Gy in 2 fractions, 12 Gy in 3 fractions or 15 Gy in 5 fractions over 1 week.

Palliative radiotherapy

Medically unfit patients not suitable for radical radiotherapy may benefit from palliative treatment to the pelvis (e.g. 8 Gy in a single fraction or 20–30 Gy, fractionated). Palliative radiotherapy is also beneficial for painful para-aortic nodes or bony metastases.

Palliative systemic anti-cancer therapy

Responses to palliative chemotherapy are generally disappointing, but agents such as cisplatin, carboplatin, topotecan, gemcitabine or paclitaxel may produce useful responses in about 30% of patients; recruitment to clinical trials should be considered. Final analysis from the GOG-0240 trial found that bevacizumab in combination with chemotherapy is associated with a significantly improved overall survival (16.6 months versus 13.3 months; $p = 0.0068$) versus chemotherapy alone (Tewari *et al.*, 2014); toxicities include GI perforation and fistula, thromboembolic events.

Special clinical problems

Cervical cancer in pregnancy

Treatment of pregnant patients depends on the gestational age. In the first and second trimesters it is usual to recommend termination of the pregnancy followed by treatment appropriate to the stage of cancer. In the third trimester, it is more common to wait until the foetus is viable before delivery and definitive treatment; a caesarean section can be combined with a radical hysterectomy (Monk and Montz, 1992).

Table 27.7 Survival for carcinoma of the cervix

FIGO stage	Approximate 5-year survival (%)
IA	100
IB	80–95
II	60–90
III	30–50
IV	5–20

Small-cell carcinoma of the cervix

Small-cell carcinoma of the cervix is a rare and aggressive tumour with a poor prognosis. Information on treatment and prognosis comes mainly from reported case series. Most patients receive chemotherapy (cisplatin and etoposide) similar to that prescribed for small-cell lung cancer (SCLC), with the addition of pelvic radiotherapy in those with localised disease. Surgery may be suitable for the few patients with small-volume early-stage disease. The incidence of brain metastases would appear to be less than that seen for SCLC.

Prognosis

Prognostic factors

Several prognostic factors have been identified for cervical cancer (International Union Against Cancer, 1995). Adverse tumour-related prognostic factors in cervical cancer include increased tumour bulk, the presence of lymph node metastases, lymphovascular space invasion, increased cancer stage and adenocarcinoma. Patient-related factors include anaemia, smoking and poor performance status. Adverse treatment-related factors include a positive surgical resection margin, a long duration of radiation treatment and no intracavitary brachytherapy treatment.

Five-year survival

Table 27.7 summarises 5-year survival figures. Selected patients with local recurrence who are treated with pelvic exenteration may achieve a 50% 5-year survival rate. Local protocols for follow-up should be adhered to, with regular history and clinical examination for 5 years.

Areas of current interest

IGBT and IMRT are becoming widely adopted. For IMRT, ongoing clinical studies are assessing tumour control and toxicity, in the adjuvant and definitive settings (Loiselle and Koh, 2010). The prescription dose is conformed to the shape of the target in three dimensions using inverse planning techniques. This targeted approach leads to the possibilities of normal tissue sparing or dose escalation to the tumour.

There is current interest in the use of monoclonal antibodies alone or in combination with chemotherapy and radiotherapy as a treatment for cervical cancer.

Ongoing clinical trials

The following open trials are currently registered with the National Cancer Research Network (http://csg.ncri.org.uk/, accessed January 2015).

DEPICT: a phase I/II, multi-centre dose escalation study of simultaneous boost IMRT for locally advanced cervical cancer.

INTERLACE: a phase III multi-centre trial of weekly induction chemotherapy followed by standard chemoradiation versus standard chemoradiation alone in patients with locally advanced cervical cancer.

MAPPING: diagnostic accuracy of MRI, diffusion-weighted MRI, FDGPET/CT and Fluoro-ethylcholine PET/CT in the detection of lymph node metastases in surgically staged endometrial and cervical carcinoma.

References

Andreyev, H. J., Benton, B., Lalji, A., et al. (2013). Algorithm-based management of patients with gastrointestinal symptoms in patients after pelvic radiation treatment (ORBIT): a randomised controlled trial. Lancet, 382, 2084–2092.

Bader, A., Winter, R., Haas J., et al. (2007). Where to look for the sentinel lymph node in cervical cancer. Am. J. Obstet. Gynecol., 197, 678.

Boon, M. E., de Graaff Guilloud, J. C., et al. (1987). Efficacy of screening for cervical squamous and adenocarcinoma: the Dutch experience. Cancer, 59, 862–866.

Buckley, S. L., Tritz, D. M., Van Le, L., et al. (1996). Lymph node metastases and prognosis in patients with stage IA2 cervical cancer. Gynecol. Oncol., 63, 4–9.

Denton, A. S., Bond, S. J., Matthews, S., et al. (2000). National audit of the management and outcome of carcinoma of the cervix treated with radiotherapy in 1993. Clin. Oncol. (R. Coll. Radiol.), 12, 347–353.

Denton, K. J., Herbert, A., Turnbull, L. S., et al. (2008). The revised BSCC terminology for abnormal cervical cytology. Cytopathology, 19, 137–157.

Ferlay, J., Bray, F., Pisani, P., et al. (2004). GLOBOCAN 2002. Cancer Incidence, Mortality and Prevalence Worldwide. IARC Cancer Base No. 5, Version 2.0. Lyon: IARC Press.

Green, J. A., Kirwan, J. M., Tierney, J. F., et al. (2001). Survival and recurrence after concomitant chemotherapy and radiotherapy for cancer of the uterine cervix: a systematic review and meta-analysis. Lancet, 358, 781–786.

Haie-Meder, C., Pötter, R., Van Limbergen, E., et al. (2005). Recommendations from Gynaecological (GYN) GEC-ESTRO Working Group (I): concepts and terms in 3D image based treatment planning in cervix cancer brachytherapy with emphasis on MRI assessment of GTV and CTV. Radiother. Oncol., 74, 235–245.

Helmerhorst, T. J. and Meijer, C. J. (2002). Cervical cancer should be considered as a rare complication of oncogenic HPV infection rather than a STD. Int. J. Gynecol. Cancer, 12, 235–236.

ICRU. (1985). Dose and Volume Specification for Intra-cavitary Therapy in Gynaecology. Report no. 38. Bethesda, MD: International Commission on Radiological Units and Measurements.

International Union Against Cancer. (1995). Prognostic Factors in Cancer, ed. P. Hermanek, M. K. Gospodarowicz, D. E. Henson, et al. Berlin: Springer-Verlag.

Jadon, R., Pembroke, C. A., Hanna, C. L., et al. (2014). A systematic review of organ motion and image-guided strategies in external beam radiotherapy for cervical cancer. Clin. Oncol. (R. Coll. Radiol.), 26, 185–196.

Keys, H. M., Bundy, B. N. and Stehman, F. B. (1999). Cisplatin, radiation and adjuvant hysterectomy compared with radiation and adjuvant hysterectomy for bulky stage 1B cervical carcinoma. N. Engl. J. Med., 340, 1154–1161.

Kelly R. S., Patnick J., Kitchener H. C., et al. (2011). HPV testing as a triage for borderline or mild dyskaryosis on cervical cytology: results from the Sentinel Sites study. Br. J. Cancer, 105, 983–988.

Lehtinen, M. and Dillner, J. (2013). Clinical trials of human papillomavirus vaccines and beyond. Nat. Rev. Clin. Oncol., 10, 400–410.

Loiselle C. and Koh W. (2010). The emerging use of IMRT for treatment of cervical cancer. J. Natl Compr. Canc. Netw., 8, 1425–1434.

Lukka, H., Hirte, H., Fyles, A., et al. (2002). Concurrent cisplatin-based chemotherapy plus radiotherapy for cervical cancer – a meta-analysis. Clin. Oncol. (R. Coll. Radiolol.), 14, 203–212.

Monk, B. J. and Montz, F. J. (1992). Invasive cervical cancer complicating intrauterine pregnancy: treatment with radical hysterectomy. *Obstet. Gynecol.*, **80**, 199–203.

Moreno, V., Bosch, F. X., Munoz, N., *et al.* (2002). Effect of oral contraceptives on risk of cervical cancer in women with human papillomavirus infection: the IARC multicentric case-control study. *Lancet*, **359**, 1085–1092.

Morris, M., Eifel, P., Lu, J., *et al.* (1999). Pelvic radiation with concurrent chemotherapy compared with pelvic and para-aortic radiation for high-risk cervical cancer. *N. Engl. J. Med.*, **340**, 1137–1143.

Nag, S., Erickson, B., Thomadsen, B., *et al.* (2000). The American Brachytherapy Society recommendations for high-dose-rate brachytherapy for carcinoma of the cervix. *Int. J. Radiat. Oncol. Biol. Phys.*, **48**, 201–211.

Nesvacil, N., Pötter, R., Sturdza, A., *et al.* (2012). Adaptive imaged guided brachytherapy for cervical cancer: a combined MRI-/CT-planning technique with MRI only at first fraction. *Radiother. Oncol.*, **107**, 75–81.

NHS Cancer Screening Programme. (2010). *Colposcopy and Programme Management for the NHS Cervical Screening Programme 2nd Edition. NHSCP publication no. 20.* Sheffield: NHS Cancer Screening Programmes.

NICE. (2003). *Guidance on the Use of Liquid-Based Cytology for Cervical Screening*, Technology Appraisal no. 69. London: National Institute for Clinical Excellence.

NICE. (2006). *High Dose Rate Brachytherapy for Carcinoma of the Cervix. Interventional Procedure Guidance 160.* London: National Institute for Clinical Excellence.

NICE. (2015). *Suspected cancer: recognition and referral. NICE guideline.* London: National Institute for Health and Care Excellence.

Percorelli, S. (2009). Revised FIGO staging for carcinoma of the vulva, cervix and endometrium. *Int. J. Gynaecol. Obstet.*, **105**, 103–104.

Peters, W. A. 3rd, Liu, P. Y., Barrett, R. J. 2nd, *et al.* (2000). Concurrent chemotherapy and pelvic radiation therapy compared with pelvic radiation therapy alone as adjuvant therapy after radical surgery in high-risk early-stage cancer of the cervix. *J. Clin. Oncol.*, **18**, 1606–1613.

Pötter, R., Haie-Meder, C., Van Limbergen, E., *et al.* (2006). Recommendations from GYN ESTRO working group (II): concepts and terms in 3D image-based treatment planning in cervix cancer brachytherapy – 3D dose volume parameters and aspects of 3D imaged-based anatomy, radiation physics, radiobiology. *Radiother. Oncol.*, **78**, 67–77.

Pötter, R., Kirisits, C., Fidarova, E. *et al.* (2008). Present status and future of high-precision image guided adaptive brachytherapy for cervix cancer. *Acta Oncol.*, **47**, 1325–1336.

Pötter, R., Georg, P., Dimopoulos, J., *et al.* (2011). Clinical outcome of protocol based image (MRI) guided adaptive brachytherapy combined with 3D conformal radiotherapy with or without chemotherapy in patients with locally advanced cervical cancer. *Radiother. Oncol.*, **100**, 116–123.

RCP and RCR. (2013). *Evidence-based indications for the use of PET-CT in the UK.* London: Royal College of Physicians and Royal College of Radiologists.

RCR. (2008). *The Timely Delivery of Radical Radiotherapy: Standards and Guidelines for the Management of Unscheduled Treatment Interruptions, Third Edition, 2008.* London: The Royal College of Radiologists.

RCR. (2009). *Implenting Image-guided Brachytherapy for Cervix Cancer in the UK.* London: Royal College of Radiologists.

Rogers, L., Siu, S., Luesley, D., *et al.* (2012). Radiotherapy and chemoradiation after surgery for early cervical cancer (Review). *Cochrane Database of Systematic Reviews*, Issue 5. Art. No.: CD007583.

Rose, P. G., Bundy, B. N., Watkins, E. B., *et al.* (1999). Concurrent cisplatin-based radiotherapy and chemotherapy for locally advanced cervical cancer. *N. Engl. J. Med.*, **340**, 1144–1153.

Sevin, B. U., Nadji, M., Averette, H. E., *et al.* (1992). Microinvasive carcinoma of the cervix. *Cancer*, **70**, 2121–2128.

Small, W., Mell, L. K., Anderson, P., *et al.* (2008). Consensus guidelines for the delineation of the clinical target volume for intensity modulated pelvic radiotherapy in the postoperative treatment of endometrial and cervical cancer. *Int. J. Radiat. Oncol. Biol. Phys.*, **71**(2), 428–434.

Smith, J. S., Herrero, R., Bosetti, C., *et al.* (2002). Herpes simplex virus-2 as a human papillomavirus cofactor in the etiology of invasive cervical cancer. *J. Natl Cancer Inst.*, **94**, 1604–1613.

Tan, L. T., Coles, C. E., Hart, C., *et al.* (2009). Clinical impact of computer tomography-based image-guided brachytherapy for cervix cancer using the tandem-ring applicator – the Addenbrooke's experience. *Clin. Oncol. (R. Coll. Radiol.)*, **21**, 175–182.

Tewari, K. S., Sill, M., Penson, R., *et al.* (2014). Final overall survival analysis of the phase III randomized trial of chemotherapy with and without Bevacizumab for advanced cervical cancer: a NRG oncology–GOG study. *Ann. Oncol.*, **25**(Suppl. 4), LBA26.

Trent Cancer Registry. (2011). *Profile of Cervical Cancer in England: Incidence, Mortality and Survival.* Sheffield: NHS Cancer Screening Programmes.

Wachter-Gerstner, N., Wachter, S., Reinstadler, E., *et al.* (2003). The impact of sectional imaging on dose escalation in endocavitary HDR-brachytherapy of cervical cancer: results of a prospective comparative trial. *Radiother. Oncol.*, **68**, 51–59.

Whitney, C. W., Sause, W., Bundy, B. N., *et al.* (1999). Randomised comparison of fluorouracil plus cisplatin versus hydroxyurea as an adjunct to radiation therapy in stage IIB/IVA carcinoma of the cervix with negative para-aortic lymph nodes: a Gynecologic Oncology and South West Oncology Group Study. *J. Clin. Oncol.*, **17**, 1339–1348.

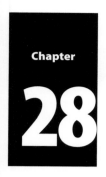

Chapter

28

Management of cancer of the vagina

Rashmi Jadon, Emma Hudson and Louise Hanna

Introduction

Primary carcinoma of the vagina is a rare condition, accounting for only 2% of gynaecological malignancies. The main risk factors are persistent human papilloma virus (HPV) infection and increasing age. Treatments are individualised, and treatment decisions are based on tumour site, size and stage, as well as involvement of adjacent anatomical structures.

Tumours affecting the vagina

Only 25% of malignant vaginal tumours arise from the vagina itself. The majority of malignant tumours affecting the vagina are tumours that have either spread from adjacent structures (cervix and vulva), are recurrent tumours originating in other genitourinary sites (cervix, rectum, bladder) or are metastases from other tumours (ovary, breast).

Table 28.1 shows the range of tumours that can affect the vagina (adapted from WHO Classification, 2003).

Anatomy

The vagina is a muscular tube approximately 8 cm long, extending upwards and backwards from the vulva to the uterus. The apex of the vagina, into which the cervix projects, is divided into four fornices: anterior, posterior and two lateral.

The relations of the vagina from superior to inferior are as follows:

- anterior – bladder, urethra;
- posterior – pouch of Douglas, rectum, perineal body (separates lower vagina from anus);
- lateral – ureter, pelvic floor and perineal muscles.

The lymphatic drainage from the upper two-thirds is to the pelvic nodes, and from the lower third to the inguinal nodes.

Table 28.1 Tumours affecting the vagina

Type	Examples
Benign	Squamous tumours (condyloma acuminatum, squamous papilloma, fibroepithelial polyp)
	Glandular tumours (müllerian papilloma, adenoma)
	Mesenchymal tumours (leiomyoma, genital rhabdomyoma, deep angiomyxoma, postoperative spindle cell nodule)
	Benign mixed tumours
	Melanocytic naevus and blue naevus
	Dermoid cyst
Malignant primary	Squamous carcinoma (keratinising, non-keratinising, basaloid, verrucous, warty)
	Adenocarcinoma (clear cell, endometrioid, mucinous, mesonephric)
	Adenosquamous carcinoma
	Other tumours (carcinoid, small cell, undifferentiated, adenoid cystic, adenoid squamous)
	Sarcomas (sarcoma botryoides, leiomyosarcoma, undifferentiated, low-grade endometrioid stromal sarcoma)
	Malignant mixed tumours (e.g. carcinosarcoma = malignant mixed müllerian tumour, adenosarcoma)
	Malignant melanoma
	Yolk sac tumour
	Ewing tumour/PNET
	Lymphoma and leukaemia

Practical Clinical Oncology, Second Edition, ed. Louise Hanna, Tom Crosby and Fergus Macbeth. Published by Cambridge University Press. © Cambridge University Press 2015.

Table 28.1 (cont.)

Type	Examples
Malignant secondary	Direct spread (from cervix, vulva, rectum)
	Metastasis (from endometrium, breast, ovary)

PNET, primitive neuroectodermal tumour. Adapted from WHO classification (2003).

Incidence and epidemiology

Vaginal cancer is rare; the annual disease incidence in the UK is 0.6 in 100,000 women. Approximately 250 new cases are diagnosed per year in England (http://www.cancerresearchuk.org/cancer-info/cancerstats/types/, accessed December 2014), and vaginal cancer accounts for approximately 1–2% of all gynaecological malignancy. The mortality-to-incidence ratio is 0.38. Incidence increases with age, with peak incidence occurring in women over 85 years of age.

Carcinoma of the vagina

Risk factors and aetiology

Vaginal cancer predominantly affects older women, with 50% affecting those above the age of 70 (Shah *et al.*, 2009). The aetiology of vaginal cancer is similar to that of cervical cancer, with HPV types 16 and 18 being of significance, as well as early coital age, multiple sexual partners and smoking (Daling *et al.*, 2002).

Vaginal intraepithelial neoplasia (VAIN), previous abnormal cervical cytology or cervical cancer and chronic vaginal trauma (e.g. procidentia) are also risk factors for squamous cell carcinoma. Exposure to diethylstilboestrol *in utero* is associated with clear cell adenocarcinoma usually in patients under the age of 40.

Pathology

As stated by the Fédération Internationale de Gynécologie et d'Obstétrique (FIGO) system, any vaginal tumour involving the cervix or vulva should be classed as cervical or vulval, respectively.

More than 80% of vaginal cancers are squamous carcinomas, and the histological features are shown in Table 28.2. Of the remaining tumours, the most common are adenocarcinomas (including clear cell carcinoma, which is associated with diethylstilboestrol exposure *in utero*), melanoma and sarcoma botryoides.

Table 28.2 Histological features of squamous vaginal carcinoma

Features	Description
Macroscopic	May be exophytic, ulcerative, annular and constricting, polypoid, sessile, indurated or fungating
	May occur anywhere in the vagina
	Size varies from microscopic to more than 10 cm
Microscopic	Typically moderately differentiated and non-keratinising
	Variants: spindle cell, warty, verrucous

Adapted from WHO classification (2003).

For squamous carcinoma, the typical precursor lesion is VAIN. Fifty per cent of invasive squamous cell carcinomas occur in the upper third of the vagina, with 20% and 30% occurring in the mid and lower vagina. The posterior vagina wall is most commonly affected.

Spread

Vaginal carcinoma spreads locally to paravaginal tissues and the pelvic side wall, the rectum and anus, and the bladder, urethra and ureter.

Lymphatic spread is to pelvic nodes (from the upper two-thirds of the vagina), inguinal and femoral nodes (from the lower third) and para-aortic nodes. Haematogenous spread is to the liver, lung and brain.

Clinical presentation

The most common presenting symptom is vaginal bleeding (postmenopausal or postcoital), although other symptoms include vaginal discharge, dysuria, pain/dyspareunia or fistula (vesico-vaginal or recto-vaginal).

Distant spread of disease may present as an inguinal lymph node mass, lymphoedema of a lower limb, pelvic pain or, uncommonly, jaundice, bone pain and shortness of breath.

Women with suspicious symptoms should be examined including a pelvic examination, and if there is an unexplained palpable mass in or at the entrance of the vagina they should be considered for referral via a 2-week suspected cancer pathway (NICE, 2015).

Investigation and staging

Diagnostic investigations

Examination under anaesthetic involves inspection of the vulva, vagina and cervix. The size and location of primary tumours should be documented, including the presence of fixity or involvement of adjacent structures.

Biopsy should be conducted, as well as cystoscopy and proctoscopy to ascertain if there is involvement of adjacent structures. Pregnancy status should be checked in premenopausal women.

Further investigations for staging

Imaging of the pelvis and abdomen should be used to assess the extent of the primary tumour, involvement of pelvic and para-aortic lymph nodes and to examine for hydronephrosis. Either CT or MRI are used; however, MRI may give more information and aid CT planning for patients having radiotherapy. T2-weighted images are particularly useful for assessing squamous cell carcinomas (Parikh et al., 2008).

The use of FDG-PET scans for staging has been reported in single institution reports (Hiniker et al., 2013), although its role not fully established.

A chest X-ray or CT chest should be performed to exclude lung metastases. If there is clinical suspicion of bone metastases, a bone scan may be performed.

Staging classification

The regional nodes for the upper two-thirds of the vagina are the pelvic nodes most commonly external, internal and common iliac nodes (Frank et al., 2005). The regional nodes for the lower third of the vagina are the inguinal and femoral nodes. Table 28.3 shows the staging classification for carcinoma of the vagina.

Treatment overview

Given the rarity of carcinoma of the vagina, no prospective randomised trials have been performed to guide management. Most of the available information is gathered from retrospective studies.

Treatment is tailored to an individual and is dependent on the location of the primary tumour within the vagina, the extent of spread and whether the patient has had a previous hysterectomy.

Radiotherapy is the mainstay of treatment for vaginal carcinoma and favourable outcomes have been

Table 28.3 Staging classification for carcinoma of the vagina

FIGO stage	Description
I	Limited to vaginal wall
II	Involved subvaginal tissue but has not extended to the pelvic wall
III	Extends to pelvic wall
IV	Beyond the true pelvis or has involved the mucosa of the bladder
IVA	Invades baldder and/or rectal mucosa and/or direct extension beyond the true pelvis
IVB	Spread to distant organs

Adapted from FIGO Committee on Gynecologic Oncology (2009).

reported (Frank et al., 2005; Blecharz et al., 2012), especially for stage I and II tumours.

Surgical treatments, if considered, are best for early-stage tumours affecting the central pelvis; however, postoperative radiotherapy may still be necessary, which may increase morbidity for the patient.

The following is an overview of the most commonly used treatment options by stage.

Stage I

Treatment options for stage I tumours include:

- radiotherapy – brachytherapy alone (for smaller and superficial tumours);
- radiotherapy – combined external beam plus brachytherapy;
- surgery ± postoperative radiotherapy.

Stages II and III

Treatment options for stage II and III tumours include:

- radiotherapy – combined external beam plus brachytherapy;
- radiotherapy – external beam alone;
- surgery ± postoperative radiotherapy (e.g. for small stage II tumours).

Stage IVa

Treatment options for stage IVa tumours include:

- radiotherapy – external beam treatment alone.;
- radiotherapy – combined external beam plus brachytherapy;
- surgery ± postoperative radiotherapy (e.g. for central tumours with fistulae).

For stages II, III and IVA concurrent chemotherapy can be considered with external beam treatment.

Stage IVb

Treatment options for stage IVb tumours include palliative radiotherapy, chemotherapy and symptom control.

Surgery

Surgery for vaginal carcinoma can be considered for stage I and small stage II tumours (local excision; radical hysterectomy ± vaginectomy). Postoperative radiotherapy can be considered in patients with positive resection margins or involved lymph nodes (Tjalma *et al.*, 2001).

For selected stage IVA tumours central pelvic exenteration can be considered, especially if a fistula is present, although this must be weighed up against considerable associated morbidity.

Radiotherapy

Frank *et al.* (2005) published guidelines for radiotherapy treatment for squamous vaginal carcinoma, based on their series of 193 patients. They suggest that treatment can be delivered in two phases as follows.

- Phase I: Initial external beam radiotherapy (EBRT) to the pelvis is recommended due to the risk of microscopic nodal disease, except for very small stage I tumours.
- Phase II: A boost is given depending on the location of the primary tumour, whether the patient has had a previous hysterectomy and the response to treatment.

  - Apical tumours –intracavitary therapy if < 0.5 cm thick; interstitial treatment or EBRT if > 0.5 cm thick. If the uterus is present, more extensive lesions may be treated with intracavitary brachytherapy.
  - Mid-vaginal tumours – interstitial treatment for small anterior or lateral tumours; EBRT for posterior or larger tumours.
  - Distal tumours – interstitial treatment for confined tumours; EBRT for larger tumours.

High-dose-rate (HDR) brachytherapy has been shown to be as effective as low-dose-rate (Nanavati *et al.*, 1993; Mock *et al.*, 2003) and more recently the addition of image guidance to brachytherapy has been demonstrated to be of value (Beriwal *et al.*, 2012).

Concurrent chemoradiotherapy

No prospective randomised trials demonstrate the benefit of chemotherapy given concurrently with radiotherapy in vaginal carcinoma. However, many centres extrapolate from the experience of other squamous carcinomas such as cervical cancer, especially in the more advanced stages of disease, and concurrent chemotherapy is given as tolerated by the individual patient.

Concurrent use of cisplatin has been demonstrated to be tolerable in retrospective series (Samant *et al.*, 2007), although no clear survival benefit has been noted as yet (Ghia *et al.*, 2011). Concurrent use of 5-FU either alone, with cisplatin or with mitomycin C has been used and a small series of 14 patients found that adding these drugs gave results comparable to previously published series using higher doses of radiation as monotherapy (Dalyrymple *et al.*, 2004).

The role of neoadjuvant chemotherapy has not been established.

Radical radiotherapy technique

Phase I: external beam radiotherapy

Patient preparation

- The patient lies supine with knees supported. A radio-opaque marker is placed to define the inferior extent of the vaginal tumour on clinical examination. Localisation tattoos are placed anteriorly and laterally.
- Patients should have a comfortably full bladder and empty rectum. Intravenous contrast is given to localise the pelvic blood vessels as a surrogate for lymph node position.
- CT scans are acquired from the level of L3 to below the vulva. If CT scanning is unavailable then orthogonal X-ray films may be used with conventional field borders.

CT planning

- The GTV is the primary tumour determined by clinical examination, EUA report, and MRI and CT scans.
- The CTV is the GTV with a 1–2 cm margin, plus the entire vagina and the regional lymph nodes depending on tumour location. For upper vaginal

tumours internal, external and common iliac as well as obturator nodes are typically included. For lower vaginal tumours the inguinal nodes and distal external iliac nodes are included. For tumours crossing the boundary between upper two thirds and lower third of the vagina, all lymph node regions are included.

Field arrangement

Conventionally, a four-field brick is used for upper vaginal tumours, although for lower vaginal tumours an anterior–posterior parallel-opposed pair is used to ensure coverage of the inguinal nodes. Conformal or, more recently, IMRT solutions are also increasingly used. It is important in these circumstances to ensure that CTV to PTV margins are adequate to account for the considerable internal organ movement that can occur.

Dose and fractionation

Typical doses include forty-five to 50.4 Gy in 25–28 fractions over 4–5+ weeks with 10 MV photons, prescribed to the ICRU reference point (e.g. midplane point). The dose of the boost will vary depending on the dose of EBRT, tumour location, extent of disease and response to EBRT (Beriwal et al., 2012).

Phase II: boost to primary tumour

There are four main techniques for boosting the primary tumour, dependent on the tumour position and size.

(1) Intracavitary treatment with an intrauterine tube:
- for tumour at the upper third of the vagina in patients with an intact uterus;
- the technique involves an intrauterine tube and ovoids or a vaginal ring, similar to the procedure for cervical cancer;
- an LDR schedule is 25–30 Gy in a single fraction to point A; the HDR schedule is typically 21–24 Gy in 3–4 fractions to point A or with an individualised image guided technique.

(2) Intracavitary treatment with a vaginal tube:
- for very superficial tumours in the lower two-thirds of the vagina;
- the technique involves placement of a vaginal cylinder;

- an LDR schedule is 20– 25 Gy in a single insertion prescribed 0.5 cm from the surface of the applicator;
- there are very few reported series for HDR e.g. 21 Gy in 3 fractions or 20 Gy in 4 fractions prescribed 0.5 cm from the surface of the applicator (Nanavati et al., 1993; Mock et al., 2003).

(3) Interstitial treatment:
- for tumour in the distal two-thirds of the lateral or anterior wall;
- the technique involves, for example, iridium hairpins or wires;
- an LDR schedule is 20–30 Gy prescribed to the 85% reference isodose;
- HDR schedules include 18–25 Gy in 3–5 fractions.

(4) External beam boost:
- for larger, posterior or deeply infiltrating tumour (e.g. tumours involving the recto-vaginal septum or bladder), a conformal technique with CT or MRI planning to minimise the dose to adjacent structures is used with a GTV–CTV margin of around 2 cm;
- doses include 18–24 Gy in 10–12 fractions.

Complications of radiotherapy

A low (3.9%) severe late complication rate has been reported following radiotherapy, with vesico-vaginal fistula and rectovaginal fistula being reported most commonly (Blecharz et al., 2012). Other complications include rectal ulceration, proctitis, urethral stricture, vaginal ulceration and necrosis, and small bowel obstruction (Chyle et al., 1996). Patients with troublesome bowel symptoms after radiotherapy are investigated via an algorithm-based approach (Andreyev et al., 2014).

Follow-up

Most locoregional recurrences and distant failures occur within the first 2 years after treatment. The following is a suggested scheme for clinical follow-up.

- Three-monthly for the first year.
- Four-monthly for the second year.
- Six-monthly for the third and fourth years.
- Then annually for 1 year.

Table 28.4 Prognosis for vaginal cancer by stage

Stage	Five-year survival (%)
I	75
II	60
III	35
IVA	20
IVB	0%

Adapted from Lilic *et al.,* (2010).

Recurrent disease

The predominant site of relapse in radically treated patients is locoregional.

Patients previously treated with radiotherapy, who develop a central recurrence in the pelvis, can sometimes be cured with pelvic exenteration.

Patients previously treated with surgery alone, who develop a localised recurrence in the pelvis, can sometimes be cured with radical radiotherapy.

Palliative treatments

Typical scenarios in patients with incurable locoregional recurrences include pelvic pain, fistula, bleeding, infection, lymphoedema, and thromboembolic disease. A multi-disciplinary approach is required. Interventions that provide a benefit include platinum-based palliative chemotherapy, palliative radiotherapy, defunctioning stoma, lymphoedema stockings and adequate pain control.

Prognosis

Table 28.4 shows the 5-year survival for different stages of vaginal cancer.

Poor prognostic factors include tumour in the lower vagina, adenocarcinoma (non-clear cell), increased tumour bulk and increased FIGO stage (Chyle *et al.,* 1996).

Favourable prognostic factors include young age (< 60), and early stage (Blecharz *et al.,* 2012). HPV-positive tumours have been shown to have a favourable outcome in one study (Larsson *et al.,* 2013). For those treated with radiotherapy, a total dose of over 70 Gy is reported to be associated with improved survival outcomes (Hiniker *et al.,* 2013).

Areas of current interest

As in other tumour sites treated with radiotherapy the use of intensity modulated radiotherapy (IMRT) is being considered for vaginal cancer, with initial positive results found in terms of tumour control and toxicity (Hiniker *et al.,* 2013); however, further data are needed to define the role of this modality.

Other areas of interest include HPV-related biomarkers as a prognostic indicator for vaginal cancers (Alonso *et al.,* 2012).

References

Alonso, I., Felix, A., Torné, A., *et al.* (2012). Human papillomavirus as a favorable prognostic biomarker in squamous cell carcinomas of the vagina. *Gynecol. Oncol.,* **125**, 194–199.

Andreyev, H. J., Benton, B., Lalji, A., *et al.* (2013). Algorithm-based management of patients with gastrointestinal symptoms in patients after pelvic radiation treatment (ORBIT): a randomised controlled trial. *Lancet,* **382**, 2084–2092.

Beriwal, S., Rwigma, J. C., Higgins, E., *et al.* (2012). Three-dimensional image-based high-dose-rate interstitial brachytherapy for vaginal cancer. *Brachytherapy,* **11**, 176–180.

Blecharz, P., Reinfuss, M., Jakubowicz, J., *et al.* (2012). Effectiveness of radiotherapy in patients with primary invasive vaginal carcinoma. *Eur. J. Gynaecol. Oncol.,* **34**, 436–441.

Chyle, V., Zagars, G. K., Wheeler, J. A., *et al.* (1996). Definitive radiotherapy for carcinoma of the vagina: outcome and prognostic factors. *Int. J. Radiat. Oncol. Biol. Phys.,* **35**, 891–905.

Daling, J. R., Madeleine, M. M., Schwartz, S. M., *et al.* (2002). A population-based study of squamous cell vaginal cancer: HPV and cofactors. *Gynecol. Oncol.,* **84**, 263–270.

Dalrymple, J. L., Russell, A. H., Lee, S. W., *et al.* (2004). Chemoradiation for primary invasive squamous carcinoma of the vagina. *Int. J. Gynecol. Cancer,* **14**, 110–117.

FIGO Committee on Gynecologic Oncology. (2009). Current FIGO staging for cancer of the vagina, fallopian tube, ovary, and gestational trophoblastic neoplasia. *Int. J. Gynaecol. Obstet.,* **105**, 3–4.

Frank, S. J., Jhingran, A., Levenback, C., *et al.* (2005). Definitive radiation therapy for squamous cell carcinoma of the vagina. *Int. J. Radiat. Oncol. Biol. Phys.,* **62**, 138–147.

Ghia, A. J., Gonzalez, V. J., Tward, J. D., *et al.* (2011). Primary vaginal cancer and chemoradiotherapy: a patterns-of-care analysis. *Int. J. Gynecol. Cancer*, **21**, 378–384.

Hiniker, S. M., Rouz, A., Murphy, J. D., *et al.* (2013). Primary squamous cell carcinoma of the vagina: prognostic factors, treatment patterns, and outcomes. *Gynecol. Oncol.* **131**, 380–385.

Larsson, G. L., Helenius, G., Andersson, S., *et al.* (2013). Prognostic impact of human papilloma virus (HPV) genotyping and HPV-16 subtyping in vaginal carcinoma. *Gynecol. Oncol.*, **129**, 406–411.

Lilic, V., Lilic, G., Filipovic, S., *et al.* (2010). Primary carcinoma of the vagina. *J. B.U.O.N.* **15**, 241–247.

Mock, U., Kucera, H., Fellner, C., *et al.* (2003). High-dose-rate (HDR) brachytherapy with or without external beam radiotherapy in the treatment of primary vaginal carcinoma: long-term results and side effects. *Int. J. Radiat. Oncol. Biol. Phys.*, **56**, 950–957.

Nanavati, P. J., Fanning, J., Hilgers, R. D., *et al.* (1993). High-dose-rate brachytherapy in primary stage I and II vaginal cancer. *Gynecol. Oncol.*, **51**, 67–71.

NICE. (2015). *Suspected cancer: recognition and referral. NICE guidance*. London: National Institute for Health and Care Excellence.

Parikh, J. H., Barton, D. P., Ind, T. E., *et al.* (2008). MR imaging features of vaginal malignancies *Radiographics*, **28**, 49–63.

Samant, R., Lau, B., E C, *et al.* (2007). Primary vaginal cancer treated with concurrent chemoradiation using cis-platinum. *Int. J. Rad. Oncol.Biol.Phys.*, **69**, 746–750.

Shah, C. A., Goff, B. A. Lowe, K., *et al.* (2009). Factors affecting risk of mortality in women with vaginal cancer. *Obstet. Gynecol.*, **113**, 1038.

Tjalma, W. A. A., Monaghan, J. M., de Barros Lopes, A., *et al.* (2001). The role of surgery in invasive squamous carcinoma of the vagina. *Gynecol. Oncol.*, **81**, 360–365.

WHO classification. (2003). In *World Health Organization Classification of Tumours: Pathology and Genetics of Tumours of the Breast and Female Genital Organs*, ed. A. Tavassoli and P. Devilee. Lyon: IARC Press, Chapter 6.

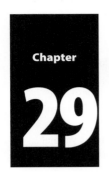

Chapter 29

Management of cancer of the vulva

Rashmi Jadon, Emma Hudson and Louise Hanna

Introduction

Carcinoma of the vulva is an uncommon disease representing only 4% of gynaecological malignancies. Effective management requires the expertise of a multidisciplinary team to support patients through the physical and psychosexual morbidity associated with radical treatment. Recent guidelines have been published jointly by the Royal College of Obstetricians and Gynaecologists and the British Gynaecological Cancer Society (RCOG/BGCS, 2014).

Range of vulval tumours

Table 29.1 shows the large range of benign and malignant tumours which may affect the vulva (adapted from WHO, 2003).

Anatomy

The vulva is the name given to the female external genitalia. The anatomical subsites are as follows.

- Mons pubis, the rounded, hair-bearing region in front of the pubis.
- Labia majora, the hair-bearing skin extending from the mons pubis.
- Labia minora, the non-hair-bearing folds of skin that meet posteriorly at the fourchette.
- Clitoris, situated in the midline at the anterior ends of the labia minora.
- Vestibule, the triangular-shaped skin between the labia minora.

Incidence and epidemiology

The annual incidence of vulval cancer in the UK is 2.5 in 100,000 women (http://www.cancerresearchuk.org/cancer-info/cancerstats/, accessed December 2014). Approximately 1200 cases are diagnosed in the UK

Table 29.1 The range of vulval tumours

Type	Examples
Benign	Squamous tumours (e.g. condylomata acuminata, keratoacanthoma)
	Glandular tumours (e.g. adenoma, Paget's disease [n.b. 10–20% invasive]); arising from anogenital mammary-like glands (e.g. papillary hydradenoma)
	Soft tissue tumours (e.g. leiomyoma, granular cell tumour)
	Melanocytic naevus
Malignant primary	Squamous carcinoma, > 90%; various types including keratinising, non-keratinising, verrucous
	Basal cell carcinoma
	Adenocarcinoma (e.g. arising from Bartholin gland; anogenital mammary-like gland; skene gland – the skene gland is the female equivalent of the prostate gland)
	Skin appendage tumour: malignant sweat gland tumour; sebaceous carcinoma
	Malignant soft tissue tumour (e.g. sarcoma botryoides, leiomyosarcoma)
	Malignant melanoma
	Lymphoma and leukaemia
	Melanoma
Malignant secondary	Direct spread from pelvic organs
	Metastasis from distant primary

Adapted from WHO (2003).

Practical Clinical Oncology, Second Edition, ed. Louise Hanna, Tom Crosby and Fergus Macbeth. Published by Cambridge University Press. © Cambridge University Press 2015.

each year. The cancer mortality to incidence ratio is around 0.3.

Disease incidence increases with age; presentation is rare in women under the age of 30, with peak incidence occurring in women over the age of 70. The highest incidence occurs in developing countries.

Carcinoma of the vulva

Risk factors and aetiology

Squamous carcinoma is the most common malignant tumour of the vulva. Key risk factors include increasing age and human papilloma virus (HPV). HPV is an important contributing factor to both invasive vulval carcinoma and vulval carcinoma *in situ*, associated with 28.6% and 87% of cases, respectively (de Sanjosé *et al.*, 2013). HPV 16 is the predominant type, although HPV 33, 18 and 45 are also important. HPV types 6 and 11 are associated with verrucous carcinoma.

Cigarette smoking, immunosuppression (e.g. renal allograft) and a history of genital warts are also significant risk factors.

Screening

There is no evidence to support the use of screening in an unselected population, but women with high-grade vulval intraepithelial neoplasia (VIN), VIN in the immunosuppressed, Paget's disease or melanoma *in situ* should be followed up in either specialist multidisciplinary vulval clinics or by gynaecological oncologists (RCOG/BGCS, 2014).

Pathology

Precursor lesions for squamous carcinoma of the vulva include the following.

- VIN associated with HPV.
- VIN not associated with HPV.
- Lichen sclerosus (6% risk of cancer).
- Chronic granulomatous vulval disease.

Table 29.2 shows the pathological features of squamous carcinoma of the vulva.

Molecular abnormalities in vulval cancer include a disruption of the PTEN and TP53 pathways. TP53 can be inactivated through binding of the HPV E6 protein.

Spread

Vulval cancer can spread locally, via lymphatics or via the bloodstream. The major route of spread

Table 29.2 Pathological features of squamous carcinoma of the vulva

Features	Description
Macroscopic	Ulcer, nodule, macule or pedunculated mass
Microscopic	Invasive neoplasm composed of malignant squamous cells of several morphological variants: • Keratinising with squamous pearls • Non-keratinising • Basaloid with nests of immature basal type cells • Warty (condylomatous) with cellular features of HPV • Verrucous, highly differentiated with rare mitotic figures and prominent inflammatory infiltrate • Kerato-acanthoma-like Variant with tumour giant cells is highly aggressive, may resemble malignant melanoma

Adapted from WHO (2003).

is locoregional, which can occur to the perineum, urethra, vagina, anus, bladder, rectum or pubic bone. Lymphatic spread is to inguinal, femoral and pelvic nodes. Approximately 30% of patients with operable vulval cancers have involved inguinal lymph nodes at the time of surgery.

Haematogenous spread is to the liver, lung and bone, although this is less common and the majority of patients who die from their disease have no clinical evidence of distant spread.

Clinical presentation

Symptoms and signs from the primary vulval cancer include an ulcer or lump, discharge, bleeding, pain, odour or pruritus vulvae, and the predominant symptoms of vulval cancer are those of locoregional spread.

Lymph node spread can present as an inguinal mass, lymphoedema of a lower limb or pelvic pain. Symptoms from metastatic disease are rare, but include jaundice, bone pain or pleural effusion.

Any woman with an unexplained lump on the vulva, vulval bleeding or ulcerated skin should be considered for referral via a 2-week suspected cancer pathway (NICE, 2015). Women with vulval pain or itching which does not settle with conservative management should also be referred.

Investigation and staging

Evaluation of the primary tumour

Diagnostic confirmation of disease involves examination under anaesthetic (EUA) and biopsy. Key assessments of the primary include size, location (in particular, distance from the midline) and fixity. Involvement of adjacent structures (urethra, vagina or anal canal) is noted at EUA, and cystoscopy and proctoscopy and a cervical smear should be performed (Hacker et al., 2012).

Evaluation of nodal stations: inguinofemoral nodes (or 'groin' nodes)

Clinical assessment of inguinofemoral nodes is not reliable. For clinically detected inguinofemoral nodes a fine-needle aspirate (FNA) can be helpful to distinguish a metastatic node from an inflammatory node.

CT scanning is not always useful for detection of involved groin nodes, and ultrasound with FNA can be more useful than CT alone (Land et al., 2006). For full surgical staging of the local lymph nodes, either an inguinofemoral groin node dissection or a sentinel node biopsy is indicated (see treatment section that follows).

Evaluation of distant disease

CT or MRI of the pelvis and abdomen is useful for detecting pelvic and para-aortic lymph nodes or hydronephrosis. Large primary tumours may also be visible. A chest X-ray or chest CT is performed to exclude lung metastases.

Staging classification

The regional nodes are the inguinal and femoral nodes. Tables 29.3 shows the TNM classification and FIGO staging groups, respectively.

Treatment overview

The cornerstone of managing vulval cancer is surgery. Techniques have evolved over recent decades, becoming less radical for early-stage disease and thus reducing morbidity for patients who are often elderly and frail.

For locally advanced disease, surgery remains the main component of treatment, although radiotherapy (with or without chemotherapy) has been used adjuvantly or neoadjuvantly.

For those unfit for surgery or with inoperable disease, primary radiotherapy is an option, with or without chemotherapy.

Those with metastatic disease are managed symptomatically, and palliative radiotherapy and chemotherapy can be considered.

Early-stage disease: stages I and II

Management of the primary

Stage IA tumours require only wide local excision because of the negligible risk of lymph node metastases in tumours with 1 mm or smaller depth of invasion (Hacker et al., 2012). The remaining vulva must be normal and a 1 cm surgical margin is required.

Stage IB to stage II tumours have previously been treated with a radical vulvectomy and bilateral groin node dissection (BGND) en bloc (butterfly incision). This approach had been replaced by a 'triple incision' procedure (Hacker et al., 1981) associated with a shorter hospital stay and less blood loss. However, in more recent years it is suggested that for early disease a radical local excision is a safe alternative to a radical vulvectomy, as recommended by a Cochrane review (Ansink et al., 2000) and this had been adopted by many centres as standard practice.

Ideally, a 15-mm margin of disease-free tissue is removed with the tumour. If, on histological examination, a resection margin of less than 10 mm is found, then further excision may be considered (RCOG/BGCS, 2014). Many patients with stage I or II disease have clear resection margins, but those with a resection margin of less than or equal to 8 mm have a 48% risk of local recurrence (compared to 0% if the margin is greater than 8 mm) and should be considered for adjuvant radiotherapy to the primary site (Faul et al., 1997).

Management of the inguinofemoral nodes

Traditionally, inguinofemoral node involvement has been surgically staged and treated with a BGND. This technique has a significant morbidity associated with it including lymphoedema (47%), lymphocysts (40%) and wound breakdown (38%) (Gaarenstroom et al., 2013).

For patients who are found to have groin node involvement, postoperative radiotherapy has a survival advantage over pelvic lymph node dissection (Holmesley et al., 1986). The indications for adjuvant

Table 29.3 Staging of carcinoma of the vulva (TNM and FIGO)

TNM	FIGO	Description
Primary tumour (T)		
Tis		Carcinoma *in situ* (preinvasive) (no longer included in FIGO)
T1		Tumour confined to vulva
T1a	IA	Lesions ≤ 2 cm in size, confined to the vulva or perineum and with stromal invasion ≤ 1.0 mm,[a] no nodal metastasis
T1b	IB	Lesions > 2 cm in size or with stromal invasion > 1.0 mm,[a] confined to the vulva or perineum, with negative nodes
T2	II	Tumour of any size with extension to adjacent perineal structures (lower third of urethra, lower third of vagina, anus) with negative nodes
T3	IVA(i)	Tumour of any size which invades any of the following: upper/proximal 2/3 of urethra, upper/proximal 2/3 of vaginal, bladder mucosa, rectal mucosa, or fixed to bone
Regional lymph nodes (N)		
N0		No regional lymph node metastasis
N1		1 or 2 regional lymph nodes with the following features:
N1a	IIIA(ii)	1 or 2 lymph node metastases of 5 mm or less
N1b	IIIA(i)	1 lymph node metastasis 5 mm or greater
N2		Regional lymph node metastasis with the following features:
N2a	IIIB	3 or more lymph node metastases each < 5 mm
N2b	IIIB	2 or more lymph node metastases 5 mm or greater
N2c	IIIC	Lymph node metastases with extracapsular spread
N3	IVA(ii)	Fixed or ulcerated regional lymph node metastasis
Distant metastasis (M)		
M0		No distant metastasis
M1	IVB	Distant metastasis (including pelvic lymph node metastasis)

[a] Depth being measured from the epithelial–stromal junction of the most adjacent superficial dermal papilla to the deepest point of invasion. Adapted from UICC (2009) and FIGO staging (Pecorelli, 2009).

radiotherapy to the groin and pelvic nodes include involvement of two or more lymph nodes or complete replacement/extracapsular spread in any node (RCOG/BGCS, 2014).

More recently, two other options have been studied: the use of unilateral lymph node dissection in place of bilateral and the use of sentinel node biopsy (SNB) which, if negative, may completely avoid a groin node dissection.

In their Cochrane review, Ansink *et al.* (2000) suggest that a unilateral lymph node dissection is safe for lateral tumours (staged at cT1 N0 M0).

Regarding SNB, a systematic review and meta-analysis of 47 studies concluded that this is an accurate staging method with a combined radioactive tracer and blue dye (Hassanzade *et al.*, 2013). The GOG-173 study of 452 patients with vulval carcinomas of at least 1 mm depth, 2–6 cm in size and no clinically detectable groin nodes found the SNB to be 91.7% sensitive with a false-negative rate of 3.7% (Levenback *et al.*, 2012).

In a prospective multicenter study of 403 patients (GROINSS-V study), those who were node-negative on SNB and did not have any further surgical management had a low groin recurrence rate (3%) and a 97% 3-year survival rate (Van der Zee *et al.*, 2008). A follow-on study, the GROINSS-V-II study, is continuing to look at the safety of observation following a negative sentinel node and studying the optimum management of patients with a positive sentinel node. Although not yet widely available, the initial success of SNB has led some to argue that this is becoming the standard of care in selected patients (Robison *et al.*, 2014).

Locally advanced disease: stages III and IVA

For patients who are known to have stage III or IVA disease prior to treatment, multimodality treatment is often planned. Treatment is individualised for this heterogeneous group of patients, and multidisciplinary team involvement is crucial. Locoregionally advanced vulval cancer is uncommon and there are very few randomised trials to guide treatment decisions.

Options for advanced disease include the following.

(1) Surgery.

- Radical vulvectomy and BGND is the most commonly adopted approach and surgery is performed if it is felt that negative margins will be achieved.
- For stage IVA disease a pelvic exenteration may be performed; this very radical procedure involves the formation of one or two stomas, and rigorous preoperative work-up and counselling are required.
- Postoperative radiotherapy to the primary may be indicated in patients with positive or close resection margins (< 8 mm) if further surgery is not possible (Heaps *et al.*, 1990; Faul *et al.*, 1997).
- Postoperative radiotherapy to the nodes is indicated in patients with two or more lymph nodes or complete replacement/extracapsular spread in any node (RCOG/BGCS, 2014).

(2) Neoadjuvant radiotherapy or chemoradiotherapy followed by surgery.

- This approach can be considered in those who have initially inoperable disease or with the aim of sphincter-sparing in patients who would otherwise require pelvic exenteration. Phase II data have shown responses to neoadjuvant chemoradiotherapy with cisplatin and 5-FU (Moore *et al.*, 1998), with 46.5% of patients having no remaining visible disease at the time of surgery.
- Cochrane reviews (van Doorn *et al.*, 2006) have suggested that this approach can reduce tumour size and improve operability rates, although it can result in severe morbidity. An updated review (Shylasree *et al.*, 2011), based on one RCT and two non-randomised studies, suggests that there is no detriment to survival with neoadjuvant chemoradiotherapy followed by surgery over surgery alone.

(3) Primary radiotherapy or chemoradiotherapy in those unfit for surgery or with very locally advanced disease. The toxicity can be considerable and caution should be advised when treating frail patients.

- There are no direct comparative studies of chemoradiotherapy compared with radiotherapy alone in these patients; however, many centres extrapolate from the use of chemoradiotherapy in cervical cancer and advocate its use. Commonly used agents include cisplatin, with or without 5-FU.
- Data on the benefit of this approach are limited to case series which suggest chemoradiotherapy results in a complete response rate of 50–60% which is frequently sustained (Russell *et al.*, 1992; Koh *et al.*, 1993; Whalen *et al.*, 1995; Cunningham *et al.*, 1997).

Radiotherapy and chemoradiotherapy techniques

Postoperative radiotherapy

Patient preparation

The patient lies supine on the couch with arms on the chest. An introital marker may be used. A planning CT is acquired, or, if not available an A–P X-ray film.

CT planning

- Postoperative radiotherapy to the vulva: the clinical target volume (CTV) includes the surgical scar and remaining vulval tissues. A boost dose can be considered to the vulva if macroscopic residual disease remains, which may be delivered using photons or electrons.
- Postoperative radiotherapy to the nodal regions: CTV includes the inguinofemoral nodes and the distal external and internal iliac nodes. If CT planning is used the nodal regions are delineated using a 7-mm margin around the blood vessels to create the CTV, expanding as necessary particularly in the inguinal regions to cover additional at-risk regions such as the tumour bed or any visible remaining nodes.

Conventional field borders for nodes

- Superior border: mid-SI joints.
- Inferior border: to cover the inferior pubic ramus. Extend the lower border down to cover the vulva if treated.
- Lateral borders: to cover the groin nodes (approximately through the long axis of the femoral shaft).

Field arrangement

Typically parallel-opposed anterior and posterior fields or a conformal plan. Bolus may be required if areas of the PTV are close to the skin surface.

Dose and fractionation

Forty-five grays in 25 fractions over 5 weeks to the mid-plane (ICRU reference point) using 6–10 MV photons.

Verification

Portal beam imaging is taken on the first 3 days of treatment and weekly thereafter for verification.

Preoperative or primary radiotherapy or chemoradiotherapy

This is given in two phases, the first phase treating the primary tumour plus nodes to a total of 45 Gy in 25 fractions. Subsequently, consideration should be given to surgical removal of residual disease if possible, or to a second phase of radiotherapy with electrons or brachytherapy to a total dose of 60–65 Gy in 1.8–2.0 Gy fractions (Board of the Faculty of Clinical Oncology, Royal College of Radiologists, 2006).

Patient preparation

The patient lies supine with arms by sides and knees supported by a wedge. An A–P X-ray film or planning CT scan is acquired.

CT planning

- Phase I: the gross tumour volume (GTV) comprises the primary tumour and any involved nodes. The CTV is the vulva, GTV plus a 2-cm margin, as well as lymph nodes. These are defined by outlining the pelvic blood vessels (in this case the distal internal and external iliac and inguinofemoral vessels) and adding a 7-mm margin, expanding as necessary, particularly in the inguinal regions to cover other visible nodes. If there is concern about lymph node involvement,

the upper internal and external iliac nodes may also be included, although this will increase toxicity.
- Phase II: the clinical target volume, e.g. with electrons: gross disease with a 2 cm margin.

Conventional field borders for phase I:

- superior border: mid SI joints, extended to sacral promontory if concern about extent of lymph node involvement;
- inferior border: 2–3 cm below the vulva;
- lateral borders: to cover groin nodes (approximately through the long axis of the femoral shaft).

Field arrangement

- For phase I, parallel-opposed anterior and posterior fields or a conformal plan are used, with bolus as necessary to sites of disease that are infiltrating skin or regions of the PTV that are close to the skin surface.
- For phase II, if electrons are used, the energy is determined by the depth of the tumour, with bolus as necessary.

Dose and fractionation

For phase I, 45 Gy in 25 fractions to the ICRU reference point (often the midplane) using 10 MV photons are given. For phase II, if surgery is not an option, a boost with electrons can be used to take the total dose to macroscopic areas of disease to 60–65 Gy in 1.8–2 Gy per fraction. If it is not possible to use electrons then megavoltage irradiation can be used. Interstitial brachytherapy can also be considered.

Verification

Portal beam images are taken on the first 3 days of treatment and weekly thereafter for verification.

Concurrent chemotherapy

Concurrent chemotherapy involves giving cisplatin 40 mg/m^2 weekly for 5 weeks or cisplatin 50 mg/m^2 days 1 and 29, and fluorouracil 1000 mg/m^2 every 24 hours for days 1–4 and 29–32.

Toxicity of chemoradiotherapy

Chemoradiotherapy toxicity is shown in Table 29.4.

Table 29.4 Toxicity of chemoradiotherapy for carcinoma of the vulva

Toxicity	Management
Acute	
Anaemia	Weekly monitoring of FBC, blood transfusion
Diarrhoea	Loperamide
Skin erythema and desquamation	1% hydrocortisone cream or Intrasite® gel Break from treatment
Fatigue	Activity pacing, goal-setting, stress management
Myelosuppression/ neutropenic sepsis	Weekly FBC, advice to monitor temperature if unwell, treat sepsis according to local protocol
Nausea and vomiting	Dexamethasone and metoclopramide with chemotherapy
Peripheral neuropathy/ renal impairment	Clinical monitoring and cisplatin dose modification
Late	
Menopause	Hormone replacement therapy
Infertility	Advice re adoption, surrogacy as appropriate
Severe radiation toxicity to bowel or bladder (risk 3–10%)	Algorithm-based approach for bowel toxicity (Andreyev et al., 2013). For bladder, pelvic floor exercises, medical/surgical management.
Vaginal shortening and narrowing	Use of vaginal dilators, lubricants

Palliative radiotherapy

This can be useful for controlling pain or bleeding, and either photons or electrons can be used. Typical doses include: 30 Gy in 10 fractions, 20 Gy in 5 fractions or a single 8–10 Gy.

Palliative chemotherapy

There are few studies to elucidate the first choice of chemotherapy agent and there is no current standard regimen. A phase II trial of 15 patients has demonstrated a 40% response rate and median overall survival of 19 months in those treated with cisplatin and vinorelbine. A combination of bleomycin, methotrexate and

CCNU (Wagenaar et al., 2001), and the use of paclitaxel have also been reported (Witteveen et al., 2009) as active in advanced vulval cancer. More recently, the use of erlotinib in vulval cancer has been suggested as potentially beneficial in a phase II trial of 41 patients (Horowitz et al., 2012).

Recurrent disease

Most recurrences occur in the perineal area (53.4%), although inguinal (18.7%), pelvic (5.7%) and distant (7.9%) recurrences can occur (Maggino et al., 2000). If the disease recurs in the vulva following limited surgery, it can often be removed with a more radical excision or pelvic exenteration. Alternatively, chemoradiotherapy has been reported to give long-term disease control in 8 of 15 patients (Thomas et al., 1989).

Recurrences in the inguinal nodes following surgery may respond to chemoradiotherapy. Surgery for groin recurrences following radiotherapy has a high complication rate.

Prognosis

Prognostic factors

The most significant prognostic factor is the presence of involved inguinofemoral lymph nodes, with 5-year survival rates reducing from 70–93% in node-negative patients to 25–41% in those who are node-positive (Gadducci et al., 2006). A tumour diameter greater than 3.5–4 cm is also associated with a poorer prognosis (Iacoponi et al., 2013; Zanvettor et al., 2014).

Prognosis

Overall mortality is approximately one-quarter of those patients diagnosed. Five-year survival rates by stage group are shown in Table 29.5 (Beller et al., 2006).

Areas of current interest

The apparent potential of SNB to spare many women with a negative sentinel node from the morbidity of groin node dissection has led to further interest in defining the management with a positive sentinel node, in particular whether those with a very small volume nodal metastasis require a full groin dissection.

As with many tumour sites, the use of IMRT is being assessed (Beriwal et al., 2008).

Pharmacological interventions are also of interest: for prevention, the use of HPV vaccine; for

Table 29.5 Five-year survival of vulval carcinoma by stage grouping, Beller *et al.,* (2006)

FIGO stage	Five-year survival (%)
I	78.5
II	58.8
III	43.2
IV	13

treatment of VIN, imiquimod, an immune stimulant, cidofovir, an antiviral agent, and photodynamic therapy; for established cancers, the use of biological agents.

Ongoing clinical trials

At the time of writing, the following trials were registered with the UK clinical research network (http://public.ukcrn.org.uk, accessed December 2014).

GROINSS-V II: GROningen INternational Study on Sentinel nodes in Vulvar cancer: assessing whether radiotherapy is as safe as surgery (± radiotherapy) in sentinel node-positive vulvar cancer where there is < 2 mm involvement.

EPIVIN: a phase II trial investigating the use of epigallocatechin-3-gallate in the treatment of VIN.

NCRN396 VE BASKET: a phase II study of vemurafenib in patients with BRAF V600 mutation-positive cancers.

RT3 VIN is a randomised phase II multicentre trial of topical treatment in women with VIN which has recently closed to recruitment and results are awaited.

References

Andreyev, H. J., Benton, B., Lalji, A., *et al.* (2013). Algorithm-based management of patients with gastrointestinal symptoms in patients after pelvic radiation treatment (ORBIT): a randomised controlled trial. *Lancet*, **382**, 2084–2092.

Ansink, A., van der Velden, J. and Collingwood, M. (2000). Surgical intervention for early squamous cell carcinoma of the vulva. *Cochrane Database Syst. Rev.*, **4**.

Beller, U, Quinn, M. A., Benedet, J. L., *et al.* (2006). Carcinoma of the vulva. FIGO 26th annual report on the results of treatment in gynecological cancer. *Int. J. Gynaecol. Obstet.*, **95**(Suppl. 1), S7–27.

Beriwal, S., Coon, D., Heron, D. E., *et al.* (2008). Preoperative intensity-modulated radiotherapy and chemotherapy for locally advanced vulvar carcinoma. *Gynecol. Oncol.*, **109**, 291–295.

Board of the Faculty of Clinical Oncology, Royal College of Radiologists. (2006). *Radiotherapy Dose-Fractionation.* London: Royal College of Radiologists.

Cunningham, M. J., Goyer, R. P., Gibbons, S. K., *et al.* (1997). Primary radiation, cisplatin and 5-fluorouracil for advanced squamous carcinoma of the vulva. *Gynecol. Oncol.*, **66**, 258–261.

de Sanjosé, S., Alemany, L., Ordi, J., *et al.* (2013). Worldwide human papillomavirus genotype attribution in over 2000 cases of intraepithelial and invasive lesions of the vulva. *Eur. J. Cancer*, **49**, 3450–3461.

Faul, C. M., Mirmow, D., Huang, Q., *et al.* (1997). Adjuvant radiation for vulvar carcinoma: improved local control. *Int. J. Radiat. Oncol. Biol. Phys.*, **38**, 381–389.

Gaarenstroom, K. N., Kenter, G. G., Trimbos, J. B., *et al.* (2003). Postoperative complications after vulvectomy and inguinofemoral lymphadenectomy using separate groin incisions. *Int. J.Gynecol. Cancer*, **13**, 522–527.

Gadducci, A., Cionini, L., Romanini, A., *et al.* (2006). Old and new perspectives in the management of high-risk, locally advanced or recurrent, and metastatic vulvar cancer. *Crit. Rev. Oncol. Hematol.*, **60**, 227–241.

Hacker, N. F., Leuchter, R. S., Berek, J. S., *et al.* (1981). Radical vulvectomy and bilateral inguinal lymphadenectomy through separate groin incisions. *Obstet. Gynecol.*, **58**, 574–579.

Hacker, N.F., Eifel, P.J. and Van der Velden, J. (2012). FIGO cancer report 2012, cancer of the vulva. *Int. J. Gynecol. Cancer*, **119**(Suppl. 2), S90–S96.

Hassanzade, M., Attaran, M., Treglia, G., *et al.* (2013). Lymphatic mapping and sentinel node biopsy in squamous cell carcinoma of the vulva: systematic review and meta-analysis of the literature. *Gynecol. Oncol.*, **130**, 237–245.

Heaps, J. M., Fu, Y. S., Montz, F. J., *et al.*(1990). Surgical–pathologic variables predictive of local recurrence in squamous cell carcinoma of the vulva. *Gynecol. Oncol.*, **38**, 309–314.

Homesley, H. D., Bundy, B. N., Sedlis, A., *et al.* (1986). Radiation therapy versus pelvic node resection for carcinoma of the vulva with positive groin nodes. *Obstet. Gynecol.*, **68**, 733–740.

Horowitz, N. S., Olawaiye, A. B., Borger, D.R., *et al.* (2012). Phase II trial of erlotinib in women with squamous cell carcinoma of the vulva. *Gynecol. Oncol.*, **127**, 141–146.

Iacoponi, S., Zapardiel, I., Diestro, M. D., *et al.* (2013). Prognostic factors associated with local recurrence in squamous cell carcinoma of the vulva. *J. Gynecol. Oncol.*, **24**, 242–248.

Koh, W. J., Wallace, H. J. 3rd, Greer, B. E., *et al.* (1993). Combined radiotherapy and chemotherapy in the management of locally–regionally advanced vulvar cancer. *Int. J. Radiat. Oncol. Biol. Phys.*, **26**, 809–816.

Land, R., Herod, J., Moskovic, E., *et al.* (2006). Routine computerized tomography scanning, groin ultrasound with or without fine needle aspiration cytology in the surgical management of primary squamous cell carcinoma of the vulva. *Int. J. Gynecol. Cancer*, **16**, 312–317.

Levenback, C. F., Ali, S. and Coleman, R. L. (2012). Lymphatic mapping and sentinel lymph node biopsy in women with squamous cell carcinoma of the vulva: a gynecologic oncology group study. *J. Clin. Oncol.*, **30**, 3786–3791.

Maggino, T., Landoni, F., Sartori, E., *et al.* (2000). Patterns of recurrence in patients with squamous cell carcinoma of the vulva. *Cancer*, **89**, 116–122.

Moore, D. H., Thomas, G. M., Montana, G. S., *et al.* (1998). Preoperative chemoradiation for advanced vulvar cancer: a phase II study of the Gynecologic Oncology Group. *Int. Radiat. Oncol. Biol. Phys.*, **42**, 79–85.

NICE. (2015). *Suspected cancer: recognition and referral. NICE guideline.* London: National Institute for Health and Care Excellence.

Pecorelli, S. (2009). Revised FIGO staging for carcinoma of the vulva, cervix, and endometrium. *Int. J. Gynecol. Obstet.*, **105**(2), 103–104.

RCOG/BGCS. (2014). *Guidelines for the Diagnosis and Management of Vulval Carcinoma.* London: Royal College Obstetricians and Gynaecologists.

Robison, K., Fiascone, S. and Moore, R. (2014). Vulvar cancer and sentinel lymph nodes: a new standard of care? *Expert Rev. Anticancer Ther.* **14**, 975–977.

Russell, A. H., Mesic, J. B., Scudder, S. A., *et al.* (1992). Synchronous radiation and cytotoxic chemotherapy for locally advanced or recurrent squamous cancer of the vulva. *Gynecol. Oncol.*, **47**, 14–20.

Shylasree, T. S., Bryant, A. and Howells, R. E. J. (2011). Chemoradiation for advanced primary vulval cancer. *Cochrane Database Syst. Rev.*, Issue 4, CD003752.

Thomas, G., Dembo, A., DePetrillo, A., *et al.* (1989). Concurrent radiation and chemotherapy in vulvar carcinoma. *Gynecol. Oncol.*, **34**, 263–267.

UICC. (2009). *TNM Classification of Malignant Tumours*, ed. L.H. Sobin, M. Gospodarowicz and Ch. Wittekind, 7th edn. Chichester: Wiley-Blackwell.

Van der Zee, A. G., Oonk, M. H., De Hullu, J. A., *et al.* (2008). Sentinel node dissection is safe in the treatment of early-stage vulvar cancer. *J. Clin. Oncol.*, **26**, 884–889.

van Doorn, H. C., Ansink, A., Verhaar-Langereis, M., *et al.* (2006). Neoadjuvant chemoradiation for advanced primary vulvar cancer. *Cochrane Database Syst. Rev.*, Jul 19;(3):CD003752.

Wagenaar, H. C., Colombo, N., Vergote, I., *et al.* (2001). Bleomycin, methotrexate, and CCNU in locally advanced or recurrent, inoperable, squamous-cell carcinoma of the vulva: an EORTC Gynaecological Cancer Cooperative Group Study. European Organization for Research and Treatment of Cancer. *Gynecol. Oncol.*, **81**, 348–354.

Wahlen, S. A., Slater, J. D., Wagner, R. J., *et al.* (1995). Concurrent radiation therapy and chemotherapy in the treatment of primary squamous cell carcinoma of the vulva. *Cancer*, **75**, 2289–2294.

WHO. (2003). *World Health Organization Classification of Tumours: Pathology and Genetics of Tumours of the Breast and Female Genital Organs*, ed. F.A. Tavassoli and P. Devilee. Lyon: IARC Press, Chapter 7.

Witteveen, P. O., Van der Velden, J. and Vergote, I. (2009). Phase II study on paclitaxel in patients with recurrent, metastatic or locally advanced vulvar cancer not amenable to surgery or radiotherapy: a study of the EORTC-GCG (European Organisation for Research and Treatment of Cancer – Gynaecological Cancer Group). *Ann. Oncol.*, **20**, 1511–1516.

Zanvettor, P. H., Falcão Filho, D. F., Soares, F. A., *et al.* (2014). Study of biomolecular and clinical prognostic factors in patients with cancer of the vulva undergoing surgical treatment. *Int. J. Gynecol. Cancer*, **24**, 766–772.

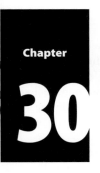

Management of gestational trophoblast tumours

Philip Savage

Introduction

Gestational trophoblast tumours (GTT) form a spectrum of rare diagnoses from the usually benign partial and complete molar pregnancies through to the aggressive malignancies of choriocarcinoma and placental site trophoblast tumour. The majority of care for the patients with molar pregnancies takes place in their local hospitals, with less than 10% of patients needing chemotherapy treatment. The cure rate for postmolar pregnancy GTT is 100% and most patients only need single-agent chemotherapy treatment. For the patients with rarer diagnoses of choriocarcinoma or placental site trophoblast tumour (PSTT), nearly all will be cured, even those presenting unwell with advanced metastatic cancer.

To provide an effective service in the UK for these rare conditions the Department of Health directly funds a national trophoblast service that cares for all patients with GTT. The trophoblast service has two specialist treatment centres, one at Weston Park Hospital in Sheffield and the other at Charing Cross Hospital in London. These centres, in addition to providing expert clinical care, also run the national human chorionic gonadotrophin (hCG) surveillance and follow-up programmes in conjunction with the Scottish follow-up centre in Dundee.

Although the main clinical care for GTT patients is centralised in the UK, it remains important for all oncologists to have a working knowledge of GTT because choriocarcinoma and PSTT can present as malignancies of unknown primary. In these patients, early involvement from the local oncology team in achieving the correct diagnosis and expediting treatment can be life-saving.

The pattern of GTT management in other countries varies; some countries have established centralised care, whereas in many other countries, patients are treated locally by doctors who are likely to only see a case every few years.

This chapter outlines the pathology, natural history and management of GTT based on the experience of the UK GTT service at Charing Cross Hospital in London.

Types of gestational trophoblast tumour

Gestational trophoblast tumours are divided into the premalignant partial and complete molar pregnancies and the malignant forms of invasive mole, choriocarcinoma and PSTT, as shown in Table 30.1. All forms of GTT constitutively produce hCG, although abnormalities of the molecule from some tumour cells can lead to false-negative results occasionally in some types of hCG assays (Cole *et al.*, 2001).

The normal range for hCG in pre menopausal women is 0–4 IU/L, while levels in postmenopausal women can reach up to 15 IU/L (Cole *et al.*, 2007). In pregnancy the hCG levels rise very rapidly and peak at around 200,000 IU/L at weeks 8–12; following this, the levels decline to 5000–50,000 IU/L by the time of delivery and should fall back to normal within 3 weeks postpartum. As a general rule, an elevated hCG level in the absence of a pregnancy can be taken as very strong evidence of a malignancy. The most frequent causes in younger women are gestational or germ cell tumours, although other types of malignancy including lung, stomach and bladder cancer can also make detectable hCG in rare cases (Stenman *et al.*, 2004). A very small number of women can have constitutively naturally elevated hCG levels generally in the range of 100–300 IU/L without any underlying pathology (Palmieri *et al.*, 2007).

Practical Clinical Oncology, Second Edition, ed. Louise Hanna, Tom Crosby and Fergus Macbeth. Published by Cambridge University Press. © Cambridge University Press 2015.

Table 30.1 Types of gestational trophoblast tumour

Premalignant	Partial hydatidiform mole
	Complete hydatidiform mole
Malignant	Invasive mole
	Choriocarcinoma
	Placental site trophoblast tumour

Premalignant forms of GTT

The premalignant forms of GTT, partial and complete molar pregnancies are rare and occur at a combined overall frequency of 1 case for every 607 viable pregnancies in the UK population (Savage *et al.*, 2013). While both occur as a result of a genetic error at the time of fertilisation, partial and complete molar pregnancies differ significantly in their clinical presentation, age-related risks, genetic make-up and their risk of malignant change.

Partial mole

In a partial molar pregnancy, the trophoblast cells are triploid with 69 chromosomes. There are two sets of paternal and one set of maternal chromosomes occurring as a result of the ovum being fertilised by two sperm. In the first trimester in an early ultrasound assessment, a partial mole may resemble a normal conception. However, the embryo, if present, becomes non-viable by week 10. Many partial moles are not suspected clinically and the diagnosis is made only after pathological review. It is likely that the partial molar pregnancies are underdiagnosed because these early cases may only show focal changes and be pathologically far less florid than complete moles. As a result, the diagnosis of a partial mole may occasionally be missed. However, as the risk of malignant change in partial moles is only 1:100, this issue rarely causes a clinical problem.

The most frequent clinical presentations of a partial mole are either via bleeding in the first trimester or more frequently as a failed pregnancy. The gynaecological management is by suction or medical evacuation and despite the low risk of malignant change, it is recommended that all patients undergo hCG follow-up and monitoring.

Complete mole

In a complete molar pregnancy, the maternal DNA is lost during the development of the ovum or at the time of fertilisation and the genetic material is entirely of male origin. Most commonly, the chromosome count is 46XX, which results from a single X sperm duplicating within an ovum that lacks the maternal chromosomes. Less frequently, the genotype can be 46XY, which occurs when an empty ovum is fertilised concurrently by two sperm.

In the UK, the majority of complete moles are diagnosed in the first trimester either following abnormal bleeding or from the first routine ultrasound, which characteristically demonstrates a complex echogenic intrauterine mass with numerous cystic spaces. The management is by suction evacuation and the histology demonstrates oedematous villi and hyperplasia, although the characteristic second-trimester textbook 'bunch of grapes' appearance is now rarely seen due to the earlier diagnosis.

In a complete molar pregnancy there is no foetal development and the risk of malignant change is significantly higher, with an overall risk of approximately 14%.

Demographics of molar pregnancies

The statistics for England and Wales for 2000–2009 show that there were 13,583 molar pregnancies compared to 8,242,511 viable conceptions, indicating an overall 1:607 risk for a molar pregnancy. Of the cases, 43% were complete moles and 57% partial moles. The risks of the two types of molar pregnancy and the subsequent risk for needing chemotherapy treatment, after the uterine evacuation, vary significantly with the maternal age, as shown in Table 30.2 (Savage *et al.*, 2013).

The international data on molar pregnancy incidence have historically shown considerable variation, with rates of up to 40.2 per 1000 births reported in the Far East. However, the more recent Korean data suggest that the reported incidence has now fallen to 2.3 per 1000, close to the European rates (Kim *et al.*, 2004). It is presently unclear whether these changes are a result of improvements in diagnostic accuracy or exogenous factors, such as changes to a Western diet.

Fortunately, the majority of women need no additional treatment after their evacuation and for those requiring chemotherapy treatment the cure rate is 100%. One of the key issues for many women is their risk of having another molar pregnancy in their next pregnancy. The data on this are reassuring, but also show an age-related trend in risk, with a risk of 1 in 80 for women aged 20–39 but rising to 1 in 32 for women

Table 30.2 The variation in the risk of having a complete (CM) or partial (PM) molar pregnancy occurring related to the maternal age. The incidence data are relative to the number of conceptions (births and terminations) within that age range. For the cases of CM and PM occurring in each age range, the risk for requiring chemotherapy is also shown

Age	CM incidence	Chemo risk for CM (%)	PM incidence	Chemo risk for PM (%)
≤19	1:926	3.7	1:1471	0.3
20–24	1:1538	8.0	1:1450	0.7
25–29	1:1620	13.8	1:1115	1.1
30–34	1:1824	17.0	1:971	1.5
35–39	1:1834	17.9	1:833	1.1
40–44	1:735	23.4	1:578	1.1
45–49	1:78	21.5	1:286	–
50+	1:7	30.5	1:100	–
Overall	1:1428	13.6	1:1057	1.1

aged 40–44 and 1 in 8 for those aged 45 and over (Savage *et al.*, 2013).

In addition to molar pregnancies with the conventional genetic structures, there is a very rare syndrome where women have recurrent molar pregnancies. In this syndrome of familial hydatidiform mole the molar pregnancies have the pathological appearance of a complete mole but contain 23 chromosomes from each partner and are termed biparental moles. This syndrome is very rare and is due to a defect in the *NALP7* gene and should be suspected in women with three molar pregnancies or a strong family history (Helwani *et al.*, 1999). Women with this syndrome are extremely unlikely to achieve a normal pregnancy, but assisted conception using egg donation appears to be a successful method to achieve pregnancy (Fisher *et al.*, 2011).

Screening after a molar pregnancy

In the majority of patients with molar pregnancy, the abnormal trophoblast cells are unable to sustain their growth and as the cells die off the hCG levels return to normal and no further treatment is required. However, in approximately 14% of complete moles and 1% of partial moles, the abnormal trophoblast cells can continue to grow, invade locally and potentially metastasise.

At present, there is no accurate way of predicting which patients with molar pregnancies will develop persistent, invasive or metastatic disease. However, as the trophoblast cells constitutively produce hCG,

monitoring the hCG level can provide an accurate assessment of regression or growth.

The UK has had a national hCG-based screening service in place for over 40 years. All patients diagnosed with a molar pregnancy are registered, and samples are sent for hCG measurement every 2 weeks. The analysis of the results allows the careful monitoring of patients with regressing disease as the hCG level falls and allows early identification of patients who require treatment before the development of any major problems.

The diagnosis of the change from a premalignant form of GTT to a malignant form is usually made clinically, based on the clinical assessment and in particular, the pattern of change of the hCG level. In contrast, information from a further biopsy in these patients is rarely of clinical value and should be avoided because these highly vascular tumours can bleed very heavily.

At Charing Cross Hospital, patients who require chemotherapy treatment after a molar pregnancy are generally referred to as having postmolar pregnancy GTT. Although the condition is scientifically a malignancy, we try to avoid using the word 'cancer' with these patients, as they have a 100% cure rate.

Indications for further treatment in molar pregnancy patients following uterine evacuation

Retrospective analysis of data from the surveillance programme has allowed the identification of some key indications for chemotherapy treatment for patients undergoing postmolar pregnancy surveillance. These data have been used to produce the current FIGO recommendations for treatment after the evacuation of a molar pregnancy (FIGO Oncology Committee, 2002):

- an hCG level plateau of four values ±10% recorded over a 3-week duration (days 1, 7, 14 and 21);
- an hCG level increase of more than 10% of three values recorded over a 2-week duration (days 1, 7 and 14);
- persistence of detectable hCG for more than 6 months after molar evacuation.

In addition to these three main indications, a number of other routinely used indications for treatment are also used at Charing Cross Hospital, including heavy PV bleeding or GI/intraperitoneal bleeding, the presence of vulval or vaginal metastases or an hCG level of greater than 20,000 IU/L more than 4 weeks after evacuation.

A small minority of these patients with indications for treatment could be cured by a second uterine evacuation, but the majority of patients will need chemotherapy. Analysis of the data from both Sheffield and Charing Cross suggests that a second uterine evacuation is rarely of benefit in patients if the hCG level is higher than 5000 IU/L and now second evacuations are only rarely recommended (Pezeshki et al., 2004; Savage and Seckl, 2005).

Malignant forms of GTT

Invasive mole

An invasive mole generally arises from a complete mole and is characterised by invasion of the myometrium, which can lead to perforation of the uterus. Histologically, an invasive mole appears similar to a complete mole, but is characterised by the ability to invade the myometrium if left untreated. With the introduction of routine ultrasound, the early evacuation of complete moles and effective hCG surveillance, the diagnosis of invasive moles has become very rare in the UK.

Choriocarcinoma

Histologically and clinically, choriocarcinoma is obviously malignant and it presents the most frequent cause of emergency medical problems in the management of trophoblast disease. Choriocarcinoma can rarely follow a complete molar pregnancy, but most frequently occurs after a term pregnancy, with an estimated frequency of 1 case per 50,000 live births. In suspected cases a tissue biopsy is often hazardous because of the risk of bleeding and is best avoided, as usually a clinical diagnosis can be made safely.

When histopathology is available, the characteristic findings of choriocarcinoma show sheets of syncytiotrophoblast or cytotrophoblast cells with haemorrhage, necrosis and intravascular growth. Genetically, choriocarcinoma contains DNA from both the mother and her partner and can have a range of gross chromosomal abnormalities but without any specific characteristic patterns.

Despite the differing genetic origins of postmolar pregnancy GTT and choriocarcinoma occurring after term pregnancy, the treatment and response are determined by the overall prognostic scores rather than by the specific histology.

Patients with choriocarcinoma can present with bleeding from the disease locally in the uterus or with a wide variety of symptoms from distant metastases, with the lungs, central nervous system and liver being the most frequent sites of distant disease.

All patients with gestational choriocarcinoma are seen urgently in view of the risk of bleeding or life-threatening pulmonary or CNS disease and similarly all PSTT patients are reviewed promptly irrespective of disease stage.

Placental site trophoblast tumour

PSTTs arise from the intermediate trophoblast cells and are the least common type of gestational trophoblast disease in that they form fewer than 2% of all cases, with an average of only two or three cases in the UK each year. Most frequently, PSTT follows a normal pregnancy, but it can rarely occur after a non-molar abortion or a molar pregnancy. The clinical presentation of PSTT can range from slow-growing disease limited to the uterus to more rapidly growing metastatic disease that is similar in behaviour to choriocarcinoma.

The average interval between the previous pregnancy and presentation of PSTT is 3.4 years and the most frequent presentations are bleeding and amenorrhoea. In PSTT, the hCG level, although elevated, is characteristically lower for the volume of disease than in the other types of GTT (Schmid et al., 2009).

Pretreatment investigations in GTT patients

For the majority of patients with GTT following a recent molar pregnancy, the only investigations routinely performed prior to consideration of chemotherapy treatment are an updated serum hCG level, a Doppler ultrasound of the pelvis and a chest X-ray. These tests allow the formal exclusion of a new pregnancy as the cause of the hCG elevation, a measurement of the uterine tumour size and an indication of the presence of any pulmonary metastases. The information is used as part of the FIGO prognostic scoring system that determines the intensity of the initial chemotherapy treatment. Additionally, the presence of pulmonary metastases on the chest X-ray is an indication that prophylactic intrathecal chemotherapy with methotrexate should be considered.

In contrast, patients presenting with choriocarcinoma or PSTT are fully staged with CT scans of the thorax, abdomen and pelvis and MRI scans of the pelvis and the brain. These patients frequently have non-pulmonary metastases and the presence of CNS or hepatic disease will alter the choice of initial chemo-therapy treatment.

Staging classification and prognostic classification

The FIGO staging classification for GTT is shown in Table 30.3. However, the value of full anatomical staging in optimising the treatment in GTT is relatively limited.

At Charing Cross and most other treatment centres, the FIGO prognostic scoring system as shown in Table 30.4 is more frequently used and is of more practical value (FIGO Oncology Committee, 2002). In this system, a number of prognostic factors are scored including the patient's age, prior pregnancy, hCG level and number and sites of metastases; the total score produced is used to place patients into either low-risk or high-risk prognostic and initial treatment groups.

For patients who fall into the low-risk prognostic group with a FIGO score of 0–6, treatment is generally commenced using relatively gentle chemotherapy with intramuscular methotrexate and folinic acid. In the high-risk prognostic group, with a FIGO score of 7 and above, historical data show that only about 10% of patients would be cured with single-agent methotrexate chemotherapy and treatment is usually started using the combination EMA-CO regimen.

Chemotherapy treatment of GTT

Low-risk disease management

The most widely used standard therapy for patients with low-risk trophoblast disease is intramuscular methotrexate given with oral folinic acid rescue, as shown in Table 30.5. At Charing Cross Hospital, the first course of treatment is given as an inpatient procedure, due to the initial high risks from bleeding at the commencement of treatment, with the subsequent courses administered closer to home.

The low-dose methotrexate chemotherapy treatment is usually well tolerated without major toxicity. Methotrexate does not cause alopecia or significant nausea, and myelosuppression is rare. The most common side effects are pleural inflammation, mucositis and hepatic toxicity, but each of these occurs only rarely and can generally be managed conservatively.

For the low-risk patients with lung metastases visible on their chest X-ray, central nervous system prophylaxis with intrathecal methotrexate (12.5 mg) is administered on three occasions, 2 weeks apart.

All patients on treatment have their hCG levels checked twice a week and following hCG normalisation, treatment is continued for another three complete

Table 30.3 FIGO staging of gestational trophoblast tumours

Stage	Description
Stage I	Tumour confined to the uterus
Stage II	Tumour extends outside of the uterus, but is limited to the genital structures (adnexa, vagina, broad ligament)
Stage III	Tumour extends to the lungs with or without genital tract involvement
Stage IV	Tumour involves all other metastatic sites

From FIGO Oncology Committee (2002).

Table 30.4 The FIGO prognostic scoring system

	Prognostic score			
Prognostic factor	0	1	2	4
Age	< 40	≥ 40	–	
Antecedent pregnancy	Mole	Abortion	Term	
Months from index pregnancy	< 4	4–6	7 to < 13	≥ 13
Pretreatment hCG (IU/L)	< 1000	1000–10,000	10,000–100,000	> 100,000
Largest tumour size	< 3 cm	3 to < 5 cm	≥ 5 cm	–
Site of metastases	Lung	Spleen, kidney	Gastrointestinal	Brain, liver
Number of metastases	–	1–4	5–8	> 8
Previous chemotherapy	–	–	Single agent	Two or more drugs

The total prognostic score is calculated by adding up individual scores for each prognostic factor. Total score of 6 or less = low risk; a score of 7 or more = high risk. From FIGO Oncology Committee (2002).

Table 30.5 Chemotherapy regimens for trophoblast tumours

Regimen	Description
Methotrexate/ folinic acid	Day 1, methotrexate 50 mg i.m. at noon
	Day 2, folinic acid 30 mg p.o. at 6 p.m.
	Day 3, methotrexate 50 mg i.m. at noon
	Day 4, folinic acid 30 mg p.o. at 6 p.m.
	Day 5, methotrexate 50 mg i.m. at noon
	Day 6, folinic acid 30 mg p.o. at 6 p.m.
	Day 7, methotrexate 50 mg i.m. at noon
	Day 8, folinic acid 30 mg p.o. at 6 p.m.
EMA-CO	*Week 1*
	Day 1, actinomycin-D 0.5 mg i.v., etoposide 100 mg/m² i.v., methotrexate 300 mg/m² i.v.
	Day 2, actinomycin-D 0.5 mg i.v., etoposide 100 mg/m² i.v., folinic acid 15 mg p.o. 12-hourly × 4 doses (starting 24 hrs after commencing methotrexate)
	Week 2
	Day 8, vincristine 1.4 mg/m² (max. 2 mg) i.v., cyclophosphamide 600 mg/m² i.v.

Table 30.6 Outcome in terms of first-line therapy success rate and overall cure rates for patients with low-risk postmolar pregnancy GTT treated initially with single-agent methotrexate and folinic acid

FIGO score	Cure rate with first-line methotrexate alone (%)	Overall cure rate including additional chemotherapy (%)
0	77	100
1	74	100
2	67	100
3	47	100
4	45	100
5	35	100
6	31	100

cycles (6 weeks) to ensure the eradication of any residual disease present below the level of serological detection. Overall, two-thirds of the low-risk patients are successfully treated with methotrexate alone, but there is a significant variation in the success rate of this gentle therapy with the change in the FIGO prognostic score, as shown in Table 30.6 (Sita-Lumsden *et al.*, 2012).

The low-risk patients who have an inadequate response to methotrexate, as shown by an hCG plateau or increase, move on to second-line therapy. For second-line therapy, treatment is changed to either single-agent actinomycin-D at 1.5 mg/m² on day 1 of a 14-day cycle or EMA-CO combination chemotherapy dependent on the hCG level at the time of change. Currently, a serum hCG level of 500 IU/L is used as the upper limit for changing to actinomycin-D. The overall survival of the low-risk treatment group is 100% and the stepwise introduction of more toxic chemotherapy as necessary minimises the long-term toxicity from

treatment in the majority of patients (Sita-Lumsden *et al.*, 2012).

Figure 30.1 shows serum hCG graphs for two patients during treatment for gestational trophoblastic dsease. The first patient (Figure 30.1(a)) was cured rapidly by methotrexate treatment alone. The second patient (Figure 30.1(b)) responded initially to methotrexate, but then required a change to EMA-CO chemotherapy to complete treatment.

High-risk disease management

Historical data from before the introduction of the modern multiagent chemotherapy schedules showed that only 10% of the high-risk prognostic group of patients would be cured with single-agent therapy (Bagshawe *et al.*, 1989).

Fortunately, the introduction of the etoposide containing combination chemotherapy treatments in the late 1970s transformed this situation, and modern series show cure rates of 94% for high-risk patients using EMA-CO chemotherapy (Alifrangis *et al.*, 2013).

The drug combination of etoposide/methotrexate/ actinomycin-D and cyclophosphamide/vincristine gives a dose-intense treatment with the five chemotherapy agents, delivered as two groups 1 week apart, as shown in Table 30.5. However, this regimen is myelosuppressive and support with G-CSF injections is frequently helpful in keeping the treatment on schedule. Fortunately, serious toxicity is rare with EMA-CO and the majority of patients tolerate treatment well. Similarly to that of low-risk patients, treatment is continued for 6 weeks after the normalisation of the hCG

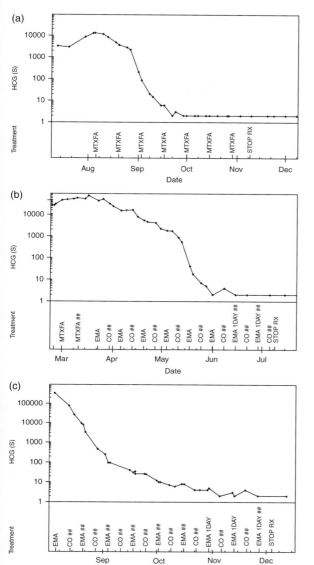

Figure 30.1 Serum hCG graphs for three patients during treatment for gestational trophoblastic disease. (a) A patient who is cured rapidly by methotrexate treatment alone. (b) A patient who responds initially to methotrexate but then requires a change to EMA-CO chemotherapy to complete treatment successfully. (c) A high-risk patient who was treated successfully with EMA-CO chemotherapy. CO, cyclophosphamide, vincristine; EMA, etoposide, methotrexate, actinomycin-D; HCG(S), serum hCG (IU/L); MTXFA, methotrexate and folinic acid; RX = treatment.

level. Figure 30.1(c) shows the treatment graph of a high-risk patient who presented 3 months after the birth of her daughter and was successfully treated with EMA-CO chemotherapy.

Of the high-risk patients treated with EMA-CO, approximately 20% develop resistance to this drug combination and require a change in treatment. In this situation the EP-EMA regimen has been the most frequently used choice, in which cisplatin and a further dose of etoposide replace the vincristine and cyclophosphamide. EP-EMA chemotherapy which may need to be combined with surgery on some occasions produces a cure rate of 90% in this relatively rare group of patients (Newlands *et al.*, 2000). However, EP-EMA is very toxic and a more modern development using a doublet combination of paclitaxel and etoposide alternating with paclitaxel and cisplatin which appears to have similar efficacy but significantly less toxicity (Wang *et al.*, 2008).

The care of high-risk choriocarcinoma patients with complex problems

Choriocarcinoma patients can be very ill at presentation and can deteriorate rapidly if not treated promptly. At Charing Cross Hospital there are facilities for emergency assessment and chemotherapy 24 hours a day and patients can, when necessary, be assessed and started on chemotherapy treatment within 1 hour of arrival.

Among the specific problems that can occur are: CNS metastases, liver metastases, respiratory compromise and life-threatening haemorrhage.

In contrast to most other malignancies in which cerebral metastases are associated with a poor prognosis, trophoblast patients with CNS disease can be routinely cured of their disease. Approximately 4% of the patients who present with trophoblast disease have cerebral metastases at the time of diagnosis.

For patients with cerebral metastases, the EMA-CO regimen is modified to contain a higher dose of methotrexate, which enhances penetration into the CNS. This modification is combined with an intrathecal methotrexate administration given the same week as the CO treatment. For patients with CNS metastases, treatment is continued for 8 weeks after a reaching a normal hCG level.

The published data examining outcomes in choriocarcinoma patients with CNS metastases treated between 1981 and 2000 indicated that 86% of the 39 patients were cured with chemotherapy treatment (Newlands *et al.*, 2002). Figure 30.2 demonstrates MRI scans in a patient with haemorrhagic brain metastases at presentation and at completion of treatment.

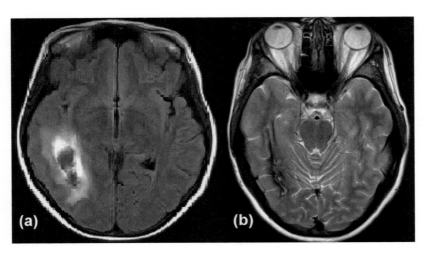

Figure 30.2 MRI scans demonstrating (a) the presence of a parietal metastasis with associated in oedema and haemorrhage in a patient with newly diagnosed choriocarcinoma with disease also in the liver and (b) the follow-up scan after completion of EMA(CNS)-EP, which indicates resolution of the mass and oedema. The patient remains in remission and is almost certainly cured.

Radiotherapy treatment is not used routinely in the care of these patients and once a normal hCG is attained, future relapse is very unusual.

Liver metastases are not seen in postmolar pregnancy GTT and are rare even in patients with choriocarcinoma. A number of publications have suggested that liver metastases are associated with a poorer prognosis and it is the policy at Charing Cross to treat patients with liver metastases with first-line cisplatin-containing chemotherapy. Generally, the EMA-EP regimen is used, although increasingly a change to the TE-TP regimen is used when toxicity becomes a problem. In patients with liver metastases, treatment is also continued for 8 weeks after reaching normal hCG levels. Despite this recent optimisation of care, the overall cure rate for patients with liver metastases is only 50% and the presence of liver disease remains a marker of poorer prognosis (Ahamed *et al.*, 2012).

In patients with multiple lung metastases, the respiratory function can be compromised by the large volume of the tumours and by tumour-associated pulmonary haemorrhage. In these patients it is prudent to start treatment urgently, but to initially use only moderate doses of chemotherapy, to minimise the risk from further bleeding that can happen with rapid tumour shrinkage. This policy introduced approximately 15 years ago has helped improve the survival of critically ill patients (Alifrangis *et al.*, 2013) and the current protocols suggest starting treatment with 1 or 2 days of low-dose etoposide and cisplatin chemotherapy using a protocol based on 1 or 2 non-bleomycin days of the BEP regimen used in germ cell tumours.

GTTs are very vascular and severe bleeding can be a major problem. In the majority of patients this usually occurs in the uterine mass, where effective control can usually be achieved by selective uterine artery embolization (McGrath *et al.*, 2012). Very occasionally, metastases at other sites can bleed heavily, usually from tumour-induced arterio-venous malformations, and embolisation or surgical intervention can be required.

Management of placental site trophoblast tumour

Placental site trophoblast tumours (PSTTs) are very rare and are treated differently from the more common types of trophoblast disease. In contrast to choriocarcinoma, the management of PSST is greatly influenced by the disease stage. In cases where the disease is limited to the uterus, hysterectomy is often curative, while in patients with metastatic disease, treatment with chemotherapy using the EP-EMA regimen, continued for 8 weeks after the normalisation of the hCG level, is recommended. Following completion of chemotherapy, a hysterectomy is recommended because viable disease can persist in the uterus despite the hCG level falling to normal values. Surgery can also be used in PSTT to resect areas of disease that are resistant to chemotherapy.

The most recent data for PSTT patients treated at Charing Cross Hospital show a 100% cure rate for those presenting within 4 years of pregnancy, but a poorer prognosis for those presenting after a longer interval (Schmid *et al.*, 2009).

Risk of relapse and late treatment complications

After the hCG level has fallen to normal, the outlook is very good for patients with trophoblast disease. At this point, the risk of relapse is less than 2.5% for patients treated for low-risk disease and 8% for high-risk patients treated with the EMA-CO regimen. Usually these recurrences happen within the first 12 months after treatment, but can occur up to 6 years later. Fortunately, trophoblast tumours remain highly curable even at relapse and a recent analysis indicated that 100% of patients who were originally in the low-risk category can be cured on relapse, with a cure rate of 90% after relapse for those initially presenting with high-risk disease (Powles *et al.*, 2006).

Subsequent fertility

Fertility is usually maintained after either low- or high-risk chemotherapy treatment and regular periods restart within 6 months of completing chemotherapy. However, there is some toxicity: the chemotherapy treatment brings menopause forward by approximately 1 year for low-risk methotrexate and 5 years for high-risk EMA-CO (Bower *et al.*, 1998).

We recommend that pregnancy be avoided for 12 months after the end of treatment to minimise any possible damaging effects on developing oocytes and to minimise the confusion over disease relapse from the hCG produced in pregnancy. Despite the patient's exposure to cytotoxic chemotherapy, there does not appear to be any significant increase in foetal abnormalities, and most women wishing to conceive are successful.

With the increasing numbers of long-term survivors following chemotherapy treatment for GTT, it has become possible to accurately estimate the impact of chemotherapy treatment on the incidence of other malignancies later in life. A recent update of the data looking at 1903 patients followed for a total of 32,244 patient years gives reassuring results. For patients treated with methotrexate and folinic acid alone there is no evidence of any impact on the risk of future cancer risk. For modern patients treated with the EMA-CO regimen there is no overall increased cancer risk, but the pattern of future malignancies is slightly altered, with less lung and breast cancer in the treated patients but a moderate increase in cases of gastrointestinal

and melanoma compared to the reference population (Savage *et al.*, 2015).

Summary

GTTs form a rare and unique group of tumours, with their aetiology, biology and responsiveness to treatment very different from those of any other form of cancer. In the UK, there is a centralised surveillance and treatment service that is a model admired in many parts of the world (Goldstein *et al.*, 2004). As a result, most UK oncologists are not routinely involved in the care of these patients. However, each year a small number of patients with choriocarcinoma present with disseminated malignancy and a delayed diagnosis can result in increased treatment-related morbidity or the patient's death before treatment can be started.

We recommend that a formal serum hCG measurement is performed in all women presenting with cancer of unknown primary and, where appropriate, that cases are discussed promptly with the teams at Charing Cross or Weston Park Hospitals.

References

Ahamed, E., Short, D., North, B., *et al.* (2012). Survival of women with gestational trophoblastic neoplasia and liver metastases: is it improving? *J. Reprod. Med.*, **57**, 262–269.

Alifrangis, C., Agarwal, R., Short, D., *et al.* (2013). EMA/CO for high-risk gestational trophoblastic neoplasia: good outcomes with induction low-dose etoposide-cisplatin and genetic analysis. *J. Clin. Oncol.*, **31**, 280–286.

Bagshawe, K. D., Dent, J., Newlands, E. S., *et al.* (1989). The role of low-dose methotrexate and folinic acid in gestational trophoblastic tumours (GTT). *Br. J. Obstet. Gynaecol.*, **96**, 795–802.

Bower, M., Rustin, G. J., Newlands, E. S., *et al.* (1998). Chemotherapy for gestational trophoblastic tumours hastens menopause by 3 years. *Eur. J. Cancer*, **34**, 1204–1207.

Cole, L. A., Shahabi, S., Butler, S. A., *et al.* (2001). Utility of commonly used commercial human chorionic gonadotropin immunoassays in the diagnosis and management of trophoblastic diseases. *Clin. Chem.*, **47**, 308–315.

Cole, L. A., Sasaki, Y. and Muller, C. Y. (2007) Normal production of human chorionic gonadotropin in menopause. *N. Engl. J. Med.*, **356**, 1184–1186.

FIGO Oncology Committee. (2002). FIGO staging for gestational trophoblastic neoplasia 2000. *Int. J. Gynaecol. Obstet.*, **77**, 285–287.

Fisher, R. A., Lavery, S. A., Carby, A., *et al.* (2011). What a difference an egg makes. *Lancet*, **378**, 1974.

Goldstein, D. P., Garner, E. I., Feltmate, C. M., et al. (2004). Comment on 'The role of repeat uterine evacuation in the management of persistent gestational trophoblastic disease.' *Gynecol. Oncol.*, **95**, 421–422.

Helwani, M. N., Seoud, M., Zahed, L.,et al. (1999). A familial case of recurrent hydatidiform molar pregnancies with biparental genomic contribution. *Hum. Genet.*, **105**, 112–115.

Kim, S. J., Lee, C., Kwon, S. Y., et al. (2004). Studying changes in the incidence, diagnosis and management of GTD: the South Korean model. *J. Reprod. Med.*, **49**, 643–654.

McGrath, S., Harding, V., Lim, A. K., et al. (2012). Embolization of uterine arteriovenous malformations in patients with gestational trophoblastic tumors: a review of patients at Charing Cross Hospital, 2000–2009. *J. Reprod. Med.*, **57**, 319–324.

Newlands, E. S., Mulholland, P. J., Holden, L., et al. (2000). Etoposide and cisplatin/etoposide, methotrexate, and actinomycin D (EMA) chemotherapy for patients with high-risk gestational trophoblastic tumors refractory to EMA/cyclophosphamide and vincristine chemotherapy and patients presenting with metastatic placental site trophoblastic tumors. *J. Clin. Oncol.*, **18**, 854–859.

Newlands, E. S., Holden, L., Seckl, M. J., et al. (2002). Management of brain metastases in patients with high-risk gestational trophoblastic tumors. *J. Reprod. Med.*, **47**, 465–471.

Palmieri, C., Dhillon, T., Fisher, R. A., et al. (2007). Management and outcome of healthy women with a persistently elevated beta-hCG. *Gynecol. Oncol.*, **106**, 35–43.

Pezeshki, M., Hancock, B. W., Silcocks, P., et al. (2004). The role of repeat uterine evacuation in the management of persistent gestational trophoblastic disease. *Gynecol. Oncol.*, **95**, 423–429.

Powles, T., Young, A., Sanitt, A., et al. (2006). The significance of the time interval between antecedent pregnancy and diagnosis of high-risk gestational trophoblastic tumours. *Br. J. Cancer*, **95**, 1145–1147.

Savage, P. and Seckl, M. J. (2005). The role of repeat uterine evacuation in trophoblast disease. *Gynecol. Oncol.*, **99**, 251–252.

Savage, P. M., Sita-Lumsden, A., Dickson, S., et al. (2013). The relationship of maternal age to molar pregnancy incidence, risks for chemotherapy and subsequent pregnancy outcome. *J. Obstet. Gynaecol.*, **33**, 406–411.

Savage, P., Cooke, R., O'Nions, J., et al. (2015). Effects of single-agent and combination chemotherapy for gestational trophoblastic tumors on risks of second malignancy and early menopause. *J. Clin. Oncol.*, **33**, 472–478.

Schmid, P., Nagai, Y., Agarwal, R., et al. (2009). Prognostic markers and long-term outcome of placental-site trophoblastic tumours: a retrospective observational study. *Lancet*, **374**, 48–55.

Sita-Lumsden, A., Short, D., Lindsay, I., et al. (2012). Treatment outcomes for 618 women with gestational trophoblastic tumours following a molar pregnancy at the Charing Cross Hospital, 2000–2009. *Br. J. Cancer*, **107**, 1810–1814.

Stenman, U. H., Alfthan, H. and Hotakainen, K. (2004). Human chorionic gonadotropin in cancer. *Clin. Biochem.*, **37**, 549–561.

Wang, J., Short, D., Sebire, N. J., et al. (2008). Salvage chemotherapy of relapsed or high-risk gestational trophoblastic neoplasia (GTN) with paclitaxel/cisplatin alternating with paclitaxel/etoposide (TP/TE). *Ann. Oncol.*, **19**, 1578–1583.

Further reading

Hancock, B. W., Seckl, M. J., Berkowitz, R. S., et al. (2009). *Gestational Trophoblastic Disease*, 3rd edn. Sheffield: International Society for the Study of Trophoblastic Diseases.

International Society for the Study of Trophoblastic Diseases (ISSTD). http://www.isstd.org/index.html (accessed December 2014).

Royal College of Obstetricians and Gynaecologists (RCOG). (2004). *The Management of Gestational Trophoblastic Neoplasia. RCOG Guideline No. 38.* London: Royal College of Obstetricians and Gynaecologists.

Seckl, M. J., Sebire, N. J. and Berkowitz, R.S. (2010). Gestational trophoblastic disease. *Lancet*, **376**, 717–729.

Chapter

31

Management of cancer of the lung

Alison Brewster and Fergus Macbeth

Introduction

Lung cancer has a significant impact on mortality in the UK, accounting for 6% of all deaths and 22% of deaths from cancer. It has one of the lowest survival outcomes of any cancer, with a 5-year survival of 7% in men and 9% in women which has changed little over the past 30 years. The last 10 years has seen a significant improvement in one-year survival, probably due to more widespread use of palliative therapies. One-year survival in the period 1990–1991 was 20.4% for men and women compared with 30.4% for men and 35.1% for women in the period 2010–2011 (http://www.cancerresearchuk.org/, accessed January 2015).

The lung cancer pathway is complex. Up to 38% of patients present as an acute medical admission compared to 23% of cancer presentations overall and this is known to be associated with a poorer outcome. Non-acute patients are assessed in rapid access clinics by chest physicians following a diagnostic CT scan. Informed of the high suspicion of lung cancer, they then undergo a series of tests to stage, establish histology and assess fitness. Specialist nurses play a key role in supporting the patient and their carers while they wait to discuss treatment options. The mean rate for surgery in England and Wales is 21.9% (range 15.1–30.8%) and for Scotland, 20.5% (Health and Social Care Information Centre, 2013). For those unfit or unwilling to undergo surgery, radiotherapy offers a possibility of cure, and high local control rates are now reported with stereotactic ablative radiotherapy (SABR) (Takeda *et al.*, 2013). Adjuvant chemotherapy can increase absolute survival rates by up to 4%, but with 70% of patients presenting with stage IIIB and IV disease, most patients are offered palliative interventions. Chemotherapy can improve symptom control, in particular systemic symptoms, and offer modest

improvements in median survival. Palliative radiotherapy is highly effective in improving symptoms such as cough, haemoptysis and pain. More recently, targeted therapies such as gefitinib offer improvements in median survival for those with EGFR mutations, and as more molecular targets are identified, there is optimism that survival outcomes in lung cancer, which has lagged far behind other malignancies such as breast cancer, may start to improve.

Incidence and epidemiology

The incidence of lung cancer in the UK is 45.1 per 100,000 population. Cancer of the breast, prostate and large bowel have a higher incidence, but lung cancer has the highest mortality with 38.3 per 100,000 population dying of the disease (EUCAN International Agency for Research on Cancer, World Health Organization, http://eco.iarc.fr/EUCAN/Country.aspx?ISOCountryCd=826, accessed October 2014). Around 40,000 cases are diagnosed each year, but although the incidence in men is falling, it continues to rise in women reflecting smoking patterns over the last three decades. Although rates in the 35–44 age group have increased by 10% since 1979, it remains a disease of the elderly, with 80% of cases diagnosed over age 60.

Screening

Defining a high-risk population (> 30 pack years and aged 55–74) and offering three annual low-dose helical CT scans compared with chest X-ray (CXR) has shown a relative risk reduction of 20% in a randomised controlled national lung screening trial (Aberle *et al.*, 2011). Overall reduction in lung cancer mortality was 6.7% and it was estimated that 320 CT scans were performed to prevent one death.

Practical Clinical Oncology, Second Edition, ed. Louise Hanna, Tom Crosby and Fergus Macbeth. Published by Cambridge University Press. © Cambridge University Press 2015.

Lack of evidence on cost-effectiveness and high false-positive rates resulting in over-investigation and anxiety mean that there are no plans to roll out a national screening programme in the UK, although this decision will be reviewed once the data from the Dutch/Belgian randomised trial (NELSON) are available (Zhao *et al.*, 2011).

Carcinoma of the lung: non-small-cell and small cell

Risk factors and aetiology

The major risk factor for lung cancer is undoubtedly cigarette smoking, which accounts for about 90% of cases. There is a clear relationship between risk and the age of smoking onset, the number of years of smoking, and the number of cigarettes smoked per day.

Smoking cessation at any age reduces the risk of lung cancer, which drops to between 30% and 50% of that of continuing smokers after 10 years. With chronic exposure to tobacco smoke, the ciliated epithelium of the respiratory mucosa undergoes squamous metaplasia, and eventually a field change can occur with the development of carcinoma *in situ* before the start of frankly invasive cancer.

Industrial exposure to nickel, chromium and some arsenic compounds is associated with increased risk. Asbestos exposure appears to increase the risk of developing lung cancer threefold in smokers and is also a risk factor for mesothelioma. 'Scar' cancers occur in areas of lung fibrosis and there is an increased risk of adenocarcinoma in patients with fibrosing alveolitis.

Anatomy

The trachea bifurcates into the right and left main bronchi at the carina. The bronchi further subdivide into the lobar bronchi (right upper, middle and lower, and left upper and lower) entering the lobes of the lung. Each lobar bronchus gives off branches called segmental bronchi which enter the bronchopulmonary segments. Each lung is attached to the mediastinum by its root, the hilum, which contains the bronchi, pulmonary vessels, lymphatics and nerves. The parietal pleura lines the thoracic wall, thoracic diaphragm and lateral mediastinum, and the visceral pleura completely covers the surfaces of the lungs extending into the fissures. These layers become continuous at the lung root (pleural reflection), and they are separated by a thin layer of fluid in a potential cavity (the pleural space).

Mediastinum

The mediastinum contains the thymic remnant, trachea, oesophagus, heart and great vessels, the thoracic duct and lymph nodes, vagus and phrenic nerves and sympathetic trunks. All these structures can therefore be involved by direct extension by lung cancer or by malignant lymphadenopathy.

Lymphatics

The lymphatic drainage from the lungs is through channels running to the hilum along the bronchi. The hilar nodes drain to the tracheobronchial group and then up via mediastinal lymph trunks to the brachiocephalic veins.

The regional lymph nodes of the thorax are defined in the 7th Edition International Association for Study of Lung Cancer TNM staging (UICC, 2009) and staging requires familiarity with the nodal stations which are shown in Figure 31.1 and described in Table 31.1 (Rusch *et al.*, 2009).

Pathology and classification

Tumours arising in the lung may be benign (e.g. papilloma, cystadenoma), primary malignant (non-small-cell, neuroendocrine, salivary gland and unclassified) or secondary (kidney, bladder, colorectal, breast, etc.)

The majority of bronchial carcinomas are 'central' in that they arise in the major airways – the main or segmental bronchi. Typically, an ulcerating mass arises within the wall, partially or sometimes completely blocking the bronchus. Upper lobe tumours are slightly more common than middle and lower lobe and right-sided than left-sided tumours. 'Peripheral' tumours arising in the more distal airways and alveoli are more often adenocarcinoma.

In recent years the importance of histological classification of NSCLC in determining treatment options and prognosis has been recognised in the 2004 WHO classification (Travis *et al.*, 2004). Lung cancer is typically heterogeneous and immunohistochemistry (IHC) is useful in characterising tumours and deciding whether the cancer is metastatic rather than primary. Small biopsies mean that IHC must be carefully chosen so that sufficient tissue is available for molecular studies, in particular with adenocarcinoma which should be tested for the presence of EGFR-sensitising mutations.

Some tumours contain mixed pathological subtypes and are designated 'combined tumour' when each

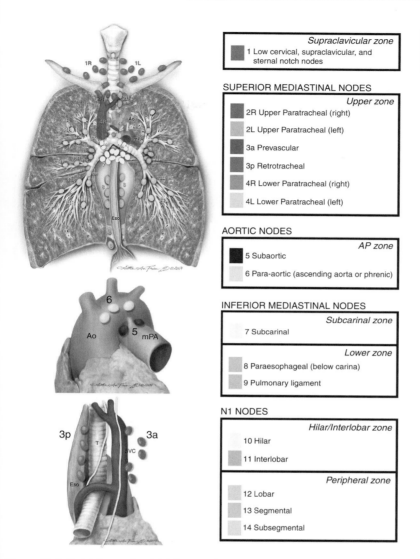

Executive Editor, Editorial Rx Press, 2009. Reprinted with permission courtesy of the International Association for the Study of Lung Cancer. © 2009 IASLC.

Figure 31.1 Nodal chart and nodal definitions; the *IASLC Staging Reference Card Series in Thoracic Oncology*, Peter Goldstraw, FRCS,

component is at least 10% of the total tumour volume. Evidence is also emerging that lung cancer can change histological subtype following treatment. Histological features are described in Table 31.2.

Spread

Lung cancer can spread locally to the mediastinum, pleura (may produce an effusion, especially adeno-carcinoma), chest wall and ribs, vertebral body or diaphragm. The disease can spread via lymph nodes to the hilar, mediastinal (pretracheal, paratracheal, para-aortic, subaortic and subcarinal) or the supracla-vicular fossa (N3) lymph nodes. It can also spread via the blood stream to the liver, adrenal gland, lung, brain, bone or skin.

Clinical presentation

Respiratory symptoms include increasing cough, breathlessness, haemoptysis or unresolving pneu-monia, all of which are symptoms that may occur in middle-aged smokers and, with a gradual onset, may be overlooked. Many patients are treated for asthma or with several courses of antibiotics before being referred for a chest X-ray or further investigation. Severe breathlessness may be due either to significant obstruction to a major airway or to a pleural effusion.

Table 31.1 Regional lymph node stations (International Association for the Study of Lung Cancer: IASLC)

Nodal status	Nodal description		IASLC station
N1	Ipsilateral hilar		10
	Ipsilateral peribronchial	Interlobar	11
	Ipsilateral intrapulmonary	Lobar	12
		Segmental	13
		Subsegmental	14
N2	Ipsilateral superior mediastinal	Upper paratracheal	2
		Prevascular/retrotracheal	3
		Lower paratracheal	4
	Aortic	Subaortic	5
		Para-aortic	6
	Ipsilateral mediastinal	Subcarinal	7
		Paraoesophageal	8
		Pulmonary ligament	9
N3	Contralateral hilar or mediastinal		
	Ipsilateral or contralateral low cervical, supraclavicular and sternal notch		1

Adapted from Goldstraw *et al.* (2007) and Rusch *et al.* (2009).

Table 31.2 Histological classification of lung cancer

Type	Classification	% (approx.)	Description
Non-small-cell carcinoma	Squamous	22	Often central, may cavitate. Keratinisation ± intracellular bridges; epithelioid sheets; coarse chromatin and dense nucleus; high-MW keratin +ve
	Adenocarcinoma	40	Generally peripheral, may arise in scar tissue
			Lepidic (formerly bronchioloalveolar), glandular and papillary architecture.CK7,CEA, TTF-1 and Napsin A +ve
			Important exceptions: thyroid tumours positive for TTF-1 and some variants of lepidic pattern express an intestinal phenotype, e.g. CK20 positive CK7 negative
	Large cell	5	No squamous or glandular patterns: often a diagnosis of default. A number of variants include LCNEC
	Adenosquamous	< 3	At least 10% of adenocarcinoma and squamous carcinoma on light microscopy
	Carcinoid	< 3	May be 'typical' with few mitosis/hpf or 'atypical' with many mitosis/hpf and necrosis
	Sarcomatoid	< 1	Poorly differentiated - can be pleomorphic containing spindle cells, sarcomatoid or sarcomatous
	Carcinoma of salivary gland	< 1%	
	Unclassified – NOS	10	Where no subtype can be defined

Table 31.2 (*cont.*)

Type	Classification	% (approx.)	Description
Small cell		15	Typically central, spreads in a submucosal fashion and crushes easily on biopsy. Usually diagnosed at light microscopy with high proliferative rate and morphologically small cells with round or oval nuclei, scant cytoplasm; lymphocyte-like cells; EM-dense IHC markers of neuroendocrine differentiation (synatophysin, chromogranin, CD56) positive. TTF-1+ve

CD56, neural cell adhesion molecule also called Cluster of Difference 56; CEA, carcino-embryonic antigen; CK, cytokeratin; EM, electron microscopy; hpf, high-powered field; IHC, immunohistochemistry; LCNEC, large cell neuroendocrine carcinoma; MW, molecular weight; TTF-1, thyroid transcription factor 1. Adapted from Travis, 2011.

Superior vena caval obstruction (SVCO) results in distended neck and arm veins, facial oedema (especially in the mornings) and the development of collateral veins on the chest wall. Lung cancer is the most common cause of SVCO in middle-aged and older patients.

A variety of different pain syndromes can occur with lung cancer.

- Mediastinal pain is very variable in site and intensity, but many patients complain of vague aching central chest pain, which can be severe and become the dominant symptom. Severe pain is usually an indication of direct mediastinal involvement.
- Chest wall pain – peripheral tumours may spread to involve the pleura and chest wall. Initially this may be poorly localised or pleuritic. With involvement of the ribs and intercostal nerve, a more characteristic severe and dysaesthetic pain may occur with dermatomal distribution.
- Back pain – direct involvement of a vertebral body may result in back pain, and if the nerve roots are affected it may also be dermatomal.
- Shoulder pain can result from direct involvement of the brachial plexus as part of the superior sulcus (Pancoast) syndrome, but it can also be due to referred pain from the diaphragm or mediastinal involvement of the phrenic nerve.
- Facial pain is a not uncommon but poorly recognised symptom, indicating mediastinal involvement. It is characteristically vague, aching and persistent and located around the ipsilateral jaw, ear or maxilla. It may be the presenting symptom and patients may be diagnosed with trigeminal neuralgia or referred for dental care

before the true cause is recognised. It is thought to be due to referred pain through the vagus.

- Metastases are common in lung cancer and are associated with a wide variety of pain syndromes. Common systemic symptoms include anorexia, fatigue, weight loss and sweats. They are often, but not always, indicators of extensive disease.

Non-metastatic syndromes include the following.

- Clubbing and hypertrophic pulmonary osteo-arthropathy (HPOA) – finger (and toe) clubbing is common. Clubbing is more often (but not always) seen in patients with NSCLC rather than SCLC. When persistent it can be associated with HPOA, resulting in joint pain (especially knees, ankles and wrists) and characteristic X-ray and bone scan appearances.
- SIADH – inappropriate ADH secretion is characterised by low serum sodium and a urine osmolality that is inappropriately concentrated compared to that in the serum. SIADH is due to tumour production of an active peptide that mimics ADH and is quite commonly found in patients with SCLC. It can occasionally occur in patients with NSCLC.
- Hypercalcaemia – high serum calcium can be caused by tumour secretion of an active peptide in the absence of bone metastases. Hypercalcaemia is unusual and most commonly occurs in patients with squamous carcinoma, but it can occur in any tumour type.
- Neurological – there are a variety of non-metastatic neurological syndromes (peripheral neuropathy, cerebellar ataxia,

417

dementia) that can occur in patients with lung cancer of any histological type. Neurological symptoms may be associated with secretion of the anti-Hu antibody. The myasthenia-like Lambert Eaton syndrome is rare and typically occurs in patients with SCLC.

- Prothrombotic tendency – many patients with lung cancer develop venous thrombosis and pulmonary embolism. There is good evidence that these patients have a prothrombotic tendency, which may be resistant to heparin.

Metastases can occur at any site; the most common are the liver, adrenals, bone and brain.

Investigations

Patients suspected of having lung cancer should be referred to a chest physician for assessment.

The following referral recommendations have been made by NICE (CG 121 2011).

- Urgent referral for a chest X-ray (CXR) should be offered when a patient presents with haemoptysis or any of the following unexplained or persistent (> 3 weeks) symptoms or signs: cough, chest/shoulder pain, dyspnoea, weight loss, chest signs, hoarseness, clubbing, features suggestive of metastases or cervical/supraclavicular lymphadenopathy.
- If CXR or CT scans suggest lung cancer (including pleural effusion and slowly resolving consolidation) patients should be offered an urgent referral to a member of the lung cancer multi-disciplinary team (MDT). Urgent referral prior to a CXR is recommended if there is persistent haemoptysis in a smoker/ex-smoker older than 40 years, signs of SVCO or stridor.
- The patient should be seen within two weeks.

Patients should also have full blood count, biochemistry and a CT scan of the thorax and upper abdomen with contrast to establish the extent of mediastinal disease and to look for metastases. Scanning also helps to establish the best way to obtain histology. Unless they are very frail, an attempt should be made to establish a histological diagnosis either at bronchoscopy or by CT-guided lung biopsy.

All patients should be discussed at the Lung MDT meeting and need full lung function and PET-CT if potentially suitable for radical treatment. Surgical candidates should be considered for cardiopulmonary testing.

If mediastinal nodes are enlarged or show increased uptake on PET, then patients should be considered for endobronchial ultrasound (EBUS) to confirm malignancy. EBUS has a high sensitivity (> 90%) but a false-negative rate of 9%. Patients may need to undergo mediastinoscopy if finding a positive node will alter management.

MRI head should also be considered before radical treatment in patients with a locally advanced NSCLC, because just under 4% of patients will be shown to have occult brain metastases (Yokoi et al., 1999).

Staging

TNM staging is used for both NSCLC and small cell lung cancer. The concept of limited and extensive stage has been dropped in favour of the consistency offered by TNM. The TNM staging system is shown in Table 31.3 and the stage groupings are shown in Table 31.4.

Radical treatment of non-small-cell lung cancer (stages I, II and III)

Surgery

Patients with NSCLC should be considered for surgery provided they are medically operable to undergo either lobectomy or pneumonectomy, depending on the site and extent of the tumour. Wedge excision is associated with poor local control and should be avoided. Survival is better for those patients who undergo complete ipsilateral mediastinal lymph node dissection compared with sampling (Manser et al., 2005).

Adjuvant chemotherapy after surgery

The NSCLC meta-analysis (Arriagada et al., 2004) suggested a 4% increase in 5-year survival following cisplatin-based adjuvant chemotherapy. This finding led to the question of whether this level of benefit (NNT = 25) is clinically useful and which groups of patients potentially gain the most benefit. A number of RCTs have since been reported, with varying results. However, a meta-analysis by the Lung Adjuvant Cisplatin Evaluation (LACE) Group (Pignon et al., 2008) looked at patient data from five large trials published since the 1995 meta-analysis and concluded that the benefit from adjuvant chemotherapy depends on the stage of disease and is greatest in patients with stage II and III disease. The need for adjuvant chemotherapy

Table 31.3 IASLC TNM classification for lung cancer which has been adopted by UICC

Stage	Description
TX	Presence of malignant cells, no visible tumour
T0	No primary detected
Tis	Carcinoma *in situ*
T1	≤ 3 cm in largest dimension surrounded by lung or visceral pleura without bronchoscopic evidence of invasion more proximal than the lobar bronchus (i.e. not in main bronchus)
	T1a ≤ 2 cm in greatest dimension
	T1b > 2 cm but ≤ 3 cm in greatest dimension
T2	Tumour > 3 cm but ≤ 7 cm or tumour with any of the following features: involves main bronchus ≥ 2 cm from carina invades visceral pleura atelectasis or obstructive pneumonitis that extends to the hilum but does not involve entire lung
	T2a Tumour > 3 cm but ≤ 5 cm greatest dimension
	T2b Tumour > 5 cm but ≤ 7 cm greatest dimension
T3	Tumour > 7 cm or directly invading chest wall (including superior sulcus tumours), diaphragm, phrenic nerve, mediastinal pleura, parietal pericardium or tumour < 2 cm from carina, or obstructive pneumonitis or atelectasis of one lung or separate tumour nodules in the same lobe as the primary
T4	Tumour with direct invasion of mediastinum, heart, great vessels, trachea, recurrent laryngeal, oesophagus, vertebrae or carina or separate nodules in a different ipsilateral lobe
Nodal	See regional lymph node status, Table 31.1.
M1a	Separate tumour nodule (s) in a contralateral lobe; tumour with pleural nodules or malignant pleural or pericardial effusion
M1b	Distant metastases

Adapted from Goldstraw *et al.*, 2007 and UICC, 2009.

Table 31.4 Stage groups for non-small-cell lung cancer according to IASLC stage

Stage	Percentage at presentation (CRUK)	Description
IA	14.5	T1aN0, T1bN0
IB		T2aN0
IIA	7.3	T1aN1, T1bN1, T2aN1, T2bN0
IIB		T2bN1, T3N0
IIIA	31.8	T4N0, T3N1, T4N1, T1-3/N2
IIIB		T4N2, T1-4N3
IV	35.8	AnyT or N but M1a or M1b
Unknown	10.5	

CRUK, Cancer Research UK; available at: http://www.cancerresearchuk.org/cancer-info/cancerstats/types/lung/survival/lung-cancer-survival-statistics#stage, accessed October 2014.

should be discussed with patients so that they can make an informed choice balancing potential risks and benefits.

Adjuvant radiotherapy after surgery

The PORT meta-analysis (PORT Meta-analysis Trialists Group, 1998) showed that adjuvant RT has a modest effect on local control and a detrimental effect on survival. There was a reduction in OS of 7% at 2 years, which was greatest in stage I and II disease. This outcome may be due to late effects on lung and heart in long-term survivors. A subgroup analysis did not show this detrimental effect in stage III disease (N2 or 3). The meta-analysis has been criticised for including mainly old trials using RT techniques and fractionation that would not be considered acceptable today. Therefore, postoperative RT may be indicated for selected patients with known residual disease following surgery.

Neoadjuvant chemotherapy before surgery

The largest randomised trial to date did not show any survival advantage from platinum based neo-adjuvant chemotherapy (Gilligan et al., 2007) and its use is not recommended.

Radical radiotherapy

In the UK, where the median age at presentation is over 70 and there is a significant risk of smoking-related (and other) comorbidity, especially emphysema, cardiovascular disease and peripheral vascular disease, a number of patients may be medically inoperable and should be considered for radical RT. There are no hard rules about the level of lung function that precludes radical RT, but any patient with an FEV-1 of less than 1.0 L or 50% of predicted should be reviewed carefully. A small apical tumour will be more safely treated than a large central or lower lobe tumour.

Patients with T1/T2a N0 peripheral tumours can be treated with stereotactic ablative radiotherapy (SABR) also referred to as SBRT. Very high biological doses with a biologically effective dose (BED) of ≥ 100 Gy delivered with multiple small fields to avoid normal tissues are associated with excellent local control rates. Senthi et al. (2012) reported a 4.9% local failure rate at 2 years, which rivals control rates achieved with surgery. Patients need to be able to lie flat for up to 45 minutes, but those with very poor lung function can be treated. 4D CT planning images are acquired as for conventional planning with the patient in a supine position and immobilised, lying comfortably with arms supported above the head, a wedge beneath the knees and foot supports. A respiratory trace, usually generated from a pressure sensor in an abdominal belt, allows the CT images to be sorted into 8–10 respiratory phases. The cancer is delineated on all respiratory phases to generate an ITV (internal target volume) which is expanded by 3–5 mm to generate a PTV. Normal tissue outlining includes oesophagus, lung, proximal bronchial tree, heart, chest wall, brachial plexus and any organ that is traversed by a treatment beam. Planning organ at risk volumes (PRV) are applied on the exported phase and normal tissue constraints adhered to, ensuring low toxicity. In SABR, unlike conventional planning where PTV dose homogeneity is critical, inhomogeneity is useful to push doses up to a maximum of 140%. Doses from 55 Gy in 3 fractions to 60 Gy in 8 fractions are prescribed to the 80% isodose to ensure rapid dose fall off outside the PTV. Delivering such high doses per fraction requires careful treatment verification, and cone

beam CT should be performed with additional checks after delivery of non-coplanar beams or if the patient moves (UK Consortium, 2014).

Patients not suitable for SABR (central tumours, T3 or any T with N1/N2 disease) are treated with conventional radiotherapy provided the volume of the PTV, which should exclude uninvolved nodes, does not exceed normal tissue constraints. The GTV is outlined using information from the diagnostic CT scan and PET which can be fused with the planning CT if necessary. Expansion to CTV (as defined by ICRU, 1999) is a clinical decision based upon likely tumour spread, clarity of tumour definition on images, barriers to spread such as arterial wall or vertebral body and respiratory movement. CTV to PTV is a geometrical construct based on the accuracy of treatment delivery and varies from 5 to 10 mm in different departments. 3D conformal lung plans are optimised with a planning algorithm such as collapsed cone that account for reduced electron transfer in lung tissue and avoid overestimating dose within the PTV. Critical normal tissue constraints include V20 (percentage total lung volume receiving > 20 Gy) which should be less than 35% to minimise risk of radiation pneumonitis (Graham et al., 1999). Dose to spinal cord (with PRV of 5 mm) should be less than 48 Gy and oesophageal constraints will be dependent on length of oesophagus treated. Off-line verification is essential ideally with cone beam CT.

If it is locally available, patients can be treated with CHART (continuous hyperfractionated accelerated radiotherapy), 54 Gy in 36 fractions over 12 days. The CHART trial showed a significant 2-year survival benefit of 29% compared to 20% for patients given 60 Gy over 6 weeks (Saunders et al., 1999). Alternative fractionation schedules include 52–55 Gy in 20 fractions over 4 weeks or 60–66 Gy in 30–33 fractions over 6 weeks. The overall 2-year survival should be in the range of 30–40%, and 5-year survival should be 15–20%.

Superior sulcus tumours should be treated with radical RT, if technically feasible, in two phases, including the whole of the adjacent vertebral bodies to the level of spinal cord tolerance because of the risk of nerve root involvement. No strong evidence exists to support combined modality approaches, although these are widely advocated.

Many UK centres are using IMRT to produce treatment plans for patients where conventional planning cannot achieve a radical dose without exceeding normal tissue constraints. Typically, this might include

Table 31.5 Side effects from radiotherapy for lung cancer

Side effect	Management
Acute	
Anorexia and nausea	Anti-emetics
Dry cough	Simple linctus, codeine linctus
Oesophagitis	Supportive: analgesia, mucilage, rarely parenteral feeding
Late	
Radiation pneumonitis	8–12 weeks after treatment: acute dyspnoea, cough and tightness; CXR can show hazy area in field Treat with oxygen, steroids: usually prednisolone up to 60 mg reduced over 2 weeks and antibiotics
Lung fibrosis	Usually asymptomatic, but may cause increased breathlessness; oxygen if needed
Myelopathy	Rare, no specific treatment

large primary tumours, N3 disease or where tumours are close to the spinal cord in the vertebral gutter.

Table 31.5 shows the side effects from radiotherapy for lung cancer.

Concurrent and sequential chemoradiotherapy

Adjuvant chemotherapy following radical radiotherapy (sequential) offers a similar survival benefit to that achieved with adjuvant chemotherapy following resection, but a meta-analysis of concomitant versus sequential chemoradiotherapy suggests that concomitant platinum-based chemoradiation may improve survival of patients with locally advanced disease (Aupérin et al., 2010). It is associated with increased but manageable grade 3/4 oesophagitis and should be considered for good performance status patients and where radiation constraints can be achieved. A randomised UK trial of concurrent compared with sequential chemoradiotherapy has reported 2-year survival rates of 50% with concurrent compared with 46% with sequential treatment (SOCCAR; Maguire et al., 2014).

Palliative treatment of non-small-cell lung cancer

Palliative radiotherapy

Palliative radiotherapy to the chest is a good option for patients who have either disease of too large a volume

for radical RT or co-morbidity. The third MRC trial (Macbeth et al., 1996) showed that for patients with good PS (0 or 1) there is a significant survival advantage to giving 39 Gy in 13 fractions (or 36 Gy in 12 fractions) compared to 17 Gy in 2 fractions. The 2-year survival was 13% compared to 9%, but with no difference in symptom control. There was a small incidence of radiation myelitis in patients receiving 39 or 17 Gy. Radiotherapy also offers a 60% chance of significant improvement in symptoms. RCTs have shown that there is no difference in symptom control or survival from radiobiologically equivalent regimens (e.g. 17 Gy in 2 fractions, 20 Gy in 5 fractions, 30 Gy in 10 fractions). Short regimens are generally preferable in that they involve fewer visits. For poor PS patients a 10 Gy single fraction is sufficient (Medical Research Council Lung Cancer Working Party, 1992). Use of 17 Gy in 2 fractions is associated with a risk of RT myelitis and either the spinal cord should be avoided by planning with oblique fields or the dose reduced to 16 Gy.

Unfortunately, many patients have obvious metastatic disease at presentation or develop it later and radiotherapy can offer useful palliation. A single fraction of 8–10 Gy can be used in bone and skin metastases. Palliative RT to brain metastases should only be considered for patients with good PS.

Palliative radiotherapy can cause side effects and patients need to be warned of these when they consent. Large fractions are associated with acute side effects such as nausea, acute chest pain, fever and rigors which can be managed with anti-emetics, analgesics and paracetamol. Asymptomatic patients can be treated when symptoms develop without detrimental effect on outcomes or palliation (Falk et al., 2002).

Systemic anti-cancer therapy (SACT)

Chemotherapy for patients with symptomatic locally advanced and metastatic disease is an option that needs to be considered carefully. Large RCTs and two meta-analyses have shown that chemotherapy in advanced disease improves survival, with an objective response rate of around 20% and with 40–50% of patients experiencing symptomatic improvement. The survival benefit is around 2 months with median survival averaging 9–10 months (Rudd et al., 2005) with a 10% increase in 1-year survival (Non Small Cell Lung Cancer Collaborative Group, 1995). In the UK, the Big Lung Trial randomised 725 patients to cisplatin-based chemotherapy or best supportive care and the median survival was increased by 9 weeks (from 5.7 to

8 months) with an improvement in 1-year survival of 9% (29% compared to 20%) (Spiro *et al.*, 2004). In the UK, the mean rate of chemotherapy treatment for stage IIIb/IV NSCLC PS 0/1 in 2012 was 57.2% and has risen from 47.8% in 2008 (LUCADA data set; Health and Social Care Information Centre, 2013).

The data on improvement in quality of life (QOL) are less robust, but it seems that overall QOL does not deteriorate and it may improve a little for patients having chemotherapy. The optimum type, number and duration of chemotherapy regimens has been extensively evaluated in RCTs and meta-analyses. In general, a two-drug combination is as effective as three drugs and less toxic. Non-platinum combinations offer no advantage over platinum-containing regimens, but overall survival is improved for adenocarcinoma patients treated with first-line pemetrexed (Scagliotti *et al.*, 2008).

A number of regimens can be used and include the following.

Cisplatin (80 mg/m^2) and vinorelbine (60 mg/m^2 orally days 1 and 8)

Cisplatin (75 mg/m^2) and gemcitabine (1250 mg/m^2 day 1 and 8)

Cisplatin (75 mg/m^2) and pemetrexed (500 mg/m^2 with vitamin B12, folic acid and dexamethasone)

The dose of cisplatin is critical. The BTOG 2 trial comparing gemcitabine combined with either cisplatin 50 mg/m^2 versus cisplatin 80 mg /m^2 versus carboplatin AUC 6 showed a lower response rate and overall survival for cisplatin 50 mg/m^2 (Ferry *et al.*, 2011).

For poor PS status patients it is reasonable to substitute carboplatin for cisplatin, as it is likely to be better tolerated causing less nausea and vomiting but more thrombocytopaenia.

Maintenance chemotherapy has been investigated in adenocarcinoma using pemetrexed and erlotinib. The PARAMOUNT trial (Paz-Ares *et al.*, 2013) suggests a 22% reduction in risk of death with maintenance pemetrexed compared with placebo after achieving stable or responding disease following a first-line pemetrexed-containing regimen. Recent NICE guidance TA190 (NICE, 2010) recommends maintenance pemetrexed only for those patients who have not received pemetrexed first-line. Maintenance erlotinib was reviewed by NICE but not found to be cost-effective (TA227; NICE, 2011).

Second line treatment can be considered with either single agent docetaxel 75 mg/m^2 if squamous or combined with nintedanib (an angiokinase inhibitor) if adenocarcinoma providing PS 0/1 (TA347;

NICE, 2015). If PS 2 then consider erlotinib (TA162; NICE, 2008).

Molecular profiling of NSCLC has resulted in highly active, well-tolerated orally available therapies for around 10% of patients in whom the cell surface EGFR demonstrates sensitising mutations which include exon 19 deletions and exon 21 L858R point mutations. Gefitinib 250 mg, afatinib 40mg or erlotinib 150 mg daily is used first line for EGFR mutation-positive patients with locally advanced or metastatic disease or on progression after other treatment.

Common side effects are manageable and include skin rash, paronychia and diarrhoea. Pulmonary fibrosis is a rare but worrying side effect.

Crizotinib is an orally available selective inhibitor of ALK receptor tyrosine kinase seen in 2–7% of patients with NSCLC. Some patients have had excellent responses, but lack of overall survival benefit compared with second-line chemotherapy means that it is not recommended (TA296; NICE, 2013).

Treatment of small-cell-lung cancer (SCLC)

Unless there is some other contraindication, good PS SCLC patients should be treated with curative intent with chemotherapy, thoracic RT and prophylactic cranial irradiation (PCI). An 18 to 20 month median survival is reported in the UK with a 3-year survival of around 15% (Thatcher *et al.*, 2005), but data from the US in which combined twice-daily concurrent chemoradiotherapy is given reports a greater than 40% 2-year survival (Turrisi *et al.*, 1999). Patients who have not relapsed after three years are unlikely to relapse subsequently, although they have an increased risk of second primary lung tumours and death from other smoking-related disease.

Chemotherapy

Patients with 'limited stage' SCLC (T1–4, N0–3, M0) with PS 0/1 should be offered 4–6 cycles of cisplatin (60 mg/m^2) and etoposide (120 mg/m^2 day 1 and 100 mg b.d. days 2 and 3). Concurrent chemoradiotherapy should be considered for fit patients where the disease can be encompassed in a radical thoracic volume aiming to give radiotherapy concomitantly with cycle one or two (NICE guideline CG121; NICE, 2011b). It is acceptable to deliver the radiotherapy as a planned volume to include involved nodal areas or as a parallel opposed pair with spinal shielding using either 40 Gy in 15 fractions o.d. or 45 Gy in 30 fractions b.d. Concurrent chemoradiotherapy has the advantage of shortening the time from initiation of chemotherapy to completion of radiotherapy which has been shown to improve 5-year survival in a systematic overview (de Ruysscher *et al.*, 2006).

Patients who are less fit or have disease that is too extensive for combined chemoradiotherapy should be offered sequential treatment.

PCI can reduce the risk of brain metastases by more than 50% and has been shown to improve overall survival at 3 years from 15% to 21% (Arriagada *et al.*, 1997). Concerns remain that it may be associated with reduction in cognitive function and should be used with caution in patients over the age of 70. Twenty-five grays in 10 fractions given as opposing lateral fields is effective and associated with few side effects.

Poor performance and metastatic patients can gain good symptomatic benefit and prolongation of survival from first-line chemotherapy with carboplatin (AUC 5) and etoposide, but patients should be properly informed of a high risk of sepsis.

Slotman *et al.* (2014) demonstrated improved survival at 2 years (13% versus 3%) for patients with extensive disease who received thoracic RT following chemotherapy. Therefore, patients with 'limited disease' who fail to achieve a good response with first-line treatment and extensive-stage patients with bulky intrathoracic disease should be considered for thoracic radiotherapy (between 30 Gy in 10 fractions and 8 Gy in 1 fraction using a parallel opposed pair of fields). PCI with 20 Gy in 5 fractions should be offered as it has been shown to prolong disease-free survival in this group of patients (Slotman *et al.*, 2007). The radiotherapy is generally given with parallel opposed fields.

Most patients relapse and, if fit enough, should be considered for further chemotherapy. If there has been a reasonable length of remission – 6 months or more – re-treating with first-line chemotherapy is appropriate. Rapid relapse is associated with a poor prognosis, but using a non-cross-resistant second-line combination may be appropriate.

Second-line regimens up to 4 cycles of either:

- CAV: day 1, cyclophosphamide 700 mg/m², doxorubicin 40 mg/m² and vincristine 1.2 mg/m² q 21 days;
- topotecan: oral 2.3 mg/m²/day (or i.v. 1.5 mg/m²/day) days 1–5 q 21 days.

Brachytherapy in lung cancer

There are a few patients for whom bronchoscopic brachytherapy may be appropriate.

- Patients with a very small, superficial and localised endoluminal T1 NSCLC who are medically inoperable.
- Patients with a symptomatic endoluminal tumour who have had previous external beam RT to the limits of the lung and/or spinal cord tolerance. An RCT comparing external beam RT with brachytherapy as a first-line palliative treatment showed external beam treatment to give better palliation of symptoms and less serious morbidity (Stout *et al.*, 2000).

Technique

Patients need to be fit enough and have adequate lung function to tolerate bronchoscopy and insertion of a fine-bore tube into the relevant bronchus. The patient is bronchoscoped, the tumour identified and its position related to the carina. A fine-bore polythene tube is passed via the suction channel into the relevant bronchus, past the site of the tumour, and the bronchoscope is then withdrawn over the catheter. The catheter is then fixed to the skin at the nasal orifice. The catheter position is confirmed by insertion of a dummy seed guide wire under fluoroscopy and the target area is outlined. An HDR afterloading technique is used with an ^{192}Ir source and so the treatment can be given as an outpatient procedure.

Dose

For palliation, a single fraction is well tolerated. The usual dose is 10–15 Gy in a single-fraction HDR at 1 cm from the centre of the source.

Brachytherapy with radical intent

The optimum regimen of radical-intent brachytherapy has not been determined. A number of fractionated regimes have been used, ranging between 22.5 and 42 Gy in 3–6 fractions, weekly. A series from the Christie Hospital also used single fractions in this group of 15 or 20 Gy with improved local control but more serious late morbidity (massive fatal haemoptysis) in the 20 Gy group.

Areas of current interest and UK clinical trials

Current areas of interests and controversy in NSCLC include the following.

- Radical radiotherapy dose escalation (I- START and IDEAL trials).

- IMRT for radical RT.
- SABR for central lung tumours.
- Adjuvant radiotherapy following surgery (LungART trial).
- Molecular profiling to identify further active agents (CRUK Stratified Medicine Project).
- Benefit of whole brain RT for patients with brain metastases (QUARTZ trial).

Rare tumour types

Bronchial carcinoid

Bronchial carcinoids are rare neuroendocrine tumours (previously described as bronchial adenomas), which comprise fewer than 5% of primary lung tumours. They tend to occur in a younger age group (≤ 40 years) and are not associated with smoking. Three types are described but they really represent a continuum:

- central carcinoid, the most common type, is polypoid and vascular and may be hormonally silent or produce ACTH. Lymph node metastases occur in 5% of patients and distant spread is rare. The 5-year survival is 70–80%;
- peripheral carcinoid usually occurs as multiple tumours, has an excellent prognosis and rarely metastasises;
- atypical carcinoids have an increased mitotic rate and exhibit nuclear hyperchromasia and necrosis. It can be difficult to differentiate atypical carcinoids from small-cell carcinoma. Lymph node spread occurs in 60% of patients, and metastases are more common.

In the absence of metastatic disease, the primary treatment for bronchial carcinoids is surgery. RT is rarely used except in palliation of metastatic disease.

Combination chemotherapy with regimens similar to those used in SCLC (e.g. carboplatin and etoposide) has been used in metastatic disease but with relatively poor results.

Carcinoid syndrome more commonly occurs in patients with metastatic GI carcinoid, but can rarely occur in bronchial carcinoid. It consists of paroxysmal flushing, bronchoconstriction, diarrhoea, abdominal pain and right heart failure. Skin lesions can also occur. These are due to secretion of serotonin and are diagnosed by elevated 5-hydroxyindoleacetic acid levels in a 24-hour urine collection. Blood chromogranin A assay can be an additional confirmatory test,

Table 31.6 The Masaoka staging system for thymoma

Stage	Description
Stage 1	No microscopic capsular invasion
Stage IIa	Microscopic invasion of capsule
Stage IIb	Microscopic invasion of mediastinal fat/pleura
Stage III	Invasion of adjacent structures
Stage IVa	Pleural and pericardial metastases
Stage IVb	Distant metastases

Adapted from Masaoka *et al.* (1981).

and octreotide (a somatostatin analogue) is useful for symptomatic relief in these cases. Carcinoid tumours are discussed further in Chapter 39.

Thymoma

Thymoma is an uncommon tumour that presents as an anterior mediastinal mass, and it arises from cells of epithelial and lymphocytic origin. The majority are benign, but 30% of tumours are thymic carcinomas. Thymomas rarely metastasise, but they can be locally invasive of the pericardium, myocardium, lung, sternum and great vessels. 'Degree of invasion' is the best indicator of overall survival, rather than the cell type, and is reflected in the Masoaka staging system (see Table 31.6).

Thymomas can be associated with the following paraneoplastic syndromes.

- Myasthenia gravis – occurs in 30–50% of patients with thymoma and 70% improve after thymectomy.
- Red cell aplasia – occurs in 5% of patients.
- Acquired hypogammaglobulinaemia – occurs in 5–10%.
- Rarely, ectopic Cushing's syndrome, polymyositis/dermatomyositis, SLE and hypertrophic pulmonary osteoarthropathy.

The main modality of treatment is surgery and completeness of resection correlates with cure rate. Non-invasive (stage 1) tumours can be treated with surgery alone, but postoperative RT should be considered for invasive tumours or incomplete excision. The usual dose is 45–50 Gy in 2 Gy fractions to the tumour bed. The role of chemotherapy is unclear, but cisplatin-based combination chemotherapy has been used in metastatic disease with some partial responses reported.

References

Aberle, D., Adams A., Berg, C., *et al.* (2011). Reduced lung-cancer mortality with low dose computed tomographic screening. *N. Engl. J. Med.*, **365**, 395–409.

Arriagada, R., Pignon, J. P., Laplanche, A., *et al.* (1997). Prophylactic cranial irradiation for small-cell lung cancer. *Lancet*, **349**, 138.

Arriagada, R., Bergman, B., Dunant, A., *et al.* (2004). Cisplatin-based adjuvant chemotherapy in patients with completely resected non-small-cell lung cancer. *N. Engl. J. Med.*, **350**, 351–360.

Aupérin, A., Le Péchoux, C., Rolland, E., *et al.* (2010). Meta-analysis of concomitant versus sequential radiochemotherapy in locally advanced NSCLC. *J. Clin. Oncol.*, **28**, 2181–2190.

de Ruysscher, D., Pijls-Johannesma, M., Vansteenkiste, J., *et al.* (2006). Systematic review and meta-analysis of randomised, controlled trials of the timing of chest radiotherapy in patients with limited-stage, small-cell lung cancer. *Ann. Oncol.*, **17**, 543–552.

Falk, S. J., Girling, D. J., White, R. J., *et al.* (2002). Immediate versus delayed palliative thoracic radiotherapy in patients with unresectable locally advanced non-small cell lung cancer and minimal thoracic symptoms: randomised controlled trial. *Br. Med. J.*, **325**, 465–472.

Ferry, D., Billingham, L., Jarrett, H. W., *et al.* (2011). S85 British Thoracic Oncology Group trial, BTOG2: Randomised phase III clinical trial of gemcitabine combined with cisplatin 50mg/m2 (GC50) vs cisplatin 80mg/m2 (GC80) vs carboplatin AUC 6 (GCB6) in advanced NSCLC. *Thorax*, **66**, A41 S85.

Gilligan, D., Nicolson, M., Smith, I., *et al.* (2007). Pre-operative chemotherapy in patients with resectable NSCLC: results of the MRC LU22/NVALT 2/EORTC 08012 multicentre randomised trial and update of systematic review. *Lancet*, **369**, 1929–1937.

Goldstraw, P., Crowley, J., Chansky, K., *et al.* (2007). The IASLC Lung Cancer Staging Project: proposals for the revision of the TNM stage grouping in the forthcoming (seventh) edition of the TNM Classification of Malignant Tumours. *J. Thoracic Oncol.*, **2**, 706–714.

Graham, M. V., Purdy, J. A., Emami, B., *et al.* (1999). Clinical dose–volume histogram analysis for pneumonitis after 3D treatment for non small cell lung cancer (NSCLC). *Int. J. Radiat. Oncol. Biol. Phys.*, **45**, 323–329.

Health and Social Care Information Centre. (2013). *National Lung Cancer Audit Report 2013. Report for the audit period 2012.* Leeds: Health and Social Care Information Centre, available at: http://www.hscic.gov.uk/catalogue/PUB12719/clin-audi-supp-prog-lung-nlca-2013-rep.pdf (accessed October 2014).

ICRU. (1999). *Prescribing, Recording and Reporting Photon Beam Therapy (Report 62): Supplement to ICRU Report 50.* Bethesda, MD: International Commission on Radiation Units and Measurements.

Macbeth, F. R., Bolger, J. J., Hopwood, P., *et al.* (1996). Randomised trial of palliative two-fraction versus more intensive thirteen fraction radiotherapy for patients with inoperable non-small cell lung cancer and good performance status. *Clin. Oncol.*, **8**, 167–175.

Maguire, J., Khan, I., McNenimin, R., *et al.* (2014) SOCCAR: A randomised phase II trial comparing concurrent chemotherapy and radical hypofractionated radiotherapy in patients with inoperable stage III non-small cell lung cancer and good performance status. *Eur. J. Cancer*, **50**, 2939–49.

Manser, R., Wright, G., Hart, D., *et al.* (2005). Surgery for early stage non small cell lung cancer. *Cochrane Database Syst Rev.*, (1) CD004699.

Masaoka, A., Monden, Y., Nakahara, K., *et al.* (1981). Follow-up study of thymomas with special reference to their clinical stages. *Cancer*, **48**, 2485–2492.

Medical Research Council Lung Cancer Working Party. (1992). A Medical Research Council (MRC) randomised trial of palliative radiotherapy with two fractions or a single fraction in patients with inoperable non-small-cell lung cancer (NSCLC) and poor performance status. *Br. J. Cancer*, **65**, 934–941.

NICE. (2008). *TA162. Erlotinib for the Treatment of Non-Small-Cell Lung Cancer.* National Institute for Health and Care Excellence, available at: http://www.nice.org.uk/guidance/ta162 (accessed October 2014).

NICE. (2010). *TA190. Pemetrexed for the Maintenance Treatment of Non-Small-Cell Lung Cancer.* National Institute for Health and Care Excellence, available at: http://www.nice.org.uk/guidance/ta190 (accessed October 2014).

NICE. (2011a). *TA227. Erlotinib Monotherapy for Maintenance Treatment of Non-Small-Cell Lung Cancer.* National Institute for Health and Care Excellence, available at: http://www.nice.org.uk/guidance/ta227 (accessed October 2014).

NICE. (2011b). *CG121. Lung Cancer: The Diagnosis and Treatment of Lung Cancer.* National Institute for Health and Care Excellence, available at: http://www.nice.org.uk/guidance/CG121 (accessed October 2014).

NICE. (2013). *TA296. Crizotinib for Previously Treated Non-Small-Cell Lung Cancer Associated with an Anaplastic Lymphoma Kinase Fusion Gene.* National Institute for Health and Care Excellence, available at: http://www.nice.org.uk/guidance/ta296 (accessed October 2014).

NICE. (2015). *TA347. Nintedanib for previously treated locally advanced recurrent non small cell lung cancer.* National Institute for Health and Care Excellence, available at: www.nice.org.uk/guidance/ta347 (accessed August 2015).

Non Small Cell Lung Cancer Collaborative Group. (1995). Chemotherapy in non-small cell lung cancer: a meta-analysis using updated data on individual patients from 52 randomised clinical trials. *Br. Med. J.*, **311**, 899–909.

Paz-Ares, L.G, de Marinis, F., Dediu, M., *et al.* (2013). Final overall survival results of the phase III study of maintenance pemetrexed versus placebo immediately after induction treatment with pemetrexed plus cisplatin for advanced nonsquamous non small cell lung cancer. *J. Clin. Oncol.*, **10**, 2895–2902.

Pignon, J. P., Tribodet, G. V., Scagliotti, J., *et al.* (2008). Lung adjuvant cisplatin evaluation: a pooled analysis by the LACE Collaborative Group. *J. Clin. Oncol.*, **26** 3552–9.

PORT Meta-analysis Trialists Group. (1998). Postoperative radiotherapy in non-small cell lung cancer: systematic review and meta-analysis of individual patient data from nine randomised controlled trials. *Lancet*, **352**, 257–263.

Rudd, R. M., Gower, N. H., Spiro, S. G., *et al.* (2005). Gemcitabine plus carboplatin versus mitomycin, ifosfamide and cisplatin in patients with stage IIIB or IV non-small cell lung cancer: a phase III randomised study of the London Lung Cancer Group *J. Clin. Oncol.*, **23**, 142–153.

Rusch, V. W., Asamura, H., Watanabe, H., *et al.* (2009). The IASLC Lung Cancer Staging Project. A proposal for a new international lymph node map in the forthcoming seventh edition of the TNM classification for lung cancer. *J. Thoracic Oncol.*, **4**, 568–577.

Saunders, M., Dische, S., Barrett, A., *et al.* (1999). Continuous hyperfractionated accelerated radiotherapy (CHART) versus conventional radiotherapy in non-small cell lung cancer: mature data from the randomised multicentre trial. *Radiother. Oncol.*, **52**, 137–148.

Scagliotti, G., Parikh, P., von Pawel, J., *et al.* (2008). Phase III study comparing cisplatin plus gemcitabine with cisplatin and pemtrexed in chemotherapy-naive patients with advanced stage non small cell lung cancer. *J. Clin. Oncol.*, **26**, 3543–3551.

Senthi, S., Lagerwaard, F. J., Haasbeek, C. J. A., *et al.* (2012). Patterns of disease recurrence after stereotactic ablative radiotherapy for early stage non-small-cell lung cancer: a retrospective analysis. *Lancet Oncol.*, **13**, 802–809.

Slotman, B., Favre-Finn, C.,Kramer, G., *et al.* (2007). Prophylatic cranial radiotherapy in extensive small-cell lung cancer. *N. Engl. J. Med.*, **357**, 664–672.

Slotman, B., von Tinteren, H., Pragg, O. G., *et al.* (2014). The use of thoracic radiotherapy for extensive stage small cell lung cancer – a phase 3 randomised controlled trial. *Lancet* published on line. http://dx.doi.org/10.1016/so140-6737(14)6105-0

Spiro, S. G., Rudd, R. M., Souhami, R. L., *et al.* (2004). Chemotherapy versus supportive care in advanced non-small cell lung cancer: improved survival without detriment to quality of life. *Thorax*, **59**, 828–836.

Stout, R., Barber, P. V., Burt, P. A., *et al.* (2000). Clinical and quality of life outcomes in the first United Kingdom randomised trial of endobronchial brachytherapy (intraluminal therapy) vs. external beam radiotherapy in the palliative treatment of inoperable non-small cell lung cancer. *Radiother. Oncol.*, **56**, 323–327.

Takeda, A., Sanuki, N., Eriguchi, T., *et al.* (2013). Stereoablative body radiotherapy for octogenarians with non small cell lung cancer. *Int. J. Radiat. Oncol. Biol. Phys.*, **86**, 257–263.

Thatcher, N., Qian, W., Clark, P., *et al.* (2005). Ifosfamide, carboplatin and etoposide with midcycle vincristine versus standard chemotherapy in patients with small cell lung cancer and good performance status: clinical and quality of life results of the British Medical Research Council multicentre randomized LU21 trial. *J. Clin. Oncol.*, **23**, 8371–8379.

Travis, L. (2011). Pathology of lung cancer. *Clin. Chest Med.*, **32**, 669–692.

Travis, W. D., Brambilla, E., Noguchi, M., *et al.* (2004). International Association for the Study of Lung Cancer/American Thoracic Society/European Respiratory/Society international multidisciplinary classification of lung adenocarcinoma. *J. Thorac. Oncol.*, **6**, 244–285.

Turrisi, A. T. 3rd, Kim, K., Blum, R., *et al.* (1999). Twice-daily compared with once-daily thoracic radiotherapy in limited small-cell lung cancer treated concurrently with cisplatin and etoposide. *N. Engl. J. Med.*, **340**, 265–271.

UICC. (2009). *TNM classification of malignant tumours (7th edition)*, ed. L. H. Sobin, M. K. Gospodarowitc and Ch. Wittekind. Oxford: Wiley-Blackwell, pp 138–146.

UK Consortium. (2014). *Stereotactic Ablative Body Radiation Therapy (SABR): A Resource*. SABR UK Consortium. v 4.1. Available at http://www.actionradiotherapy.org/ (accessed October 2014).

Yokoi, K., Kamiya, N., Matsuguma, H., *et al.* (1999). Detection of brain metastasis in potentially operable non-small cell lung cancer: a comparison of CT and MRI. *Chest*, **115**, 714–719.

Zhao, Y., Xie, X., deKonig, H., *et al.* (2011). NELSON lung screening study. *Cancer Imag.*, **11**(1A), S79–84.

Management of mesothelioma

Louise Hanna, Jason Lester and Fergus Macbeth

Introduction

Mesothelioma is a challenging disease for patients, relatives and doctors. It is strongly linked to exposure to asbestos and, despite a ban on the use of asbestos in the 1960s in the UK, its incidence is continuing to rise because of the long latent period between exposure and development of the disease. The incidence of mesothelioma is expected to peak around 2020 (Peto *et al.*, 1995). High-quality clinical research evidence to guide treatment decisions is lacking, and there is an urgent need to identify and evaluate new chemotherapeutic agents and treatment strategies.

Of all mesotheliomas, 94.5% affect the pleura, 5.1% affect the peritoneum and 0.4% affect the pericardium alone (Yates *et al.*, 1997). Mesotheliomas may also rarely arise in the tunica vaginalis.

Types of pleural tumour

The most common tumours affecting the pleura are metastatic from other sites. Table 32.1 shows the types of tumour that affect the pleura.

Anatomy of the pleura

The pleural surfaces surround both lungs and each is divided into two parts. The parietal pleura lines the cavity bounded by the thoracic wall, diaphragm and lateral mediastinum. The visceral pleura covers the surface of the lungs and extends into the interlobular fissures. The two layers are separated by a small amount of pleural fluid, which reduces friction during respiration.

The parietal pleura is divided into regions: cervical, costal, diaphragmatic and mediastinal. The costal pleura is supplied by intercostal nerves and are sensitive to pain and touch.

Table 32.1 Types of tumour affecting the pleura

Type	Examples
Benign	Solitary fibrous tumour (occasionally behaves in malignant way) Adenomatoid tumour
Malignant primary	Malignant mesothelioma (usually diffuse, rarely localised) Well-differentiated papillary mesothelioma Lymphoma Mesenchymal tumours (e.g. angiosarcoma, synovial sarcoma) Desmoplastic small round cell tumour of the pleura (aggressive) Calcifying tumour of the pleura (rare, slow growing)
Malignant secondary	Frequently adenocarcinoma (e.g. from ovary, breast, lung)

Adapted from Travis *et al.*, 2004.

Pleural mesothelioma

Incidence and epidemiology

The incidence of mesothelioma is 5.2 in 100,000 per year for males and 0.8 in 100,000 per year for females (www.cancerresearchuk.org, accessed October 2014). Approximately 2600 cases are diagnosed per year in the UK. The male-to-female ratio for the disease is 5.5:1, and the mortality-to-incidence ratio is 0.88 for males and 1.0 for females. The incidence rates have increased significantly since the 1970s and it is predicted that they will peak in the 2020s and then decrease.

Practical Clinical Oncology, Second Edition, ed. Louise Hanna, Tom Crosby and Fergus Macbeth. Published by Cambridge University Press. © Cambridge University Press 2015.

Risk factors and aetiology

Asbestos exposure

Exposure to asbestos is the single most important aetiological factor in mesothelioma and around 90% of patients with mesothelioma report a history of occupational exposure (Yates *et al.*, 1997).

The risk of developing mesothelioma is related to the level of exposure and to the type of asbestos fibre; 1 in 10 workers heavily exposed early in their working life may die of mesothelioma (Peto *et al.*, 1982). The latent interval between exposure and diagnosis is often very long; the mean latent interval between asbestos exposure and death is 41 years (Yates *et al.*, 1997). The use of asbestos has now been banned in the UK for construction and refurbishment, but asbestos is still present in many buildings.

There are two types of asbestos: amphibole and chrysotile. The most carcinogenic are the amphibole fibres: crocidolite (blue asbestos) and amosite (brown asbestos). The less carcinogenic type is chrysotile (white asbestos).

Asbestos-containing products include the following.

- Roofing materials.
- Fire protection materials, including blankets and curtains.
- Electrical casings.
- Water pipe products.

Occupational exposure to asbestos can occur in construction, renovation and demolition workers; ship builders and dock workers; carpenters and electricians; or manufacturers of asbestos products. Non-occupational exposure can occur in people who wash their partner's work clothes, from contaminated soil, from proximity to naturally occurring asbestos or from proximity to industrial plants where asbestos is used.

Clinical effects of asbestos exposure include the following.

- Asbestosis – lung fibrosis.
- Pleural plaques.
- Diffuse pleural fibrosis.
- Pleural effusion.
- Mesothelioma.
- Lung cancer.

Asbestos is also a possible aetiological factor in the development of other cancers such as laryngeal, oropharyngeal, gastrointestinal and renal.

Table 32.2 Pathological features of malignant mesothelioma

Features	Description
Macroscopic	Diffuse: multiple small nodules in early stages becoming confluent, fusing the visceral and parietal pleurae, encasing and contracting the lung
	Localised: has features of diffuse mesothelioma but appears as a localised nodule
Microscopic	Epithelioid – tubulopapillary, adenomatoid or sheet like
	Sarcomatoid – spindle cells resembling fibrosarcoma or malignant fibrous histiocytoma
	Desmoplastic –dense collagen stroma separated by atypical cells in > 50% of the tumour
	Biphasic – combined epithelial and sarcomatoid, each comprising at least 10% of the tumour; greater tumour sampling increases the ability to detect biphasic pattern

Adapted from Travis *et al.* (2004).

The mechanism of carcinogenesis is not fully understood, but asbestos fibres are known to induce DNA and chromosome damage. Simian virus 40 (SV 40) may act as a co-factor via transforming activity of two viral proteins, large T and small t antigens (Jaurand and Fleury-Feith, 2005).

Other possible aetiological factors

Other possible aetiological factors for mesothelioma include (Hubbard, 1997):

- erionite rock (in central Turkey);
- sugar cane;
- ionising radiation;
- pleural scars;
- SV 40 that accidentally contaminated millions of polio vaccines in the late 1950s and early 1960s.

Pathology

The main pathological types of mesothelioma are epithelioid, sarcomatoid and biphasic (Travis *et al.*, 2004). The term desmoplastic refers to sarcomatoid mesothelioma with dense collagen stroma. The pathological features of mesothelioma are shown in Table 32.2.

Table 32.3 Spread of pleural mesothelioma

Route of spread	Sites
Local	Chest wall, intercostal nerves, ribs
	Mediastinum, including pericardium and oesophagus
	Vertebral body
	Diaphragm and liver
Lymph node	Mediastinal nodes
	Internal mammary nodes
	Cervical nodes
Metastatic	Bone
	Contralateral lung
	Liver
	Brain

Immunohistochemistry

It can be difficult to differentiate epithelioid mesothelioma from adenocarcinoma on morphological appearance, and immunohistochemistry may be helpful.

Immunohistochemical markers which are positive in mesothelioma (and negative in adenocarcinoma) include calretinin, pan-cytokeratin, CK 5/6, thrombomodulin and WT1. Markers positive in adenocarcinoma and negative in mesothelioma include TTF-1 MOC-31, Ber-EP4 and CEA. The pathological diagnosis of a diffuse malignant mesothelioma is not always straightforward, and interpretation should always be taken in context, with full knowledge of the clinical history, examination findings and radiological appearance.

Spread

The predominant mode of spread is local. However, distant metastases do commonly occur as a late event, but are frequently asymptomatic. Routes of mesothelioma spread are shown in Table 32.3.

Clinical presentation

Typically, mesothelioma presents with symptoms and signs relating to the primary tumour (Parker and Neville, 2003):

- chest pain, which can be dull, diffuse or pleuritic and may have a neuropathic component;
- shortness of breath, often multifactorial, caused by pleural fluid, pleural thickening, thoracic restriction and lung encasement or comorbid conditions (e.g. airflow obstruction, cardiac dysfunction);

- incidental finding of pleural effusion or pleural thickening;
- weight loss;
- finger clubbing;
- profuse sweating.

Other, less common clinical features of mesothelioma include the following (BTS Statement, 2001):

- chest wall mass;
- abdominal pain or ascites;
- cervical lymphadenopathy;
- haemoptysis;
- hoarseness of voice;
- superior vena cava obstruction;
- dysphagia;
- cardiac tamponade.

Investigation and staging

Techniques for imaging and pathological confirmation of mesothelioma can be found in the BTS Statement (2007).

Imaging

A chest X-ray may show pleural thickening, a pleural-based mass, or effusion. Other features of asbestos exposure may be present. Ultrasound of the chest can be used to distinguish between solid and fluid lesions. A CT or MRI scan demonstrates invasion of the chest wall and enlarged mediastinal lymph nodes. Features suggestive of mesothelioma include nodular pleural thickening, thickening of the mediastinal pleura, constriction of the hemithorax and loss of lung volume. It can be difficult to quantify the amount of disease from a CT scan, an important issue when assessing response to treatment.

Pathological confirmation

Cytological examination of pleural fluid and appropriate immunocytochemistry may confirm the diagnosis, but it can be difficult to distinguish mesothelioma from highly reactive benign cells. Blind biopsy techniques such as Abrams' punch biopsy are quick to perform but are less effective for reaching a diagnosis than an ultrasound- or CT-guided percutaneous biopsy. In difficult cases, a thoracoscopic or open biopsy may be needed.

Staging classification

The TNM staging classification is shown in Table 32.4 (UICC, 2009).

Table 32.4 The TNM staging system for pleural mesothelioma

Stage	Description
T1	Tumour involves ipsilateral parietal pleura, with or without focal involvement of visceral pleura
T1a	Tumour involes ipsilateral parietal (mediastinal, diaphragmatic) pleura. No involvement of visceral pleura
T1b	Tumour involves ipsilateral parietal (mediastinal, diaphragmatic) pleura, with focal involvement of the visceral pleura
T2	Tumour involves any of the following ipsilateral pleural surfaces, with at least one of the following: • confluent visceral pleura tumour (including the fissure) • invasion of diaphragmatic muscle • invasion of lung parenchyma
T3[a]	Tumour involves any ipsilateral pleural surfaces, with at least one of the following: • invasion of endothoracic fascia • invasion into mediastinal fat • solitary focus of tumour invading soft tissues of the chest wall • non-transmural involvement of the pericardium
T4[b]	Tumour involves any ipsilateral pleural surfaces, with at least one of the following: • diffuse or multifocal invasion of soft tissues of chest wall • any involvement of rib • invasion through diaphragm to peritoneum • invasion of any mediastinal organ(s) • direct extension to contralateral pleura • invasion into the spine • extension to internal surface of pericardium • pericardial effusion with positive cytology • invasion of myocardium • invasion of brachial plexus
N1	Metastases in ipsilateral bronchopulmonary and/or hilar lymph nodes
N2	Metastases in subcarinal lymph node(s) and/or ipsilateral internal mammary or mediastinal lymph node(s)
N3	Metastases in contralateral mediastinal, internal mammary, or hilar node(s) and/or ipsilateral or contralateral supraclavicular or scalene lymph node(s)
M0	No distant metastases
M1	Distant metastases present

Adapted from UICC (2009). [a]T3 describes locally advanced, but potentially resectable tumour. [b]T4 describes locally advanced, technically unresectable tumour.

Treatment overview

Malignant pleural mesothelioma is generally considered an incurable disease, however treated.

Patients should be managed by a specialist multidisciplinary team. There is an emphasis on symptomatic and supportive treatments aimed at controlling the pleural effusion, pain and breathlessness. Patients of good performance status should be considered for palliative chemotherapy.

Patients and relatives should be informed of the possibilities for financial compensation.

The British Thoracic Society has recommended that radical surgery should be considered only within a randomised trial (BTS Statement, 2007).

Deaths due to mesothelioma must be reported to the coroner, and a postmortem examination is usually required.

Surgery

For more information on surgical procedures, see the BTS Statement (2007).

Radical surgery

Extrapleural pneumonectomy

Extrapleural pneumonectomy (EPP) is radical surgery that involves the removal of lung, and parietal and visceral pleura, together with the hemi-diaphragm and part of the pericardium. EPP is almost always carried out as part of a multimodality approach (see section below). It has an operative mortality of around 5% and a morbidity of around 50%, which has led to recommendations that it should be carried out only in the context of a clinical trial (Scherpereel et al., 2010). EPP is now rarely carried out in the UK following publication of the MARS trial (see below).

Radical/total pleurectomy

Radical (also called 'total' pleurectomy) can be carried out using video-assisted thorascopic surgery (VATS) or as an open procedure. It is less morbid than EPP and the aim of the surgery is complete macroscopic resection of all disease. The MARS 2 trial is a feasibility study looking at the role of extended pleurectomy decortication in patients given chemotherapy.

Palliative surgery

Debulking/cytoreductive surgery

- Removal of as much of the tumour as possible in a debulking operation can prevent recurrence of the pleural effusion and allow re-expansion of the lung. It is almost always carried out using VATS, which is associated with low operative morbidity and mortality.
- The MesoVATS trial randomly allocated patients to VATS pleurectomy, which involved partial parietal pleurectomy and decortication of the visceral pleura or talc pleurodesis. VATS pleurectomy did not improve overall survival and was associated with a higher complication rate, leading the authors to conclude that talc pleurodesis might be preferable (Rintoul et al., 2014).

Management of pleural effusion

Thoracoscopy

Thoracoscopy allows complete drainage of the pleural space followed by talc poudrage. It can be performed under conscious sedation (medical thoracoscopy) or under general anaesthesia (when VATS is used). It is a very effective way of controlling pleural effusions.

Talc pleurodesis

If the patient is too frail to undergo thoracoscopy or a firm diagnosis has already been made, talc slurry pleurodesis may be performed via an intercostal drain. Talc pleurodesis is a well-tolerated procedure and reduces fluid accumulation, but is not as effective as a thoracoscopic approach in controlling pleural effusion.

Pleuroperitoneal shunt

Pleuroperitoneal shunts can be used when pleurodesis has failed and for trapped lung, but there is a high incidence of shunt blockage and peritoneal seedlings. Their use is diminishing.

Palliative radiotherapy

Wide-field radiotherapy using parallel-opposed fields to a dose of 30 Gy in 10 fractions can improve pain in around 60% of patients (Bissett et al., 1991), but the effect is generally short-lived. Breathlessness does not improve.

Obvious and symptomatic chest wall masses and localised pain may be treated with short courses of palliative radiotherapy (e.g. 8–10 Gy in a single fraction or 16–17 Gy in 2 fractions).

Chemotherapy

In a randomised phase III trial of 456 patients with pleural mesothelioma, pemetrexed plus cisplatin resulted in a 3-month improvement in median survival when compared to cisplatin alone (Vogelzang et al., 2003). Pemetrexed plus cisplatin also resulted in an improvement in lung function, and was better at controlling dyspnoea and pain than cisplatin alone. As a result, chemotherapy is now offered routinely to good performance patients, and pemetrexed plus cisplatin has become the standard first-line regimen for fitter patients.

There has only been one phase III trial randomised controlled trial of active symptom control (ASC) with or without chemotherapy in the first-line setting. MS01 randomised patients to ASC, MVP (mitomycin, vinblastine and cisplatin) or vinorelbine (Muers et al., 2007). There was no benefit from chemotherapy, although the trial design was modified to compensate for a fall in recruitment once the Vogelzang results became known, and the trial was probably underpowered as result.

Sarcomatoid mesothelioma is generally viewed as resistant to chemotherapy; only about 10% of patients in the Vogelzang trial had the sarcomatoid variant, and they did not seem to benefit from the combination regimen.

Currently, there are no licensed, NICE-approved treatments in the second-line setting for patients with pleural mesothelioma.

Multimodality treatment

Multimodality treatment is defined as at least two of chemotherapy, surgery and radiotherapy. The attraction of a multimodality approach is that clinical trials have shown that treatment results with any single modality are disappointing.

For many years, highly selected, retrospective surgical case series have reported long-term survival in fit patients with low-volume epithelioid disease undergoing EPP. In an attempt to improve outcomes, Sugarbaker et al. (1996) treated 120 patients with EPP followed by combination chemotherapy and radiotherapy, and showed an overall survival of 45% at 2 years and 22% at 5 years, with a 5% operative mortality rate. Postoperative radiotherapy was part of the original protocol described by Sugarbaker and has remained an integral part of EPP protocols which recently have included neoadjuvant chemotherapy. Most protocols describe delivering 45–54 Gy to the ipsilateral hemithorax. Rusch et al. (2001) reported a phase II trial of postoperative radiotherapy in 54 patients who had undergone EPP. The local recurrence rate was observed to be much lower than expected in patients undergoing surgical resection alone.

Given the large volumes needed to treat the affected hemithorax and normal structures adjacent to the treatment volume, IMRT might be expected to improve dose distribution. Forster et al. (2003) described an IMRT technique with a CTV that was defined with the help of the thoracic surgeon. All spaces that had been entered surgically were included within the CTV with a 5–10-mm margin, as well as the ipsilateral mediastinum above the heart. The CTV was expanded by 5 mm to form the PTV. They found that IMRT allowed higher doses to large, complex target volumes with acceptable doses to normal tissues compared to conventional 3D conformal radiotherapy. Subsequently, IMRT has been mandated in almost all studies of multimodality treatment in mesothelioma, and evidence suggests that IMRT may result in improved local control over more traditional ways of delivering radiotherapy.

In a feasibility study for a randomised trial investigating multimodality treatment, the MARS trial randomly allocated patients to EPP plus hemithorax radiotherapy or no EPP following induction cisplatin-based chemotherapy. It took 3 years to randomise 50 patients, and only 8/24 patients allocated to surgery underwent EPP and completed postoperative radiotherapy as planned; the authors concluded that a larger study of EPP was not feasible (Treasure et al., 2011). The trial was not designed to detect a difference in survival between the two arms, but median survival was 14.4 months for the EPP group and 19.5 months for the no-EPP group. This result has led many experts to question the benefit of multimodality treatment in malignant mesothelioma.

In summary, there are no randomised trials showing benefit for a multimodality approach in the management of malignant mesothelioma. There are case series in selected patients that report impressive long-term survival, but these are subject to selection bias, and further evidence is needed to best define the optimum approach to this difficult disease. At present, therefore, multimodality treatment is not considered part of routine practice.

Symptomatic treatments

For the treatment of dyspnoea, consider breathing exercises, relaxation, home oxygen, opiates and benzodiazepines and exclude a pleural effusion.

For chest pain, consider analgesics according to the WHO ladder, non-steroidal anti-inflammatory drugs, tricyclic antidepressants or anticonvulsants.

For cough, consider simple linctus, codeine linctus, oral steroids and opiates or saline nebulisers for sticky sputum.

Prognosis

Survival

The median survival of patients with mesothelioma is around 8 months (Van Gelder et al., 1994) and the 5-year survival is 4.7% (Gatta et al., 2006).

Prognostic factors

There are several prognostic models in use. A review of the best-known prognostic scoring systems from the EORTC and CALGB (both based on multivariate analysis) has shown that the most important predictors of poor prognosis are likely to be:

- poor performance status;
- non-epithelioid histology;
- male gender;
- low haemoglobin;

- high platelet count;
- high white blood cell count;
- high lactate dehydrogenase (LDH).

The EORTC model was validated in a group of 145 UK patients treated in chemotherapy trials. Those having the best EORTC prognosis had a median survival of 19.2 months compared to 9.9 months for those in the worst group (Steele *et al.*, 2005).

Compensation

Patients and relatives should be given advice about compensation and benefits for mesothelioma patients.

Information can be obtained from the clinical nurse specialist, social worker or solicitor. Possibilities for benefits are listed here (see Macmillan; http://www.macmillan.org.uk/Cancerinformation/Cancertypes/Mesothelioma/ or Mesothelioma UK; http://www.mesothelioma.uk.com/, accessed August 2014).

- Industrial Injuries Disablement Benefit – a weekly allowance for patients with mesothelioma who can show they were occupationally exposed to asbestos.
- Civil law personal injury claim against the previous employer.
- Pneumoconiosis Worker's Compensation or, more recently, the 2008 Diffuse Mesothelioma Scheme or the Diffuse Mesothelioma Payment Scheme if the employer has gone out of business.
- Statutory Sick Pay for those with adequate National Insurance contributions, paid for a maximum of 28 weeks.
- The Employment and Support Allowance is for people who are unable to work due to illness or disability. It has now been replaced by the Universal Credit in certain parts of the UK.
- The Disability Living Allowance has been replaced by the Personal Independence Payment.
- Attendance Allowance.
- Constant Attendance Allowance.
- For carers, the Carer's Allowance is for looking after someone with substantial caring needs and the Carer's Credit helps build entitlement to a state pension.

Areas of current interest and current clinical trials

Malignant mesothelioma is refractory to most treatments, and the only treatment shown to prolong life is chemotherapy with pemetrexed plus cisplatin. There is an urgent need for new therapeutic agents, but, unlike with many other solid tumours, there are no targeted systemic treatments currently in routine clinical use. There are, however, several potential molecular targets that are currently undergoing evaluation in clinical trials.

STAT3 is signal transduction protein active in malignant mesothelioma. The randomised RUXSAC trial is investigating the role of the STAT3 inhibitor ruxolitinib in combination with chemotherapy.

Arginine deprivation is a new anti-metabolite strategy for the treatment of arginine-dependent cancers that exploits differential expression and regulation of key urea cycle enzymes. The recent phase II study of the arginine depletor ADI-PEG20 in mesothelioma (ADAM trial) showed longer progression-free survival in heavily pretreated patients compared to placebo. A phase I combination trial (TRAP) is now open in the UK.

Mesothelioma is molecularly characterised by the loss of tumour suppressor genes rather than the gain of function mutations. The observation that BRCA-associated protein 1 (BAP1) is inactivated in around a quarter of mesothelioma cancers has raised the possibility that this subset may harbour a therapeutic target (Bott *et al.*, 2011).

Another tumour suppressor gene that is often inactivated is neurofibromatosis type 2 (NF2), with NF2 loss occurring in around 40% of patients. NF2 encodes for the protein merlin, which in turn interacts with more than 30 other intracellular proteins. Drug classes that may be active on the basis of these interactions include MTOR inhibitors, and the use of dual PI3K/MTOR inhibitors, in view of the compensatory upregulation of PI3K seen with MTOR inhibition alone. A phase I trial of the PI3K/MTOR inhibitor GDC0980 showed some activity in a subset of patients with mesothelioma (Wagner *et al.*, 2011).The role of FAK inhibitors is being investigated, because of the negative regulation of FAK by an intact merlin protein via FAK phosphorylation.

Prophylactic radiotherapy to drainage or biopsy sites

The use of less-invasive diagnostic procedures (such as CT-guided biopsies instead of open biopsies) has led to a fall in the incidence of intervention site mesothelioma seeding. A pooled analysis of trials looking at the affect of prophylactic irradiation found no significant reduction in the frequency of procedure track metastases. There are currently two larger randomised UK trials looking at the role of prophylactic intervention site radiotherapy in a contemporary mesothelioma population (PIT and SMART). Until the results of these trials are known, prophylactic radiotherapy to drainage or biopsy sites is not recommended unless in the context of a trial.

Clinical trials

The following trials were among those listed as open by the UK Clinical Research Network (http://public.ukcrn.org.uk, accessed August 2014).
Prophylactic Irradiation of Tracts in Mesothelioma (PIT): a phase III randomised trial of prophylactic irradiation of tracts in patients with malignant pleural mesothelioma following invasive chest wall intervention.
COMMAND: a phase II randomised double-blind, placebo-controlled, multicentre study of VS-6063 in subjects with malignant pleural mesothelioma.
VE-BASKET: an open-label, phase II study of vemurafenib in patients with BRAF V600 mutation-positive cancers.
NCRN–2509: a phase II, randomised, double-blind study comparing tremelimumab to placebo in second- or third-line treatment of subjects with unresectable pleural or peritoneal malignant mesothelioma.
Mesothelioma and Radical Surgery Trial (MARS2): a study to determine if it is feasible to recruit into a randomised trial comparing (extended) pleurectomy decortication versus no pleurectomy decortication in the multimodality management of patients with malignant pleural mesothelioma.

References

Bissett, D., Macbeth, F. R. and Cram, I. (1991). The role of palliative radiotherapy in malignant mesothelioma. *Clin. Oncol. (R. Coll. Radiol.)*, **3**, 315–317.

Bott, M., Brevet, M., Taylor, B. S., *et al.* (2011). The nuclear deubiquitinase *BAP1* is commonly inactivated by somatic mutations and 3p21.1 losses in malignant pleural mesothelioma. *Nat. Genet.*, **43**, 668–672.

BTS Statement. (2007). Statement on malignant mesothelioma in the UK. *Thorax*, **62**, ii1–ii19.

Forster, K. M., Smyth, W. R., Starkschall, G., *et al.* (2003). Intensity-modulated radiotherapy following extrapleural pneumonectomy for the treatment of malignant mesothelioma: clinical implementation. *Int. J. Radiat. Oncol. Biol. Phys.*, **55**, 606–616.

Gatta, G., Ciccolallo, L., Kunkler, I., *et al.* (2006). Survival from rare cancer in adults: a population-based study. *Lancet Oncol.*, **7**, 132–140.

Hubbard, R. (1997). The aetiology of mesothelioma: are risk factors other than asbestos exposure important? *Thorax*, **52**, 496–497.

Jaurand, M. C. and Fleury-Feith, J. (2005). Pathogenesis of malignant pleural mesothelioma. *Respirology*, **10**, 2–8.

Muers, M., Stephens, R. J., Fisher, P., *et al.* (2007). Active symptoms control with or without chemotherapy in the treatment of patients with malignant pleural mesothelioma (MS01): a multicentre randomised trial. *Lancet*, **371**, 1685–1694.

National Statistics. (2005). *Cancer Statistics and Registrations*, Series MB1 no. 34. London: Office for National Statistics.

Parker, C. and Neville, E. (2003). Lung cancer 8: management of malignant mesothelioma. *Thorax*, **58**, 809–813.

Peto, J., Hodgson, J. T., Matthews, F. E., *et al.* (1995). Continuing increase in mesothelioma mortality in Britain. *Lancet*, **345**, 535–539.

Peto, J., Seidman, H. and Selikoff, I. J. (1982). Mesothelioma mortality in asbestos workers: implications for models of carcinogenesis and risk assessment. *Br. J. Cancer*, **45**, 124–135.

Rintoul, R. C., Ritchie, A. J., Edwards, J. G., *et al.* (2014). Efficacy and cost of video-assisted thoracoscopic partial pleurectomy versus talc pleurodesis in patients with malignant pleural mesothelioma (MesoVATS): an open-label, randomised, controlled trial. *Lancet*, **384**, 1118–1127.

Rusch, V. W., Rosenzweig, K., Venkatraman, E., *et al.* (2001). A phase II trial of surgical resection and adjuvant high-dose hemithoracic radiation for malignant pleural mesothelioma. *J. Thorac. Cardiovasc. Surg.*, **122**, 788–795.

Scherpereel, A., Astoul, P., Baas, T., *et al.* (2010). Guidelines of the European Respiratory Society and the European Society of Thoracic Surgeons for the management of malignant pleural mesothelioma. *Eur. Resp. J.*, **35**, 279–495.

Steele, J. P., Klabatsa, A., Fennell, D. A., *et al.* (2005). Prognostic factors in mesothelioma. *Lung Cancer*, **49**, S49–52.

Sugarbaker, D. J., Garcia, J. P., Richards, W. G., *et al.* (1996). Extrapleural pneumonectomy in the multimodality therapy of malignant pleural mesothelioma. Results in 120 consecutive patients. *Ann. Surg.*, **224**, 288–294.

Travis, W. D., Brambilla, E., Muller-Hermelink, H. K., *et al.* (2004). *World Health Organization Classification of Tumours. Pathology and Genetics, Tumours of the*

Lung, Pleura, Thymus and Heart. Lyon: IARC Press, pp. 125–144.

Treasure, T., Lang-Lazdunski, L., Waller, D., *et al.* (2011). Extra-pleural pneumonectomy versus no extra-pleural pneumonectomy for patients with malignant pleural mesothelioma: clinical outcomes of the Mesothelioma and Radical Surgery (MARS) randomised feasibility study. *Lancet Oncol.*, **12**, 763–772.

UICC (2009). *TNM Classification of Malignant Tumours*, ed. L. H. Sobin, M. K. Gospodarowicz and Ch. Wittekind, 7th edn. Chichester, Wiley-Blackwell, pp. 147–150.

Van Gelder, T., Damhuis, R. A. and Hoogsteden, H. C. (1994). Prognostic factors and survival in malignant pleural mesothelioma. *Eur. Respir. J.*, **7**, 1035–1038.

Vogelzang, N. J., Rusthoven, J. J., Simanowski, J., *et al.* (2003). Phase III study of pemetrexed in combination with cisplatin versus cisplatin alone in patients with malignant pleural mesothelioma. *J. Clin. Oncol.*, **21**, 2636–2644.

Wagner, A. J., Bendell, J. C., Dolly, S., *et al.* (2011). A first-in-human phase I study to evaluate GDC-0980, an oral PI3K/mTOR inhibitor, administered QD in patients with advanced solid tumors. *J. Clin. Oncol.*, **29**, abstr. 3020.

Yates, D. H., Corrin, B., Stidolph, P. N., *et al.* (1997). Malignant mesothelioma in south east England: clinicopathological experience of 272 cases. *Thorax*, **52**, 507–512.

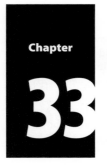

Chapter 33

Management of soft tissue and bone tumours in adults

Owen Tilsley

Soft tissue sarcoma

Introduction

Soft tissue sarcomas are mesenchymally derived malignant tumours that may arise virtually anywhere in the body. They are rare, with an incidence of 45 per million (http://www.cancerresearchuk.org/, accessed January 2015). The overall survival is approximately 50% at 5 years. Treatment is largely surgical with adjuvant radiotherapy offered where there is deemed to be a significant risk of local relapse. Of patients with intermediate or high-grade tumours, 50% develop metastatic disease, usually by haematogenous spread to the lungs or in the case of sarcomas draining to the portal vein, the liver. Palliative chemotherapy may be offered, usually with single agent doxorubicin. Response rates are low at around 20%, although a further 20% achieve disease stabilisation. UK and ESMO European guidance on the management of soft tissue sarcoma tumours exist (Grimer et al., 2010b; The ESMO and European Sarcoma Network Working Groups, 2012b). American NCCN Guidelines are also available after free registration at the NCCN website. The National Institute for Health and Clinical Excellence has published Improving Outcomes Guidance for people with sarcoma (NICE, 2006).

Types of soft tissue tumour

Over 100 different morphology codes relating to sarcoma are present within the ICD-O-3 and World Health Organisation (WHO) classifications of sarcomas, but they can be grouped into the subtypes leiomyosarcoma, liposarcoma, fibrosarcoma, synovial sarcoma, vascular sarcoma, nerve sheath tumours, malignant phylloides tumours, sarcoma not-otherwise-specified and others. This chapter will not deal with GIST, which is covered in Chapter 18, rhabdomyosarcoma (covered in Chapter 40), and Kaposi's sarcoma (in Chapter 36). Ewing sarcoma of soft tissue and bone are treated identically and is covered in the bone sarcoma section of this chapter.

Incidence and epidemiology

A detailed analysis of the epidemiology of soft tissue sarcoma in England has been published recently by the West Midlands Cancer Intelligence Unit and is available online as 'Soft Tissue Sarcoma Incidence and Survival Tumours Diagnosed in England Between 1985 and 2009' (Dennis et al., 2012). The age-standardised soft tissue sarcoma incidence rates in England is around 45 cases per million, similar to the rates found in other registries outside the UK. Incidence rates have increased significantly over the 25-year period examined from 34 cases per million in 1985 to 48 cases per million in 2009. This increase may simply be due to improved diagnostic techniques and more accurate recording. Historically, the incidence of sarcoma has been difficult to ascertain accurately as the ICD-10 classification of cancers is dependent on location rather than morphology.

After a small peak in children aged 0–4 years, the number of soft tissue sarcomas diagnosed increases gradually with age. A similar pattern is seen in males and females. Patients with a bone or soft tissue sarcoma diagnosis tend to be younger than the majority of cancer patients. Of sarcomas, 16% are diagnosed in patients less than 30 years of age, compared to around 2% of all cancers, and 37% of bone or soft tissue sarcoma patients are aged less than 50 years compared with 11% of all cancer patients. Soft tissue sarcomas are most likely to arise in the limbs (23%) and the connective tissues of the trunk (13%), although they can occur at any site of the body. Incidence rates for each

Practical Clinical Oncology, Second Edition, ed. Louise Hanna, Tom Crosby and Fergus Macbeth. Published by Cambridge University Press. © Cambridge University Press 2015.

436

anatomical cancer site vary with age; with sarcomas arising in the brain and CNS being most common in patients under the age of 10 years, and sarcomas of the limbs being most common in patients aged between 10 and 29 and 80 years and over. Soft tissue sarcomas arising within the head, face and neck are also more prominent in patients aged under 20 years. Tumours of the retroperitoneum, on the other hand, are very rarely diagnosed in patients less than 40 years old.

Risk factors and aetiology

In most cases, the cause of soft tissue sarcoma is unclear. Exposure to radiation and vinyl chloride monomer, dioxins and chlorophenols are known to increase the incidence of sarcoma, but do not account for the overwhelming majority of tumours. With improved cancer survival, treatment-induced second tumours including sarcoma are becoming more frequent. Chronic lymphoedema may lead to the development of angiosarcoma (Stewart Treves syndrome). A number of inherited conditions are known to be associated with soft tissue sarcomas. Neurofibromatosis type I is associated with a range of benign and malignant tumours of neural origin, including malignant peripheral nerve sheath tumours and plexiform neurofibromata which run an 8–12% lifetime risk of malignant change. Li Fraumeni syndrome is associated with a wide range of soft tissue and bone sarcomas. Familial retinoblastoma – a germ-line mutation of the RB1 gene – carries a 10% risk of sarcoma. Gardner's syndrome consists of adenomatous polyps of the gastrointestinal tract and a number of benign and malignant tumours including desmoids. Tuberous sclerosis gives rise to angiomyolipomas, which are, however, generally considered to be benign.

Anatomy and pathology

Malignant tumours may develop a pseudo- or false capsule via compression of surrounding tissue, but tumour cells may be found in the peritumoural oedema even some centimetres away from the visible primary. This oedema extends by the path of least resistance, usually axially in a limb, and it respects fascial and compartmental boundaries. Approximately half of soft tissue sarcomas arise in limbs, 20% are retroperitoneal, 15% are visceral and 10% occur in the head and neck. Completeness of excision, grade, size and, to a lesser extent, the depth of a tumour guide the choice of further treatment, admittedly without a strong evidence base. These indicators are often of more use than the histological subtype in determining treatment. Benign tumours outnumber malignant ones by at least 100 to 1, and even for lumps excised and sent for histology, the ratio is 20 to 1, which has been a challenge for the centralisation and optimisation of sarcoma services. A number of grading systems are in common use internationally. In Europe, including the UK, the Trojani system is widely used. This system divides sarcomas into grades 1–3 based on a scoring system of differentiation, mitoses and necrosis, with scores of 2–3 being classed as grade 1, 4–5 as grade 2, and 6+ as grade 3.

Spread

Sarcomas may spread by local invasion, which usually respects fascial boundaries, or by haematogenous spread to the lung or to the liver for organs that drain into the portal vein. Sarcoma metastases are often limited in number, leading some to propose metastectomy in certain circumstances. Sarcomas rarely spread via the lymphatic system.

Clinical presentation

Any patient with a soft tissue mass that is increasing in size, has a size greater than 5 cm or is deep to the deep fascia, whether or not it is painful, should be referred to a diagnostic centre as a suspected soft tissue sarcoma.

Investigation and staging

Suspected soft tissue sarcomas should be referred to a specialist sarcoma unit. Triple assessment with clinical history, imaging and several cores should be obtained by wide-needle biopsy. Occasionally, incisional or planned excisional biopsy may be the most practical especially for superficial lesions. The biopsy must be planned so that the track will be easily removed at the time of definitive surgery to reduce the risk of seeding. Fine-needle aspiration (FNA) is not recommended, as it provides only limited information on tumour morphology, and can at times be misleading. Confirmed cases of sarcoma require a CT thorax and local imaging of the primary, usually by MRI. The Royal College of Radiologists' 'Evidence based indications for the use of PET-CT in the United Kingdom 2012' recommends ^{18}F-FDG PET for high-grade sarcomas if distant disease has not been already been discovered or where the decision for amputation or metastectomy would be altered by the discovery of distant disease (The

Table 33.1 TNM classification of soft tissue sarcoma

Stage	Description
T1	Tumour ≤ 5 cm
T2	Tumour > 5 cm
N0	No regional lymph node metastasis
N1	Regional nodes involved
M0	No distant metastases
M1	Distant metastases

Adapted from UICC, 2009.

Royal College of Physicians and the Royal College of Radiologists, 2013).

Staging classification

The TNM classification of malignant soft tissue tumours is shown in Table 33.1. The T stage may be further subclassified a or b if the primary tumour is superficial (a) or deep (b) to the deep fascia. The regional lymph nodes are defined as those nodes most appropriate to the primary tumour site, and they vary with the location of the tumour (UICC, 2009).

Treatment overview

Patients should be managed by a specialist multidisciplinary team. The aim of treatment is to maximise the chance of a cure while safely minimising treatment-related morbidity. Soft tissue sarcoma is incurable without surgery. Appropriate limb-sparing operations have the same local control and cure rates as amputation: surgery should be undertaken by specialists. Radiotherapy halves the recurrence rate of large high-grade tumours. The role of adjuvant chemotherapy remains uncertain, but in limb sarcoma the preliminary results of a recent EORTC large randomised trial showed no benefit. Doxorubicin and fairly high-dose ifosfamide are the most active agents against advanced disease, but they are toxic and have response rates of only 20%, and so palliative care alone may be appropriate. The newer agents trabectedin and pazopanib have also shown activity. Recently, gemcitabine and docetaxel were compared against doxorubicin as first-line therapy in metastatic disease in the UK with final results awaited.

Local disease: surgical treatments

The primary tumour should be excised with a 1-cm margin, although the optimum margin has not been investigated in a clinical trial. The wider margins that have been historically recommended are no longer felt necessary and excision beyond fascial boundaries is not needed. A randomised trial of limb salvage surgery with RT versus amputation revealed a salvageable reduction in local control but no difference in disease-free or overall survival (Rosenberg et al., 1982). The functional loss from arm amputation is considerably more than that from leg amputation, and limb salvage should always be considered. Below the knee, the functional outcome from amputation and limb-sparing surgery are the same, but patient well-being and satisfaction, although high for both, is greater with limb salvage.

A preoperative scan, good operative notes, clips at areas of concern, and photographs, diagrams, or annotated explanations of the operative procedure are helpful in planning radiotherapy.

Local disease: radiotherapy

Postoperative radiotherapy

Poor, possibly inadvertent, surgery results in a high local relapse rate, and, where feasible, re-excision should be undertaken. Sometimes limb salvage means accepting close or involved margins – for example, where a tumour abuts the sciatic nerve. For large tumours, a randomised trial has shown a halving in the risk of local relapse with postoperative adjuvant external beam RT (Yang et al., 1998). Another trial has shown the same for brachytherapy for high-grade tumours (Pisters et al., 1996). Neither trial showed an effect on overall survival. However, quality of life and limb function depend on local control; if it is thought that there is an appreciable risk of local recurrence RT should be given.

The recently closed UK Vortex Trial of radiotherapy margin size advised re-excision or RT in all cases if the surgical margin was less than 10 mm, and RT for all T2b (> 5 cm and deep) tumours and for high-grade T1b (≤ 5 cm and deep) tumours with margins less than 20 mm. Traditionally the majority of oncologists apply a 5-cm margin to both the surgical scar and the tumour bed when planning. Historically, even wider margins of 7–15 cm have been advocated. However, the radial margin of 2 cm and longitudinal margin of 4 cm in a brachytherapy trial gave equivalent local control. It is common practice to use a shrinking field, with a 5-cm margin to 50 Gy and a 2-cm margin to 60–66 Gy, but because the majority of local relapses occur in the high-dose volume, the shrinking field may not be necessary. In an attempt to clarify the size of the required margin, the Vortex Trial was conducted. This was a randomised trial with the standard-arm first-phase CTV defined as the larger of either 5 cm around the preoperative GTV or 1 cm around the postoperative scar, and the phase 2 CTV being 2 cm around the preoperative GTV. A dose of 50 Gy is given to the phase 1 volume and 66 Gy to the phase 2 volume. The experimental arm treats only the phase 2 volume to 66 Gy. Its results are awaited. The optimum dose remains controversial. Local relapse appears unacceptably high with a dose below 50 Gy and the functional outcome is worse after 66 Gy than after 60 Gy. Most oncologists currently prescribe 66 Gy to the ICRU reference point. High-quality surgery is particularly important in areas such as the retroperitoneum, where adjuvant RT to a dose of even 50 Gy may be impossible. Postoperative adhesions can pose a problem of bowel toxicity. A spacer (e.g. a breast prosthesis) inserted at the time of operation and clips at particular areas of concern can be helpful.

Primary (preoperative) radiotherapy

The optimum time for RT is controversial, but preoperative RT is becoming increasingly common in the UK. Preoperative RT has not been compared with surgery alone in a randomised trial but has been compared with postoperative RT. This study was ended prematurely at a planned interim analysis, when a statistically significant increase in wound healing problems was found after 50 Gy preoperatively. Continued follow-up has shown a marginal but significant improvement in overall survival with preoperative RT, but has shown no effect on local control, and longer-term poorer functional outcome with 66 Gy given postoperatively (Davis et al., 2005). Because of the lower dose and smaller volumes than those used for postoperative RT, this approach is thought to be particularly useful in sites where wound healing is not usually a problem, and in sites such as the retroperitoneum, where normal tissue tolerance may limit the safe dose.

Definitive radiotherapy

Long-term local control can be achieved in as many as 30% of patients with RT alone and may be considered where surgery is not possible. Palliative RT may also be given.

Radiotherapy delivery technique

Patient preparation, position and immobilisation

For limbs, appropriate limb positioning is essential for RT planning; for example, placing the arm away from the trunk for a forearm sarcoma, abducting and externally rotating the hip into a frog leg position for anterior thigh treatment, or raising one leg above another for a calf treatment. However, the patient needs to be comfortable to ensure reproducibility of the set-up. Limb immobilisation, for example, with a plastic shell or vacuum bag, should always be considered, but is not always needed for proximal tumours. A photograph of the position helps record the exact position. For other sites such as the head and neck region, an immobilisation shell is required.

Localisation and target volume

Delineating the CTV can be difficult following surgery and requires a good understanding of limb anatomy. Historically, sarcoma radiotherapy was planned on a simulator, but modern radiotherapy is undertaken with CT planning. CT scanning may, however, constrain the positioning and immobilisation of the limb because the patient, the limb and the immobilisation device all need to fit through the aperture of the CT scanner. A diagnostic scanner typically has an aperture of 60 cm and CT simulators are usually wider, but even an aperture 100 cm wide can be limiting. With reference to all available information, such as preoperative scans and operation notes, the target volumes are planned. The phase 1 CTV for limbs typically comprises the operative bed plus 5 cm longitudinally and 2 cm radially and includes the scar and biopsy sites. The phase 2 CTV has only a 2 cm longitudinal margin. An additional margin dependent on the confidence of set-up accuracy, typically 0.5–1 cm is added to form the PTV. Individualised shielding may be required – for example, of pelvic structures during RT to the upper leg – and is usually achieved by conformal 3D radiotherapy planning. A strip of skin should always be spared in limbs to minimise the late complication of lymphoedema, and if possible long bone dose should be kept below 50 Gy to reduce radiation-induced osteopenia.

Plan

Frequently limbs can be treated with a parallel-opposed pair of fields, where the use of wedges and tissue compensators helps to achieve a uniform dose distribution. RT to other sites usually requires multiple beam arrangements, and IMRT may deliver a more acceptable plan. In the UK, the IMRiS (Intensity Modulated Radiotherapy in Sarcoma) trial, a comparison of this and conventional 3D conformal planning, is proposed.

Verification

Given the possibility of quite large set-up errors, often in excess of 1 cm, it is desirable to verify treatment delivery. However, field sizes exceeding the size of the portal imager and the angle of the RT fields may make portal imaging difficult to take or interpret. It may be difficult to confirm and correct set-up with portal image containing only a long bone. Cone beam CT or small field portal images of the isocentre may be necessary.

Dose, energy and fractionation

In phase 1, the dose is 50 Gy in 25 fractions over 5 weeks to the ICRU reference point. In phase 2, the dose is 10–16 Gy in 5–8 fractions over 1–1.5 weeks to the ICRU reference point. Sites such as the retroperitoneum and pelvis are generally prescribed a lower dose. Because of small bowel tolerance, the phase 1 dose is usually 45 Gy in 25 fractions over 5 weeks, and the phase 2 dose, if given, is individualised to stay within organ tolerance. The use of preoperative rather than postoperative RT for retroperitoneal tumours should always be considered. Sarcomas in para-spinal locations may be considered for proton therapy.

Preoperative radiotherapy technique

The most obvious differences between preoperative and postoperative planning volumes are that the tumour is still *in situ* and, apart from the biopsy site, there is no scar. Because of this, the volumes tend to be smaller than those for postoperative RT. GTV to CTV margins are typically 5 cm longitudinally and 2 cm radially. The dose is 50 Gy in 25 fractions.

Adjuvant chemotherapy

Adjuvant chemotherapy in soft tissue sarcoma has been tested in a number of clinical trials with conflicting results. The two largest trials were conducted by the EORTC. The first EORTC study (Bramwell *et al.*, 1994) trialled a combination of cyclophosphamide, vincristine, doxorubicin and dacarbazine (CYVADIC), a regime not now regarded as particularly effective, against no chemotherapy. This showed no significant improvement in survival, but an improvement in local control. A meta-analysis reached a similar

conclusion, but was dominated by this first EORTC trial (Sarcoma Meta-analysis Collaboration, 1997). The second EORTC study (Woll *et al.*, 2012) trialled ifosfamide at 10 g/m² (with mesna) over 4 days and single-dose doxorubicin at 25 mg/m² over 3 days against no chemotherapy and showed no difference, but local control rates in both were higher than would have been expected historically. A pooled analysis of adjuvant doxorubicin-based chemotherapy showed no survival advantage in any pathological subgroup (Le Cesne *et al.*, 2014). A trial is currently underway in Italy looking at chemotherapy tailored to the specific subtype of soft tissue sarcoma. Uterine leiomyosarcoma has shown high response rates with gemcitabine and docetaxel (Hensley *et al.*, 2002), and a trial of adjuvant chemotherapy with these drugs is under way in the UK.

Metastatic disease

Metastectomy, usually pulmonary, may be curative, but the effectiveness of this strategy has been questioned, and although a randomised trial has been considered, there are concerns about the willingness of patients or doctors to accept randomisation. No trial has tested immediate versus delayed chemotherapy in soft tissue sarcoma, but observational studies have shown similar outcomes.

First-line chemotherapy

Single-agent doxorubicin at a dose of 60–75 mg/m² is currently the standard of care. Doxorubicin probably does improve survival, because although it has never been tested against best supportive care, it showed improved survival compared to brostallicin in a randomised trial (Gelderblom *et al.*, 2014). Epirubicin has shown similar activity to doxorubicin in two randomised trials and in some countries is used in preference to doxorubicin. Single-agent ifosfamide in high doses with mesna is also active. Reported response rates are higher with doses in excess of 6 g/m² (van Oosterom *et al.*, 2002). A randomised trial showed ifosfamide at 6 g/m² over 3 days to be as effective as doxorubicin but more toxic (Lorigan *et al.*, 2007). A trial of the combination of ifosfamide and doxorubicin against doxorubicin alone showed an improved response rate, but no improvement in survival, suggesting sequential doxorubicin then ifosfamide is as effective (Judson *et al.*, 2014). Gemcitabine and docetaxel appear particularly effective in uterine leiomyosarcoma (Hensley *et al.*, 2002). A UK randomised trial of this regimen against doxorubicin (GeDDiS, 'gemcitabine and docetaxel compared with doxorubicin in sarcoma') has recently completed accrual. Preliminary results present at ASCO suggest equivalence (Seddon *et al.*, 2015). A trial of trabectedin first-line in a range of sarcomas showed equivalent activity to doxorubicin (Blay *et al.*, 2014). Darcarbazine has activity in sarcoma. Paclitaxel is active in advanced angiosarcoma.

Second- and subsequent line chemotherapy

Trabectedin, dacarbazine and pazopanib have all demonstrated activity in soft tissue sarcoma. Trabectedin has not been compared to observation in second and subsequent line chemotherapy, but a regimen of 3-weekly trabectedin at 1.5 mg/m^2 showed improved progression-free but not overall survival over a weekly schedule (Demetri *et al.*, 2009) and is approved by NICE when treatment with anthracyclines and ifosfamide has failed, is poorly tolerated or contraindicated (NICE, 2010). Pazopanib has shown improved progression-free but not overall survival over placebo in non-lipomatous sarcomas (van der Graaf *et al.*, 2012) and is currently approved for use in England and Wales but not Scotland. Dacarbazine improved survival when added to gemcitabine in second-line therapy (García-del-Muro *et al.*, 2011). Eribulin inhibits microtubule formation and a trial of this compared with dacarbazine is under way in patients previously treated with an anthracycline. The alkylating agent bendamustine has shown activity in otherwise refractory sarcoma.

Prognosis

Soft tissue sarcoma 5-year relative survival rates have improved significantly in the last 25 years from 48% in 1985–1989 to 56% in 2000–2004. Five-year relative survival rates are similar in males and females.

Clinical trials

A variety of clinical trials are looking at soft tissue sarcomas. For more information, see http://csg.ncri.org.uk/ (accessed January 2015).

The EORTC is conducting a randomised phase II trial of cabazitaxel or prolonged infusional ifosfamide in metastatic or inoperable locally advanced dedifferentiated liposarcoma and a phase II trial of preoperative radiotherapy plus surgery versus surgery alone in patients with retroperitoneal sarcoma.

Axi-STC is a phase II study of axitinib in patients with advanced angiosarcoma and other soft tissue sarcomas.

Bone tumours

Introduction

Bone cancer is rare and in the UK care is best directed by one of the five UK reference centres with the cooperation of the regional cancer centre, as recommended in NICE guidance 'Improving Outcomes for People with Sarcoma' (NICE, 2006). Additionally, the management of Ewing sarcoma of bone is directed by an internet virtual MDT. UK and ESMO (Grimer *et al.*, 2010a; The ESMO and European Sarcoma Network Working Groups, 2012a) guidance on the management of bone tumours exists. American NCCN Guidelines are also available after free registration at the NCCN website (www.nccn.org, accessed February 2015).

Range of tumours

The commonest bone tumour is a secondary, and the commonest primary bone malignancy in adults is myeloma. This chapter confines itself to the mesenchymally derived primary tumours, osteosarcoma, Ewing sarcoma, chondrosarcoma, chordoma and other bone sarcomas.

Incidence and epidemiology

A detailed analysis of the epidemiology of bone sarcoma in England has recently been published by the West Midlands Cancer Intelligence Unit (NCIN, 2012). SEER monographs for children (Gurney *et al.*, 1999) and young adults (Mascarenhas *et al.*, 2006) provide detailed accounts of the epidemiology of bone cancers in the USA at the stated ages. The average annual incidence of bone sarcoma in England over the period 1985–2009 is around 7.9 per million persons. This has increased in more recent years to around 10 per million persons, but this may reflect improved diagnostic techniques and reporting rather than a true increase in incidence. In England there were 437 new diagnoses of bone sarcoma in 2009; 131 (30%) were osteosarcomas, 161 (37%) were chondrosarcomas, 62 (14%) were Ewing sarcomas and 28 (6%) were chordomas. They are all more common in males. There have been no significant improvements in bone sarcoma 5-year relative survival rates for patients diagnosed between

1985 and 2004. At around 54%, relative survival rates in England are low when compared with those calculated using other international databases, such as the SEER programme. Differences in the age distribution of patients included in the two cohorts and the variants included in the analyses could explain some of these differences. Osteosarcoma has a peak age at 15, with a second peak in the elderly. Osteosarcoma is uncommon before puberty. Ewing sarcoma has a peak incidence at age 15. It has a broader age range, but becomes increasingly uncommon beyond 30.

Risk factors and aetiology

A genetic predisposition to osteosarcoma is found in patients with hereditary retinoblastoma, Rothmund–Thomson and Li–Fraumeni syndromes. Osteosarcoma is associated with Paget's disease of bone, and has also been associated with solitary or multiple osteochondroma, solitary enchondroma or enchondromatosis (Ollier's disease), multiple hereditary exostoses, fibrous dysplasia, chronic osteomyelitis, sites of bone infarcts, sites of metallic prostheses and sites of prior internal fixation and ionizing radiation including historic use of Thorotrast and in radium workers. Exposure to alkylating agents may also contribute to its development independent of the administration of radiotherapy. There are no known risk factors for Ewing sarcoma, although it is less common in US populations of Black and Chinese ethnicity, suggesting genetic factors might play a role. Chondrosarcoma may arise from benign cartilaginous tumours such as osteochondromas and chondromas, and high-grade chondromas may arise by dedifferation of a low-grade chondrosarcoma. It is associated with Maffucci's syndrome, a combination of multiple enchondromas that usually affect the hands and angiomas. Chordomas are rare cancers that arise from embryonic notochord remnants along the length of the neuraxis.

Spread

Osteosarcoma commonly metastasises to lung, and less commonly to bone. Skip metastases may be seen as non-contiguous deposits in the same or neighbouring bone. Ewing sarcoma presents with metastases in around 25% of patients, but with a dismal 5% cure rate in the era before chemotherapy it is probably a systemic illness almost from the start. Metastases occur most commonly to the lungs, liver, bone and bone marrow.

Anatomy and pathology

Osteosarcoma is commonest in the diaphysis of long bones. The diaphysis is that part of the metaphysis (the middle) close to the epiphyseal growth plate from which the diaphysis/metaphysis and epiphyses (the ends of the bone) grow. It occurs most commonly on either side of the knee, and away from the elbow, so with reducing frequency, the commonest sites are the distal femur, proximal tibia, proximal humerus and distal radius or ulna.

Ewing sarcoma occurs in both membranous and long bones. The incidence roughly mirrors the mass of bone, but it is commoner in the diaphyseal regions of the long bones of the leg.

Osteosarcoma is a spindle cell sarcoma characterised by the presence of osteoid in the tumour-associated stroma. Spindle cell sarcomas that do not produce osteoid cannot be called osteosarcoma, but behave similarly and are treated identically. Ewing sarcoma is a 'small round blue cell tumour of childhood', and can look very similar to rhabdomyosarcoma, lymphoma and in younger patients neuroblastoma. The presence of the t(11;22) EWS-FLI1 gene translocation in 85% of patients and the t(21;22) EWS-ERG gene translocation in 10% has become useful in identifying Ewing sarcoma. Extraskeletal Ewing sarcomas also contain the translocation.

Clinical presentation

The commonest symptom of a primary bone tumour is non-mechanical or night pain. A mass may be apparent. A plain X-ray is the correct first investigation, and bone destruction, new bone formation and periosteal or soft tissue swelling suggest the presence of a tumour. If a primary bone tumour is suspected direct referral to a UK reference centre should occur. The usual delay between the onset of symptoms and referral is typically 3 months, but can exceed twice that.

Investigation and staging

A biopsy is essential. The presentation of bone sarcoma, especially Ewing sarcoma, can be very similar to osteomyelitis. Biopsy of the involved bone should be undertaken by a specialist orthopaedic oncology service at a tertiary referral centre.

Plain radiographs of the involved area may show the characteristic Codman's triangle of osteosarcoma and are helpful in assessing the risk of pathological fracture.

MRI of the entire length of the involved bone is required. Special planar reconstructions may be helpful in planning conservative surgery if the tumour is close to neurovascular structures. CT may occasionally be helpful in providing additional anatomical information.

Other staging investigations include the following.

- CXR and CT lung are used for assessing for pulmonary secondaries.
- Bone scan for bone secondaries.
- Routine bloods. Alkaline phosphatase has some limited use as a tumour marker.
- A bone marrow sample in patients with Ewing sarcoma.

Staging classification

Two staging systems are used in bone cancer, the Enneking (Jawad and Scully, 2010) and the TNM system (UICC, 2009). Neither has gained universal acceptance or usage. The Enneking system is based on tumour grade (low/high), breach of bone cortex and the presence of metastases, whereas the TNM system is based on tumour grade, size, presence of non-contiguous primary, lymph nodes (very rare in bone tumours) and metastases. Tables 33.2 and 33.3 show the TNM and Enneking staging systems, respectively.

Treatment overview

Complete surgical excision is the preferred treatment of chondrosarcoma, with radiotherapy where excision is incomplete or impossible. A large majority of chondrosarcomas are low-grade and have low metastatic potential, and chemotherapy is generally regarded as ineffective and unnecessary. Higher-grade dedifferentiated and mesenchymal variants may be treated, respectively, with osteosarcoma and Ewing sarcoma type chemotherapy.

Complete surgical excision is also the preferred treatment of chordoma, but as the majority arise in the clivus or sacrum, this may not be possible, and radiotherapy may be given, ideally to a dose of 70 Gy. Given the proximity of critical structures this may not be possible without the use of advanced radiotherapy techniques, including protons.

Localised chordoma treated with curative intent, skull base chondrosarcoma and spinal and paraspinal bone (and soft tissue) sarcomas are included in the National Specialised Commissioning Team list of approved diagnoses for referral abroad for protons (National Specialised Commissioning Team, 2011).

Table 33.2 The TNM classification of bone tumours

Stage	Description
T1	Tumour ≤ 8 cm in greatest dimension
T2	Tumour > 8 cm in greatest dimension
T3	Discontinuous tumours in the primary bone site
N0	No regional lymph node metastases
N1	Regional lymph node metastases
M0	No distant metastases
M1	Distant metastais
M1a	Lung
M1b	Other distant sites

Adapted from UICC, 2009.

Table 33.3 The Enneking stage groupings for bone cancer

Stage	Description
IA	Low-grade: intracompartmental (periosteum intact)
IB	Low-grade: extracompartmental (periosteum breached)
IIA	High-grade: intracompartmental (periosteum intact)
IIB	High-grade: extracompartmental (periosteum breached)
III	Any grade: regional or distant metastasis

Adapted from Jawad and Scully, 2010.

Spindle cell sarcomas of bone including fibrosarcoma, malignant fibrous histiocytoma, leiomyosarcoma and undifferentiated sarcoma may be treated as osteosarcoma.

The treatment of osteosarcoma and Ewing sarcoma both involve sandwich chemotherapy and local therapy, but the details differ appreciably and so they are discussed separately.

Treatment of osteosarcoma

Chemotherapy

The published institutional cure rates of osteosarcoma rose in the 1970s from around 20% to around 60%. This coincided with the introduction of adjuvant chemotherapy, but also improved local surgery, the wider use of pulmonary metastectomies and upstaging with pulmonary CT scanning, so at the time the importance of chemotherapy was contested, but two randomised trials of methotreaxate or multi-agent chemotherapy demonstrated an improvement in disease-free, and eventually overall survival (Link *et al.*, 1986; Eilber *et al.*, 1987). A small, possibly under-powered trial demonstrated the equivalence of neoadjuvant and postoperative chemotherapy (Goorin *et al.*, 2003). As neoajuvant chemotherapy will allow time for the planning of complex surgery, possibly with a custom-made endoprosthesis, neoadjuvant and postoperative 'sandwich' chemotherapy has become standard. The European Osteosarcoma Intergroup randomised studies in osteosarcoma have shown that cisplatin and doxorubicin is as effective as Rosen T10 (a complex multi-agent regimen) and in later trials that the addition of methotrexate or fortnightly administration with G-CSF did not improve survival (Craft, 2010). The lack of a survival advantage with methotrexate may have been due to a compensatory reduction and delay in administration of cisplatin and doxorubicin, and despite the lack of randomised evidence it remains part of standard therapy and the evidence for its use had been reviewed by the Cochrane Collaboration (van Dalen *et al.*, 2011). In the USA, the Children's Oncology Group (COG) showed no benefit to the addition of ifosfamide (Meyers *et al.*, 2005). The use of sandwich chemotherapy permits dose intensification in those with a poor histological response, often with the addition of ifosfamide and etoposide. Such an approach is common in the USA, but not in Europe. A European and American study, Euramos1, tested these two approaches and preliminary results showed equivalent survival but increased toxicity with treatment intensification (Marina *et al.*, 2014). Thus, the current standard treatment is with MAP. In those over the age of 40, a phase 2 trial of cisplatin and doxorubicin and ifosfamide with methotrexate intensification in poor responders has shown outcomes similar to younger patients but with appreciable toxicity (Ferrari *et al.*, 2009).

Radiotherapy

In the 1930s Sir Stanford Cade advocated 60 Gy fractionated radiotherapy to the primary and observation for 6–9 months, with excision of the primary if pulmonary metastases did not develop, thus avoiding 'futile mutilation'. The strategy was largely unsuccessful as local tumour recurrence occurred despite radiotherapy in those developing secondaries, often necessitating a palliative amputation (Sweetnam *et al.*, 1971). This lead to a belief that radiotherapy is ineffective in osteosarcoma. However, it can effectively palliate bone secondaries, and modern radiotherapy techniques including protons have reported high local control rates where surgery is incomplete or impossible. Suggested indications for radiotherapy have included a bulky primary, poor response to chemotherapy, incomplete or marginal excision, pathological fracture and the presence of pulmonary metastases, but no consensus exists.

Immunotherapy

Immunotherapy in osteosarcoma remains contentious. The use of a number of immunomodulatory manoevres, including interferon, was reported in the 1970s and interferon became part of standard adjuvant therapy at the Karolinska Institute in the 1970s and 1980s. Two randomised studies of immunomodulators have been performed, one with mifamurtide, a component of mycobacterial cell wall, and the other with pegylated interferon. The COG compared the addition of ifosfamide and/or mifamurtide to standard methotrexate/doxorubicin/cisplatin chemotherapy in a 2×2 factorial design, and found no improvement from the addition of ifosfamide but a significant 8% increase in overall survival with the addition of mifamurtide, but only in the ifosfamide arm (Meyers *et al.*, 2008). Its efficacy has been accepted on the strength of this by the European Medicines control agency, but not the FDA. NICE and the SMC have approved its use in the UK (NICE, 2011; SMC, 2011). The favourable responders to MAP chemotherapy in Euramos1 were randomised to continued MAP chemotherapy ± pegylated interferon. Preliminary results report a non-significant 3% increase in 3-year disease-free survival with interferon (Bielack *et al.*, 2013).

Recurrent disease

Around 30% of patients with localised disease and 80% of the patients presenting with metastatic disease will relapse. A solitary metastasis, late relapse and resectability are associated with better survival. Patients not amenable to surgery and those with a second or third recurrence have a poor prognosis. Chemotherapy at relapse has not been standardised, and should take account of what has been administered previously. It may include ifosfamide and etoposide or gemcitabine and docetaxel.

Prognostic factors and prognosis in osteosarcoma

In osteosarcoma, raised lactate dehydrogenase and alkaline phosphatase or the presence of metastatic disease (particularly non-pulmonary) at diagnosis, poor histologic response to chemotherapy, pelvic tumour site, male gender and age greater than 18 are associated with a poorer outcome. Modern series report 5-year survivals ranging from 55% to 70%.

Future directon

Pilot studies with zoledronic acid and trastuzumab have been performed and a second international trial, Euramos2, is being planned, with MAP as the standard arm.

Treatment of Ewing sarcoma

Over the last 40 years, the survival in Ewing sarcoma has improved to 60% but was only 6% in the era before the use of multi-agent chemotherapy with patients dying of metastatic disease. The use of chemotherapy in Ewing sarcoma was first reported in the early 1960s with cyclophosphamide and subsequently vincristine as well. In 1974 the use of these agents combining with actinomycin-D and doxorubicin (VACD) marked the beginning of the era of multi-modality therapy in a range of paediatric tumours including Ewing sarcoma (Rosen et al., 1974).

The first Intergroup Ewing's Sarcoma Study (IESS-1; 1973–1978) showed a 5-year disease survival of 60% with the addition of doxorubicin compared to 24% with vincristine, actinomycin-D, cyclophosphamide (VAC). The addition of prophylactic whole-lung radiotherapy to VAC also improved outcome, although not as much as the addition of doxorubicin (Nesbit et al., 1990). The second trial, IESS-, (1978–1982) demonstrated that higher doses of VAC plus doxorubicin (150% increase in the initial weeks of therapy) was superior to continuous moderate dose therapy with these agents (Evans et al., 1991).

Subsequent trials showed improved outcomes with the addition of either etoposide, ifosfamide or both. In the UK, 5-year survival was 44% in the Ewing's Tumour ET-1 study, using VAC and doxorubicin but was 62% in ET-2 using vincristine, actinomycin-D, doxorubicin and ifosfamide (Craft et al., 1998). The first American Intergroup Ewing's trial randomised patients to VACD with or without ifosfamide and etoposide (IE). Survival in localised disease was improved with IE, but remained poor at 22% in metastatic disease (Grier et al., 2003).

The second American Intergroup trial investigated dose intensity with randomisation to a treatment protocol of either 30 or 48 weeks with cumulative doses of agents similar in both arms and similar outcomes (Womer et al., 2012). However, increasing dose intensity by giving chemotherapy 2-weekly with G-CSF improved 5-year event-free survival from 65% on the standard arm to 73% in the 2-weekly arm without increased toxicity in the latter, and is the current standard of care in the USA.

EICESS-92 randomised non-metastatic Ewing sarcoma to vincristine, doxorubin, actinomycin-D and either cylophosphamide or ifosfamide (VAIA or VACA), and found that cyclophosphamide seemed to have similar effects as ifosfamide but was associated with increased toxicity. In high risk patients, the randomised addition of etoposide to VAIA seemed to be beneficial but was not statistically significant (Paulusson et al., 2008).

The European EuroEWING99 trial closed to accrual in 2014. All patients received 6 cycles of vincristine, doxorubicin, ifosfamide and etoposide 3-weekly (VIDE), and those without metastastses and a resulting tumour volume below 200 cm^3 were randomised to 8 cycles of vincristine, actinomycin-D and either ifosfamide or cyclophosphamide (VAI vs VAC) to test the relative toxicity of these regimens in the better-risk patients. Patients with residual tumours greater than 200 cm^3 were randomised to either VAI or high-dose busulfan and melphalan chemotherapy and peripheral blood stem cell transplantation. Those with non-pulmonary metastases at presentation all received high-dose chemotherapy because the outcome with conventional chemotherapy is poor in this group with survival below 20%. Those with post-VIDE tumours less than 200 cm^3 and solely pulmonary metastases were randomised to either high-dose chemotherapy or VAI and whole-lung radiotherapy to see if the benefit seen in IESS-1 remains with a more modern chemotherapy regimen containing doxorubicin and ifosfamide. Results are awaited and in the meantime the EuroEWING2012 trial has opened in the UK.

Definitive radiotherapy in Ewing sarcoma

Ewing sarcoma is seldom cured without effective local therapy, which may be with either surgery or radiotherapy or both. Although never tested in a randomised fashion, it is widely believed that complete excision is superior, although radiotherapy tends to be reserved for the larger, central, more challenging and inoperable primaries. An analysis of the EICESS92 study, the precursor to EuroEWING99, revealed a worse outcome in the UK compared to Germany. The cause of this remains uncertain, but fewer German patients received just radiotherapy and have led to the belief that aggressive local management is important (Cotterill *et al.*, 2000). The dose is 55 Gy in 30 fractions.

Recurrent disease

Recurrent and locally relapsed Ewing sarcomas are seldom curable. The treatment of recurrent Ewing sarcoma has not been standardised, but palliative radiotherapy and drugs including temozolomide, irinotecan and topotecan can cause tumour shrinkage and symptom relief.

Prognosis of Ewing sarcoma

Modern series report 5-year survivals ranging from 55% to 70% in localised Ewing sarcoma, 20% with pulmonary metastases and less than 10% with metastases elsewhere. Large tumours, axial tumours and increasing age are associated with a poorer outcome.

Current clinical trial

The EuroEWING2012 trial has recently opened. It will examine several areas:

- a comparison between the European standard of VIDE induction and VAI/VAC consolidation with the American standard of VDC/IE induction and IE/VC consolidation;
- whether the addition of a bisphosphonate during and after consolidation improves the outcome of good responders;
- whether high-dose therapy with BuMel followed by stem cell rescue improves the outcome of patients with poor response to induction chemotherapy;
- whether high-dose therapy improves the outcome of patients with pulmonary and/or pleural metastases at diagnosis.

The use of radiotherapy in benign conditions of the soft tissues and bones

Ankylosing spondylitis

Ankylosing spondylitis is an inflammatory arthritis of the spine and sacro-iliac joints, predominantly affecting young males.

Small radiotherapy fields are used to treat affected joints, or in 12 × 8 cm fields to the whole spine in stages. The recommended dose is 10 Gy in 10 fractions with orthovoltage.

The response is dose-dependent, but 60–90% of those treated report a good response.

The incidence of leukaemia is increased 9.5-fold, with 52 reported cases out of 14,000 treated. There are some reports of reactivated TB.

Heterotopic bone formation (HBF)

HBF is postoperative ossification which can develop 3–6 weeks after surgery and calcify within about 8 weeks. It occurs in up to 43% of patients who have a hip replacement, but is only clinically significant in 9% (Balboni *et al.*, 2006).

The dose is 8 Gy in a single fraction within 4 days of surgery or 4–6 hours before re-operation.

Radiotherapy prevents recurrent HBF in 52–98% cases.

Long-term risks are quoted as 1 in 3000–5000, but risks will depend on age, treatment site and reproductive status.

Desmoid tumours

Desmoid tumours are also known as aggressive fibromatosis where low-grade invasive non-metastasising tumours arise in connective tissue. They tend to merge into local structures, and resection margins are often positive, resulting in high rates of local recurrence.

The recommended dose is 50 Gy in 2 Gy fractions after local resection. There is a 70% local control rate and regression can continue to occur up to 2 years after radiotherapy.

Synovitis

Synovitis is an inflammatory reaction, affecting synovial lining of joints, of variable aetiology.

Treatment is with an intra-arterial injection of ^{90}Y to give 185 MBq. Response rates appear to be comparable with surgical synovectomy. Radiotherapy for synovitis should be restricted to those patients in whom other measures have failed.

Arterial restenosis

Restenosis of coronary arteries after balloon angioplasty can occur. Postangioplasty intravascular brachytherapy is given using 15–20 Gy with ^{192}Ir.

Radiotherapy gives a reduction of restenosis incidence from 54% to between 17% and 25%. Several clinical trials are in progress to confirm preliminary findings.

References

Balboni, T. A., Gobezie, R. and Mamon, H. J. (2006). Heterotropic ossification: pathophysiology, clinical features and the role of radiotherapy for prophylaxis. *Int. J. Radiat. Oncol. Biol. Phys.*, **65**, 1289–1299.

Bielack, S.S., Smeland, S., Whelan, J., et al. (2013). MAP plus maintenance pegylated interferon {alpha}-2b (MAP-IFN) versus MAP alone in patients (pts) with resectable high-grade osteosarcoma and good histologic response to preoperative MAP: first results of the EURAMOS-1 good response randomization. *J. Clin. Oncol.*, **31**(Suppl.); abst. LBA10504.

Blay, J. Y., Leahy, M. G., Nguyen, B. B., et al. (2014). Randomised phase III trial of trabectedin versus doxorubicin-based chemotherapy as first-line therapy in translocation-related sarcomas. *Eur. J. Cancer*, **50**, 1137–1147.

Bramwell, V., Rouesse, J., Steward, W., et al. (1994). Adjuvant CYVADIC chemotherapy for adult soft tissue sarcoma – reduced local recurrence but no improvement in survival: a study of the European Organization for Research and Treatment of Cancer Soft Tissue and Bone Sarcoma Group. *J. Clin. Oncol.*, **12**, 1137–1149.

Cotterill, S. J., Ahrens, S., Paulussen, M., et al. (2000). Prognostic factors in Ewing's tumor of bone: analysis of 975 patients from the European Intergroup Cooperative Ewing's Sarcoma Study Group. *J. Clin. Oncol.*, **18**, 3108–3114.

Craft, A. W. (2010). Osteosarcoma: the European Osteosarcoma Intergroup (EOI) perspective. *Paediatr. Adol. Osteosarcoma Cancer Treat. Res.*, **152**, 263–274.

Craft, A., Cotterill, S., Malcolm, A., et al. (1998). Ifosfamide-containing chemotherapy in Ewing's sarcoma: the Second United Kingdom Children's Cancer Study Group and the Medical Research Council Ewing's Tumor Study. *J. Clin. Oncol.*, **16**, 3628–3633.

Davis, A. M., O'Sullivan, B., Turcotte, R., et al. (2005). Late radiation morbidity following randomization to preoperative versus postoperative radiotherapy in extremity soft tissue sarcoma. *Radiother. Oncol.*, **75**, 48–53.

Demetri, G. D., Chawla, S. P. Von Mehren, M., et al., (2009). Efficacy and safety of trabectedin in patients with advanced or metastatic liposarcoma or leiomyosarcoma after failure of prior anthracyclines and ifosfamide: results of a randomized phase II study of two different schedules. *J. Clin. Oncol.*, **27**, 4188–4196.

Dennis, N., Francis, M., Lawrence, G., et al. (2012). *Soft Tissue Sarcoma Incidence and Survival – Tumours Diagnosed in England Between 1985 and 2009. Report Number R12/06.* Birmingham: West Midlands Cancer Intelligence Unit. (http://www.wmciu.nhs.uk/documents/ReportR1205_BoneSarcomaIncidenceAndSurvival.pdf, accessed January 2015.)

Eilber, F. R., Giuliano, A., Eckardt, J., et al. (1987). Adjuvant chemotherapy for osteosarcoma: a randomized prospective trial. *J. Clin. Oncol.*, **5**, 21–26.

Evans, R. G., Nesbit, M. E., Gehan, E. A., et al. (1991). Multimodal therapy for the management of localized Ewing's sarcoma of pelvic and sacral bones: a report from the second intergroup study. *J. Clin. Oncol.*, **9**, 1173–1180.

Ferrari, S., Smeland, S., Bielack, S., et al. (2009). A European treatment protocol for bone sarcoma in patients older than 40 years. *J. Clin. Oncol.*, **27**(15Suppl.), abstr. 10516.

García-del-Muro, X., López-Pousa, A., Maurel, J., et al. (2011). Randomized phase II study comparing gemcitabine plus dacarbazine versus dacarbazine alone in patients with previously treated soft tissue sarcoma: a Spanish Group for Research on Sarcomas study. *J. Clin. Oncol.*, **29**, 2528–2533.

Gelderblom, H., Blay, J. Y., Seddon, B. M., et al. (2014). Brostallicin versus doxorubicin as first-line chemotherapy in patients with advanced or metastatic soft tissue sarcoma: a European Organisation for Research and Treatment of Cancer Soft Tissue and Bone Sarcoma Group randomised phase II and pharmacogenetic study. *Eur. J. Cancer*, **50**, 388–396.

Goorin, A. M., Scwartsentruber, D. J., Devidas, M., et al. (2003). Presurgical chemotherapy compared with immediate surgery and adjuvant chemotherapy for nonmetastatic osteosarcoma: Pediatric Oncology Group Study POG-8651. *J. Clin. Oncol.*, **21**, 1574–1580.

Grier, H. E., Krailo, M. D., Tarbell, N. J., et al. (2003). Addition of ifosfamide and etoposide to standard chemotherapy for Ewing's sarcoma and primitive neuroectodermal tumor of bone. *N. Engl. J. Med.*, **348**, 694–701.

Grimer, R., Athanasou, N., Gerrand, C., et al. (2010a). UK guidelines for the management of bone sarcomas. *Sarcoma*, 317462.

Grimer, R., Judson, I., Peake, D., et al. (2010b). Guidelines for the management of soft tissue sarcomas. *Sarcoma*, 506182.

Gurney, J. G., Swensen, A. R. and Bulterys, M. (1999). Malignant bone tumours. In *Cancer Incidence and Survival among Children and Adolescents: United States SEER Program 1975–1995*, ed. L. Ries, M. Smith, J. Gurney, et al. NIH Pub. No. 99–4649, Bethesda: National Cancer Institute.

Hensley, M. L., Maki, R., Venkatraman, E., *et al.* (2002). Gemcitabine and docetaxel in patients with unresectable leiomyosarcoma: results of a phase II trial. *J. Clin. Oncol.*, **20**, 2824–2831.

Jawad, M. U. and Scully, S. P. (2010). In brief: classifications in brief: Enneking classification: benign and malignant tumors of the musculoskeletal system. *Clin. Orthop. Relat. Res.*, **468**, 2000–2002.

Judson, I., Verweij, J., Gelderblom, H., *et al.* (2014). Doxorubicin alone versus intensified doxorubicin plus ifosfamide for first-line treatment of advanced or metastatic soft-tissue sarcoma: a randomised controlled phase 3 trial. *Lancet Oncol.*, **15**, 415–423.

Le Cesne, A., Ouali, M., Leahy, M.G. *et al.* (2014). Doxorubicin-based adjuvant chemotherapy in soft tissue sarcoma: pooled analysis of two STBSG-EORTC phase III clinical trials. *Ann. Oncol.*, **25**, 2435–32.

Link, M. P., Goorin, A. M., Miser, A. W., *et al.* (1986). The effect of adjuvant chemotherapy on relapse-free survival in patients with osteosarcoma of the extremity. *N. Engl. J. Med.*, **314**, 1600–1606.

Lorigan, P., Verweij, J., Papai, Z., *et al.* (2007). Phase III trial of two investigational schedules of ifosfamide compared with standard-dose doxorubicin in advanced or metastatic soft tissue sarcoma: a European Organisation for Research and Treatment of Cancer Soft Tissue and Bone Sarcoma Group Study. *J. Clin. Oncol.*, **25**, 3144–3150.

Marina, N., Smeland, S., Bielack, S. S., *et al.* (2014). MAPIE vs MAP as post-operative chemotherapy in patients with a poor response to preoperative chemotherapy for newly-diagnosed osteosarcoma: results from EURAMOS-1 Connective Tissue Oncology Society, 2014 Annual Meeting, Final Program, Oct. 15–18, 2014, paper 032, p. 96.

Mascarenhas, L., Siegel, S., Spector, L., *et al.* (2006). Malignant bone tumours. In *Cancer Epidemiology in Older Adolescents and Young Adults 15 to 29 Years of Age, Including SEER Incidence and Survival: 1975–2000.* NIH Pub. No. 06-5767, Bethesda, MD: National Cancer Institute.

Meyers, P. A., Schwartz, C. L., Krailo, M., *et al.* (2005) Osteosarcoma: a randomized, prospective trial of the addition of ifosfamide and/or muramyl tripeptide to cisplatin, doxorubicin, and high-dose methotrexate. *J. Clin. Oncol.*, **23**, 2004–2011.

Meyers, P. A., Schwartz, C. L., Krailo, M. D., *et al.* (2008). Osteosarcoma: the addition of muramyl tripeptide to chemotherapy improves overall survival – a report from the Children's Oncology Group. *J. Clin. Oncol.*, **26**, 633–638.

National Specialised Commissioning Team. (2011). *Guidance for the Referral of Patients Abroad for NHS Proton Treatment.* Version 2.3. July 2011. London: National Specialised Commissioning Team. (Available at http://www.england.nhs.uk/wp-content/uploads/2014/09/guidance-referral-pat-abroad-nhs-proton.pdf, accessed February 2015.)

NCIN. (2012). *Bone Sarcoma Incidence and Survival. Tumours Diagnosed Between 1985 and 2009. Report Number R12/05.* Birmingham: West Midlands Cancer Intelligence Unit. (Available at http://www.ncin.org.uk/publications/reports/reports_archive, accessed January 2015.)

Nesbit, M. E., Gehan, E. A., Burgert, E. O., *et al.* (1990). Multimodal therapy for the management of primary, nonmetastatic Ewing's sarcoma of bone: a long-term follow-up of the First Intergroup study. *J. Clin. Oncol.*, **8**, 1664–1674.

NICE. (2006). *Improving Outcomes for People with Sarcoma. The Manual.* London: National Institute for Health and Clinical Excellence.

NICE. (2010). *Trabectedin for the Treatment of Advanced Soft Tissue Sarcoma. NICE Technology Appraisal Guidance 185.* London: National Institute for Health and Care Excellence.

NICE. (2011). *Mifamurtide for the Treatment of Osteosarcoma. NICE Technology Appraisal Guidance 235.* London: National Institute for Health and Care Excellence.

Paulussen, M., Craft, A. W., Lewis, I., *et al.* (2008). Results of the EICESS-92 Study: two randomized trials of Ewing's sarcoma treatment – cyclophosphamide compared with ifosfamide in standard-risk patients and assessment of benefit of etoposide added to standard treatment in high-risk patients. *J. Clin. Oncol.*, **26**, 4385–4393.

Pisters, P. W., Harrison, L. B., Leung, D. H., *et al.* (1996). Long-term results of a prospective randomized trial of adjuvant brachytherapy in soft tissue sarcoma. *J. Clin. Oncol.*, **14**, 859–868.

Rosen, G., Wollner, N., Tan, C., *et al.* (1974). Disease-free survival in children with Ewing's sarcoma treated with radiation therapy and adjuvant four-drug sequential chemotherapy. *Cancer*, **33**, 384–393.

Rosenberg,S. A., Tepper, J., Glatstein, E., *et al.* (1982). The treatment of soft-tissue sarcomas of the extremities: prospective randomized evaluations of (1) limb-sparing surgery plus radiation therapy compared with amputation and (2) the role of adjuvant chemotherapy. *Ann. Surg.*, **196**, 305–315.

Sarcoma Meta-analysis Collaboration. (1997). Adjuvant chemotherapy for localised resectable soft-tissue sarcoma of adults: meta-analysis of individual data. *Lancet*, **350**, 1647–1654.

Seddon, B. M., Whelan, J., Strauss, S. S., *et al.* (2015). GeDDis: a prospective randomised controlled phase

III trial of gemcitabine and docetaxel compared with doxorubicin as first-line treatment in previously untreated advanced unresectable or metastatic soft tissue sarcomas (EudraCT 2009-014907-29). *J. Clin. Oncol.* **33**, 2015 (suppl; abstr 10500).

SMC. (2011). *SMC No. 621/10. Mifamurtide.* Glasgow: Scottish Medicines Consortium.

Sweetnam, R., Knowelden, J. and Seddon, H. (1971). Bone sarcoma: treatment by irradiation, amputation, or a combination of the two. *Br. Med. J.*, **2**(5758), 363–367.

The ESMO and European Sarcoma Network Working Groups. (2012a). Bone sarcomas: ESMO Clinical Practice Guidelines for diagnosis, treatment and follow-up. *Ann. Oncol.*, **23**(Suppl. 7), vii100–vii109.

The ESMO and European Sarcoma Network Working Groups. (2012b). Soft tissue and visceral sarcomas: ESMO Clinical Practice Guidelines for diagnosis, treatment and follow-up. *Ann. Oncol.*, **23** (Suppl. 7), vii92–vii99.

The Royal College of Physicians and the Royal College of Radiologists. (2013). *Evidence Based Indications for the Use of PET - CT in the UK.* London: The Royal College of Physicians and The Royal College of Radiologists.

UICC. (2009). *TNM Classification of Malignant Tumours*, ed. L. H. Sobin, M. K. Gospodarowicz and Ch. Wittekind. Chichester: Wiley-Blackwell.

Van Dalen, E. C., van As, J. W. and de Camargo, B. (2011). Methotrexate for high-grade osteosarcoma in children and young adults. *Cochrane Database Syst. Rev.*, 11 May 2011.

van der Graaf, W. T. A., Blay, J-Y., Chawla, S. P., *et al.* (2012). Pazopanib for metastatic soft-tissue sarcoma (PALETTE): a randomised, double-blind, placebo-controlled phase 3 trial. *Lancet*, **379**, 1879–1886.

van Oosterom, A. T., Mouridsen, H. T., Nielson, O. S., *et al.* (2002). Results of randomised studies of the EORTC Soft Tissue and Bone Sarcoma Group (STBSG) with two different ifosfamide regimens in first- and second-line chemotherapy in advanced soft tissue sarcoma patients. *Eur. J. Cancer*, **38**, 2397–2406.

Woll, P. J., Reichardt, P., Le Cesne, A., *et al.* (2012). Adjuvant chemotherapy with doxorubicin, ifosfamide, and lenograstim for resected soft-tissue sarcoma (EORTC 62931): a multi-centre randomised controlled trial. *Lancet Oncol.*, **13**, 1045–1054.

Womer, R. B., West, D. C., Krailo, M. D., *et al.* (2012). Randomized controlled trial of interval-compressed chemotherapy for the treatment of localized Ewing sarcoma: a report from the Children's Oncology Group. *J. Clin. Oncol.*, **30**, 4148–4154.

Yang, J. C., Chang, A. E., Baker, A. R., *et al.* (1998). Randomized prospective study of the benefit of adjuvant radiation therapy in the treatment of soft tissue sarcomas of the extremity. *J. Clin. Oncol.*, **16**, 197–203.

Management of the lymphomas and myeloma

Eve Gallop-Evans

Introduction

The incidence of lymphoma is rising, and current attention is focused not just on improving cure rates, but also on minimising late effects of treatment. Patients should be managed by multidisciplinary teams that bring together the appropriate expertise of haematologists, oncologists, radiologists, pathologists and specialist nurses. Management guidelines are produced by the British Committee for Standards in Haematology (BCSH) and are a useful resource.

Lymphomas

Introduction

The World Health Organisation (WHO) classification of neoplasms of the hematopoietic and lymphoid tissues was first published in 2001 and updated in 2008 (Table 34.1: Swerdlow *et al.*, 2008). This distinguishes more than 60 specific entities on the basis of morphologic, immunophenotypic, genetic, molecular and clinical features, stratified according to cell lineage and derivation from precursor or mature lymphoid cells.

Non-Hodgkin lymphoma (NHL) is the sixth most common cancer in the UK, with over 12,000 patients diagnosed each year, accounting for 4% of all new cases of cancer. The incidence is related to age, with the majority of cases diagnosed over the age of 65 years. Nearly half of all cases diagnosed in the UK are diffuse large B cell lymphoma (DLBCL, 48%). Marginal zone lymphomas (MZL) and follicular lymphoma (FL) account for 20% and 19%, respectively, with T cell lymphomas (6%), mantle cell lymphoma (MCL, 5%) and Burkitt lymphoma (2%) making up the remainder. Crude incidence rates in the UK range from 0.2 to 9 cases per 100,000.

Hodgkin lymphoma (HL) accounts for 0.6% of all cancer cases, with a relatively stable incidence of

around 1700 cases per year. In children under 14 years of age, lymphoma is the third most common cancer after leukaemia and brain tumours. Lymphomas are the most common cancer in teenagers and young adults, accounting for 21% of cancers in this age group, with two-thirds of these being HL.

Aetiology

The aetiology of lymphoma is not clearly understood and appears to be multifactorial. The most significant risk factor is immune dysfunction which may be secondary to viral infection (e.g. HIV, HBV, HCV, EBV, HTLV-1), autoimmune disease or iatrogenic immunosuppression (Roman and Smith, 2011). Mucosa-associated lymphoid tissue (MALT) lymphomas are associated with antigenic stimulation by infectious agents including *Helicobacter pylori*, *Chlamydia psittaci* and *Borrelia burgdorferi*.

Clinical presentation

One of the most common presentations is painless lymphadenopathy, and NICE guidance for investigation of unexplained lymphadenopathy advises sending FBC, blood film and ESR, plasma viscosity or CRP (NICE, 2011). Persistent or enlarging lymph nodes greater than 2 cm should be investigated further. Patients may describe systemic or 'B' symptoms in the 6 months before diagnosis, including fever higher than 38°C, drenching night sweats and weight loss of more than 10% of the original body weight though the suffixes A and B are now only used in Hodgkin lymphoma (Cheson *et al.*, 2014).

Investigations and staging

Accurate diagnosis and staging are essential for planning management, including eligibility for clinical

Practical Clinical Oncology, Second Edition, ed. Louise Hanna, Tom Crosby and Fergus Macbeth. Published by Cambridge University Press. © Cambridge University Press 2015.

Table 34.1 WHO classification of the mature B cell, T cell and NK cell neoplasms, 2008

Mature B cell neoplasms

Chronic lymphocytic leukaemia/small lymphocytic lymphoma

B cell prolymphocytic leukaemia

Splenic marginal zone lymphoma

Hairy cell leukaemia

Splenic lymphoma/leukaemia, unclassifiable

Lymphoplasmacytic lymphoma

Waldenstrom macroglobulinemia

Heavy chain diseases

Plasma cell myeloma

Solitary plasmacytoma of bone

Extramedullary plasmacytoma

Extranodal marginal zone B cell lymphoma of mucosa associated lymphoid tissue (MALT lymphoma)

Nodal marginal zone B cell lymphoma (MZL)

Follicular lymphoma

Primary cutaneous follicle centre lymphoma

Mantle cell lymphoma

Diffuse large B cell lymphoma (DLBCL), not otherwise specified

T cell/histiocyte-rich large B cell lymphoma

DLBCL associated with chronic inflammation

Epstein–Barr virus (EBV)+ DLBCL of the elderly

Lymphomatoid granulomatosis

Primary mediastinal large B cell lymphoma

Intravascular large B cell lymphoma

Primary cutaneous DLBCL, leg type

ALK+ large B cell lymphoma

Plasmablastic lymphoma

Primary effusion lymphoma

Large B cell lymphoma arising in HHV8-associated multicentric Castleman disease

Burkitt lymphoma

B cell lymphoma, unclassifiable, with features intermediate between diffuse large B cell lymphoma and Burkitt lymphoma

B cell lymphoma, unclassifiable, with features intermediate between diffuse large B cell lymphoma and classical Hodgkin lymphoma

Hodgkin lymphoma

Nodular lymphocyte-predominant Hodgkin lymphoma

Classical Hodgkin lymphoma

Nodular sclerosis classical Hodgkin lymphoma

Lymphocyte-rich classical Hodgkin lymphoma

Mixed cellularity classical Hodgkin lymphoma

Lymphocyte-depleted classical Hodgkin lymphoma

Mature T cell and NK cell neoplasms

T cell prolymphocytic leukaemia

T cell large granular lymphocytic leukaemia

Chronic lymphoproliferative disorder of NK cells

Aggressive NK cell leukaemia

Systemic EBV-positive T cell lymphoproliferative disease of childhood

Hydroa vacciniforme-like lymphoma

Adult T cell leukaemia/lymphoma

Extranodal NK/T cell lymphoma, nasal type

Enteropathy-associated T cell lymphoma

Hepatosplenic T cell lymphoma

Subcutaneous panniculitis-like T cell lymphoma

Mycosis fungoides

Sézary syndrome

Primary cutaneous CD30-positive T cell lymphoproliferative disorders

Lymphomatoid papulosis

Primary cutaneous anaplastic large cell lymphoma

Primary cutaneous gamma-delta T cell lymphoma

Primary cutaneous CD8-positive aggressive epidermotropic cytotoxic T cell lymphoma

Primary cutaneous CD4-positive small/medium T cell lymphoma

Peripheral T cell lymphoma, NOS

Angioimmunoblastic T cell lymphoma

Anaplastic large cell lymphoma, ALK-positive

Anaplastic large cell lymphoma, ALK-negative

Adapted from Swerdlow *et al.* (2008).

trials. History and examination will allow assessment of systemic symptoms, performance status and any palpable disease. A full excision biopsy of an affected lymph node is always recommended to allow comprehensive molecular and histopathological examination including assessment of architecture, and a formal haematopathology review is essential. Further investigations should include FBC, ESR, biochemical evaluation including renal and liver function, lactate dehydrogenase (LDH) and β2-microglobulin, HIV, HCV and HBV serology, CT scans of the neck, chest, abdomen, and pelvis.

A bone marrow examination (aspirate, immunophenotyping and trephine) is recommended for most cases of NHL, although PET-CT is a valid method of assessing bone marrow involvement in Hodgkin lymphoma and high-grade NHL (El-Galaly *et al.*, 2012; Khan *et al.*, 2013). CSF should be sent for flow cytometry and cytology in patients suspected of or at high risk of CNS involvement.

The standard staging system used for HL was proposed at the Ann Arbor Conference in 1971 and modified at the Cotswolds Meeting in 1988 (Table 34.2). It is also used in NHL despite the different pattern of disease, with a greater chance of discontiguous nodal, extranodal and bone marrow involvement. The criteria for defining disease bulk and thus higher risk disease is set at 10 cm for HL, 6 cm for FL and 6–10 cm for DLBCL (Cheson *et al.*, 2014).

Lymph node regions

The lymph node regions are as follows.

- Right and left cervical (including cervical, supraclavicular, occipital and pre-auricular).
- Right and left axillary.
- Right and left infra-clavicular.
- Mediastinal.
- Right and left hilar.
- Para-aortic.
- Mesenteric.
- Right and left pelvic.
- Right and left inguinal/femoral.

Pretreatment assessment

Fertility preservation options should be discussed and offered to all patients if appropriate. Baseline cardiac assessment should be performed before anthracycline use, particularly for patients with cardiac risk factors. Lung function testing may be required before treatment with bleomycin.

The risk of tumour lysis syndrome should be considered if the patient has bulky disease and an elevated LDH, and allopurinol 300 mg once daily started as prophylaxis. When there is evidence of tumour lysis occurring with an elevated serum uric acid, rasburicase should be given. Rasburicase may be indicated as prophylaxis in patients allergic to allopurinol or in patients with impaired renal function before starting chemotherapy.

PET scanning in lymphoma

The International Working Group (IWG) criteria includes use of FDG-PET-CT for staging, interim response assessment and post-treatment evaluation (Cheson *et al.*, 2014). The impact of PET-CT on clinical outcome in different settings is being tested in prospective trials. Contrast-enhanced PET-CT is better than CT for staging of HL and NHL with respect to sensitivity, specificity, negative and positive predictive value. PET-CT can detect bone marrow involvement even in patients with a negative iliac crest bone marrow biopsy, and may replace the need for a biopsy in HL and DLBCL (El-Galaly *et al.*, 2012; Khan *et al.*, 2013). The usefulness of PET-CT in staging indolent lymphoma is less clear. Follicular lymphoma appears to be avid on PET scanning though with lower standardised uptake values than high grade lymphomas, whereas CLL/SLL

Table 34.2 Ann Arbor staging system with Cotswold modification

Stage I	Involvement of a single lymph node region or single lymphoid structure, such as spleen or Waldeyer ring or a single extranodal site (IE)
Stage II	Involvement of two or more lymph node regions or lymphoid structures on the same side of the diaphragm (II) or localised involvement of an extralymphatic site (IIE)
Stage III	Involvement of lymph node regions or lymphoid structures on both sides of the diaphragm (III), or localised involvement of an extralymphatic site (IIIE), or spleen (IIIS) or both (IIIES)
Stage IV	Involvement of one or more extralymphatic organs (e.g. lungs, liver or bone marrow) irrespective of lymph node involvement
Extranodal disease	A single site of extralymphatic involvement due to limited direct extension from an adjacent nodal site
Systemic symptoms	Fever >38°C with no evident cause for 3 consecutive days, night sweats and unexplained weight loss > 10% of body weight Patients are divided according to the presence (B) or not (A) of these symptoms
Bulky disease	Applies to nodal masses measuring ≥ 10 cm on cross-sectional imaging, or to a mediastinal mass on CXR, when the maximum width is ≥ one-third of the internal transverse diameter of the thorax at the level of T5–T6

Adapted from Lister *et al.* (1989).

and MZL, especially at extranodal sites, are less often avid, and T-cell lymphomas are more heterogeneous (Meignan *et al.*, 2014).

There is good correlation between the results of post-treatment scanning and outcome, and so PET-CT can be used to detect any residual active disease. Patients with a negative post-treatment PET scan result have an excellent outcome, and several studies have shown that FDG-PET performed after treatment is highly predictive of progression-free and overall survival in HL and high-grade NHL.

Interval PET-CT scanning after the start of chemotherapy may have a role in determining the prognosis of patients with HL (Hutchings *et al.*, 2006; Safar *et al.*, 2012), but it is unclear whether changing therapy in the light of PET-CT results improves outcomes. Following salvage treatment for relapse, a positive PET-CT before autologous stem-cell transplantation predicts a poor outcome, and patients should be considered for alternative treatments.

Diffuse large B-cell lymphoma (DLBCL)

This is the most common lymphoma subtype in the UK with a median age at diagnosis of 64 years. Gene expression profiling can distinguish two major subtypes, germinal centre B cell-like (GCB) and activated B cell-like (ABC), representing different stages of B cell differentiation. Patients with GCB DLBCL appear to have a significantly better overall survival than those with ABC-DLBCL, even since the introduction of R-CHOP treatment.

Clinical presentation

Patients usually present with nodal or extranodal disease and B symptoms; 10% have bone marrow involvement.

Prognostic index

The International Prognostic Index (IPI) is shown in Table 34.3 and is based on a study of more than 2000 patients with high-grade NHL treated with anthracycline-containing regimens, and defines five factors that independently predicted outcome and remain valid for DLBCL since the introduction of R-CHOP (Ziepert *et al.*, 2010).

Treatment

The addition of the anti-CD20 monoclonal antibody rituximab (R) to standard 3-weekly CHOP

Table 34.3 International Prognostic Index (IPI) for DLBCL

No. of risk factors	Risk group	5-year overall survival (%)
0–1	Low	73
2	Low intermediate	51
3	High intermediate	43
4–5	High	26

Risk factors are: age > 60 years; PFS 2 to 4; stage 3–4; LDH above normal; > 1 extranodal site. Adapted from Shipp, 1993.

(cyclophosphamide, doxorubicin, vincristine, prednisolone) chemotherapy has significantly improved outcomes in DLBCL. The GELA study of patients aged 60–80 years compared 8 cycles of R-CHOP with CHOP alone and showed 2-year survival rates of 76% compared to 63% in favour of R-CHOP, with similar benefits seen at 5 years (Feugier *et al.*, 2005). The MInT study for patients below the age of 60 with low-risk IPI scores showed that the addition of rituximab to anthracycline-based chemotherapy improved 6-year progression-free survival from 55.8% to 74.3% (Pfreundschuh *et al.*, 2011). RT (30–40 Gy) was given to initial sites of disease larger than 5 cm. Bulky disease larger than 7.5 cm was found to be an independent poor prognostic factor. Attempts to improve survival with dose intensification using two-weekly R-CHOP-14 rather than three-weekly R-CHOP-21 showed no significant difference (Cunningham *et al.*, 2013), and 6 cycles of R-CHOP-21 may be considered the current standard treatment for all except stage I non-bulky DLBCL. No survival benefit has yet been shown with high-dose chemotherapy consolidation in first remission in the R-CHOP era (Stiff *et al.*, 2013). In the future, determination of high-risk molecular phenotypes may identify patients for whom intensification may be beneficial.

Combined modality treatment

- A SWOG study in which 70% of patients had low-risk IPI scores compared eight cycles of CHOP to three cycles of CHOP with involved-field radiotherapy (IFRT) of 40–55 Gy (Miller *et al.*, 1998). The CHOP plus IFRT arm had higher rates of 5-year progression-free (76% versus 67%) and overall survival (82% versus 74%). An ECOG study randomised patients with early-stage disease in complete remission between eight cycles of CHOP alone, and CHOP combined with 30 Gy IFRT (Horning *et al.*, 2004). Patients in partial remission received 40 Gy IFRT. Ten-year follow-up showed that the addition of RT in complete responders improved 10-year disease-free survival (57% versus 46%) but not overall survival (64% versus 60%). Short-course chemotherapy and radiotherapy is an alternative treatment option for patients not fit for or not tolerating an extended course of chemotherapy.

- There are no long-term follow-up data from prospective RCTs of the role of consolidation RT for patients with initial bulky masses or for patients with residual masses in the R-CHOP and PET-CT era. The GHSG RICOVER-60 trial was a randomised study of CHOP-14 in patients aged between 61 and 80, testing the addition of rituximab as well as number of cycles (Held *et al.*, 2014). 36 Gy of consolidation radiotherapy was given to extranodal sites and initial bulk ≥ 7.5 cm. Six cycles of R-CHOP-14 was found to be the most effective arm, and subsequent patients received this regimen but without RT. A per protocol analysis comparing patients who did and didn't receive RT showed that RT significantly improved progression-free and overall survival although this benefit was not seen in an intention-to-treat analysis. Subsequently, the GHSG UNFOLDER study randomised patients over 60 years to either R-CHOP-21 or R-CHOP-14. Patients in complete remission underwent a second randomisation between RT to bulky (> 7.5 cm) and/or extranodal sites or no further treatment. An interim analysis found an unacceptable rate of relapses in the no RT arm, which was closed early (Held *et al.*, 2014). Outside a clinical trial, radiotherapy is not routinely recommended for patients in complete metabolic remission following full-course R-CHOP but may be considered for patients over the age of 60 years with initial bulky disease. The UK BNLI dose trial for consolidation IFRT in high-grade lymphomas found no advantage to 40 Gy over 30 Gy in 2 Gy fractions (Lowry *et al.*, 2011). The role of combination and consolidation RT as part of first-line therapy in the management of patients with advanced stage DLBCL remains unclear. Biopsy of residual PET-positive masses is advised to enable individualised treatment decisions.

Treatment recommendation:

- stage 1A non-bulky or stage IIA less-fit elderly patients – 3 cycles of R-CHOP-21 and 30 Gy IFRT/ISRT;
- stage 1A bulky and above – 6 cycles of R-CHOP-21;
- patients not fit for anthracyclines can be treated with R-CVP or a gemcitabine-based regimen, R-GCVP.

Primary testicular lymphoma

This is a DLBCL with a propensity for CNS spread. Treatment of fit patients, even with early-stage disease, consists of definitive chemotherapy with 6 cycles of R-CHOP, intrathecal prophylaxis and contralateral testicular irradiation with 30 Gy (Vitolo *et al.*, 2011). A current IELSG study is investigating the role of systemic CNS prophylaxis.

Primary mediastinal B-cell lymphoma

This can be distinguished from DLBCL by unique clinical and molecular features. It is more common in adolescents and young adults, with a median age at presentation in the fourth decade. The cells express CD20 and CD79a, but do not express surface immunoglobulin. Gene expression profiling shows an overlap between PMBCL and nodular sclerosing HL, with a further distinct entity intermediate between the two, the newly defined 'grey zone lymphoma'.

Clinical presentation

Patients usually present with a bulky mediastinal mass and pericardial and pleural effusions.

Treatment

The current standard treatment is six cycles of R-CHOP, although response rates may be poorer than those for DLBCL. Mediastinal RT is usually recommended because of initial bulky disease, but the effectiveness of this approach for complete responders is currently the subject of the IELSG-36 trial. There are limited data to suggest that dose-adjusted R-EPOCH (etoposide, prednisolone, vincristine, cyclophosphamide, doxorubicin) is effective without the need for mediastinal radiotherapy (Dunleavy *et al.*, 2013).

Prognosis

The 5-year overall survival ranges from 0% to 65%, depending on the patient's IPI score.

CNS prophylaxis in lymphoma

CNS relapse occurs in fewer than 3% of patients with DLBCL treated in the R-CHOP era and may involve the brain parenchyma, spinal cord, leptomeninges, or eyes. Risk factors include high IPI scores, particularly more than one extranodal site, and para-meningeal or testicular involvement. In most cases, CNS relapse is associated with systemic relapse and a very poor prognosis. Isolated CNS relapse is much less common but may be treatable. The median time to CNS relapse is 1.8 years and median overall survival is 1.6 years. As the incidence is relatively low, effort has gone into trying to define a high-risk group. Patients with Burkitt lymphoma have a very high risk of CNS relapse and both intrathecal and systemic high-dose methotrexate (HD-MTX) are an integral part of the standard regimen, R-CODOX-M/R-IVAC. The optimal prophylaxis regimen for other high-grade lymphomas has not been defined, but BCSH guidelines recommend 3–6 doses of intrathecal MTX given weekly or with each cycle of systemic chemotherapy (McMillan *et al.*, 2013).

Treatment for relapsed/refractory disease

High-dose chemotherapy, the most widely used regimen being BEAM (BCNU, etoposide, cytarabine, melphalan) with an autologous stem cell transplant has been shown to improve progression-free and overall survival for patients with chemosensitive disease. The PARMA study randomised patients responding to second-line chemotherapy with DHAP (dexamethasone, cytarabine, cisplatin) to receive either high-dose chemotherapy with autologous stem cell transplant (HDC/ASCT) or four further cycles of DHAP (Philip *et al.*, 1995). At eight years, both event-free and overall survival was better in the HDC/ASCT group (36% versus 11%, and 47% versus 27%, respectively). The most effective conditioning regimen has not been established, and includes GDP (gemcitabine, dexamethasone, cisplatin), DHAP, ESHAP (etoposide, cisplatin, cytarabine, methyprednisolone) and ICE (ifosfamide, carboplatin, etoposide), usually given with rituximab (Gisselbrecht *et al.*, 2010). Poor prognostic factors include chemorefractory disease and a short duration of remission, especially for patients treated with R-CHOP.

Primary CNS lymphoma (PCNSL)

DLBCL account for 90% of primary central nervous system lymphoma (PCNSL), although these comprise only 1% of NHL cases and 4% of all brain tumours. Most cases of non-HIV-related PCNSL are diagnosed in patients between 45 and 70 years of age, with a median age at diagnosis in the fifth decade. Men and women are equally affected, with an annual incidence of 0.47 per 100,000.

Clinical presentation

Patients may present with progressive neurological signs, cognitive and personality changes, fits, raised intracranial pressure or cranial neuropathies. In immunocompetent patients, single or multiple periventricular enhancing lesions are typical, whereas ring-enhancing lesions are seen in immunodeficient patients. The most common sites of involvement are the frontal lobes, followed by the basal ganglia and thalamus. PCNSL can also spread across the corpus callosum, giving a typical butterfly pattern. Empiric treatment with corticosteroids may cause prolonged remission of clinical signs and symptoms as well as imaging findings; however, spontaneous remission can also occur.

Investigation

A biopsy is required for diagnosis, but there is no benefit from surgical resection. Recommended investigations include brain MRI and whole body CT, stereotactic biopsy, lumbar puncture, ophthalmological examination, serum LDH and viral serology.

Management

There is a relapse rate of 60% following treatment with whole-brain RT (WBRT) alone, with a median survival of 12–18 months. Chemotherapy regimens with high CNS penetration are required in patients fit enough to tolerate them, and HD-MTX has always been the standard. A phase 2 study showed improved response rates with the addition of high-dose cytarabine (HD-AC) to HD-MTX (Ferreri *et al.*, 2009). Seventy-nine patients aged up to 75 years were randomised and all patients received WBRT following chemotherapy – those ≤ 60 years and in complete remission received 36 Gy. Patients with less than complete response received 36 Gy WBRT followed by a tumour bed boost of 9 Gy. Of patients receiving HD-MTX and HD-AC, 46% had a complete response to treatment compared with 18% of patients receiving HD-MTX alone. Following radiotherapy, the complete remission rates increased to 64% and 30%, respectively. The follow-up study IELSG 32 has shown an improvement in progression-free and overall survival with the addition of rituximab and thiotepa (MATRIX regimen) and is also examining the use of high-dose chemotherapy as consolidation instead of WBRT (Ferreri et al., 2015).

The major drawback of WBRT in conjunction with HD-MTX-based chemotherapy is the high incidence of cognitive impairment and white matter damage, especially in patients over 60 years. Neurotoxicity may manifest as a rapidly progressive dementia characterised by psychomotor slowing, executive and memory dysfunction, behavioural changes, gait ataxia and incontinence. Optimising chemotherapy regimens may allow reduction of WBRT dose whilst maintaining efficacy, though the long term effects of this approach is unknown (Morris et al., 2013).

WBRT is recommended following a partial response or stable disease with first-line chemotherapy.

For patients with a poor performance status consider best supportive care, with or without steroids. Palliative radiotherapy may be appropriate in patients with a good performance status who are not fit for HD-MTX-based chemotherapy or for patients who relapse following first-line chemotherapy.

HIV-associated PCNSL

The incidence of PCNSL has reduced since the introduction of highly active antiretroviral therapy (HAART; 1.2 versus 3.0 cases per 1000), and the median survival is improving. Patients may be able to receive similar HD-MTX-based regimens as immunocompetent patients. Comprehensive guidelines for the treatment of HIV-associated malignances are available on the British HIV Association website (http://www. bhiva.org/, accessed November 2014).

Whole-brain radiotherapy

The standard treatment volume includes the whole brain, eyes and optic nerves, while shielding the anterior chamber and lens. 3D CT planning is standard, otherwise left and right lateral equally weighted opposed-fields can be used, treating with 6–10 MV photons. The posterior two-thirds of the orbits should be shielded after 30 Gy, or 36 Gy in the case of intraocular involvement. The inferior border should encompass the vertebral body of C2. Patients with intraocular lymphoma should receive WBRT due to the high risk of CNS relapse. If required, the boost volume encompasses residual tumour with a 1–2-cm margin.

Acute side effects are tolerable and include fatigue, headaches, hair loss and skin dryness and/or erythema.

In patients with significant mass effect, corticosteroids should be prescribed to avoid worsening cerebral oedema, but the dose can be reduced reasonably quickly. Acute symptoms of confusion are usually mild and transient.

Delayed symptoms, such as somnolence syndrome occurring within 7–40 days of radiotherapy, are thought to result from inhibition of myelin synthesis. Patients should be warned about the possibility and evaluated carefully, as this can be misinterpreted as disease progression.

Dose

Curative treatment following a complete or partial remission to induction multiagent chemotherapy: 23.4–36 Gy in 1.8 Gy fractions, depending on the chemotherapy regimen used with it.

Palliation: 23.4–30 Gy in 1.8–2 Gy fractions.

Follicular lymphoma (FL)

Follicular lymphoma is the most common indolent lymphoma and accounts for 20% of all cases of NHL. It is characterised by a relapsing and remitting pattern, with progressive shortening of the intervals between treatments. Apart from patients who present with non-bulky stage IA disease, FL is considered incurable. The median age at diagnosis is 60 years, and median survival is between 8 and 12 years.

FL is a nodal lymphoma with a follicular growth pattern and arises from a mature B cell in the germinal centre of the lymph node. FL is graded from 1 to 3 according to the number of large centroblasts per high-power field. Grade 3 can be further subdivided into 3a and 3b; the latter resembles de novo DLBCL and is generally treated as such. Almost all FL carry breaks at 18q21, with approximately 85% having the t(14;18) translocation. This results in the juxtaposition of the BCL-2 gene on chromosome 18 with the immunoglobulin heavy-chain locus on chromosome 14, leading to overexpression of the anti-apoptotic BCL-2. Tumour cells show light chain restriction.

Clinical presentation

Patients commonly present with advanced-stage disease, bulky lymphadenopathy and bone marrow involvement. In patients with early-stage disease, detection of a low-level B cell clone in the bone marrow of uncertain significance would not necessarily alter management.

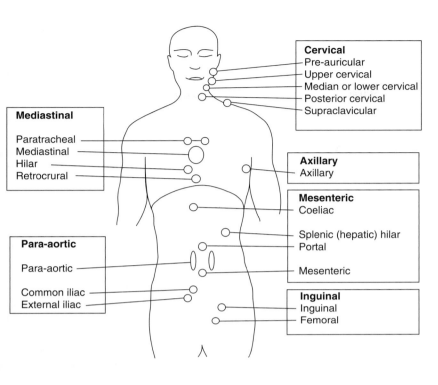

Cervical
- Pre-auricular
- Upper cervical
- Median or lower cervical
- Posterior cervical
- Supraclavicular

Mediastinal
- Paratracheal
- Mediastinal
- Hilar
- Retrocrural

Axillary
- Axillary

Mesenteric
- Coeliac
- Splenic (hepatic) hilar
- Portal
- Mesenteric

Para-aortic
- Para-aortic
- Common iliac
- External iliac

Inguinal
- Inguinal
- Femoral

Others: Epitrochlear, popliteal

Table 34.4 Follicular Lymphoma International Prognostic Index 2 (FLIPI-2)

No. of risk factors	Risk group	3-year PFS (%)	3-year OS (%)
0	Low	91	99
1–2	Intermediate	69	96
3–5	High	51	84

Risk factors are: age > 60 years; β2 microglobulin > normal; Hb < 120 g/L; bone marrow involvement; dimension of largest involved node > 6 cm. Adapted from Federico *et al.*, 2009.

Prognostic factors

The Follicular Lymphoma International Prognostic Index (FLIPI) allows for a score of 1 point for each of the following:

- age > 60 years;
- stage III or IV;
- five or more nodal sites involved (see Figure 34.1);
- LDH > normal;
- Hb < 120 g/L.

The prognosis based on FLIPI category (score) and 10-year survival (10YS) can be good (0–1; 10YS = 71%), intermediate (2; 10YS = 51%) or poor (3–5; 10YS = 36%).

A subsequent evaluation (FLIPI-2) of 832 patients, the majority of whom were treated with immunochemotherapy, defined five prognostic factors (Federico *et al.*, 2009) (Table 34.4). However, these prognostic scores are not used to determine need for treatment at diagnosis.

Treatment of stage IA non-bulky FL

Local radiotherapy can give progression-free survival rates of approximately 50% (Guadagnolo *et al.*, 2006; Pugh *et al.*, 2010). The UK BNLI dose trial showed 24 Gy in 12 fractions equivalent to 40 Gy in 20 fractions (Lowry *et al.*, 2011), while the FoRT trial showed that 24 Gy in 12 fractions is more effective than 4 Gy in 2 fractions and remains the standard (Hoskin *et al.*, 2013a). An EORTC trial of IFRT alone or IFRT followed by CVP (cyclophosphamide, vincristine, prednisolone) showed progression-free but no overall survival advantage with the addition of chemotherapy (Somers *et al.*, 1987).

Treatment of advanced FL

For asymptomatic patients, there is no survival benefit for immediate treatment compared with a 'watch-and-wait' approach, although early treatment with rituximab induction and maintenance may defer the need for chemotherapy (Ardeshna *et al.*, 2010). The impact of early treatment with rituximab on subsequent treatment response is unknown, so this approach remains experimental. Radiotherapy may be helpful for symptomatic disease sites in the absence of widespread progression and may delay the need for systemic therapy; response rates with 24 Gy or 4 Gy in 2 Gy fractions are 81–74% respectively, with a higher 2-year progression-free rate in the 24 Gy arm (94% versus 80%; Hoskin *et al.*, 2013a). Indications for systemic treatment include bulky disease, impaired organ function, or progressive symptoms, and first-line regimens incorporate rituximab with CVP, CHOP, chlorambucil or bendamustine (Marcus *et al.*, 2008; McNamara *et al.*, 2011). In the pre-rituximab era, the addition of an anthracycline improved response rates but not overall survival, and R-bendamustine appears to be as effective as R-CHOP, but with less toxicity (Rummel *et al.*, 2013).

The PRIMA study randomised FL patients with at least a partial response to rituximab plus chemotherapy to either observation or rituximab maintenance every 2 months for 2 years (Salles *et al.*, 2011). With a median follow-up of 3 years, the progression-free survival in those responding to induction was 75% in the rituximab maintenance group and 58% in the observation group. Time to next treatment was also significantly longer in the maintenance arm. NICE subsequently approved the use of rituximab maintenance in patients responding to first-line induction therapy.

Treatment of relapsed disease

At relapse, a repeat biopsy to exclude transformation to high-grade disease is recommended. Factors influencing management include age, duration of remission, previous treatment, burden of FL, symptoms and performance status. With increasing use of maintenance rituximab, relapse during this period will label a patient as 'rituximab-refractory', but if the patients are asymptomatic, surveillance may still be appropriate. The purine analogue fludarabine can give useful responses in pretreated patients, but will reduce the ability to harvest stem cells, an important consideration in younger patients. In addition, fludarabine can result in prolonged lymphopenia, increasing the risk of opportunistic infections and transfusion-related graft-versus-host disease necessitating life-long use of irradiated blood products. Bendamustine is another active drug for rituximab-refractory patients, given on days 1 and 2 of a 28-day cycle. Maintenance rituximab can be used after second-line induction treatment if appropriate, and a three-monthly schedule is commonly used. In young, fit patients with short remissions, more intensive induction regimens such as R-CHOP may be considered, with discussion of transplant options for consolidation.

HDC/ASCT may improve disease-free survival, but most patients eventually relapse as FL is not a chemo-curable lymphoma. The only potentially curative treatment is allogeneic SCT using a reduced-intensity approach, if a suitable donor is available. Lower relapse rates are offset by treatment-related mortality rates of up to 30% and this is only considered for younger patients with short remissions.

Radioimmunotherapy (^{90}Y anti-CD20 or ^{131}I anti-CD20) can give overall response rates of about 75% and complete response rates of up to 40% in heavily pretreated patients and may be a good option for some patients.

The main cause of death of patients with FL is transformation to high-grade lymphoma, usually DLBCL, but sometimes Burkitt lymphoma. The prognosis was considered to be poorer than for patients who present *de novo* with these lymphomas, but recent data suggests that outcomes have improved over time. Patients responding to salvage chemotherapy should be considered for consolidation with HDC/ASCT.

Mantle cell lymphoma

Mantle cell lymphoma (MCL) accounts for around 5% of NHL. The median age of diagnosis is 65 years, and the male-to-female ratio is 4:1. Mantle cell lymphoma arises from CD5+ cells that populate the mantle zone of follicles. It is characterised by the chromosomal translocation t(11;14) which results in overexpression of the cell cycle protein cyclin D1 and deregulation of cell cycle progression. Rare cases of cyclin D1-negative MCL can occur. A diffuse growth pattern and high proliferation rate (Ki-67 > 30%) are associated with a worse prognosis. MCL is characteristically described as having the worst features of both high- and low-grade NHL in that it is an incurable lymphoma with an aggressive clinical course, and the median survival is 4–5 years.

Clinical presentation

Most patients present with advanced disease with nodal and extranodal involvement (bone marrow in 90%, spleen, liver, gastrointestinal tract). CNS involvement is rare. There is a spectrum of pathology from low-grade, especially with a leukaemic presentation that seems to carry a better prognosis, to a blastoid variant with a very poor prognosis. Observation alone is a reasonable strategy for asymptomatic patients.

Treatment

A meta-analysis of three RCTs involving 260 patients with MCL concluded that the addition of rituximab to chemotherapy improved overall survival. The prognosis of younger patients under 65 years has improved with the use of high-dose cytarabine in induction chemotherapy before consolidation with HDC/ASCT (McKay *et al.*, 2012). However, the majority of patients with MCL are not fit for intensive treatment options. An RCT for older patients compared R-CHOP with rituximab, fludarabine, cyclophosphamide (R-FC), followed by a second randomisation to maintenance with rituximab or IFN-alpha. The best results were obtained with R-CHOP followed by rituximab maintenance.

A new treatment currently under investigation is ibrutinib, with early-phase trials showing high response rates in relapsed refractory MCL. Bruton's tyrosine kinase (BTK) is a mediator of B cell receptor signalling, essential for normal B-cell development. Ibrutinib is an oral BTK inhibitor, and has been shown to be effective in the treatment of CLL.

Extranodal marginal zone B-cell lymphoma (MALT type)

Extranodal marginal zone B-cell lymphoma has an annual incidence of 0.6 in 100,000 patients and represents 8% of NHL. The median age at diagnosis is 60 years. MALT lymphoma is a clinicopathologically distinct entity arising within acquired mucosa-associated lymphoid tissue (MALT) of extranodal sites such as the stomach, salivary glands, conjunctiva, orbits, lung, breast and thyroid. It is frequently associated with a pre-existing inflammatory or infective condition. Gastric MALT lymphoma is associated with *H. pylori* infection in up to 90% of cases.

Management

Local treatments such as surgery or radiotherapy appear to be as effective as chemotherapy, and so one needs to weigh up the morbidity of treatment against performance status and comorbidities of the patient. Surgery (e.g. gastrectomy) is not usually recommended although an excision biopsy leaving no residual disease means that surveillance might be appropriate. Local radiotherapy is usually convenient, quick and well tolerated. Remission following radiotherapy may take up to 24 months and can be confirmed by a repeat biopsy, although the interpretation of lymphoid infiltrates in post-treatment gastric biopsies can be very difficult.

Helicobacter pylori eradication

H. pylori eradication therapy must be given to all patients with gastric MALT lymphomas, irrespective of stage or histological grade, and may lead to complete and prolonged histological remission in up to 70% of patients. A urea breath test (or a monoclonal stool antigen test) can be used to assess response 6 weeks or more following eradication therapy and at least 2 weeks after PPI withdrawal. *H. pylori* eradication therapy includes omeprazole 20 mg b.d., metronidazole 400 mg b.d. and amoxicillin 1 g b.d. (clarithromycin 500 mg b.d. if allergic) for 14 days. This is less likely to be successful if there is full-thickness invasion of the gastric wall, lymph node involvement or a t(11;18) genetic abnormality. However, patients with t(11;18) may rarely transform to DLBCL.

Chemotherapy

Chemotherapy is also effective, although the t(11;18) translocation seems to predict for poor response to alkylating agents as sole treatment. The addition of rituximab to chlorambucil has been shown to improve 5-year event-free but not overall survival, which was 89% at 5 years for both arms (Zucca *et al.*, 2013).

Local radiotherapy

Radiotherapy is the treatment of choice for stage 1A extranodal MALT lymphoma, as it results in good long-term control rates with minimal toxicity (Goda *et al.*, 2010).

CTV definition

Gastric MALT – the whole stomach

Salivary glands – the whole gland

Orbital MALT – this may be due to involvement of the lacrimal gland, which then should be included the CTV, but with bulky tumours and posterior extension, the CTV should include the whole orbit. For conjunctival MALT, superficial X-rays may be used.

Dose: 24–30 Gy in daily 2 Gy fractions.

Prognosis

The disease remains localised for prolonged periods and prognosis is generally good; 5-year disease-free survival rates are higher than 90%.

T- and NK-cell NHL

These account for approximately 12% of NHL. EBV-associated extranodal NK-/T-cell lymphoma is a specific entity seen more commonly in the Far East and causes destructive lesions in the nasal or paranasal areas. A study of 82 patients with localised disease (stage IE to IIE) showed that early radiotherapy was the only independent prognostic factor and that 5-year overall survival was significantly better for patients receiving > 54 Gy. The optimal dose is at least 50 Gy to the nasal cavity and both antra. The use of chemoradiotherapy for localised disease showed improved results compared to historical controls treated with radiotherapy alone. Reported responses to CHOP vary, and current treatment regimens are testing the incorporation of L-asparaginase (Dearden et al., 2011; Tse and Kwong, 2013).

Radiotherapy

PET and MRI staging are very helpful when planning RT, and uninvolved nodes are not routinely included.

IMRT may allow sparing of the parotid glands.

CTV–GTV plus whole nasal cavity and both maxillary antra, or 1–2 cm beyond any soft tissue extension, depending on the accuracy and quality of staging imaging, respecting anatomical boundaries.

Upfront radiotherapy before chemotherapy is recommended, but neoadjuvant chemotherapy for bulky tumours can reduce the need for re-planning rapidly shrinking volumes on treatment (Jiang et al., 2012).

Dose: 50–56 Gy in 1.8–2 Gy fractions.

Cutaneous T-cell lymphomas

Cutaneous lymphomas are characterised by malignant lymphocytes, most often of T-cell origin (CTCL),

Table 34.5 Predictive factors for the Cutaneous Lymphoma International Prognostic Index (CLIPi) in mycosis fungoides and Sézary syndrome

	No. of risk factors	Risk	10-year survival (%)
Early stage	0–1	Low	90.3
	2	Intermediate	76.2
	3–5	High	48.9
Late stage	0–1	Low	53.2
	2	Intermediate	19.8
	3–5	High	15.0

Risk factors for early-stage (IA–IIA) disease are: male gender; age > 60 years, presence of plaques, folliculotropic MF; palpable nodes, uninvolved (N1/Nx). Risk factors for late stage (IIB– IVB) are: male gender; age > 60 years; node-positive; > 5% circulating tumour cells (B1/B2); visceral involvement (M1). Adapted from Benton et al. (2013).

localised to the skin. The most common type is mycosis fungoides (MF) with Sézary syndrome (SS) accounting for 5%. The diagnosis can be difficult to make in the early stages, with patients presenting with an eczematous skin rash for a median of 6 years before the histological diagnosis. Distinct clinical stages are seen, with cutaneous patches and plaques progressing later to bulkier tumours. No treatments have been shown to influence survival but the clinical course of MF can be indolent over several years, and some patients never progress. The revised International Society for Cutaneous Lymphomas/EORTC TNM-Blood staging system is used. The median survival is not reached at 35.5 years for stage IA, and is 21.5 years for stage IB, 4.7 years for stage IIB, 3.4 years for stage IIIB, 2.1 years for stage IVA and 0.9 years for stage IVB. Sézary syndrome is defined by the presence of erythroderma, lymphadenopathy and Sézary cells in peripheral blood and is associated with a poor median survival of only 32 months from diagnosis. Survival data from a UK cohort of 1502 patients, validated for a similar cohort of US patients, allowed analysis of predictive factors (Table 34.5) which formed the basis of the Cutaneous Lymphoma International Prognostic Index (CLIPi; Benton et al., 2013).

Management

It is reasonable to simply observe the patient until he/she becomes symptomatic, and then skin-directed treatment can be used such as topical steroids, psoralen and ultraviolet A (PUVA) or UVB therapy (Willemze *et al.*, 2013). Palliative radiotherapy is useful for persistent or symptomatic lesions. The target volume when treating patches, plaques and tumours is the clinically defined lesion (GTV) with a PTV margin of 0.5–1.0 cm. Patches and plaques can be treated to a depth of 7–9 mm in the skin, but thicker tumours require greater depth doses. Doses depend on the size of the treatment field and may range from single 4–6 Gy fractions, 8 Gy in 2 daily fractions, 15 Gy in daily 3 Gy fractions, to 30 Gy in 2 Gy fractions. Low doses are effective and allow retreatment or overlapping fields.

Low-energy superficial or orthovoltage X-rays are convenient but electrons are better if a steeper dose drop off is required to minimise toxicity. Bolus is used to increase the dose to the skin surface to 95%; typically 1 cm of bolus is needed for a 10×10 cm field using 6 MeV electrons to give a surface dose of > 95% and a depth dose of 90% at 8–9 mm. Large areas such as on the scalp may require complex matched electron and photon techniques, intensity-modulated radiotherapy or mould brachytherapy (Morris, 2012).

Chemotherapy is often used for advanced disease although response durations are short and multi-agent regimens such as CHOP give no additional benefit over single agents (methotrexate, liposomal doxorubicin, gemcitabine). Biological response modifiers such as IFN-α may help, although prominent side effects include fatigue and flu-like symptoms. Bexarotene is a synthetic retinoid available for the treatment of advanced-stage CTCL refractory to at least one systemic treatment. It is well tolerated but causes central hypothyroidism and hyperlipidaemia, which should be controlled before starting treatment (Scarisbrick *et al.*, 2013).

Total skin electron beam therapy (TSEBT)

A meta-analysis of predominantly retrospective studies of TSEBT has shown that response rates are related to cancer stage, dose and energy. Complete response rates vary from 96% in early stages to 60% in stage III disease. Knowing when to offer TSEBT can be a difficult decision, and it is best managed by an experienced team including oncologists, physicists, radiographers, nurses and dermatologists, using a modification of the original Stanford technique. A 6-MeV Linac is used in high-dose electron mode, with angled dual fields to treat the patient in different positions to allow maximum skin exposure. The patient stands on a TSEB frame 3.5 m from the linear accelerator head, which rotates to two gantry angles of 17.5° above and below the beam axis to produce the dual fields. A Perspex

screen is placed in front of the patient to attenuate and scatter the incident electrons, resulting in an electron energy of 4 MeV at the skin surface. EORTC recommendations are that the 80% isodose should be at least 4 mm deep to the surface of the skin, and the dose at 20 mm deep should be less than 20% of the maximum dose at the skin surface. Eyes and nails are shielded and some areas of the skin, including the top of the scalp, soles, palms, perineum and infra-mammary areas may be underdosed and require additional treatment. The standard Stanford schedule treats to 30–36 Gy in 2 Gy fractions spread over 9–10 weeks, with a treatment gap if necessary but lower doses may give useful responses and are well tolerated.

Acute complications of TSEBT include erythema, dry desquamation, hair and nail loss and reduced sweating. Late complications include secondary skin cancers and skin changes, such as hyperpigmentation and telangiectasia. Although TSEBT is not curative, it can produce prolonged palliation, and recurrences may be limited in penetration and extent (Morris *et al.*, 2013). Low-dose TSEBT can be repeated after 1 year or more if other disease-control measures fail and patients have had an initial good response.

Hodgkin lymphoma

The incidence of HL is bimodal. In developing countries, the first peak occurs in childhood, whereas in developed countries, it is seen in young adults. The second peak occurs in older adults, and the male-to-female ratio of disease incidence is 1.5:1. Epidemiological studies suggest a link with EBV, although the exact mechanism of association is unknown. Of patients, 95% have classic HL, in which the tumour cells express CD30 and CD15, and lack B-cell antigens. In nodular lymphocyte-predominant HL (5%), B-cell markers such as CD20 are expressed, and CD30 and CD15 are absent. However, in both types, the malignant Reed–Sternberg cells appear to be clonally derived germinal-centre B cells.

Management of early-stage (I to IIA) disease

Patients with early-stage HL may be divided into two groups, depending on the presence or absence of risk factors, as shown in Table 34.6. These are used for risk stratification in clinical trials, and differ between trial groups.

Table 34.6 German Hodgkin Study Group definition of risk factors in early-stage HL.

GHSG risk factors
Bulky mediastinal mass
≥ 3 nodal areas
ESR ≥ 50
Extranodal site

Adapted from Eich *et al.*, 2010.

Combined-modality treatment based on ABVD chemotherapy (doxorubicin, bleomycin, vinblastine, dacarbazine) followed by radiotherapy to initially involved sites is the standard of care for early stage HL. The GHSG HD10 trial for patients with stage I–IIA disease with no risk factors found no difference with the number of cycles of ABVD chemotherapy (two versus four) or involved field radiation dose (20 versus 30 Gy; Engert *et al.*, 2010). For patients with risk factors, the best results are obtained with 2 cycles of escalated BEACOPP and 2 cycles of ABVD, followed by 30 Gy IFRT, although this approach is more toxic than 4 cycles of ABVD and 30 Gy IFRT, which remains the UK standard (Eich *et al.*, 2010; von Tresckow *et al.*, 2012).

Trials undertaken in the pre-PET era with a chemotherapy-only arm show that omission of radiotherapy increases the relapse rate but as salvage treatment is often successful, overall survival is usually similar for both arms (Meyer *et al.*, 2005; Thomas *et al.*, 2004). The UK RAPID study for stage I–IIA patients without mediastinal bulk used a centrally reviewed interim PET scan after 3 cycles of ABVD to see if radiotherapy could be omitted (Radford *et al.*, 2015). Seventy-five percent of patients had a Deauville score of 1 or 2, and were randomised between 30 Gy IFRT or no further treatment. All other patients completed treatment with one further cycle of ABVD followed by 30 Gy IFRT. Five patients randomised to IFRT died of chemotherapy complications prior to starting radiotherapy. In the intention to treat analysis, the 3-year progression-free survival rate was 94.6% in the radiotherapy group and 90.8% in the group that received no further therapy. On a per-protocol basis, the 3-year progression-free survival rate was 97.1% in the RT group versus 90.8% for no further therapy. Omitting radiotherapy therefore is associated with a slightly higher risk of relapse. Older patients or those for whom salvage therapy is not an option may be best treated with combined modality therapy, whereas a young female patient with mediastinal involvement may have better long term outcomes with a chemotherapy-alone approach. This study provides data for an informed discussion with the patient. It is important that if a chemotherapy-alone approach is planned, the PET scan should be done after cycle 3 and the response criteria based on that used in the study.

Treatment recommendation for early-stage HL:

No risk factors: 2 cycles ABVD and 20 Gy ISRT.

GHSG risk factors: 4 cycles ABVD and 30 Gy ISRT.

Stage I-IIA, non-bulky: 3 cycles ABVD followed by PET scan to determine need for RT. If the score is 1–2, no further treatment; if the score is 3–4 then one further cycle of ABVD and 30 Gy ISRT is needed.

Management of advanced disease (stage IIB and higher)

ABVD has been the standard regimen in the UK for many years. Analysis of over 5000 patients with advanced HL treated with ABVD or an equivalent regimen found 7 prognostic factors associated with a reduction of 7–8% in tumour control at 5 years (Hasenclever *et al.*, 1998). The International Prognostic Score (IPS) correlates with 5-year progression-free survival, which was 74% for patients with 0–2 factors and 47% for those with 4 or more.

- Age > 45 years.
- Male.
- Serum albumin < 40 g/L.
- Hb < 105 g/L.
- Stage IV disease.
- Leucocytosis > 15×10^9/L.
- Lymphopenia < 0.6×10^9/L or < 8% WBC count.

More intensive combinations have been developed in the last decade to improve outcome. Randomised trials showed superior disease-free but not overall survival for escalated BEACOPP over ABVD, due to the use of salvage with HDC/ASCT for ABVD failures. Escalated BEACOPP is associated with higher rates of acute haematological toxicity, secondary myelodysplastic syndromes and/or acute leukaemias, and infertility, particularly in patients over 65 years. An early interim PET scan after 2 cycles of ABVD appears to be predictive of outcome, but whether treatment adaptation at this point can improve survival is currently the subject of clinical trials (Gallamini *et al.*, 2007).

Role of radiotherapy in advanced HL

Outside clinical trials, consolidation radiotherapy is the current standard treatment after chemotherapy for patients with bulky mediastinal or residual PET positive masses, 30–40 Gy in 1.8–2 Gy fractions.

Paediatric Hodgkin lymphoma

Patients are divided into low-, intermediate- or high-risk groups according to prognostic factors which include stage, tumour volume and ESR. Two cycles of induction chemotherapy with OEPA (vincristine, etoposide, prednisolone and doxorubicin) are followed by an interim PET-CT scan. Patients with a positive PET scan receive radiotherapy at the end of chemotherapy. Patients in the low-risk group have no further chemotherapy, while those in the intermediate- and high-risk groups receive two or four cycles of COPDAC (cyclophosphamide, vincristine, dacarbazine and prednisolone), respectively. Radiotherapy consists of a modified IFRT technique, with a standard dose of 19.8 Gy in 11 fractions and a 10 Gy boost if required. Delineation guidelines have also been published for paediatric Hodgkin lymphoma (Hodgson *et al.*, 2013).

Management of relapsed/refractory Hodgkin lymphoma

Patients with refractory, progressive or relapsed HL can be successfully treated with salvage chemotherapy followed by HDC/ASCT. Second-line chemotherapy regimens include IGEV (ifosfamide, gemcitabine, prednisolone, vinblastine), miniBEAM or ESHAP. Published studies show progression-free survival of up to 61% at 5 years. Poor prognostic factors include relapse within a year, chemorefractory disease, extranodal relapse and B symptoms. Achieving a metabolic complete response before HDC is associated with better outcomes (Moskowitz *et al.*, 2012).

Monoclonal antibodies against CD30 have been shown to be ineffective in clinical trials as single agents, but, when combined with an anti-tubulin agent (MMAE), brentuximab vedotin showed significant activity in relapsed and refractory HL following ASCT. The overall response rate was 75% with complete remission in 34% of patients. The median progression-free survival was 5.6 months, and the median duration of response for those in complete remission was 20.5 months (Younes *et al.*, 2012). Brentuximab is currently licensed for patients who have relapsed following ASCT or after more than two lines of chemotherapy, as a bridge to allogeneic SCT. Clinical trials are currently testing its use in first-line treatment regimens.

Allogeneic SCT using reduced intensity conditioning can be effective in relapsed HL after HDC/ASCT.

Nodular lymphocyte-predominant Hodgkin lymphoma (NLPHL)

NLPHL may present as slowly progressive lymphadenopathy at a peripheral site such as the neck, axilla or groin over a period of several years. It is more common in men in the third or fourth decade, and rarely affects the mediastinum. Expert haematopathology review is essential, as it can transform to T cell-rich B cell lymphoma. Local radiotherapy gives durable control, and given the predominantly peripheral sites involved, late effects are rare (Nogová *et al.*, 2006; Chen *et al.*, 2010; Eichenauer *et al.*, 2015). Although the clinical behaviour of NLPHL resembles that of a low-grade B-cell lymphoma, higher stages have traditionally been treated as for classical HL. As NLPHL is CD20-positive, rituximab has been used in combination with chemotherapy regimens such as R-ABVD, R-CVP or R-CHOP, though this has not been tested in a randomised trial.

Paediatric treatment guidelines recommend a watch-and-wait strategy in patients who are PET-negative after surgical excision, and the current EuroNet-L1 study is also testing the use of a non-anthracycline-based chemotherapy regimen for early-stage patients below the age of 18 years.

Recommendation

Stage IA on PET-CT, non-bulky: IFRT/ISRT alone, 30 Gy in 15 fractions.

Stage IIA – non-bulky: 2 cycles ABVD and 20 Gy IFRT/ISRT.

Stages I–IIA bulky: 4 cycles ABVD and 30 Gy IFRT/ISRT.

Stages III–IV: 6 cycles ABVD, CVP or CHOP, with/without rituximab.

Myeloma and solitary plasmacytoma

Myeloma

Incidence and epidemiology

The annual incidence of myeloma in the UK is 60–70 per million, with a median age at presentation of 70 years.

Table 34.7 Screening and diagnostic tests for multiple myeloma

Screening tests	Diagnostic tests
FBC	Serum albumin
Serum urea, electrolytes, calcium	Serum uric acid
Serum protein electrophoresis	Bone marrow aspirate and trephine, to include cytogenetic studies
Serum immunoglobulins	β_2-microglobulin
ESR or plasma viscosity	LDH
Urine sample for Bence–Jones proteins.	Serum paraprotein and urinary light chain excretion
Skeletal survey	Serum-free light chains

Table 34.8 Diagnosis and new definitions of myeloma and related diseases

MGUS	Asymptomatic myeloma	Symptomatic myeloma
M-protein in serum < 30 g/L	M-protein in serum ≥ 30 g/L and/or	M-protein in serum and/or urine
Bone marrow clonal plasma cells < 10%	Bone marrow clonal plasma cells ≥ 10%	Bone marrow clonal plasma cells or biopsy-proven plasmacytoma
No end-organ damage including bone lesions or symptoms	No end-organ damage including bone lesions or symptoms	Myeloma-related organ impairment or bone lesions

Adapted from Bird et al., 2011.

Myeloma has a higher incidence in Afro-Caribbean ethnic groups, but there are few other distinctive epidemiological features. The majority of cases present *de novo*, but it is now recognised that myeloma is preceded by an asymptomatic monoclonal gammopathy of undetermined significance (MGUS) in almost all patients. The natural history of myeloma is variable, with survival times ranging from a few weeks to over 20 years.

Pathology

A neoplastic clone of plasma cells in the bone marrow produces monoclonal (M) protein, usually IgG, IgA with excess light chains or free light chain only, and more rarely IgD. A few myelomas are non-secretory by standard assay. Light chains appear in the urine as Bence–Jones proteins. Overproduction of IL-6 appears to be an important factor in the pathogenesis of myeloma and the high expression of vascular endothelial growth factor receptors (VEGFR) makes them a useful target for therapy with anti-angiogenesis drugs such as thalidomide and lenalidomide.

Clinical presentation

The main presenting symptoms are due to bone destruction causing pain or pathological fractures, myelosuppression leading to anaemia and recurrent infections, hypercalcaemia, renal failure or amyloid deposition.

Investigation and staging

Investigation of a patient with suspected myeloma includes screening and diagnostic tests (Table 34.7). Serum-free light chain assessment is indicated where there is a strong suspicion of myeloma but serum protein electrophoresis is negative. A diagnosis of myeloma should be confirmed by bone marrow assessment (Table 34.8). Analysis of prognostic factors is essential when comparing outcomes in clinical trials. The Durie/Salmon staging system has been superseded by the International Staging System which defines three risk groups based on albumin and β_2-microglobulin levels (Greipp et al., 2005; Table 34.9). Additional information comes from cytogenetics, and patients with 17p deletion, t(14;16), and t(14;20) are considered to have high-risk myeloma. Patients with t(4;14) translocation are considered intermediate-risk, while all others are considered standard-risk.

Treatment overview

Patients with asymptomatic myeloma ('smouldering myeloma') do not require chemotherapy but should have long-term monitoring for signs of organ or tissue damage. Patients with active disease require chemotherapy. Patients may be very unwell at presentation with dehydration, hypercalcaemia, renal failure, anaemia, infection and severe pain and may require full supportive care, including bisphosphonates,

Table 34.9 International Staging System (ISS) for multiple myeloma

Stage	Criteria	Median survival in months
I	Serum β_2 microglobulin < 3.5 mg/L and serum albumin ≥ 35 g/L	62
II	Neither I or III	45
III	Serum β_2 microglobulin ≥ 5.5 mg/L	29

Adapted from Bird *et al.*, 2011.

transfusions and analgesia. Plasma exchange may be necessary for symptomatic hyperviscosity.

Hypercalcaemia

Up to 30% of patients present with hypercalcaemia and may have central nervous system symptoms and signs, muscle weakness, pancreatitis, constipation, thirst, polyuria, shortening of the Q-T interval on ECG and acute renal insufficiency. Treatment of hypercalcaemia and the underlying myeloma should be initiated immediately to minimize long-term renal damage. Mild hypercalcaemia (corrected calcium 2.6–2.9 mmol/L) may be corrected with oral and/or intravenous rehydration. Moderate to severe hypercalcaemia (corrected calcium ≥ 2.9 mmol/L) requires intravenous rehydration with normal saline. All patients with moderate to severe hypercalcaemia should receive a bisphosphonate, preferably zoledronate. The treatment of hypercalcaemia is discussed in Chapter 8.

Chemotherapy

The treatment aims are to control disease, maximise quality of life and prolong survival if possible and consist of three phases: induction, consolidation and maintenance. Although HDC/ASCT may improve progression-free survival, not all patients will be suitable due to advanced age, comorbidities or poor performance status. If HDC/ASCT is a possible option, the aim of induction treatment is to induce remission rapidly with minimal toxicity and to preserve haemopoietic stem cell function for successful mobilisation of peripheral blood stem cells. The MRC Myeloma IX trial showed that induction chemotherapy with CTD (cyclophosphamide, thalidomide and dexamethasone) was more effective than CVAD (cyclophosphamide, vincristine, doxorubicin and dexamethasone)

(Morgan *et al.*, 2011). The Myeloma XI trial compares the current standard of CTD with cyclophosphamide, lenalidomide and dexamethasone.

Bone disease in myeloma

Patients commencing first-line treatment of myeloma should also receive zoledronate together with oral calcium and vitamin D supplements. This confers a survival benefit, although it is associated with a risk of osteonecrosis of the jaw (Morgan *et al.*, 2010). Kyphoplasty should be considered for symptomatic vertebral compression fractures. Orthopedic consultation should be sought for long-bone fractures, spinal cord compression and vertebral column instability.

Radiotherapy in myeloma

Indications for RT include pain, impending or actual pathological fracture and spinal cord compression. Patients with bone involvement at high risk of fracture should be referred for surgical stabilisation and treated postoperatively to improve pain and local control. Patients with spinal cord compression should have a neurosurgical opinion.

A single 8-Gy fraction can give good palliation of pain. For patients with spinal cord compression, 30 Gy in 10 fractions is recommended in view of the possibility of long-term disease control, but 20 Gy in 5 fractions is also acceptable.

Solitary plasmacytoma

A localised proliferation of malignant plasma cells may arise in a bone as a solitary bone plasmacytoma (SBP) or less frequently at an extramedullary site as a solitary extramedullary plasmacytoma (SEP). The male-to-female incidence ratio is 2:1, and the median age of patients is 50–55 years. Solitary plasmacytoma accounts for fewer than 5% of plasma cell malignancies.

The investigations are the same as for the diagnosis and staging of multiple myeloma, which needs to be excluded (Soutar *et al.*, 2004; Table 34.7). Criteria for diagnosis include the following.

- Histologically confirmed single lesion.
- Normal bone marrow biopsy (< 10% plasma cells).
- Negative skeletal survey.
- Normal haemoglobin, renal function and calcium. Low levels of a serum paraprotein may be present in up to 70% patients, but a level greater than 20 g/L suggests a diagnosis of myeloma.

The impact of improved diagnostic and staging techniques such as flow cytometry, molecular detection of heavy and light chain gene rearrangements in clonal plasma cells and MRI scans is unclear.

Solitary bone plasmacytoma

The most common site for SBP is in the axial skeleton, including the spine (most commonly thoracic and lumbar vertebrae), skull, ribs and sternum. Patients usually present with pain, or less commonly with spinal cord or nerve root compression, or with a pathological fracture. MRI of the whole spine is required to delineate the extent of the tumour and to exclude possible disease at other sites. More than 75% of patients progress to multiple myeloma in a median time of 2–4 years, giving a median survival of 7–11 years.

Management

- Surgery has a role where there is structural instability due to a fracture or rapidly progressive symptoms from spinal cord compression, but is not a definitive treatment, even if the diagnostic biopsy appears to have achieved a complete excision.
- Radical radiotherapy is the treatment of choice for SPB, although there have been no randomised trials. The largest retrospective study included 206 patients with SPB (Knobel *et al.*, 2006). Treatments included radiotherapy alone (169 patients), radiotherapy and chemotherapy (32 patients), and surgery alone (4 patients). For patients treated with radiotherapy alone, 10-year rates of overall survival, disease-free survival, and local control were 51%, 21% and 78%, with a 71% progression rate to myeloma. There is little evidence for a dose-response effect over 40 Gy even for tumours > 5 cm (Tsang *et al.*, 2001). Local control rates of over 85% can be achieved, but progression to myeloma remains the main problem.
- Radiotherapy techniques and beam energies will vary with treatment sites. The CTV should include tumour visible on MRI with a margin of at least 2 cm, or in the case of vertebral involvement, both adjacent vertebrae. If a surgical procedure has been performed, care must be taken to include any areas within the surgical field that may be at risk from tumour contamination. There is no benefit from irradiating the entire medullary cavity of a long bone, or regional lymph nodes.

Solitary extramedullary plasmacytoma

Of SEPs, 90% occur in the head and neck, especially the upper respiratory tract, and produce local compressive symptoms. PET-CT may be helpful in staging for regional node involvement, which occurs in up to 50% of SEPs in the head and neck. MRI is important for the assessment of tumour extent and can help in radiotherapy planning.

Management

- Surgery can give high rates of local control, but complete excision may be difficult to achieve depending on the site of the tumour.
- Radiotherapy is the primary treatment of choice, giving 5-year local control rates of 88–100%, but there are no prospective study data to determine the optimal treatment field and dose.
- A retrospective single institution analysis of 67 consecutive patients who received radiotherapy (median dose 50 Gy) for EMP of the head and neck reported 5- and 10-year local control rates of 95% and 87%, respectively. The 5- and 10-year disease-free survival rates were 56% and 54%, respectively (Sasaki *et al.*, 2012). The optimal dose of radiotherapy is considered to be between 45 and 50 Gy. A report of 17 patients found that doses of 45 Gy or greater were associated with 5-year local control rates of 100% compared with 90% for doses of 40 Gy and greater, and 40% for doses below 40 Gy (Tournier-Rangeard *et al.*, 2006).
- The primary tumour should be encompassed with a margin of at least 2 cm, and involved nodes included. The role of elective nodal irradiation is unclear. Only one of 51 patients who received radiotherapy to the tumour alone recurred in regional lymph nodes; there were no regional nodal recurrences seen in 16 patients who received radiotherapy to the primary tumour and regional nodes (Sasaki *et al.*, 2012).
- The role of adjuvant chemotherapy is uncertain, but it may be considered in patients with high-grade extramedullary tumours, or for tumours larger than 5 cm.
- Recommendation: solitary bone or extramedullary plasmacytoma: 40–50 Gy in 1.8–2.0 Gy fractions, depending on site and size.

Stem cell transplantation in lymphoma

Allogeneic stem cell transplantation (SCT) has the advantage of using a tumour cell-free graft, and can result in a significant graft-versus-lymphoma effect. This can produce long-term remissions, even equating to a cure for some patients. Conditioning regimens may be myeloablative or reduced-intensity (RIC). RIC can be as effective as myeloablative regimens in terms of stable hematopoietic engraftment and remission induction but with significantly less toxicity, making it a feasible option for a larger number of patients. Patients who relapse after allogeneic SCT may be successfully treated with donor lymphocyte infusions due to the graft-versus-lymphoma effect.

Total-body irradiation

Total body irradiation (TBI) is usually combined with chemotherapy as conditioning before SCT. The purpose is to eradicate tumour cells, particularly from sanctuary sites, and to ablate the bone marrow before engraftment of transplanted stem cells. Cyclophosphamide plus TBI (CyTBI) and busulfan plus cyclophosphamide (BuCy) are both commonly used conditioning regimens before allogeneic SCT.

Standard TBI technique

The target volume is the entire body, treated within a single field at an extended source–skin distance (SSD; usually 4 m). Set-up techniques vary considerably, but important considerations are dose homogeneity, accurate delivery, reproducibility, ease of set-up and local constraints on field and room size. Thermoluminescent dosimeters are placed at set locations on both sides of the body to calculate the dose received. Doses vary along the body contour, and compensators are required. The dose-limiting toxicities are interstitial pneumonitis and hepatic veno-occlusive disease, which are more common with single-fraction regimens. Most parts of the body will receive within 10% of the dose delivered at the mid-plane.

Helical tomotherapy is a feasible approach for a more conformal form of TBI with the potential to reduce the dose to organs at risk, and possibly allow for dose escalation. However, the clinical data are still limited, with only small numbers of patients treated to date.

The standard dose regimen is 14.4 Gy in 8 fractions over 4 days, with a minimum 6-hour interval between fractions. In reduced intensity allogeneic SCT, a single 2 Gy fraction may be used.

Acute side effects include fatigue, nausea, mucositis, parotitis and diarrhoea. Late effects additional to those caused by chemotherapy include hypothyroidism, interstitial pulmonary fibrosis and cataracts. Secondary cancers, infections and organ dysfunction can cause late deaths, and there are international guidelines for screening and health improvement initiatives in survivors (Majhail et al., 2012).

Radiotherapy techniques in lymphoma

Three different techniques can be used:
- involved node radiotherapy (INRT),
- involved site radiotherapy (ISRT), and
- involved field radiotherapy (IFRT).

They are described in more detail below.

Involved node radiotherapy (INRT)

This concept was first proposed by the EORTC group (Girinsky et al., 2006), and aims to treat only the initial involved node as the CTV. Following a complete response to chemotherapy, the CTV outlined encompasses the pre-chemotherapy extent of the disease without a margin, and respects anatomical boundaries. If there is a residual lymph node remnant, this is contoured and forms the GTV. A boost to the GTV may be considered. INRT requires good-quality pretreatment imaging, ideally in the radiotherapy position, and contrast-enhanced planning scans. The CTV to PTV margin will vary, but 1 cm is considered acceptable. If initially involved nodes are more than 5 cm apart, separate fields are recommended. However, different study groups use the term INRT variably and the conditions required for accurate delineation and delivery are hard to achieve in practice. This was acknowledged in a follow-up publication (Girinsky et al., 2008), and led to the development of the ISRT concept which takes these factors into account (Hoskin et al., 2013b).

Involved site radiotherapy (ISRT)

The aim of ISRT is to include initially involved nodes, and differs from INRT by incorporating a safety margin, but unlike IFRT does not include uninvolved nodes in the whole lymphatic region (Specht et al.,

2014; Illidge *et al.*, 2014). If the extent of initial involvement is uncertain, the default should be to use IFRT. A 3D conformal technique is recommended, although in some cases, an AP/PA arrangement may be preferable to reduce doses to normal tissues.

GTV

This refers to a visible residual mass, but does not apply where there has been a complete radiological response.

CTV

In the axial dimension this includes the pretreatment extent adapted to anatomical boundaries, including GTV where required, while in the cranio-caudal dimension it includes the extent of pretreatment disease with a 1.5-cm safety margin. CTV to PTV margins are as defined locally.

Involved field radiotherapy (IFRT)

IFRT refers to irradiation of the entire lymph node regions initially involved with lymphoma as defined in the Ann Arbor staging system. However, definitions for IFRT vary and were based on anatomical field borders used in conventional simulator planning (Yahalom and Mauch, 2002). Extrapolation of these boundaries to volumes defined on 3D planning CT scans may increase the size of the radiotherapy field. The volume of irradiated normal tissue can be reduced in the mediastinum and para-aortic regions, where the post-chemotherapy volume is treated with lateral margins of 1.0–1.5 cm. These field definitions offer guidance only; review of staging and post-treatment contrast-enhanced CT and PET-CT is required. Where possible, involved lymph node regions are irradiated within a single field.

Target delineation

Standard 3D conformal planning using contrast-enhanced planning CT is recommended, although in some cases, AP/PA fields may help to reduce doses to normal tissues, e.g. breast tissue in young women.

Neck

To treat ipsilateral cervical and supraclavicular nodes:
Superior border: tip of mastoid process.
Inferior border: 1 cm below the head of the clavicle.
Lateral border: junction of the medial 2/3 and outer 1/3 of the clavicle.
Medial border: ipsilateral edge of the spinal canal, with half beam block if appropriate.

Supraclavicular fossa

To treat ipsilateral supraclavicular and lower cervical nodes:
Superior border: hyoid.
Inferior border: 1 cm below the head of the clavicle.
Lung apices should be shielded if possible.

Waldeyer's ring

To treat all the lymphoid tissue of the nasopharynx, tonsils and base of tongue:
The whole oropharynx should be outlined including the submental, bilateral submandibular, pre-auricular, nuchal and upper cervical nodes.
IMRT may allow sparing of the superficial parotid glands.

Axilla

Superior border: above the clavicle (covering the axillary vessels).
Inferior border: 2 cm below the lowest axillary node.
Medial border: include head of clavicle.
Lateral border: to include axillary space.
The lung apex and the acromio-clavicular joint should be shielded if possible.

Mediastinum

Superior border: upper margin of the first rib or hyoid if supraclavicular nodes are involved.
Lateral superior border: junction of the medial 2/3 and outer 1/3 of the clavicle.
Lateral inferior border: 1 cm from mediastinal contours, including the hilae.
Inferior border: 3 cm below any nodal involvement or the carina, whichever is lower.

Para-aortic nodes

Superior border: T10/11 junction or 2 cm above the pre-chemotherapy volume.
Inferior border: L4/5 junction or 2 cm below the pre-chemotherapy volume.
Lateral border: edge of the transverse processes and 1.5 cm from post-chemotherapy volume.

Spleen

Include spleen and splenic hilum.
The whole spleen is outlined as the CTV with a PTV margin of 1.5 cm axially and 2–2.5 cm sup-inf.

Iliac

Ipsilateral iliac and pelvic nodes.

Superior border: L4/5 interspace and 3 cm above involved nodes.

Inferior border: inferior edge of the obturator foramen.

Lateral border: 2 cm around post-chemotherapy volume.

Inguinal/femoral

Ipsilateral inguinal, femoral and external iliac nodes.

Superior border: middle of the sacro-iliac joint.

Inferior border: 5 cm below the lesser trochanter or 2 cm below nodes.

Lateral border: greater trochanter or 2 cm lateral to initially involved nodes.

Medial border: medial edge of the obturator foramen or 2 cm medial to involved nodes.

Extranodal sites

There are published guidelines for treating extranodal sites (Yahalom et al., 2015).

Maxillary antrum: CTV – whole ipsilateral antrum, or 1 cm beyond soft tissue extension outside the antrum

Bone involvement: Treat the involved site with margins of 2 cm.

Skin: This will depend on the histology and treatment intent, and GTV to CTV margin may vary from 1–2 cm (Specht et al., 2015).

Doses may range from 24 Gy for radical treatment of localised cutaneous lymphoma (FL or marginal zone lymphoma, or cutaneous CD30+ lymphoproliferative lesions), to 4 Gy for palliation or where there are multiple lesions (Hoskin et al., 2013a).

Late complications of radiotherapy for lymphoma

Subclinical hypothyroidism develops in about a third of patients who have irradiation to the bilateral neck, and annual thyroid function monitoring is needed. The development of subfertility impairment and hormonal failure depends on the sites irradiated and is made worse by the use of alkylating chemotherapy, particularly high-dose chemotherapy. Mediastinal irradiation increases the risk of coronary artery disease and valvular abnormalities, and when combined with anthracyclines, increases the risk of cardiac failure. Patients should be warned about additional risk factors such as smoking, hyperlipidaemia and hypertension. Second malignancies include myelodysplasia, leukaemia, NHL and solid tumours, particularly of the breast, thyroid and lung. It is clear that the risk of breast cancer is inversely related to age at treatment, and directly related to increasing dose.

The risk is relatively high for patients under the age of 25 years treated with supradiaphragmatic radiotherapy for HL, particularly with mantle fields (Swerdlow et al., 2012). The current strategy of using smaller field sizes and lower radiation doses should reduce this risk without compromising survival. Current guidelines recommend screening women who were treated for HL under the age of 36 years, starting 8 years after radiotherapy, using either mammography or MRI, depending on the patient's age and breast density.

References

Ardeshna, K. M., Smith, P., Qian, W., et al. (2010). An Intergroup randomised trial of rituximab versus a watch and wait strategy in patients with Stage II, III, IV, asymptomatic, non-bulky gollicular lymphoma (Grades 1, 2 and 3a). A Preliminary Analysis. *ASH Annual Meeting Abstracts*, available at https://ash.confex.com/ash/2010/webprogram/Paper27692.html (accessed December 2014).

Benton, E. C., Crichton, S., Talpur, R., et al. (2013). A cutaneous lymphoma international prognostic index (CLIPi) for mycosis fungoides and Sezary syndrome. *Eur. J.Cancer*, **49**, 2859–2868.

Bird, J. M., Owen, R. G., D'Sa, S.,et al. (2011). Guidelines for the diagnosis and management of multiple myeloma 2011. *Br. J. Haematol.*, **154**, 32–75.

Chen, R. C., Chin, M. S. Ng, A. K., et al. (2010). Early-stage, lymphocyte-predominant Hodgkin's lymphoma: patient outcomes from a large, single-institution series with long follow-up. *J. Clin. Oncol.*, **28**, 136–141.

Cheson, B. D., Fisher, R. I., Barrington, S. F., et al. (2014). Recommendations for initial evaluation, staging and response assessment of Hodgkin and non-Hodgkin lymphoma: the Lugano Classification. *J. Clin. Oncol.* **32**, 3059–3068.

Cunningham, D., Hawkes, E. A., Jack, A., et al. (2013). Rituximab plus cyclophosphamide, doxorubicin, vincristine, and prednisolone in patients with newly diagnosed diffuse large B-cell non-Hodgkin lymphoma: a phase 3 comparison of dose intensification with 14-day versus 21-day cycles. *Lancet*, **381**, 1817–1826.

Dearden, C. E., Johnson, R., Pettengell, R., et al. (2011). Guidelines for the management of mature T-cell and NK-cell neoplasms (excluding cutaneous T-cell lymphoma). *Br. J. Haematol.*, **153**, 451–485.

Dunleavy, K., Pittaluga, S., MaedaL, S., et al. (2013). Dose-adjusted EPOCH-rituximab therapy in primary mediastinal B-cell lymphoma. *N. Engl. J. Med.*, **368**, 1408–16.

Eich, H. T., Diehl, V., Görgen, H., et al. (2010). Intensified chemotherapy and dose-reduced involved-field radiotherapy in patients with early unfavorable Hodgkin's lymphoma: final analysis of the German Hodgkin Study Group HD11 Trial. *J. Clin. Oncol.*, **28**, 4199–4206.

Eichenauer, D., Plutschow, A., Fuchs, M., *et al.* (2015). Long-term course of patients with Stage IA nodular lymphocyte-predominant Hodgkin lymphoma: a report from the German Hodgkin Study Group *J. Clin. Oncol.*, DOI: 10.1200/JCO.2014.60.4363.

El-Galaly, T. C., d'Amore, F., Mylam, K. J., *et al.* (2012). Routine bone marrow biopsy has little or no therapeutic consequence for positron emission tomography/ computed tomography-staged treatment-naive patients with Hodgkin lymphoma. *J. Clin. Oncol.*, **30**, 4508–4514.

Engert, A., Plütschow, A., Eich, H. T., *et al.* (2010). Reduced treatment intensity in patients with early-stage Hodgkin's lymphoma. *N. Engl. J. Med.*, **363**, 640–652.

Federico, M., Bellei, M., Marcheselli, L., *et al.* (2009). Follicular Lymphoma International Prognostic Index 2: a new prognostic index for follicular lymphoma developed by the International Follicular Lymphoma Prognostic Factor Project. *J. Clin. Oncol.*, **27**, 4555–4562.

Ferreri, A. J., Cwynarski, K., Pulczynski, E., *et al.* (2015). Addition of thiotepa and rituximab to antimetabolites significantly improves outcomes in primary CNS lymphoma: first randomization of the IELSG32 trial. *Haematol. Oncol.*, **33**, Supplement S1:1-20, abstract 009.

Ferreri, A. J., Reni, M., Foppoli, M., *et al.* (2009). High-dose cytarabine plus high-dose methotrexate versus high-dose methotrexate alone in patients with primary CNS lymphoma: a randomised phase 2 trial. *Lancet*, **374**, 1512–1520.

Feugier, P., Van Hoof, A., Sebban, C., *et al.* (2005). Long-term results of the R-CHOP study in the treatment of elderly patients with diffuse large B-Cell lymphoma: a study by the Groupe d'Etude des Lymphomes de l'Adulte. *J. Clin. Oncol.*, **23**, 4117–4126.

Gallamini, A., Hutchings, M., Rigacci, L., *et al.* (2007). Early interim 2-[18F]fluoro-2-deoxy-D-glucose positron emission tomography is prognostically superior to international prognostic score in advanced-stage Hodgkin's lymphoma: a report from a joint Italian-Danish study. *J. Clin. Oncol.*, **25**, 3746–3752.

Girinsky, T., van der Maazen, R. and Specht, L. (2006). Involved-node radiotherapy (INRT) in patients with early Hodgkin lymphoma: concepts and guidelines. *Radiother. Oncol.*, **79**, 270–277.

Girinsky, T., Specht, L., Ghalibafian, M., *et al.* (2008). The conundrum of Hodgkin lymphoma nodes: to be or not to be included in the involved node radiation fields. The EORTC-GELA lymphoma group guidelines. *Radiother. Oncol.*, **88**, 202–210.

Gisselbrecht, C., Glass, B., Mounier, N., *et al.* (2010). Salvage regimens with autologous transplantation for relapsed large B-Cell lymphoma in the rituximab era. *J. Clin. Oncol.*, **28**, 4184–4190.

Goda, J. S., Gospodarowicz, M., Pintilie, M., *et al.* (2010). Long-term outcome in localized extranodal mucosa-associated lymphoid tissue lymphomas treated with radiotherapy. *Cancer*, **116**, 3815–3824.

Greipp, P. R., Miguel, J. S., Durie, B. G. M., *et al.* (2005). International staging system for multiple myeloma. *J. Clin. Oncol.*, **23**, 3412–3420.

Guadagnolo, B., Li, S., Neuberg, D., *et al.* (2006). Long-term outcome and mortality trends in early-stage, Grade 1–2 follicular lymphoma treated with radiation therapy. *Int. J. Radiat. Oncol. Biol. Phys.*, **64**, 928–934.

Hasenclever, D., Diehl, V., Armitage, J. O., *et al.* (1998). A prognostic score for advanced Hodgkin's disease. International Prognostic Factors Project on Advanced Hodgkin's Disease. *N. Engl. J. Med.*, **339**, 1506–1514.

Held, G., Murawski, N., Ziepert, M., *et al.* (2014). Role of radiotherapy to bulky disease in elderly patients with aggressive B-Cell lymphoma. *J. Clin. Oncol.*, **32**, 1112–1118.

Hodgson, D. C., Dieckmann, K., Terezakis, S., *et al.* (2014). Implementation of contemporary radiation therapy planning concepts for pediatric Hodgkin lymphoma: guidelines from the International Lymphoma Radiation Oncology Group. *Pract. Radiat. Oncol.*, **5**, 85–92.

Horning, S. J., Weller, E., Kim, K., *et al.* (2004). Chemotherapy with or without radiotherapy in limited-stage diffuse aggressive non-Hodgkin's lymphoma: Eastern Cooperative Oncology Group Study 1484. *J. Clin. Oncol.*, **22**, 3032–3038.

Hoskin, P., Kirkwood, A., Popova, B., *et al.* (2013a). FoRT: a phase 3 multi-center prospective randomized trial of low dose radiation therapy for follicular and marginal zone lymphoma. *Int. J. Radiat. Oncol. Biol. Phys.*, **85**, 22.

Hoskin, P. J., Diez, P., Williams, M., *et al.* (2013b). Recommendations for the use of radiotherapy in nodal lymphoma. *Clin. Oncol. (R. Coll. Radiol.)*, **25**, 49–58.

Hutchings, M., Loft, A., Hansen, M., *et al.* (2006). FDG-PET after two cycles of chemotherapy predicts treatment failure and progression-free survival in Hodgkin lymphoma. *Blood*, **107**, 52–59.

Illidge, T., Specht, L., Yahalom, J., *et al.* (2014). Modern radiation therapy for nodal non-Hodgkin lymphoma-target definition and dose guidelines from the International Lymphoma Radiation Oncology Group. *Int. J. Radiat. Oncol. Biol .Phys.*, **89**, 49–58.

Jiang, M., Zhang, H., Jiang, Y., *et al.* (2012). Phase 2 trial of 'sandwich' L-asparaginase, vincristine, and prednisone chemotherapy with radiotherapy in newly diagnosed, stage IE to IIE, nasal type, extranodal natural killer/T-cell lymphoma. *Cancer*, **118**, 3294–3301.

Khan, A. B., Barrington, S. F., Mikhaeel, N. G., *et al.* (2013). PET-CT staging of DLBCL accurately identifies and provides new insight into the clinical significance of bone marrow involvement. *Blood*, **122**, 61–67.

Knobel, D., Zouhair, A., Tsang, R. W., *et al.* (2006). Prognostic factors in solitary plasmacytoma of the bone: a multicenter Rare Cancer Network study. *B. M. C. Cancer*, **6**, 118.

Lister, T. A., Crowther, D., Sutcliffe, S. B., *et al.* (1989). Report of a commettee convened to discuss the evaluation and staging of patients with Hodgkin's disease: Cotswold meeting. *J. Clin. Oncol.*, **7**, 1630–1636.

Lowry, L., Smith, P., Qian, W., *et al.* (2011). Reduced dose radiotherapy for local control in non-Hodgkin lymphoma: a randomised phase III trial. *Radiother. Oncol.*, **100**, doi: 10.1016/j.radonc.2011.05.013. Epub 2011 Jun 12.

Majhail, N. S., Rizzo, J. D., Lee, S. J., *et al.* (2012). Recommended screening and preventive practices for long-term survivors after hematopoietic cell transplantation. *Bone Marrow Transpl.*, **47**, 337–341.

Marcus, R., Imrie, K. and Solal-Celigny, P. (2008). Phase III study of R-CVP compared with cyclophosphamide, vincristine, and prednisone alone in patients with previously untreated advanced follicular lymphoma. *J. Clin. Oncol.*, **26**, 4579–4586.

McKay, P., Leach, M., Jackson, R., *et al.* (2012). Guidelines for the investigation and management of mantle cell lymphoma. *Br. J. Haematol.*, **159**, 405–426.

McMillan, A., Ardeshna, K. M., Cwynarski, K., *et al.* (2013). Guideline on the prevention of secondary central nervous system lymphoma: British Committee for Standards in Haematology. *Br. J. Haematol.*, **163**, 168–181.

McNamara, C., Davies, J., Dyer, M., *et al.* (2011). Guidelines on the investigation and management of follicular lymphoma. *Br. J. Haematol.*, **156**, 446–467.

Meignan, M., Barrington, S., Itti, E., *et al.* (2014). Report on the 4th International Workshop on Positron Emission Tomography in Lymphoma held in Menton, France, 3–5 October 2012. *Leuk. Lymphoma*, **55**, 31–37.

Meyer, R. M., Gospodarowicz, M. K., Connors, J. M., *et al.* (2005). Randomized comparison of ABVD chemotherapy with a strategy that includes radiation therapy in patients with limited-stage Hodgkin's lymphoma: National Cancer Institute of Canada Clinical Trials Group and the Eastern Cooperative Oncology Group. *J. Clin. Oncol.*, **23**, 4634–4642.

Miller, T. P., Dahlberg, S., Cassady, J. R., *et al.* (1998). Chemotherapy alone compared with chemotherapy plus radiotherapy for localized intermediate- and high-grade non-Hodgkin's lymphoma. *N. Engl. J. Med.*, **339**, 21–26.

Morgan, G. J., Davies, F. E., Gregory, W. M., *et al.* (2010). First-line treatment with zoledronic acid as compared with clodronic acid in multiple myeloma (MRC Myeloma IX): a randomised controlled trial. *Lancet*, **376**, 1989–1999.

Morgan, G. J., Davies, F. E., Gregory, W. M., *et al.* (2011). Cyclophosphamide, thalidomide, and dexamethasone (CTD) as initial therapy for patients with multiple myeloma unsuitable for autologous transplantation. *Blood*, **118**, 1231–1238.

Morris, P., Correa, D., Yahalom, J., *et al.*, (2013). Rituximab, methotrexate, procarbazine, and vincristine followed by consolidation reduced-dose whole-brain radiotherapy and cytarabine in newly diagnosed primary CNS lymphoma: final results and long-term outcome. *J. Clin. Oncol.*, **31**, 3971–3979.

Morris, S. L. (2012). Skin lymphoma. *Clin. Oncol. (R. Coll. Radiol.)*, **24**, 371–385.

Morris, S. L., McGovern, M., Bayne, S., *et al.* (2013). Results of a 5-week schedule of modern total skin electron beam radiation therapy. *Int. J. Radiat. Oncol. Biol. Phys.*, **86**, 936–941.

Moskowitz, C. H., Matasar, M. J., Zelenetz, A. D., *et al.* (2012). Normalization of pre-ASCT, FDG-PET imaging with second-line, non–cross-resistant, chemotherapy programs improves event-free survival in patients with Hodgkin lymphoma. *Blood*, **119**, 1665–1670.

NICE. (2011). *Referral Guidelines for Suspected Cancer. NICE Clinical Guideline 27. Issued June 2005, last modified April 2011.* London: National Institute for Health and Care Excellence.

Nogová, L., Rudiger, T. and Engert. A. (2006). Biology, clinical course and management of nodular lymphocyte-predominant Hodgkin lymphoma. *Hematology*, **2006**, 266–272.

Pfreundschuh, M., Kuhnt, E., Trümper, L., *et al.* (2011). CHOP-like chemotherapy with or without rituximab in young patients with good-prognosis diffuse large-B-cell lymphoma: 6-year results of an open-label randomised study of the MabThera International Trial (MInT) Group. *Lancet Oncol.*, **12**, 1013–1022.

Philip, T., Guglielmi, C., Hagenbeed, A., *et al.* (1995). Autologous bone marrow transplantation as compared with salvage chemotherapy in relapses of chemotherapy-sensitive non-Hodgkin's lymphoma. *N. Engl. J. Med.* **333**, 1540–1545.

Pugh, T. J., Ballonoff, A., Newman, F., *et al.* (2010). Improved survival in patients with early stage low-grade follicular lymphoma treated with radiation. *Cancer*, **116**, 3843–3851.

Radford, J., Illidge, T., Counsell, N., *et al.* (2015). Results of a trial of PET-directed therapy for early-stage Hodgkin's lymphoma. *N. Engl. J. Med.*, **372**, 1598–1607.

Roman, E. and Smith, A. G. (2011). Epidemiology of lymphomas. *Histopathology*, **58**, 4–14.

Rummel, M. J., Niederle, N., Maschmeyer, G., *et al.* (2013). Bendamustine plus rituximab versus CHOP plus rituximab as first-line treatment for patients with indolent and mantle-cell lymphomas: an open-label, multicentre, randomised, phase 3 non-inferiority trial. *Lancet*, **381**, 1203–1210.

Safar, V., Dupuis, J., Itti, E., *et al.* (2012). Interim [18F] fluorodeoxyglucose positron emission tomography scan in diffuse large B-Cell lymphoma treated with anthracycline-based chemotherapy plus rituximab. *J. Clin. Oncol.*, **30**, 184–190.

Salles, G., Seymour, J. F., Offner, F., *et al.* (2011). Rituximab maintenance for 2 years in patients with high tumour burden follicular lymphoma responding to rituximab plus chemotherapy (PRIMA): a phase 3, randomised controlled trial. *Lancet*, **377**, 42–51.

Sasaki, R., Yasuda, K., Abe, E., *et al.* (2012). Multi-institutional analysis of solitary extramedullary plasmacytoma of the head and neck treated with curative radiotherapy. *Int. J. Radiat. Oncol. Biol. Phys.*, **82**, 626–634.

Scarisbrick, J. J., Morris, S., Azurdia, R., *et al.* (2013). U.K. consensus statement on safe clinical prescribing of bexarotene for patients with cutaneous T-cell lymphoma. *Br. J. Dermatol.*, **168**, 192–200.

Shipp, M. A. (1993). A predictive model for aggressive non-Hodgkin's lymphoma. *N. Engl. J. Med.*, **329**, 987–994.

Solal-Céligny, P., Roy, P., Colombat, P., *et al.* (2004). Follicular Lymphoma International Prognostic Index. *Blood*, **104**, 1258–1265.

Somers, R., Burgers, J. M., Qasim, M., *et al.* (1987). EORTC trial non-Hodgkin lymphomas. *Eur. J. Cancer Clin. Oncol.*, **23**, 283–293.

Soutar, R., Lucraft, H., Jackson, G., *et al.* (2004). Guidelines on the diagnosis and management of solitary plasmacytoma of bone and solitary extramedullary plasmacytoma. *Clin. Oncol. (R. Coll. Radiol.)*, **16**, 405–413.

Specht, L., Dabaja, B., Illidge, T., *et al.* (2015). Modern radiation therapy for primary cutaneous lymphomas: field and dose guidelines from the International Lymphoma Radiation Oncology Group. *Int. J. Radiat. Oncol. Biol. Phys.*, **92**, 32–39.

Specht, L., Yahalom, J., Illidge, T., *et al.* (2014). Modern radiation therapy for Hodgkin lymphoma: field and dose guidelines from the International Lymphoma Radiation Oncology Group (ILROG). *Int. J. Radiat. Oncol. Biol. Phys.*, **89**, 954–962.

Stiff, P. J., Unger, J. M., Cook, J. R., *et al.* (2013). Autologous transplantation as consolidation for aggressive non-Hodgkin's lymphoma. *N. Engl. J. Med.*, **369**, 1681–1690.

Swerdlow, A. J., Cooke, R., Bates, A., *et al.* (2012). Breast cancer risk after supradiaphragmatic radiotherapy for Hodgkin's lymphoma in England and Wales: a National Cohort Study. *J. Clin. Oncol.*, **30**, 2745–2752.

Swerdlow, S. H., Campo, E., Harris, N. L., *et al.* (2008). *WHO Classification of Tumour of Haematopoietic and Lymphoid Tissues*. Lyon: IARC Press.

Thomas, J., Ferme, C., Noordijk, E., *et al.* (2004). Six cycles of EBVP followed by 36 Gy involved-field irradiation vs. no irradiation in favourable supradiaphragmatic clinical stages I–II Hodgkin's lymphoma: the EORTC-GELA strategy in 771 patients. *Eur. J. Haematol.*, **73**(Suppl. 64), Abstr. 40.

Tournier-Rangeard, L., Lapeyre, M., Graff-Caillaud, P., *et al.* (2006). Radiotherapy for solitary extramedullary plasmacytoma in the head-and-neck region: a dose greater than 45 Gy to the target volume improves the local control. *Int. J. Radiat. Oncol. Biol. Phys.*, **64**, 1013–1017.

Tsang, R. W., Gospodarowicz, M. K., Pintilie, M., *et al.* (2001). Solitary plasmacytoma treated with radiotherapy: impact of tumor size on outcome. *Int. J. Radiat. Oncol. Biol. Phys.*, **50**, 113–120.

Tse, E. and Kwong, Y. L. (2013). How I treat NK/T-cell lymphomas. *Blood*, **121**, 4997–5005.

Vitolo, U., Chiappella, A., Ferreri, A. J. M., *et al.* (2011). First-line treatment for primary testicular diffuse large B-cell lymphoma with rituximab-CHOP, CNS prophylaxis, and contralateral testis irradiation: final results of an international phase II trial. *J. Clin. Oncol.*, **29**, 2766–2772.

von Tresckow, B., Plütschow, A., Fuchs, M., *et al.* (2012). Dose-intensification in early unfavorable Hodgkin's lymphoma: final analysis of the German Hodgkin Study Group HD14 Trial. *J. Clin. Oncol.*, **30**, 907–913.

Willemze, R., Hodak, E., Zinzani, P. L., *et al.* (2013). Primary cutaneous lymphomas: ESMO Clinical Practice Guidelines for diagnosis, treatment and follow-up. *Ann. Oncol.*, **24**(Suppl. 6), vi149–vi154.

Yahalom, J., Illidge, T., Specht, L., *et al.* (2015). Modern radiation therapy for extranodal lymphomas: field and dose guidelines from the International Lymphoma Radiation Oncology Group. *Int. J. Radiat. Oncol. Biol. Phys.*, **92**, 11–31.

Yahalom, J. and Mauch, P. (2002). The involved field is back: issues in delineating the radiation field in Hodgkin's disease. *Ann. Oncol.*, **13**, 79–83.

Younes, A., Gopal, A. K., Smith, S. E., *et al.* (2012). Results of a pivotal phase II study of brentuximab vedotin for patients with relapsed or refractory Hodgkin's lymphoma. *J. Clin. Oncol.*, **30**, 183–189.

Ziepert, M., Hasenclever, D. and Kuhnt, E. (2010). Standard International prognostic index remains a valid predictor of outcome for patients with aggressive CD20+ B-Cell lymphoma in the rituximab era. *J. Clin. Oncol.*, **28**, 2373–2380.

Zucca, E., Conconi, A., Laszlo, D., *et al.* (2013). Addition of rituximab to chlorambucil produces superior event-free survival in the treatment of patients with extranodal marginal-zone B-cell lymphoma: 5-year analysis of the IELSG-19 randomized study. *J. Clin. Oncol.*, **31**, 565–572.

Chapter

35

Management of cancers of the central nervous system

Sean Elyan

Introduction

This chapter describes the management of tumours in adults in the following anatomical areas: cerebral convexity and cerebral hemispheres, the skull base, the pituitary, the pineal region and the spinal cord.

Central nervous system (CNS) tumours are heterogeneous. The terms malignant and benign are not very useful because:

- even small slowly growing tumours can cause severe symptoms because the brain is enclosed in a rigid skull;
- surgery can be difficult because many tumours are infiltrating and often lie close to critical structures;
- most of these tumours rarely, if ever, metastasise outside the CNS;
- slow-growing tumours may transform into a much more aggressive variant.

This chapter does not deal with metastatic disease to the CNS that is considered in other relevant chapters, although management of cerebral metastases that require specialist neuro-oncology input is discussed briefly. CNS tumours in children are considered in Chapter 40.

Anatomy

The tentorium separates the supratentorial from the infratentorial areas of the brain. The motor and sensory cortices lie at the central sulcus. Broca's area (frontal above the lateral sulcus) is responsible for expressive speech, and Wernicke's area (temporal, posterior end of the lateral sulcus) is responsible for receptive speech. The ventricular system is lined with ependymal cells. CSF travels from the third to the fourth ventricle through the cerebral aqueduct and from the fourth ventricle to the subarachnoid space through the foramina of Magendie (median) and Luschka (lateral).

The anterior and intermediate lobes of the pituitary arise from Rathke's pouch. The cavernous sinuses transmit cranial nerves IIV, IV, VI and the maxillary branch of V.

Incidence and epidemiology

Primary brain and CNS tumours are fairly common. The incidence of disease is approximately 15 in 100,000 per annum. In 2011, 9365 primary tumours of the brain and CNS were registered in the United Kingdom, where brain tumours account for 3% of all cancers. Approximately 5000 deaths occur per year in the UK that are attributable to primary brain and CNS tumours. (http://www.cancerresearchuk.org/cancer-info/cancerstats/, accessed October 2014). On an average, GPs in England see one patient with a brain tumour every 7 years.

For high-grade brain tumours the peak disease incidence occurs in the 70–80-year-old age group. There has been an increase in recent years, probably because of increased investigation.

There may be a significant under-registration of intracranial tumours: perhaps as many as half are not being recorded in cancer registries (Pobereskin and Chadduck, 2000).

Risk factors and aetiology

The risk of developing a primary CNS tumour is related to increasing age, male gender and higher socio-economic status. There is, in general, a lower incidence in less developed countries.

The acquired immune deficiency syndrome (AIDS) is a well-recognised cause of cerebral lymphoma (Beral et al., 1991). The only other certain causative factors are inherited cancer syndromes and ionising radiation. A number of familial autosomal dominant syndromes

Practical Clinical Oncology, Second Edition, ed. Louise Hanna, Tom Crosby and Fergus Macbeth. Published by Cambridge University Press. © Cambridge University Press 2015.

Table 35.1 Inherited syndromes and their associated tumours

Syndrome	Nervous system effects	Chromosome involved
Neurofibromatosis type 1	Neurofibromas, malignant nerve sheet tumours, optic nerve gliomas, astrocytomas	17q12-22
Neurofibromatosis type 2	Bilateral acoustic schwannomas, multiple meningiomas, astrocytomas, glial hamartomas	22q
Von Hippel–Lindau syndrome	Haemangioblastomas	3p13-14, 3p25-26
Tuberous sclerosis	Subependymal giant cell astrocytoma	9q32-34, 11q
Li–Frameni	Astrocytomas/PNET	17p (p53)
Cowden's disease	Dysplastic gangliocytoma of the cerebellum	10q22–23
Turcot's syndrome	Medulloblastoma, glioblastoma	5q
Naevoid basel cell carcinoma syndrome (Gorlin syndrome)	Medulloblastoma	1q22, 9q31

PNET, primitive neuroectodemal tumour.

give rise to an increased rise of CNS tumours, which include neurofibromatosis types 1 (incidence 1 in 3000) and 2 (1 in 40), von Hippel–Lindau syndrome, tuberous sclerosis, Li–Fraumeni syndrome Cowden's disease, Turcot's syndrome and naevoid basal cell carcinoma (Gorlin) syndrome.

Table 35.1 summarises these syndromes and associated tumours.

Pathology

For some patients a tissue diagnosis is not possible. As a result, unlike most other tumour groups, the final diagnosis may depend on the results of imaging rather than a biopsy.

The classification of CNS tumours is complex. The World Health Organisation (WHO) produced a clarification in 1993, most recently updated in 2007 (Louis *et al.*, 2007), which is now widely used (Table 35.2).

The term 'high-grade' includes III and IV and 'low-grade' includes grade I and II tumours. The terms 'benign' and malignant' are best avoided.

- WHO grade I includes tumours with low proliferative potential, frequently discrete and with the possibility of a cure following surgical resection alone.
- WHO grade II includes tumours that are generally infiltrating and have few mitoses, but that can recur. Some tumour types may progress to higher grades of malignancy.
- WHO grade III includes tumours with histological evidence of malignancy, generally in the form

Table 35.2 The WHO classification of CNS tumours

Type	Examples
Neuroepithelial tumours	Gliomas Astrocytoma Oligodendroglioma Ependymoma Neuronal and mixed neuronal–glial tumours Gangliocytoma Paraganglionoma Nonglial tumours Pineal parenchymal tumour
Meningeal tumours	Meningioma
Germ cell tumours	Germinoma Teratoma
Tumours of sellar region	Pituitary adenoma Craniopharyngioma
Primary CNS lymphoma	
Tumours of peripheral nerves that affect the CNS	Schwannoma
Metastatic tumours	

Adapted from Louis *et al.*, 2007.

of mitotic activity, clear signs of infiltration and anaplasia.

- WHO grade IV includes tumours that are mitotically active, necrosis-prone, and generally associated with a rapid pre- and postoperative growth.

The majority of pituitary tumours (95%) are adenomas. The remainder include craniopharyngiomas, Rathke's cleft cysts and meningiomas.

There is a wide variety of tumours of the base of the skull, ranging from slow-growing to very malignant. The most common tumour occurring at this site is the schwannoma, a low-grade and usually slow-growing tumour that arises from the acoustic nerve.

Tumours involving the pineal gland are very unusual. There are three main histological types: germ-cell tumours (GCTs), astrocytomas and pineal parenchymal tumours which include pineocytomas and pineoblastomas.

In this chapter, tumours are divided by their anatomical site and subdivided using the WHO histopathological classification.

Molecular markers in neuro-oncology

The histological classification of primary brain tumours remains the mainstay of pathological diagnosis. However, the increasing knowledge and use of molecular diagnostic techniques will undoubtedly have an increasing influence on predicting prognosis and determining treatment. The most widely quoted examples of this are MGMT promoter methylation in glioblastomas particularly in elderly people, and 1p and 19q co-deletions in anaplastic oligodendroglial tumours. MGMT promoter methylation is associated with an improved prognosis because patients are unable to inactivate chemotherapeutic agents such as temozolomide. Co-deletion of 1p and 19q in anaplastic oligodendroglioms is also associated with an improved prognosis.

Other markers such as EGFR expression are not as yet used in routine practice but may become important as their role in predicting prognosis and guiding treatment becomes clearer.

Table 35.3 shows some prognostic biomarkers in CNS tumours.

Spread

Tumours of the CNS rarely metastasise outside the CNS axis. Table 35.4 shows the main modes of spread. Malignant glial tumours typically spread via white matter tracts and knowledge of these routes is important in planning radiotherapy.

Clinical presentation

Patients with primary CNS tumours present with signs and systems attributable to the mass effect of

Table 35.3 Prognostic biomarkers in CNS tumours

Marker	Example
Proliferation index	Ki-67
DNA studies	Flow cytometry
Activation of oncogenes	RAS
Inactivation of suppressor genes	PTEN
Allelic loss	19q
Cytokine dysregulation	EGFR
Chromosomal aberration	Chromosome 19
Other	MGMT methylation

EGFR, epidermal growth factor receptor; Ki-67, marker of proliferation Ki-67; MGMT, O^6 methylguanine-DNA methyltransferase; PTEN, phosphatase and tensin homolog; RAS, rat sarcoma oncogene. Adapted from AJCC, 2010.

Table 35.4 Routes of spread of CNS tumours

Route	Site	Examples
Local invasion	To involve contiguous structures	Gliomas
Local pressure	To compromise local structures	Pituitary adenomas
CSF spread	To ventricles and spine	PCNSL, medulloblastoma, ependymoma
Haematogenous spread (rare)	To lungs, liver, bones	Medulloblastoma

CSF, cerebrospinal fluid; PCNSL, primary central nervous system lymphoma.

the tumour. Patients may initially present to a general practitioner, as an acute medical admission, or through a range of specialties including ophthalmology, neurology and gynaecology.

For intracranial tumours, the main symptoms are headaches, seizures, changes of mental state, unilateral deafness and progressive neurological deficit and hormone dysfunction (particularly for pituitary tumours).

For spinal tumours, the main symptoms are pain and a progressive loss of neurological function.

The finding of new neurological signs together with symptoms is more suggestive of pathology than symptoms alone. New neurological symptoms in patients with a past history of cancer suggest metastatic disease.

Some tumours may cause cognitive, expressive and psychological problems and the patient may not be able to explain his or her symptoms fully. Therefore, it may be very important to get a history from a friend or relative. Many patients need a lot of psychological, social and physical support and, because of the poor prognosis of many CNS tumours, management should be aimed at maximising the patient's quality of life.

General principles of management

- All patients must be discussed at a neurosciences multidisciplinary team (MDT) meeting.
- Early referral to a key worker is essential to ensure coordinated care.
- All patients must have a tissue diagnosis unless deemed unsafe at the specialist MDT.
- No patients should have radical treatment without a histological diagnosis.
- Careful consideration should be given to the balance of active intervention with quality of life.

Investigation and staging

All patients with CNS tumours should have their investigations and management plan coordinated by a neuro-oncology MDT in the forum of a multidisciplinary meeting.

The key investigations include routine blood tests, including HIV status where relevant, imaging, angiography, other laboratory tests and biopsy.

Neuroradiological imaging is used, particularly CT scanning and MRI. Where biopsy would be too risky or in cases where the age or performance status of the patients would preclude biopsy or tumour resection, a presumptive diagnosis of a primary CNS tumour may need to be made on radiological grounds alone.

A CT scan should reliably exclude a tumour in the majority of cases, but may miss early tumours, especially in the temporal lobes and posterior fossa. MRI should be performed as an initial investigation in a patient who has persisting symptoms despite a normal CT scan. MRI also gives useful information for planning surgery and radiotherapy.

Angiography may be useful in planning surgical treatment for some CNS tumours (e.g. spinal tumours).

Other laboratory tests may be performed, such as an assessment of pituitary function, CSF cytology in lymphomas or serum tumour markers of primary GCTs.

Imaging has a high sensitivity for identifying the presence of a tumour but is unreliable in identifying grade and type. Wherever possible, a histopathological specimen should be obtained to classify the tumour, plan appropriate treatment and determine prognosis. Sometimes a diagnosis can be made by cytological examination of the CSF or, for pineal GCTs, simply by finding raised tumour markers.

Tissue can be obtained either by biopsy or tumour resection via one of the following methods.

- Stereotactically guided biopsy.
- Radiologically guided needle biopsy.
- Radiologically guided open biopsy and/or resection.
- Endoscopic biopsy.
- Electrophysiologically guided resection

There should be a preoperative discussion with the neurosurgeon, neuropathologist and neuroradiologist about the best approach to surgery and the processing of tissue specimens.

Intraoperative histopathological diagnosis is particularly valuable during needle biopsy and helps to ensure that enough of the right tissue is obtained. It can also provide information that will influence the course of the operation.

Various other tests include the following.

- Molecular diagnostics tests such as loss of chromosomes 1p and 19q and MGMT expression, which are expected to become more important (Cairncross et al., 1998; Stupp et al., 2005).
- Pituitary function.
- Visual field assessment (pituitary).
- Ophthalmology review (primary CNS lymphoma [PCNSL]).
- Tumour markers (primary GCTs).
- Other imaging techniques, including MR spectroscopy, single photon emission computed tomography (SPECT), and positron emission tomography (PET), which are currently predominantly research tools and are not in day-to-day use.

Certain groups of patients, for example those with neurofibromatosis types 1 and 2, are at particular risk of developing intradural spinal tumours. These patients require monitoring and early resection if the tumours enlarge or cause symptoms.

Patients with skull base tumours also may require the following assessments before treatment.

- Audiological testing.
- Auditory-evoked brain stem responses testing.
- Vestibular testing.
- Prosthetic assessment to establish the need for ocular, aural or skull bone replacement.
- Speech and language therapy assessment and explanation to the patient of likely postoperative impairment.
- Dietetic assessment.

TNM staging for brain tumours has been withdrawn following publication of the fourth edition of the AJCC manual for staging of cancer and does not contribute to the management of most primary CNS tumours. Chang staging does determine treatment protocols in the medulloblastoma.

Treatment of brain tumours

The general principals of treating tumours in the various anatomical sites are described, followed by a detailed discussion of radiotherapy.

Treatment of low-grade glioma (WHO grades I and II)

Low-grade gliomas account for approximately 15% of all adult brain tumours. Up to 40% of low-grade gliomas (LGGs) diagnosed on imaging are found to have high-grade histopathological features and so all patients need to have a confirmed diagnosis unless a biopsy would be too risky for the patient or is otherwise inappropriate.

The options for initial management are either watchful waiting or immediate surgery. The EORTC criteria (Pignatti *et al.*, 2002) can help identify patients who are at an increased risk of rapid deterioration and who may benefit from early intervention. Radiotherapy may be used in the following situations.

- Patients with persisting neurological symptoms and significant residual tumour.
- Patients with regrowth following surgery.
- Patients with evidence of tumour progression from low to high grade.

Radiotherapy improves survival but the benefit is evident, whether it is given initially or on progression (van den Bent *et al.*, 2005).

Chemotherapy with agents such as temozolomide is increasingly being explored as an alternative to radiotherapy. The EORTC 22033–26033 trial recently reported at ASCO showed no survival difference between patients treated with radiotherapy or temozolomide. As the exact role of molecular markers becomes clearer, chemotherapy may become the treatment of choice for some of these patients (Baumert *et al.*, 2013).

Treatment of high-grade glioma (WHO grades III and IV)

High-grade gliomas (HGGs) include glioblastoma, anaplastic astrocytoma, anaplastic oligodendrogliomas and anaplastic ependymomas. The important prognostic factors are age, performance status and comorbidity, tumour type and grade and presence or absence of seizures (Bleehen and Stenning, 1991). Molecular markers can identify some patients with better prognosis particularly in the elderly (Wick *et al.*, 2012).

The principles of treatment are to increase survival while maximising the patient's functional capability and quality of life. It is important to identify patients who need urgent surgery (e.g. emergency decompression or shunt insertion for hydrocephalus) and patients suitable for elective surgery to debulk the tumour. Some patients are unfit for any intervention.

Radical radiotherapy may be considered after a histopathological diagnosis has been confirmed.

Adjuvant chemotherapy has been shown to have a small but significant survival advantage (Stewart, 2002), but is currently not widely used in the UK.

Both the use of carmustine implants in combination with surgical resection (Westphal *et al.*, 2003) and of adjuvant postoperative temozolomide (Stupp *et al.*, 2009) concurrently with radiotherapy in patients with a newly diagnosed HGG have been shown to improve survival by approximately 2–3 months.

For good performance status patients with grade IV astrocytomas, combined temozolomide and radiotherapy is the standard of care.

Treatment of meningioma

Meningiomas most commonly arise in the skull vault, are usually low-grade tumours (WHO grade 1) and have an indolent course. Disease management depends on signs, symptoms, the patient's fitness and the tumour site and size. Watching and waiting are appropriate for patients with small, incidental meningiomas. In patients with skull vault meningiomas, surgical resection can prevent both further disease progression and the associated deterioration in neurological function, although recurrence may occur.

The indications for radiotherapy (following histopathological confirmation) are as follows.

- WHO histopathological grade II/III tumour.
- Invasion by tumour of the adjacent structures.
- Relapsed disease.
- Surgical contraindications.

Treatment of primary CNS lymphoma (PCNSL)

Primary CNS lymphoma is discussed in Chapter 34.

Treatment of medulloblastoma

Medulloblastoma is a rare tumour found in adults, and probably fewer than 50 patients present annually in England and Wales. This type of tumour usually occurs in the posterior fossa and is associated with cerebellar symptoms and raised intracranial pressure. It commonly spreads through the craniospinal axis.

Patients need to have MRI imaging of the brain and whole spine before surgery. Surgery to remove as much tumour as possible, followed by radiotherapy to the whole neuraxis, is the most appropriate treatment.

The role of chemotherapy in addition to surgery and radiotherapy in the management of adults is not established but is increasingly being used (Brandes *et al.*, 2010).

Treatment of ependymoma

Ependymoma usually occurs in association with the ventricles and patients may present with an obstruction or a mass lesion. There is a tendency for ependymoma to spread via the CSF throughout the neuraxis, but less commonly than for medulloblastoma.

Patients need to have an MRI of the brain and whole spine before surgery. Standard treatment depends on the type and grade of the tumour and the details remain controversial. Surgery is commonly used to remove as much tumour as possible and this may be followed by radiotherapy, sometimes to the whole neuraxis. The role of chemotherapy following surgery and radiotherapy in the management of adults is not established.

Treatment of pineal tumours

Patients with pineal tumours most commonly present with symptoms and signs of raised intracranial pressure. Treatment varies according to the tumour type, the level of tumour marker and CSF cytology status. Many GCTs and pineal parenchymal tumours are curable with appropriate management. GCTs occurring elsewhere with the CNS are managed according to principles similar to those used in the pineal region.

Surgical options include stereotactic or endoscopic biopsy, CSF diversion or resection for parenchymal tumours. The diagnosis of GCTs may be confirmed in some cases by the measurement of hormonal markers (αFP and βhCG). When positive, no biopsy is required; in marker-negative patients, a biopsy is necessary.

Radiotherapy may be needed, especially for GCTs but only once the diagnosis has been confirmed from the histopathological evaluation of biopsy material. Craniospinal axis irradiation may be needed for patients with pineoblastoma and metastatic GCTs.

Stereotactic radiotherapy may be appropriate for low-grade pineocytomas.

Chemotherapy forms part of the management plan of GCTs but has no proven role in the treatment of other pineal tumours.

Treatment of metastases

Metastases in the brain occur in 20–40% of patients who have other primary cancers and are usually associated with a poor prognosis. The majority of patients require appropriate palliative support and treatments depending on the site of the primary tumour. In the following circumstances, involvement of the neuro-oncology team should be considered.

- When cerebral metastases are the first sign of malignant disease.
- When the imaging findings suggestive of metastases are in doubt.
- For patients with solitary metastases and with a prognosis that warrants considering neurosurgical intervention, in whom complete surgical excision should be considered but only when the risk of unacceptable complications is low (Patchell *et al.*, 1990).
- Following the resection of solitary metastases, when postoperative radiotherapy may reduce the likelihood of intracranial relapse (Patchell *et al.*, 1998).
- When stereotactic radiotherapy is considered as an alternative to surgery in patients with small (< 3 cm) solitary (or occasionally multiple) tumours for which the histopathological diagnosis is known.

Treatment of pituitary and pituitary-related tumours

All patients with pituitary mass lesions should be referred to an endocrinologist who specialises in pituitary dysfunction and the patient's case should be discussed by an MDT so that a management plan can be agreed on. Following the appropriate investigation and management of hyposecretion (with replacement therapy) or hypersecretion (e.g. somatostatin analogues and dopamine agonists for acromegaly), patients should be considered for surgery or radiotherapy. The role of both has decreased with the increased use of endocrinological treatments.

The indications for surgery are to control the tumour mass effect and manage hypersecretions. Most operations are via the trans-sphenoid route. Transcranial and subfrontal approaches are reserved for those patients with tumours extending above the optic apparatus.

The indications for radiotherapy are in patients who are unfit for surgery, following tumour regrowth after surgery, and when there is persistent hormonal hypersecretion. Stereotactic approaches are now being used in patients with small functioning tumours (Mondok *et al.*, 2005).

Patients treated for pituitary tumours require follow-up in the form of regular assessment by an endocrinologist, regular assessment of the visual fields by perimetry with access to a neuro-ophthalmologist as clinically indicated and MRI imaging.

Treatment of skull base tumours

All patients benefit at presentation from discussion by a specialist MDT to agree on a management plan. Biopsy, either endoscopically or under CT guidance, is usually required depending on the site involved. Open intracranial biopsy is sometimes necessary.

Surgery, often with a variety of expertise (e.g. neurosurgery, ENT, maxillofacial), is normally the treatment of choice. Complete excision may not be possible because of involvement of the surrounding structures. Ventricular shunting or draining may be required for large tumours. Some vascular tumours require embolisation.

Proton beam therapy should be considered for appropriate patients including skull base and spinal chordomas, skull base chondrosarcomas and spinal and paraspinal bone and soft tissue sarcomas.

Radiotherapy may be considered where complete excision is not possible, or for consolidation. External beam conformal radiotherapy is well established and there is increasing evidence of a role for stereotactic techniques, particularly for patients with small acoustic schwannomas.

Treatment of spinal cord tumours

Intradural spinal cord tumours may either be within the spinal cord (intramedullary) or outside the cord (extramedullary).

Extramedullary tumours account for 70% of intradural tumours: with few exceptions, they are histologically benign. Extramedullary tumours include nerve sheath tumours (schwannoma, neurofibroma). Metastases are more unusual.

Intramedullary tumours arise from glial cells in 80% of cases. The primary glial tumours include astrocytomas, ependymomas, gangliogliomas and oligodendrogliomas. Haemangioblastomas, metastases, nerve sheath tumour, melanocytomas and vascular tumours account for the remainder.

In patients with low-grade tumours, the main aim of treatment is to prevent further neurological deterioration. Most intradural tumours can be treated with surgery alone and can be completely excised. However, excision of intramedullary glial tumours can cause further damage to the spinal cord without any survival advantage if the lesion is high grade. For this reason, intraoperative pathology is essential. In addition, intraoperative neurophysiological recording helps minimise the risk of spinal cord injury.

Radiotherapy is an appropriate treatment for patients with incomplete resection and high-grade histology. Craniospinal axis irradiation should be considered for the treatment for high-grade spinal ependymona.

There is currently no proven role for the use of chemotherapy in adult patients with primary spinal tumours.

Radiotherapy techniques

Brain

For patient preparation, positioning and immobilisation, the principles of radiotherapy for brain tumours are the same regardless of the primary tumour type. The patient is positioned supine or prone depending on

Table 35.5 Radiotherapy GTV, PTV and dose/fractionation for different CNS tumours

Tumour type	GTV	PTV	Dose/fractionation
High-grade glioma (radical)	Enhancing preoperative tumour	3 cm margin	60 Gy in 30 fractions
High-grade glioma (palliative)	Enhancing tumour	3 cm margin	30 Gy in 6 fractions
Low-grade glioma	Preoperative tumour mass	2 cm margin	45–50.4 Gy in 25–28 fractions
Meningioma, low-grade	Preoperative tumour mass	2 cm margin	45–50 Gy in 25 fractions
Meningioma, high-grade	Preoperative tumour mass	3 cm margin	60 Gy in 30 fractions
Pineocytoma	Preoperative tumour mass	1 cm margin	45–50 Gy in 25 fractions
Pituitary adenoma	MRI mass	1 cm margin	45 Gy in 25 fractions
Skull base	As for histological type		
Craniospinal axis (e.g. medulloblastoma, pineoblastoma, high-grade ependymona)	Craniospinal axis Boost	2 cm margin	34 Gy in 18 fractions 11 Gy in 6 fractions
Spinal cord	MRI tumour mass	2–3 cm margin	45–50 Gy in 25 fractions

the locality of the tumour. Immobilisation is achieved with a Perspex® or thermoplastic shell.

Treatment for brain tumours is localised using CT planning, ideally with 3D conformal capabilities, and for patients with longer survival times receiving radical radiotherapy IMRT should be considered, including those with high-grade gliomas. The additional information from the preoperative cross-sectional imaging is essential and pre- and postoperative image co-registration should be used. Axial slices at appropriate intervals, depending on the tumour size and proximity of surrounding critical structures, of 0.2–0.5 cm are taken through the areas of interest. Radio-opaque markers in the sagittal and coronal plane facilitate localisation of fields from the CT scan baseline marked on the shell.

The GTV is defined on each slice and the PTV is grown manually or automatically. The GTV and PTV are defined for different situations in Table 35.5 (Burnet *et al.*, 2004). The same treatment principles apply for patients receiving palliative hypofractionated radiotherapy for HGGs (Ford *et al.*, 1997). Critical structures are outlined including the optic chiasm, optic nerves, eyes, brain stem and pituitary. Where IMRT is being used, planning organ at risk volumes (PRV) of 2–5 mm should be outlined. Table 35.6 summarises tolerance doses. Figure 35.1 shows (a) typical IMRT plan for a grade III glioma and (b) a DVH for OARs.

Table 35.6 Organs at risk – brain

Structure	Dose
Spinal cord PRV	Max. 1 cm^3 > 48 Gy
Brainstem PRV	Max. 54 Gy organ 1 cc < 59 Gy max
Optic Chiasm PRV	Max. < 55 Gy
Optic Nerve PRV	Max. < 55 Gy
Retina PRV	Max. 45 Gy
Cochlea PRV	Mean < 40 Gy

The radiotherapy dose is prescribed to the ICRU reference point and delivered using a three- to four-field technique. Each field should be treated daily, Monday to Friday. The PTV minimum should be no less than 95% and the PTV maximum should be no more than 107% of the dose prescribed to the ICRU reference point. No point outside the PTV should receive more than 105%.

For lateralised tumours, the treatment is usually planned using a two- or three-field technique.

The plan should be verified in the simulator using lateral digital reconstructed radiographs (DRRs) reconstructed from CT scans before starting treatment; at least one portal image should be taken in the first three fractions on the linear accelerator and weekly throughout treatment thereafter.

(a)

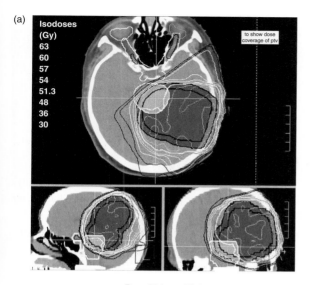

Dose Volume Histogram

(b)

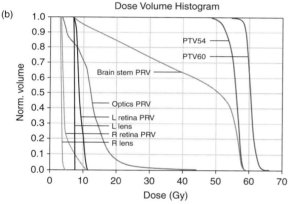

Figure 35.1 An IMRT radiotherapy plan for grade III astrocytoma is shown in (a) and the DVH set for the OARs is shown in (b). Note how the dose has been adjusted ensure that while the main part of the PTV receives 60 Gy, the isodoses are contoured so that the brain stem receives 54 Gy.

The toxicity of brain radiotherapy is shown in Table 35.7.

Spine

Patient preparation, positioning and immobilisation for spinal tumours involve the patient lying prone on a vacuum bag.

For spinal tumours, treatment is localised using CT planning, ideally with 3D conformal capabilities as for brain tumours. Lateral and midline tattoos are placed to position the patient. The additional information from the preoperative cross-sectional imaging (particularly MRI) is essential and where available pre- and

Table 35.7 Toxicity of radiotherapy to the brain

Effect	Management
Acute	
Tiredness	Advice about fatigue (e.g. goal-setting, treat anxiety/ depression, moderate exercise if tolerable)
Skin reaction	Emollient
Nausea and vomiting	Anti-emetics
Hairloss	Prosthetic
Late	
Memory loss	Neuropsychology
Pituitary hypofunction	Endocrine review in relevant patients
Second malignancies (1% approx.; Bliss *et al.*, 1994)	Warn patient
Optic chiasm damage (< 1%)	Warn patient

Table 35.8 Toxicity of radiotherapy to the spine and craniospinal axis

Effect	Management
Acute	
Tiredness	Advice about fatigue (as in Table 35.7)
Skin reaction	Emollient
Nausea and vomiting	Anti-emetics
Hairloss	Prosthetic
Diarrhoea	Loperamide
Myelosuppression	Regular FBC: G-CSF
Late	
Memory loss	Neuropsychology support
Pituitary hypofunction	Endocrine review in relevant patients
Second malignancies (1% approx.)	Warn patient
Optic chiasm damage (< 1%)	Warn patient
Ovarian failure	Avoid ovaries with planning
Spinal cord damage	Warn patient

postoperative image co-registration should be used. Axial slices at appropriate intervals, depending on the tumour size and proximity of surrounding critical structures, of 0.3–0.5 cm are taken through the area of interest. The GTV is defined on each slice and the PTV is grown manually or automatically. The GTV and PTV are defined for different situations in Table 35.5.

Care must be taken in treatment planning to avoid exit beams passing through renal tissue and ovaries.

Dose is prescribed to the ICRU reference point and verification is as for brain tumours.

The treatment plan usually involves a two-field technique with wedged oblique fields.

The toxicity of spinal radiotherapy is shown in Table 35.8.

Craniospinal axis

Patient preparation, positioning and immobilisation for craniospinal axis irradiation are complex. The principles are the same regardless of the primary tumour type. The patient is positioned prone. Immobilisation is achieved with a Perspex® or thermoplastic shell and with the patient lying in a vacuum-formed bag. Skull rotation is corrected by aligning outer canthus markers, and the spine is screened on the simulator with central tattoos to enable correct positioning.

The patient is CT-scanned in the treatment position. The whole brain is treated, down to the third cervical vertebra. Shielding to the orbit, nasopharynx and pharynx can be delineated using lateral films or from outline on the CT planning scan. Where appropriate, the boost PTV is outlined, as in Table 35.5. This composite target area is drawn on the central slice, and an outline is taken through the central volume.

Dose is prescribed to the ICRU reference point and verification is a for brain tumours.

The treatment plan is done with lateral skull fields. Centring the field on the outer canthus avoids beam divergence through the contralateral eye. Gantry twist to match the beam divergence from the upper spinal field enabled easier field matching. The spine is treated with two fields matched at the C3 level and normally the mid- to lower thoracic spine. The cervical and thoracic junction should be moved by 1 cm every 10 Gy, which is achieved by increasing or reducing the field size accordingly. Homogeneous dose distribution can often be best achieved by utilising a mixture of photons and electrons for the spinal fields. Boost volumes are planned as mentioned earlier.

The plan should be verified in the simulator using lateral DRRs reconstructed from a CT scan before starting treatment, and at least one portal image should be taken in the first three fractions on the linear accelerator and weekly, thereafter. The toxicity of radiotherapy is shown in Table 35.8.

Table 35.9 Prognosis for CNS tumours

Tumours	Five-year survival (%)
All malignant brain tumours	17
Grade IV glioma	5
Grade III glioma	25
Grade II glioma	65

Recurrent disease

The prognosis for patients with recurrent CNS tumours is generally poor. For patients with gliomas, a number of options are available.

- Repeat surgery with consideration given to use of chemotherapy implants.
- Administer chemotherapy using either combination treatment or single-agent temozolomide. Oligodendrogliomas appear to be more chemosensitive than other types of glioma (van den Bent et al., 2003).
- Use either of these chemotherapy regimens:
  - probarbazine 200 mg/m^2 days 1–10;
  - CCNU 200 mg/m^2 day 1;
  - vincristine 1.4 mg/m^2 (max. 2 mg) day 1;
  - repeated every 42 days

or

  - temozolomide 200 mg/m^2 days 1–5;
  - repeated every 28 days.

Radiotherapy can be considered for small recurrences in previously irradiated patients, although suitable patients are rare. Recurrent pituitary, skull base and pineal tumours may in some instances be managed surgically.

Prognosis

The prognosis for CNS tumours varies very widely. Some tumours such as pituitary adenomas may not affect long-term survival at all, whereas elderly patients with an HGG have a median survival of 3 months or less. Table 35.9 shows prognosis for some CNS tumours.

- Radical radiotherapy for HGGs prolongs survival by about 6 months.
- Adjuvant chemotherapy prolongs survival by about 2 months.
- Concurrent chemotherapy for HGGs prolongs survival by about 2.5 months in addition to radiotherapy alone.

Prognostic factors

The prognosis of gliomas is determined by the tumour grade, the patient age, the extent of surgery, the presence of fits and the patient's performance status at presentation (Bleehen and Stenning, 1991) Similar factors have been shown to influence the prognosis in other tumour types. For medulloblastoma, stage, the presence of metastases, subtotal resection of less that 75% of the tumours and positive CSF cytology after surgery have been shown to affect prognosis (Laurent *et al.*, 1985).

Areas of current interest and current clinical trials

Prognosis

Molecular indicators of prognosis in CNS tumours are being used more often (see Table 35.3). An association between a profile of loss on chromosomes 1 p and 19q in anaplastic oligodendrogliomas has been identified as predictive of chemotherapy responsiveness.

Downregulation of the *MGMT* gene may also be a predictor of chemoresponsiveness to alkylating agents such as temozolomide in HGGs.

Radiotherapy

Dose

For HGGs in the brain, the optimum dose of radiotherapy has been the point of investigation. Although there is some evidence that dose escalation can increase the control of tumours, it also increases the risk of radionecrosis. The data with regard to stereotactic boosting are uncertain.

Stereotactic radiotherapy

Stereotactic radiotherapy is increasingly being used as an alternative to surgery for solitary cerebral metastases and in the treatment of some pituitary and skull base tumours. This treatment has not been subjected to randomised controlled clinical trials.

Use of systemic therapy

Chemotherapy

Carmustine implants

Implantable chemotherapy wafers, used at the time of the initial radical resection and on subsequent relapse after conventional first-line treatment, have been investigated

in two small randomised clinical trials. The evidence suggests that these treatments delay relapse, but the impact on the patient's quality of life remains uncertain.

Temozolomide

The BR14 trial is assessing the use of concurrent and adjuvant temozolomide chemotherapy in 1p/19q intact anaplastic glioma.

Biological therapies

A number of biological therapies are currently being investigated. The EORTC 26091 and 26101 trails are assessing the significance of bevacizumab in recurrent gliomas. Other studies are in progress to explore novel agents in first-line and recurrent treatment. At present these agents are not recommended outside well-conducted clinical trials.

The use of radiotherapy in cerebral arteriovenous malformation (AVM)

An AVM is a benign network of arterial channels which bypass the capillaries and shunt oxygenated blood into the venous system. Intraluminal hypertension can occur and result in aneurysm formation. AVMs account for 1–2% of strokes, and can cause headache, epilepsy, cranial nerve palsy and raised intracranial pressure.

The recommended dose is 15–30 Gy to the 50% isodose using stereotactic radiosurgery. Complete obliteration is seen in 71–90% of cases within 2 years. Results are best when the lesion is 1–2 cm in size and all feeder vessels are irradiated.

References

AJCC. (2010) *AJCC Cancer Staging Manual.* Ed. S. Edge, D. R. Byrd. C. C. Compton, *et al.* 7th edn. New York: Springer.

Baumert, B. G., Mason, W. P., Ryan, G., *et al.* (2013). Temozolomide chemotherapy versus radiotherapy in molecularly characterized (1p loss) low-grade glioma: a randomized phase III intergroup study by the EORTC/NCIC-CTG/TROG/MRC-CTU (EORTC 22033–26033). *J. Clin. Oncol.*, **31** (Suppl.; abstr 2007).

Beral, V., Peterman, T., Berkelman, R., *et al.* (1991). AIDS-associated non-Hodgkin lymphoma. *Lancet*, **337**, 805–809.

Bleehen, N. M. and Stenning, S. P. (1991). A Medical Research Council trial of two radiotherapy doses in the treatment of grades 3 and 4 astrocytoma. The Medical

Research Council Brain Tumour Working Party. *Br. J. Cancer*, **64**, 769–774.

Bliss, P., Kerr, G. R. and Gregor, A. (1994). Incidence of second brain tumours after pituitary irradiation in Edinburgh 1962–1990. *Clin. Oncol. (R. Coll. Radiol.)*, **6**, 361–363.

Brandes, A. A., Franceschi, E., Tosoni, A., *et al.* (2010). Efficacy of tailored treatment for high- and low-risk medulloblastoma in adults: A large prospective phase II trial. *J. Clin. Oncol.*, **28**:182s (Suppl.; abstr 2003).

Burnet, N. G., Thomas, S. J., Burton, K. E., *et al.* (2004). Defining the tumour and target volumes for radiotherapy. *Cancer Imaging*, **4**, 153–161.

Cairncross, J. G., Ueki, K., Zlatescu, M. C., *et al.* (1998). Specific genetic predictors of chemotherapeutic response and survival in patients with anaplastic oligodendrogliomas. *J. Natl Cancer Inst.*, **90**, 1473–1479.

Ford, J. M., Stenning, S. P., Boote, D. J., *et al.* (1997). A short fractionation radiotherapy treatment for poor prognosis patients with high grade glioma. *Clin. Oncol. (R. Coll. Radiol.)*, **9**, 20–24.

Laurent, L. P., Chang, C. H. and Cohen, M. E. (1985). A classification system for primitive neuroectodermal tumors (medulloblastoma) of the posterior fossa. *Cancer*, **56**, 1807–1809.

Louis, D. N., Ohgaki, H., Wiestler, O. D., *et al.* (2007). The 2007 WHO classification of tumours of the central nervous system. *Acta Neuropathol.*, **114**, 97–109.

Mondok, A., Szeifert, G. T., Mayer, A., *et al.* (2005). Treatment of pituitary tumors: radiation. *Endocrine*, **28**, 77–85.

Patchell, R. A., Tibbs, P. A., Walsh, M. D., *et al.* (1990). A randomized trial of surgery in the treatment of single metastases to the brain. *N. Engl. J. Med.*, **322**, 494–500.

Patchell, R. A., Tibbs, P. A., Regine, W. F., *et al.* (1998). Postoperative radiotherapy in the treatment of single metastases to the brain: a randomized trial. *J. Am. Med. Ass.*, **280**, 1485–1489.

Pignatti, F., van den Bent, M., Curran, D., *et al.* (2002). Prognostic factors for survival in adult patients with cerebral low-grade glioma. *J. Clin. Oncol.*, **20**, 2076–2084.

Pobereskin, L. H. and Chadduck, J. B. (2000). Incidence of brain tumours in two English counties: a population based study. *J. Neurol. Neurosurg. Psychiatry*, **69**, 464–471.

Stewart, L. A. (2002). Chemotherapy in adult high-grade glioma: a systematic review and meta-analysis of individual patient data from 12 randomised trials. *Lancet*, **359**, 1011.

Stupp, R., Mason, W. P., van den Bent, M. J., *et al.* (2005). Radiotherapy plus concomitant and adjuvant temozolomide for glioblastoma. *N. Engl. J. Med.*, **352**, 987–996.

Stupp, R., Hegi, M. E., Mason, W. P., *et al.* (2009). Effects of radiotherapy with concomitant and adjuvant temozolomide versus radiotherapy alone on survival in glioblastoma in a randomised phase III study: 5-year analysis of the EORTC-NCIC trial. *Lancet Oncol.*, **10**, 459.

van den Bent, M. J., Chinot, O. L. and Cairncross, J. G. (2003). Recent developments in the molecular characterization and treatment of oligodendrogial tumors. *Neuro. Oncol.*, **5**, 128–138.

van den Bent, M. J., Afra, D., de Witte, O., *et al.* (2005). Long-term efficacy of early versus delayed radiotherapy for low-grade astrocytoma and oligodendroglioma in adults: the EORTC 22845 randomised trial. *Lancet*, **366**, 985–990.

Westphal, M., Hilt, D. C., Bortey, E., *et al.* (2003). A phase 3 trial of local chemotherapy with biodegradable carmustine (BCNU) wafers (Gliadel wafers) in patients with primary malignant glioma. *Neuro. Oncol.*, **5**, 79.

Wick, W., Platten, M., Meisner, C., *et al.* (2012). Temozolomide chemotherapy alone versus radiotherapy alone for malignant astrocytoma in the elderly: the NOA-08 randomised, phase 3 trial. *Lancet Oncol.*, **13**, 707.

Management of skin cancer other than melanoma

Sankha Suvra Mitra

Introduction

Non-melanoma skin cancer is the commonest cancer in the UK. It is usually caused by ultraviolet radiation from chronic sun exposure in a fair-skinned population. Basal cell carcinoma is the most frequent variety (74%), and presents as a superficial tumour that very rarely metastasises. Squamous cell carcinoma (23%) can spread to regional lymph nodes.

Surgical excision is the treatment of choice for the majority of tumours. Non-surgical treatment options include radiotherapy, curettage, imiquimod cream, photodynamic therapy and topical 5-FU therapy. Radiotherapy is an important treatment option for older patients and is preferred to surgery for large superficial tumours, multiple tumours, and in areas around the eye, nose and ear where the cosmetic results may be better and function can be preserved. The radiotherapy technique involves treatment with either superficial X-rays (SXR) or electron therapy. Cure rates are about 95% at 5 years.

The National Institute for Health and Clinical Excellence has published service guidance on the care of these patients (NICE, 2006).

Range of tumours

In the differential diagnosis, the tumour could be benign or malignant, and a malignant tumour could be either primary or secondary.

Premalignant conditions

Premalignant conditions include the following (Soutar and Robertson, 2001):

- actinic keratosis;
- Bowen's disease;
- erythroplasia of Queyrat;
- Paget's disease.

Benign tumours

Benign tumours include the following:

- benign naevus;
- sebaceous cyst;
- epidermal cyst;
- basal cell papilloma (seborrhoeic keratosis);
- vascular angioma;
- keratoacanthoma;
- dermatofibroma.

Malignant tumours

Primary malignant tumours include:

- basal cell carcinoma;
- squamous cell carcinoma;
- Merkel cell carcinoma;
- malignant eccrine porocarcinoma;
- amelanotic melanoma;
- cutaneous T-cell lymphoma;
- primary cutaneous B-cell lymphoma;
- Kaposi's sarcoma;
- angiosarcoma;
- lymphangiosarcoma;
- atypical fibroxanthoma.

Secondary malignant tumours can arise from any primary site, but occur most commonly from breast cancer, lung cancer, colon cancer and melanoma.

Incidence and epidemiology

There were about 100,000 cases of non-melanoma skin cancer in the UK in 2010. This comprises about 20% of all new cancers and there are about 500 deaths annually. More than 5% of the population over age 60 will develop a non-melanoma skin cancer (American Cancer Society, 2003).

Practical Clinical Oncology, Second Edition, ed. Louise Hanna, Tom Crosby and Fergus Macbeth. Published by Cambridge University Press. © Cambridge University Press 2015.

Risk factors and aetiology

Risk factors for skin cancer include the following (Soutar and Robertson, 2001):

- Chronic sun exposure and ultraviolet radiation. Premalignant conditions include actinic keratosis and Bowen's disease.
- Phototherapy with ultraviolet A or B radiation.
- Immunosuppression in transplant patients CML, CLL, and AIDS.
- Ionising radiation from radiotherapy (voluntary exposure by early pioneer radiologists and children treated with radium for ringworm of the scalp) or atomic fallout. Cancers include squamous cell cancer, angiosarcoma and lymphangiosarcoma.
- Chemical carcinogenesis from nitrates, arsenicals in tonics and pesticides, oral methoxsalen, soot (chimney sweeps' SCC of the scrotum), mineral oils (yarn workers lubricating spinning mules) and coal tar.

Genetic predisposition

Naevoid basal cell carcinoma syndrome (Gorlin's syndrome) is an autosomal familial cancer syndrome in which multiple basal cell carcinomas appear at an early age. The gene responsible (PTCH, patched gene) is on chromosome 9q22–31. Other features of the syndrome include bone cysts of the mandible that are visible on orthopantomograms, abnormalities of the ribs, short fourth metacarpal, coloboma at birth or cataracts in later life, and an increased risk of both medulloblastoma and meningioma. A skull X-ray shows calcification of the falx cerebri in 90% of cases by the age of 12 years.

Bazex's syndrome is a rare X-linked syndrome that predisposes individuals to multiple basal cell carcinomas. This disease is linked to chromosome Xq24–27.

Xeroderma pigmentosa is a rare autosomal recessive genetic disease associated with non-melanoma skin cancer due to defective DNA repair (nucleotide-excision repair).

Ferguson–Smith disease is a familial disease presenting as self-healing squamous cell carcinoma.

Muir–Torre syndrome is an autosomal dominant disease with sebaceous or adnexal gland tumours usually associated with colonic tumours (Soutar and Robertson, 2001).

Chronic inflammation

Erythroplasia of Queyrat is a chronic inflammatory premalignant condition, which can develop into squamous cell cancer of the glans penis. This is similar to Bowen's disease.

Chronic scar

The cancer from a chronic scar is called Marjolin's ulcer, and it may occasionally complicate chronic leg ulcers.

Basal cell carcinoma and squamous carcinoma

Basal cell carcinoma

Basal cell carcinoma accounts for 80% of all non-melanoma skin cancers.

The major cause is exposure to ultraviolet radiation. Recreational exposure to the sun during childhood and adolescence poses a significant risk. Fair complexion, red or blonde hair, and light eye colour are also independent risk factors (Rubin et al., 2005).

Clinical presentation

Basal cell carcinoma characteristically arises in body areas exposed to the sun. The most common site is the head and neck, followed by the trunk.

Basal cell carcinomas (also known as rodent ulcers) tend to grow very slowly over years, and eventually result in itching, bleeding and discomfort. They very rarely metastasise, unlike other cancers, but if neglected, they will infiltrate locally and cause adjacent tissue destruction.

The classic form is the nodular basal cell cancer, which presents as a pearly papule, nodule, or cyst with overlying telangiectasia and a rolled border, with central crusting or ulceration. Occasionally, nodular basal cell cancers may resemble enlarged pores or pits on the sebaceous skin of the central portion of the face. Superficial spreading basal cell carcinoma presents as a scaly erythematous patch or plaque. Both of these forms may have a brownish colour due to melanin pigmentation. The morphoeic form appears as an indurated, whitish, scar-like plaque with indistinct margins. Other variants include micro-nodular, mixed, basosquamous, adamantinoid and clear cell types.

Molecular pathogenesis

Inappropriate activation of the hedgehog (HH) signalling pathway in 90% of basal cell cancers results in secreted sonic HH protein binding to a tumour-suppressor gene and preventing its suppression of transmembrane proteins and downstream targets. The GLI family of transcription factors is activated. Mutations in TP53 are found in about 50% of cases (Rubin *et al.*, 2005).

Squamous carcinoma

Unlike basal cell carcinoma, there may be a clear progression through dysplasia, carcinoma *in situ*, or Bowen's disease to frankly invasive squamous cell carcinoma. Solar damage causes red scaly patches that persist for several years and are termed actinic keratoses. Actinic keratoses are premalignant, but only an estimated 1% transform into a squamous cell carcinoma and up to 25% resolve spontaneously. The patches usually overlie a superficial ulcer; any induration or infiltration suggests that the tumour has progressed to frank malignancy. Another typical picture is a rapidly growing ulcer with a rolled edge and an indurated margin. Sometimes there can be exophytic growth resulting in a cauliflower-like mass (Soutar and Robertson, 2001).

Secondary spread occurs first to the regional lymph nodes. The ear, lip and columella are sites that have a higher incidence of metastases (approximately 5–7%).

Keratoacanthoma is histologically similar to squamous cell carcinoma but the history is of a tumour that grows rapidly over 4–6 weeks that subsequently undergoes spontaneous regression, leaving a small pitted scar on the surface.

Poor prognostic factors

Risk factors for extensive subclinical spread include a tumour size greater than 2 cm, poorly defined borders, location on the central part of the face and ears, long-standing duration, incomplete excision, recurrent cancer, site of previous radiotherapy, an aggressive histological pattern of growth including morphoeaform, sclerosing, mixed infiltrative, micro-nodular features, baso-squamous metatypical features and perineural or perivascular involvement. Patients with known immunosuppression also tend to develop more rapidly growing and invasive tumours (Rubin *et al.*, 2005).

Table 36.1 The TNM staging classification for carcinomas of the skin (excuding eyelid, vulva and penis)

Stage	Description
T1	Tumour ≤ 2 cm
T2	Tumour > 2 cm
T3	Tumour with invasion of deep structures, e.g. muscle, bone, cartilage, jaws, and orbit
T4	Tumour with direct or perineural invasion of skull base or axial skeleton
N0	No regional lymph node metastasis
N1	Metastasis in a single lymph node ≤ 3 cm in greatest dimension
N2	Metastasis in a single lymph node, > 3 cm but ≤ 6 cm in greatest dimension, or in multiple lymph nodes ≤ 6 cm in greatest dimension
N3	Metastasis in a lymph node > 6 cm in greatest dimension
M0	No distant metastasis
M1	Distant metastasis

Adapted from UICC (2009).

Staging classification for skin carcinomas

The TNM staging classification for skin carcinomas is shown in Table 36.1.

Assessment of the patient

History

It is important to consider the patient's age, ethnic background, occupation and geographic factors (Diepgen and Mahler, 2002). The patient should be asked about any past high sun exposure (e.g. life in the tropics or outdoor work), about topical treatment used in the past, history of chemical exposure, or previous irradiation to the involved area. Enquire about symptoms from the tumour, its duration and rate of growth. If the tumour has been present for years and slowly growing, then it is likely to be a basal cell cancer; if it has grown over a few months, then it is likely to be a squamous cell cancer; and if it has been growing rapidly over a few weeks, then it is likely to be a keratoacanthoma.

Clinical examination

Examine the tumour with a magnifying glass under a bright light. The margins of the tumour should be determined by careful palpation and the depth of the tumour assessed to determine the type of radiation and energy to be used. It may be difficult to assess the depth accurately in the embryonic folds such as the inner canthus, nasolabial fold, ala nasi, tragus and postauricular areas, because palpation may underestimate the depth of the tumour. Regional lymph node areas must be examined, particularly in patients with squamous cell carcinomas. Large ulcerative tumours of the scalp may need assessment of bony involvement by palpation.

Investigation

Tumour diagnosis is confirmed by scrapings, punch biopsy, or excisional biopsy.

Large tumours may need to be assessed for deep involvement (e.g. with X-ray and CT scans) if they appear fixed to underlying tissues. Perineural involvement may require MRI.

Treatment overview

The majority of BCCs carry no risk to survival and many patients with uncomplicated tumours can be managed in the community (see NICE, 2010 for further details). Patients with other tumour types are referred to specialist teams.

Surgery

Mohs micrographic surgery

Mohs micrographic surgery is a specialised technique of surgical excision method that requires special training. It is indicated for sites that have a high initial treatment failure rate when traditional methods are used (e.g. periorbital area, nasolabial fold, etc.) and for recurrent tumours. It involves rapid examination of horizontal frozen-section samples, which are processed to examine all the peripheral and deep surgical margins and to determine whether further excision is required. Cure rates at 5 years approach 99% (Thomas and Amonette, 1998; Malhotra et al., 2004).

Surgical excision

Surgery is indicated for small tumours that can be excised and the defect closed directly. This single procedure results in a good cosmetic result and a high probability of cure. An advantage of this over radiation is that complete removal can be confirmed histologically, avoiding the need for long-term follow-up (Avril et al., 1997).

Patients younger than 60 years should be offered surgical excision rather than radiotherapy because the cosmetic results are better. Surgery is also indicated for recurrent tumours, those with uncertain or incomplete margins, those involving cartilage, tendon, bone or joint and large, bulky tumours. Keratoacanthoma is usually treated by surgical excision, curettage or cautery.

Curettage and electro-desiccation and cryosurgery

Curettage and electro-desiccation and cryosurgery are indicated for tumours such as small well-defined primary tumours on the neck, trunk, arms and legs. Close follow-up is required. Cure rates are 95% at 5 years.

Non-surgical treatments

Imiquimod 5%

Imiquimod 5% is a topical immune modulator licensed for biopsy-proven, small, primary, superficial basal cell cancers on the trunk, neck, arms or legs of adults with normal immune systems. A course of treatment involves once-daily administration of imiquimod 5 days per week for 6 weeks. Cure rates are approximately 85% (Tran et al., 2003; Lebwohl et al., 2004).

Photodynamic therapy

Photodynamic therapy, using either systemic or topical porphyrins, is only of value in treating superficial tumours. Methyl aminolaevulinic acid is a photoactivated agent applied topically under occlusive foil to enhance tissue penetration and reduce side effects of bleaching and other systemic effects. Deeper penetration is poor. It is especially useful for small, superficial basal cell carcinomas at cosmetically tricky sites such as the central face and the 'V' of the neck.

Topical 5-fluorouracil therapy

Topical 5-fluorouracil is available for superficial cancers in strengths of 2% or 5% and is usually applied twice daily to the tumour and its margins (Dabski and Helm, 1988).

Radiotherapy

Radiotherapy is an important treatment option for older patients who are less concerned about long-term cosmesis. It is also preferred to surgery for large superficial or extensive tumours and for multiple tumours because the cosmetic results are better and function can be preserved. Tumours at sites where surgical excision is difficult or which are unresectable should also be treated by radiotherapy. Patients who refuse surgery, who are unfit or who are on anticoagulant therapy should be offered radiotherapy. Cure rates are about 95% at 5 years (Lovett *et al.*, 1990; Caccialanza *et al.*, 2003).

Radiotherapy is contraindicated for patients with xeroderma pigmentosum and the basal cell naevus syndrome because it may induce more tumours in the treated area. Sites of previous radiotherapy, areas of vascular insufficiency, skin overlying the shin and malleoli of the lower leg, the middle third of the upper eyelid and the dorsum of the hand should not be irradiated as they tolerate radiotherapy poorly.

Squamous cell carcinomas of the lower lip can be treated by surgery, external beam radiation with electrons or X-rays, or with interstitial radiotherapy.

Radical radiotherapy

Informed consent must first be obtained after full discussion with the patient. Acute effects include dry, red, inflamed skin like a mild sunburn, moist skin breakdown, scabbing and ulceration. Intermediate effects include slow healing over 4–8 weeks, tiredness and watery eyes (epiphora due to nasolacrimal duct oedema and stenosis which can be treated by recanalisation) if the inner canthus area is being treated. Late effects include chronic radiation dermatitis with pale, thin skin with red dots (telangiectasis), fibrosis, permanent hair loss in the scalp, eyebrow and eyelash tumours, dry eyes due to lacrimal gland damage, upper eyelid conjunctival keratinisation, delayed radiation necrosis and secondary cutaneous malignancies. Assessment of disease is by clinical examination with imaging if relevant.

Mould room preparation. A customised lead cut-out is made, 1.5 mm thick for 90–150 kV superficial X-ray therapy (SXR) and 4 mm thick for electron therapy. For electron beam therapy, wax bolus is added over the cut-out area to increase the surface dose to the 90% isodose which should cover the entire PTV. The thickness of the wax depends on the electron energy to be used and the field size, and is determined from the depth dose chart.

Definition of target volume. A margin is drawn around the gross tumour to allow for any subclinical extension and the penumbra of the beam. For a cystic, superficial, basal cell cancer with well-defined margins, a 0.5-cm margin is adequate for SXR. For large,

morphoeic, or poorly defined basal cell cancers and squamous cell cancers, a 1-cm margin is required for SXR. For electron therapy, a wider circumferential margin of 1.5 cm is required to account for bowing of the isodoses. For large infiltrative tumours with an unknown deep extension or when treating with beam energies greater than 6 MeV electrons or 100 kV SXR over critical structures like brain (for scalp cancers), a CT plan is recommended for accurate assessment of extension and depth (Solan *et al.*, 1997).

Shielding. A lead shield must be used to protect the eye when the eyelids and inner or outer canthus are treated. This protects the conjunctiva, cornea, and lens. An internal eye shield, shaped like a large contact lens with a screw thread on the anterior surface, is used when the target volume involves both eyelids. An external spade-shaped eye shield is placed under the upper or lower eyelid when only one eyelid is included in the target volume. Internal eye shielding can only be done if the patient is not driving themselves to and from the appointment. The patient is warned that the local anaesthetic drops sting and a dose of one to two drops of 0.5% amethocaine eye drops is instilled into the eye. The eye shield is aseptically withdrawn from the sterile solution and is rinsed in sterile normal saline. The inner surface is coated with liquid paraffin to reduce friction with the cornea and the eyelid is pulled in one direction to introduce the eye shield. Both eyelids are usually taped together over the internal eye shield, whereas the external eye shield is usually taped over the other eyelid. The patient has to wear an eye pad for 2 hours afterwards, until the effects of the local anaesthetic have worn off and the corneal reflex is back to normal.

Intranasal shielding. An intranasal lead shield is used to protect the nasal mucosa and cartilage of the nasal septum while treating tumours of the ala nasi. This shield is wrapped in wet gauze before it is inserted into the nostril. For electron treatments, any shielding that is placed internally (e.g. gum or nostril shielding) or, for example, behind the ear requires aluminium or wax coating to reduce the backscatter caused by secondary electrons produced in the lead.

Intraoral shielding. An intraoral lead gum shield is used to protect the gums and mucosa when squamous cell cancers of the lower lip are treated with electron therapy. The lead is usually anteriorly coated with aluminium (surface facing the beam) to reduce the backscatter from secondary electrons released in the lead (Solan *et al.*, 1997).

Table 36.2 Percentage depth doses for 95 kV photons

Applicator size (cm)	–	1.5 circle	2 circle	2.5 circle	3 circle	3.5 circle	4 circle	5 circle	6 circle	7 circle	8 circle	10 circle	14 circle	17 circle	5 × 15
Equivalent diameter (cm)	1	1.5	2	2.5	3	3.5	4	5	6	7	8	10	14	17	8.4
Depth (cm)															
0	100.0	100.0	100.0	100.0	100.0	100.0	100.0	100.0	100.0	100.0	100.0	100.0	100.0	100.0	100.0
0.5	80.8	82.5	84.1	85.3	86.5	87.3	88.1	89.2	91.2	91.7	92.1	92.6	93.5	94.0	92.2
1	65.7	68.2	70.7	72.8	74.8	75.7	76.6	78.4	81.8	82.7	83.5	84.5	86.2	87.1	83.7
2	44.3	47.0	49.7	51.9	54.1	55.6	57.1	59.5	64.8	66.0	67.1	68.8	71.1	72.3	67.4
3	31.0	33.2	35.4	37.4	39.4	40.9	42.3	44.6	50.0	51.4	52.7	54.7	57.1	58.2	53.1
4	22.3	24.3	26.2	27.6	28.9	30.0	31.1	33.0	38.4	39.9	41.3	43.5	46.1	47.3	41.7
5	15.9	17.2	18.5	19.8	21.1	22.1	23.1	24.8	29.7	31.0	32.3	34.3	37.0	38.3	32.7
6	11.7	12.8	13.8	14.8	15.8	16.6	17.4	18.8	23.0	24.2	25.3	27.3	30.0	31.2	25.7
7	8.7	9.6	10.4	11.2	11.9	12.6	13.2	14.5	18.0	19.2	20.3	22.2	24.9	26.2	20.7
8	6.4	7.1	7.8	8.4	9.0	9.6	10.2	11.2	14.2	15.2	16.1	17.8	20.4	21.7	16.4
9	4.8	5.3	5.8	6.3	6.8	7.3	7.8	8.8	11.4	12.3	13.2	14.6	16.6	17.7	13.5
10	3.6	4.0	4.4	4.9	5.3	5.7	6.1	6.9	9.2	9.9	10.6	11.8	13.4	14.3	10.8

HVL, half value layer = 3.0 Al; diameter ≤ 5 cm; SSD, source–skin distance = 20 cm; other applicators, SSD = 30 cm. Permission to print has been obtained from Mr David Prior, Physicist, Sussex Cancer Centre and Dr David Bloomfield, Head, Sussex Cancer Centre. Disclaimer: this table is for academic purposes only and applies to a specific machine and cancer centre. It should not be used to guide treatment for any patient.

Table 36.3 Percentage depth doses for 195 kV photons

Applicator size (cm)	–	5 circle	–	6 circle	–	7 circle	6 × 8	7 × 7	8 circle
Side of eq. square (cm) / Depth (cm)	4	4.5	5	5.4	6	6.3	6.9	7	7.2
0	100.0	100.0	100.0	100.0	100.0	100.0	100.0	100.0	100.0
0.5	95.6	96.1	96.6	96.8	97.2	97.3	97.6	97.6	97.6
1	90.3	91.0	91.7	92.1	92.7	92.9	93.4	93.5	93.6
2	78.5	79.5	80.5	81.2	82.2	82.6	83.4	83.5	83.8
3	66.5	68.0	69.5	70.4	71.8	72.4	73.5	73.7	74.0
4	55.7	57.3	58.8	59.8	61.3	62.0	63.3	63.5	63.9
5	46.6	48.1	49.5	50.5	52.0	52.7	54.0	54.2	54.6
6	38.8	40.1	41.4	42.4	43.8	44.5	46.0	46.2	46.6
7	32.1	33.4	34.6	35.6	37.1	37.8	39.3	39.5	39.9
8	26.3	27.6	28.8	29.7	31.1	31.7	33.0	33.2	33.6
9	22.0	23.0	24.0	24.8	26.1	26.6	27.6	27.8	28.2
10	18.2	19.2	21.0	20.9	22.1	22.6	23.6	23.8	24.2
11	15.1	16.0	16.8	17.5	18.6	19.1	20.1	20.3	20.6
12	12.5	13.4	14.2	14.8	15.7	16.2	17.1	17.3	17.6
13	10.2	11.0	11.8	12.4	13.2	13.6	14.4	14.5	14.7
14	8.5	9.2	9.9	10.4	11.2	11.6	12.3	12.4	12.6
15	7.2	7.7	8.2	8.6	9.3	9.6	10.1	10.2	10.4
16	6.0	6.5	6.9	7.3	7.9	8.1	8.6	8.7	8.9
17	4.9	5.4	5.8	6.1	6.6	6.8	7.3	7.4	7.6
18	4.1	4.5	4.8	5.1	5.6	5.8	6.1	6.2	6.4
19	3.4	3.7	4.0	4.3	4.7	4.9	5.2	5.3	5.4
20	2.8	3.1	3.4	3.6	4.0	4.2	4.5	4.5	4.6

HVL, half value layer = 1.0 mm Cu; SSD, source–skin distance = 50 cm; closed applicators; eq. square = equivalent square. Permission to print has been obtained from Mr David Prior, Physicist, Sussex Cancer Centre and Dr David Bloomfield, Head, Sussex Cancer Centre. Disclaimer: this table is for academic purposes only and applies to a specific machine and cancer centre. It should not be used to guide treatment for any patient.

Choice of radiation: tumours smaller than 4 cm. Tumours that are less than 4 cm in diameter and less than 5 mm thick are appropriate for SXR therapy. Tumours around the face, particularly in small concave areas like the inner canthus and ala nasi, obtain excellent cosmetic results from SXR therapy. Different superficial machines have different depth doses depending on the use of different filters in the head of the beam. Usually 90–150 kV is adequate to treat to a depth of a few millimetres. Tumours on both sides of the pinna have a thickness of about 6 mm and 160 kV is adequate to treat this through a single field.

Radiotherapy should be withheld if the cartilage is directly involved. Percentage depth dose tables for 95 and 195 kV photons are shown in Tables 36.2 and 36.3, respectively.

Choice of radiation: tumours larger than 4 cm. Tumours that are more than 4 cm in diameter and more than 1 cm thick should be treated by electron therapy. With smaller tumours, beam flatness is lost. Tumours on the scalp are treated by low-energy electrons to reduce the exit dose to the brain. Flat tumours on the trunks and limbs are suitable for electron therapy but lower-leg tumours are usually better treated

Table 36.4 Electron depth dose table for 95 cm source–surface distance (SSD), showing the depth in mm of percentage isodoses for different size applicators

% Dose	6 MeV					8 MeV				
	3 © 7 cm²	4 © 12 cm²	5 © 20 cm²	6 © 28 cm²	10 □ 100 cm²	3 © 7 cm²	4 © 12 cm²	5 © 20 cm²	6 © 28 cm²	10 □ 100 cm²
90	2	4	4	4	5	0	0	0	0	4
100	11	13	13	13	13	12	15	16	17	17
90	16	18	18	18	18	20	22	24	24	24
80	19	20	20	20	20	23	25	26	26	27
50	23	24	24	24	25	29	31	32	32	33
30	26	27	27	27	27	34	35	35	35	36
10	31	31	31	31	31	40	40	40	40	41
Surface dose	89%	87%	86%	86%	84%	94%	92%	91%	90%	88%

% Dose	15 MeV						18 MeV	
	5 © 20 cm²	6 © 28 cm²	7 © 38 cm²	8 © 50 cm²	10 □ 100 cm²	14 □ 196 cm²	5 © 20 cm²	6 © 28 cm²
90	0	0	0	0	0	0	0	0
100	9	14	20	23	25	27	4	7
90	36	38	43	43	44	44	39	43
80	42	45	48	48	49	49	48	52
50	55	57	59	59	59	59	64	67
30	62	63	64	64	65	65	74	76
10	72	72	73	73	73	73	86	87
Surface dose	99%	98%	96%	96%	94%	92%	100%	99%

© = cm circle; □ = cm square. Permission to print has been obtained from Mr David Prior, Physicist, Sussex Cancer Centre and Dr David Bloomfield, Head, Sussex Cancer Centre. Disclaimer: this table is for academic purposes only and applies to a specific machine and cancer centre. It should not be used to guide treatment for any patient.

with surgery. It is advisable to avoid electron therapy near the eyes; wide margins of 1.5 cm are required because of bowing of the isodoses, and lateral scatter of radiation makes eye shielding difficult. However, if there is a 3-cm thick tumour between the eyes, then tighter field margins with electrons can be used with lead skin collimation. Electron therapy should also be avoided near complicated air spaces like the nasal cavities, sinuses, and mastoid air cells because of the uncertain dose distribution due to tissue inhomogeneity.

Determining the electron energy. Once the thickness and diameter of the tumour and diameter of the field are established, an equivalent square calculation is made for the field size. In conjunction with the physicist, the electron depth dose chart is consulted for that field size. If the tumour is 2-cm thick, then a margin of 0.5 cm is usually added posteriorly and a 0.5–1 cm wax/Perspex® bolus is required anteriorly to increase the skin dose to 90%. Multiplying this total thickness by 3 usually gives the approximate electron energy (9 MeV) that will treat the PTV to a 90% isodose. The total dose is prescribed to the 100% isodose (equivalent to the ICRU reference point for photons). If the total dose is prescribed to the 90% isodose, then the total dose to the PTV will be 10% greater and the equivalent ICRU

10 MeV					12 MeV					
3© 7 cm²	4© 12 cm²	5© 20 cm²	6© 28 cm²	10□ 100 cm²	3© 7 cm²	4© 12 cm²	5© 20 cm²	6© 28 cm²	10□ 100 cm²	14□ 196 cm²
0	0	0	0	3	0	0	0	0	0	3
11	17	19	21	22	11	16	18	21	25	25
22	27	29	29	30	25	29	32	33	35	35
26	30	32	33	33	29	33	36	37	39	39
35	38	39	39	40	38	43	45	45	46	46
41	43	44	44	44	45	49	50	50	50	50
48	49	50	50	50	54	55	55	55	56	56
97%	95%	94%	93%	88%	98%	97%	97%	95%	91%	88%

20 MeV									
7© 38 cm²	8© 50 cm²	10□ 100 cm²	14□ 196 cm²	5© 20 cm²	6© 28 cm²	7© 38 cm²	8© 50 cm²	10□ 100 cm²	14□ 196 cm²
0	0	0	0	0	0	0	0	0	0
16	22	26	30	5	9	13	17	22	30
50	52	54	54	39	43	52	54	57	59
58	59	60	60	50	55	62	63	65	66
71	71	71	71	70	73	77	78	79	79
78	78	78	78	81	83	86	86	87	87
88	88	88	88	95	96	97	97	97	97
98%	98%	96%	94%	100%	99%	98%	98%	97%	94%

reference point at the 100% will also receive a higher dose than originally intended. The electron depth dose tables for 95 and 100 cm SSD for different field sizes are shown in Tables 36.4 and 36.5, respectively. Electron depth dose curves are shown in Figure 36.1.

Plan calculation. The SSD is increased by the 'stand off' between the applicator and the tumour whereas the SSD is decreased by 'stand in'. In both cases, corrections must be made for the change in output with variation in SSD according to the inverse-square law.

Dose. Some radiotherapy dose schedules are as follows.

- For small basal cell cancers (< 3 cm), give 35 Gy in 5 fractions over 5 days to the 100% isodose (National Comprehensive Cancer Network, 2005). (In very frail elderly patients, a single fraction of 18–20 Gy to the 100% isodose may be used.)

- For large basal cell cancers (> 3 cm) and squamous cell cancers, give 45 Gy in 10 fractions over 2 weeks or 55 Gy in 20 fractions over 4 weeks to the 100% isodose.

- For very large, thick squamous cell cancers, give 64 Gy in 32 fractions over 6.5 weeks to the 100% isodose.

Table 36.5 Electron depth dose table for 100 cm SSD, showing the depth in mm of percentage isodoses for different size applicators

% Dose	6 MeV					8 MeV				
	3© 7 cm²	4© 12 cm²	5© 20 cm²	6© 28 cm²	10□ 100 cm²	3© 7 cm²	4© 12 cm²	5© 20 cm²	6© 28 cm²	10□ 100 cm²
90	3	5	6	6	6	0	3	5	5	5
100	11	13	13	13	13	12	16	17	17	17
90	17	18	18	18	18	20	23	24	24	24
80	19	20	20	20	20	24	26	27	27	27
50	24	25	25	25	25	30	32	32	32	32
30	27	27	27	27	27	35	35	36	36	36
10	31	31	31	31	31	40	40	40	40	41
Surface dose	87%	83%	82%	82%	82%	91%	88%	85%	85%	85%

% Dose	15 MeV						18 MeV		
	5© 20 cm²	6© 28 cm²	7© 38 cm²	8© 50 cm²	10□ 100 cm²	14□ 196 cm²	5© 20 cm²	6© 28 cm²	7© 38 cm²
90	0	0	0	0	0	0	0	0	0
100	19	22	23	23	25	27	18	23	25
90	38	40	43	43	44	44	44	47	51
80	44	46	48	48	49	49	51	55	58
50	56	57	58	58	59	59	67	69	71
30	63	64	64	64	64	64	75	77	78
10	72	72	72	72	72	72	86	87	87
Surface dose	93%	93%	92%	92%	92%	92%	94%	94%	94%

© = cm circle; □ = cm square. Permission to print has been obtained from Mr David Prior, Physicist, Sussex Cancer Centre and Dr David Bloomfield, Head, Sussex Cancer Centre. Disclaimer: this table is for academic purposes only and applies to a specific machine and cancer centre. It should not be used to guide treatment for any patient.

- For adjuvant radiotherapy, give 50 Gy in 20 fractions over 4 weeks or 60 Gy in 30 fractions over 6 weeks to the 100% isodose.

* For interstitial radiotherapy, 45 Gy in 10 fractions with HDR brachytherapy is suitable although a more prolonged fractionation of the lower limb may be advisable (Coyle, 2005).

Skin reaction clinic. The patient should be advised to wash the area with plain running water in a shower or bath every day and to pat it dry gently afterwards. Shaving and use of artificial deodorants and soaps should be avoided because they could sensitise the skin to radiation (heavy metals increase the photo-electric effect) and cause a radiation burn. A cream such as E45® is applied and sun exposure should be avoided by using sun barrier cream and hats.

Follow-up. After the radiotherapy reaction has healed, patients with basal cell carcinomas are usually discharged. Patients with squamous cell carcinomas should be followed up for 5 years.

Areas of current interest

Vismodegib, a cyclopamine-competitive antagonist of the smoothened receptor (SMO) which is part of the HH signaling pathway is licensed for the treatment of both locally advanced and metastatic basal cell carcinoma (BCC). SMO inhibition causes GLI 1 and 2 to remain inactive preventing expression of tumour-mediating genes. Based on a phase II trial there was a 43% response rate in locally advanced BCC with approximately 21% complete response and a 30% response in metastatic BCC (Sekulic et al., 2012).

10 MeV					12 MeV					
3 ©	4 ©	5 ©	6 ©	10 □	3 ©	4 ©	5 ©	6 ©	10 □	14 □
7 cm²	12 cm²	20 cm²	28 cm²	100 cm²	7 cm²	12 cm²	20 cm²	28 cm²	100 cm²	196 cm²
0	0	3	4	5	0	0	0	2	2	3
15	18	20	21	21	16	18	22	23	24	25
24	27	29	30	30	26	30	33	34	35	35
27	31	33	33	33	30	35	37	38	39	39
36	39	39	40	40	41	44	46	46	46	46
42	43	44	44	44	47	50	50	50	50	50
49	49	50	50	50	56	56	56	56	56	56
92%	90%	87%	87%	86%	93%	92%	90%	89%	89%	88%

			20 MeV					
8 ©	10 □	14 □	5 ©	6 ©	7 ©	8 ©	10 □	14 □
50 cm²	100 cm²	196 cm²	20 cm²	28 cm²	38 cm²	50 cm²	100 cm²	196 cm²
0	0	0	0	0	0	0	0	0
25	25	25	16	17	22	22	22	28
52	54	54	46	49	54	55	57	59
59	60	60	55	59	63	64	65	66
71	71	71	72	75	78	78	79	79
78	78	78	82	84	86	86	87	87
87	87	87	95	96	96	96	97	97
94%	94%	94%	95%	95%	95%	95%	95%	94%

Updated results in 2013 showed a response rate of 60.3% in locally advanced BCC and 48.5% in metastatic BCC, with a median duration of response of 20.3 and 14.7 months, respectively (Sekulic *et al.*, 2013). The dose is 150 mg capsules once a day, swallowed whole, with the side effects being muscle spasms, hair loss, weight loss, nausea, diarrhoea, change of taste and tiredness.

Merkel cell carcinoma

Merkel cell carcinoma is a highly malignant tumour that develops satellite tumours and lymph node metastases and occurs mainly in elderly patients. The cells are thought to be of neuroendocrine origin from the APUD (amine precursor uptake and decarboxylation) system. It can present as a painless, red, indurated nodule or an ulcer, usually in the region of the head and neck. Sentinel lymph node biopsy (SLNB) with appropriate immunohistochemical analysis and wide local excision is the main treatment, but local recurrence rates are high and lymph node metastases can occur in about 40–65% of cases. Therefore, SLNB+ve patients should be considered for nodal dissection followed by adjuvant radiotherapy, because it reduces the risk of local and regional relapse (Lewis *et al.*, 2006). The use of adjuvant chemotherapy is not routinely recommended, but can be considered in select clinical circumstances (NCCN Guidelines, 2013, available at http://www.merkelcell.org/usefulInfo/documents/ NCCNMCC2013.pdf, accessed Janaury 2015). Patients with metastatic disease often respond to chemotherapy

(a)
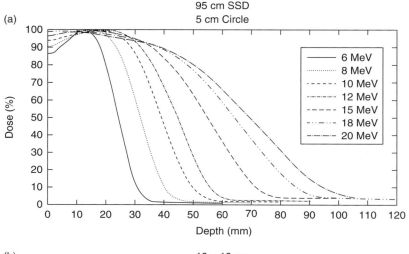

(b)
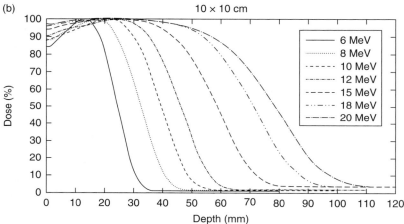

Figure 36.1 Electron depth dose curves for a 5 cm circle and 10 × 10 cm square at 95 cm SSD. Permission to print has been obtained from Mr David Prior, Physicist, Sussex Cancer Centre and Dr David Bloomfield, Head, Sussex Cancer Centre. Disclaimer: these graphs are for academic purposes only and apply to a specific machine and cancer centre. They should not be used to guide treatment for any patient. SSD, source–skin distance.

with carboplatin and etoposide, but the duration of response is short.

Malignant porocarcinoma and eccrine carcinoma

The adnexal structures include the eccrine sweat glands, hair follicles, sebaceous and apocrine glands, and the APUD system. The majority of tumours are benign. Eccrine carcinoma is histologically like an anaplastic squamous cell carcinoma, infiltrates locally and may metastasise. Some tumours may resemble salivary gland tumours and show features of adenoid cystic carcinoma. Malignant sebaceous gland tumours are rare but most frequently found in the eyelids. Surgical excision with a wide margin is the preferred treatment (Soutar and Robertson, 2001).

Kaposi's sarcoma

There are four different types of Kaposi's sarcoma (Safai, 1997):

- HIV-related Kaposi's sarcoma is the most common malignancy in people with AIDS. Treatment is almost always palliative. Kaposi's sarcoma can occur in the absence of HIV positivity;
- classical Kaposi's sarcoma occurs as an indolent condition most commonly affecting the lower limbs in elderly Ashkenazi Jews. It also occurs in patients from Mediterranean countries. There may be a link to immunosuppression because patients also have an increased incidence of non-Hodgkin lymphoma;
- endemic Kaposi's sarcoma is mainly found in sub-Saharan Africa, where it is more aggressive, occurs in children of both sexes, and causes

fulminant lymphadenopathy. Some men present with a benign nodular form of the disease; and

- Kaposi's sarcoma also occurs in immunosuppressed patients with a 400-fold increase in renal transplant recipients who are on long-term immunosuppressive therapy.

The clinical presentation is with small, painful, reddish or purple papules, nodules or plaques on the face, hard palate, gums, shins, lower legs and soles of the feet. The oral tumours can cause ulceration, haemorrhage and dental instability. Sometimes there can be marked oedema in the limbs, scrotum or face. Pulmonary and gastrointestinal involvement is common and all internal organs can be affected except the brain.

A symptomatic patient with Kaposi's sarcoma referred for palliative radiotherapy should be immediately referred to colleagues who specialise in HIV for HIV counselling and testing. If the patient is found to be HIV-positive, he or she is usually treated with highly active antiretroviral therapy (HAART). The patient should be reassessed in the radiotherapy department after 3 months of HAART, by which time some of the tumours may have resolved. If a tumour has not resolved by then, the patient should be offered palliative radiotherapy.

Nodular localised disease in the limbs can be treated with a single 8 Gy fraction with SXR or electron therapy depending on the site, size and thickness of the tumour. This procedure can be repeated if necessary and multiple tumours can also be treated.

Mucosal tumours in the mouth, palate, and conjunctiva are treated with 20 Gy in 10 fractions over 2 weeks to avoid acute radiotherapy reactions, which are more severe in patients with HIV-associated Kaposi's sarcoma.

Classic non-HIV-related disease is usually treated with 16 Gy in 4 fractions given over 8 days.

Palliative chemotherapy improves more than 50% of patients with more extensive disease. Liposomal doxorubicin (Safai, 1997) and paclitaxel are licensed for use in AIDs-related Kaposi's sarcoma. Reponses have also been seen with daunorubicin or vinorelbine.

Skin lymphomas

Mycosis fungoides

Mycosis fungoides is discussed in Chapter 34.

Primary cutaneous B-cell lymphoma

SXR or electrons may be used as appropriate. The PTV is typically the GTV plus a 2–3 cm margin. Appropriate doses include 15 Gy in 5 fractions over 1 week or 20 Gy in 5 fractions.

Malignant fibrous histiocytoma

Malignant fibrous histiocytoma is the most common soft tissue sarcoma in adults. It usually presents as a nodule, but the histological appearance is of a high-grade sarcoma. The prognosis is related to the size of the primary tumour, and it is best treated by wide local excision (Soutar and Robertson, 2001).

Dermatofibrosarcoma protuberans

Dermatofibrosarcoma protuberans is a slowly growing multinodular low-grade sarcoma that typically affects the trunk in young black males. Local recurrence is a major problem, whereas metastases are very rare. Wide local surgical excision is the treatment of choice using Mohs micrographic surgery (Soutar and Robertson, 2001).

Angiosarcoma and lymphosarcoma

Angiosarcomas without lymphoedema almost always occur on the face and scalp of adults over 50 years. Nodules or ulcerated areas occur within blue–red discoloured skin. Local recurrence and distant metastases to the lungs are both common. Postoperative radiotherapy is usually offered after surgery, but the prognosis is very poor.

Angiosarcoma with lymphoedema, or lymphangiosarcoma, may arise in the chest and breast following radiotherapy or in the upper limb following a history of chronic lymphoedema.

Lymphangiosarcoma can occur in postmastectomy lymphoedema and it is known as Stewart–Treves syndrome. Rapid lymphatic and haematogenous metastases occur, with a poor prognosis. Radical surgery with amputation is often undertaken in conjunction with postoperative radiation. Isolated limb perfusion is also used (Soutar and Robertson, 2001).

Secondary metastases

Secondary metastases can cause pain, bleeding or fungation. A single fraction of 8 Gy or 20 Gy in 5 fractions over 5 days with SXR therapy or electron therapy usually provides prompt symptomatic relief. Single fractions can frequently be repeated after several months.

The use of radiotherapy for keloid scar

A keloid is a benign fibrous overgrowth associated with scar formation.

Patients are treated with a 6 Gy single exposure with 100 kV photons if less than 2 cm. Larger keloids have a higher risk of recurring and so in these cases a dose schedule of 12 Gy in 3 fractions with 6–8 MeV electrons is recommended. Consider using 1 cm wet gauze to increase dose to skin. Use a minimal margin around the scar and include sutures. Alternatively, use an iridium implant giving 20 Gy at 2.5 mm, over 24 hours.

Radiotherapy is effective in 80% cases.

The procedure first requires careful excision of the existing scar first and then radiotherapy within 1–10 days.

References

American Cancer Society. (2003). *Cancer Facts and Figures.* Atlanta: American Cancer Society.

Avril, M. F., Auperin, A., Margulis, A., et al. (1997). Basal cell carcinoma of the face: surgery or radiotherapy? Results of a randomized study. *Br. J. Cancer*, **76**, 100–106.

Caccialanza, M., Piccinno, R., Moretti, D., et al. (2003). Radiotherapy of carcinomas of the skin overlying the cartilage of the nose: results in 405 lesions. *Eur. J. Dermatol.*, **13**, 462–465.

Coyle, C. (2005). The role of brachytherapy at miscellaneous sites: skin. In *Radiotherapy in Practice: Brachytherapy*, ed. P. Hoskin and C. Coyle. Oxford: Oxford University Press.

Dabski, K. and Helm, F. (1988). Topical chemotherapy. In *Skin Cancer: Recognition and Management*, ed. R. A. Schwartz. New York: Springer-Verlag, pp. 378–389.

Diepgen, T. L. and Mahler, V. (2002). The epidemiology of skin cancer. *Br. J. Dermatol.*, **146** (Suppl. 61), 1–6.

Lebwohl, M., Dinehart, S., Whiting, D., et al. (2004). Imiquimod 5% cream for the treatment of actinic keratosis: results from two phase III, randomised, double-blind, parallel group, vehicle-controlled trials. *J. Am. Acad. Dermatol.*, **50**, 714–721.

Lewis, K. G., Weinstock, M. A., Weaver, A. L., et al. (2006). Adjuvant local irradiation for Merkel cell carcinoma. *Arch. Dermatol.*, **142**, 693–700.

Lovett, R. D., Perez, C. A., Shapiro, S. J., et al. (1990). External irradiation of epithelial skin cancer. *Int. J. Radiat. Oncol. Biol. Phys.*, **19**, 235–242.

Malhotra, R., Huilgol, S. C., Huynh, N. T., et al. (2004). The Australian Mohs database, part II. Periocular basal cell carcinoma outcome at 5-year follow-up. *Ophthalmology*, **111**, 631–636.

National Comprehensive Cancer Network. (2005). Basal and squamous cell skin cancer guideline. In *The Complete Library of NCCN Clinical Practice Guidelines in Oncology, version 1*. Jenkintown, PA: National Comprehensive Cancer Network (CD-ROM).

NICE. (2006). *Improving Outcomes for People with Skin Tumours Including Melanoma*. London: National Institute for Health and Clinical Excellence.

NICE. (2010). *Improving Outcomes for People with Skin Tumours Including Melanoma (update): The Management of Low-risk Basal Cell Carcinomas in the Community*. London: National Institute for Health and Clinical Excellence.

Rubin, A. I., Chen, E. H. and Ratner, D. (2005). Basal-cell carcinoma. *N. Engl. J. Med.*, **353**, 2262–2269.

Safai, B. (1997). Kaposi's sarcoma and acquired immunodeficiency syndrome. In *AIDS: Epidemiology, Diagnosis, Treatment and Prevention*, ed. V. T. DeVita, S. Hellman and S. Rosenberg, 4th edn. Philadelphia, PA: Lippincott-Raven, pp. 295–358.

Sekulic, A., Migden, M. R., Oro, A. E., et al. (2012). Efficacy and safety of Vismodegib in advanced basal cell carcinoma. *N. Engl. J. Med.*, **366**, 2171–2179.

Sekulic, A., Migden, M. R., Baset-Seguin, N., et al. (2013). Long term safety and efficacy of vismodegib in patients with advanced basal cell carcinoma (aBCC): 18 month update of the pivotal ERIVANCE BCC study. *J. Clin. Oncol.*, **31** (Suppl.; abstr. 9037).

Solan, M. J., Brady, L. W., Binnick, S. A., et al. (1997). Skin. In *Principles and Practice of Radiation Oncology*, ed. C. A. Perez and L. W. Brady, 3rd edn. Philadelphia, PA: Lippincott-Raven, pp. 723–744.

Soutar, D. S. and Robertson, A. G. (2001). Skin cancer other than melanoma. In *Oxford Textbook of Oncology*, 2nd edn. Oxford: Oxford University Press, pp. 1235–1243.

Thomas, R. M. and Amonette, R. A. (1998). Mohs micrographic surgery. *Am. Fam. Physician*, **37**, 135–142.

Tran, H., Chen, K. and Shumack, S. (2003). Summary of actinic keratosis studies with imiquimod 5% cream. *Br. J. Dermatol.*, **149** (Suppl. 66), 37–39.

UICC. (2009). *TNM Classification of Malignant Tumours*, ed. L. H. Sobin, M. Gospodarowicz and Ch. Wittekind, 7th edn. Chichester: Wiley-Blackwell, pp. 165–168.

Chapter 37

Management of melanoma

Satish Kumar and Julie Martin

Introduction

Melanocytes originate in the neural crest of the embryo and migrate widely during development to locations such as the basal layer of the epidermis and the uveal tract. As a result, malignant melanoma (MM) can affect sites other than the skin, including the central nervous system (e.g. meninges and uveal tract) and the aerodigestive and genitourinary tracts (e.g. nasopharynx, oral cavity and vagina). Cutaneous melanoma has one of the fastest rising cancer incidences worldwide. In the UK it is the fifth commonest cancer and the second commonest cancer in the 15–34 year age group, with about 27% of cases occurring below the age of 50 (http://www.cancerresearchuk.org/, accessed February 2015).

Mortality rates have also increased over time, but less so than the increase in incidence because of improvements in the chance of survival from melanoma. Mortality rates appear to have stabilised in some countries, most notably Australia. A shift to proportionately more *in situ* and thin melanomas being diagnosed in the same period suggests that this reduction in mortality may be due to earlier detection (Coory *et al.*, 2006).

This chapter focuses on cutaneous melanoma, but will also cover some of the main features of the rarer subtypes such as mucosal and ocular melanoma.

Cutaneous melanoma

Types of cutaneous melanoma

The main clinicopathological varieties of cutaneous MM are superficial spreading, nodular, acral lentiginous and lentigo maligna melanoma.

Incidence and epidemiology

The annual age-standardised disease incidence of cutaneous melanoma in the UK is 17 per 100,000. Approximately 11,500 new cases are diagnosed per year in England and Wales, comprising 4% of all new cancer cases. Around 2000 deaths from melanoma occur annually in the UK (from Cancer Research UK, http://www.cancerresearchuk.org/, accessed February 2014).

The incidence of cutaneous melanoma has continued to rise worldwide for the last 40 years. The annual increase varies between populations, but in general has been in the order of 3–7% per year for fair-skinned Caucasian people. Some of this increase may be due to increased surveillance and therefore earlier detection, as well as changes in diagnostic criteria. However, most of the increase is considered real, and linked to changes in lifestyle resulting in excessive recreational exposure to sunlight (Lens and Dawes, 2004).

There is a wide geographical variation in incidence (see Table 37.1), and the diagnosis is 10-fold more common among whites than non-whites. Melanoma incidence increases with age, rising to a peak in incidence in the fourth and fifth decades.

Risk factors and aetiology

UV exposure

Excessive sun exposure, especially during childhood and leading to sunburn, is associated with an increased risk of developing MM. It has been estimated that two-thirds of the cases worldwide may be related to sun exposure. Just one episode of severe sunburn doubles the risk of developing MM. However, the complex association between genetic and environmental factors is

Table 37.1 World age-standardised incidence rates per 100,000 population (2008 estimates)

Population	Incidence (per 100,000 population)
Asian	4.8
Western Europe	22.6
United States	28.3
Australia and New Zealand	73

Adapted from Cancer Research UK (www.cancerresearchuk. org/cancer-info/cancerstats/types/skin/incidence/uk-s kin-cancer-incidence-statistics). Accessed September 2013.

Table 37.2 Risk factors for developing melanoma

Risk factor	Odds ratio for melanoma
11–50 common moles > 2 mm	1.7–1.9
51–100 common moles > 2 mm	3.2–3.7
> 100 common moles > 2 mm	7.6–7.7
Family history of melanoma	1.8
Presence of 1–4 atypical moles	1.6–7.3

Adapted from Roberts *et al.*, (2002).

shown by the fact that, unlike non-melanomatous skin cancers, patients do not necessarily develop tumours in sites of maximum sun exposure.

UV radiation through sunbed use is also a significant risk factor for developing MM. A recent meta-analysis has shown that sunbed use for the first time before age 35 increases the risk of MM by 59%, and use at any age increases MM risk by 20–25% (Boniol *et al.*, 2012).

Skin type

The risk of developing MM is higher in fair-skinned people with blond or red hair, who have a tendency to burn.

Melanocytic naevi

The number of common naevi, as well as the presence of atypical (dysplastic) naevi on a person's body correlates well with the risk of developing MM, as shown in Table 37.2.

Other risk factors

People with a family history of MM (particularly in a first-degree relative) have an increased risk of developing the disease. A genetic predisposition probably accounts for 5–10% of all cases. The major high-risk inherited susceptibility gene for MM is CDKN2A. The lifetime MM risk in carriers of mutations from families with germline mutations in CDKN2A is over 60%.

The inherited condition xeroderma pigmentosa is a risk factor.

Immunosuppressed people have an increased risk of developing MM. Patients receiving immunosuppressive therapy following organ transplant are at a threefold increased risk.

Extensive treatment with PUVA (psoralens and UVA therapy) is associated with the development of MM many years after treatment.

There have been reports of increased risk in patients developing MM during pregnancy and while on the oral contraceptive pill. These findings have not been confirmed in extensive studies, although reports of changes in moles during pregnancy have been recorded, and prompt diagnosis of suspicious areas should be made.

Vitamin D

There is some evidence that vitamin D may be protective against malignant transformation of melanocytes, and that lower levels contributed to by reduced sun exposure may predispose to MM as well as adverse effects on bone and cardiovascular health.

Screening and prevention

Early detection

There is no MM screening programme for the general population in the UK. For patients at a high risk of melanoma, various strategies are available, such as regular self-examination or examination by suitably qualified health professionals. Serial recording of images using conventional or digital photography can help in long-term monitoring.

Prevention

Based on current evidence, it seems sensible to avoid prolonged periods of direct sun exposure and to protect children from the same. If out in the sun, it is important to avoid sunburn by wearing loose-fitting clothing with generous cover, wide-brimmed hats and sunglasses. Additionally, sunscreen should be applied generously to exposed parts of the body such as the face, arms and legs and it should be remembered that the use of sunscreen should not lead to spending longer time in the sun than necessary.

Cancer Research UK's SunSmart campaign recommends the following (SunSmart, http://www.sunsmart.org.uk/, accessed October 2014).

- Spend time in the shade between 11 am and 3 pm.
- Avoid getting sunburnt.
- Cover up with a hat, t-shirt and sunglasses.
- Take extra care with sun protection for children.
- Use at least an SPF 15 sunscreen.

Pathology

By definition, MM involves atypical melanocytes that infiltrate into the dermis. There may be features of neighbouring dysplastic or benign pigmented lesions. There are four main types of MM with distinct clinicopathological characteristics. Breslow thickness and the presence or absence of ulceration primarily determine stage and treatment (surgery, adjuvant therapy and follow-up). Other features commonly reported in pathological data sets are number of mitoses, lymphovascular invasion and regression.

Superficial spreading melanoma (SSM)

Superficial spreading melanoma occurs in approximately 70% of cases; it accounts for the changing epidemiology in recent decades, usually arising from a dysplastic naevus. Macroscopically, SSMs are pigmented lesions that are often flat or with slight elevation. Typically they have an irregular border and irregular pigmentation. Microscopically, there is predominantly horizontal growth. Cytological variations occur (e.g. epithelioid, spindle cell, small naevoid-like, or giant cell).

Nodular melanoma (NM)

Nodular melanomas make up approximately 15% of cases; they form raised, nodular lesions which may vary in colour from blue–grey to completely amelanotic, and they are often associated with ulceration and/or bleeding. Microscopically they have no or minimal horizontal growth but extensive dermal invasion.

Acral lentiginous melanoma (ALM)

Acral lentiginous melanomas make up approximately 10% of cases; they occur on the palms, soles, subungual regions (most commonly great toe or thumb) and mucosal surfaces. ALMs are probably genetically distinct from SSM and less related to UV light exposure. Mucosal lesions are often diagnosed later. Microscopically there is acanthosis of the epidermis, atypical melanocytes with branching dendritic processes, and frequent spindle cells with marked desmoplastic reaction.

Lentigo maligna melanoma (LMM)

Lentigo maligna melanomas make up approximately 5% of cases; they occur in older patients, usually on the skin of the face, and they are almost certainly related to chronic sun exposure. The precursor condition, lentigo maligna (Hutchinson's freckle), is slow-growing with a long radial growth phase. About 5% progress to invasive LMM, which may be indicated by localised thickening of the lesion. Microscopically, there is lentiginous proliferation of atypical melanocytes, which is often associated with solar atrophy of the epidermis.

Depth of invasion

Cutaneous melanoma can be defined by its depth of invasion, which has important prognostic significance. The Breslow thickness is the depth in millimetres from the granular layer of the epidermis to the deepest identifiable tumour cells (Breslow, 1970). Clark's classification also defines melanoma by the depth of invasion, but is used less commonly than Breslow thickness (Clark et al., 1969; Table 37.3).

Spread

The skin, subcutaneous tissues and lymph nodes tend to be the first site of metastatic disease. Recurrences tend to occur most commonly in the first two years for thicker MMs, and thinner types tend to recur several years after diagnosis.

Local spread

After undergoing malignant transformation, melanoma becomes invasive by penetrating into and beyond the dermis. Initially there is a variable horizontal growth phase, followed by a vertical growth phase invading through dermis and into the surrounding structures.

Lymphatic spread

Satellite nodules and in-transit metastases

The observation that recurrences may develop in the scar or a short distance away from the original area

Table 37.3 Clark's classification for melanoma (level of invasion)

Level	Definition
I	Lesions involving only the epidermis (*in situ* melanoma); not an invasive lesion
II	Invasion of the papillary dermis but does not reach the papillary–reticular dermal interface
III	Invasion fills and expands the papillary dermis but does not penetrate the reticular dermis
IV	Invasion into the reticular dermis but not into the subcutaneous tissue
V	Invasion through the reticular dermis into the subcutaneous tissue

Adapted from Clark *et al.,* 1969.

Table 37.4 Clinical features suggestive of melanoma

Scheme	Description
Revised seven-point checklist	*Major features*
	Change in size of lesion
	Irregular pigmentation
	Irregular border
	Minor features
	Inflammation
	Change in sensation
	Largest diameter 7 mm or greater
	Oozing, crusting, or bleeding
ABCDE rule	A Asymmetry
	B irregular Border
	C irregular Colour
	D Diameter > 5 mm
	E Elevation

Adapted from MacKie (1989) and Fitzpatrick *et al.* (1988).

following primary excision is consistent with spread within lymphatics. Satellite nodules are defined as cutaneous or subcutaneous nodules that occur less than 2 cm from the primary tumour, in-transit lesions are beyond 2 cm but not beyond the draining lymph nodes. Satellite lesions and in-transit lesions signify dermal lymphatic involvement and represent stage 3 disease.

Lymph nodes

Regional lymph nodes are the most common sites of spread beyond the skin.

Metastatic spread

Haematogenous spread to the lungs, liver, bone, brain and skin occurs particularly with more invasive or thicker lesions. Melanomas can also disseminate to unusual locations such as the small bowel causing intussusception, the meninges, gallbladder and the adrenals.

Clinical presentation

The main clinical features of cutaneous melanoma are a pigmented lesion with an irregular edge and irregular pigmentation. Over 95% of patients report a change in size, shape or colour, whereas fewer than 50% describe a change in sensation or bleeding (Roberts *et al.*, 2002). Occasionally, melanoma present first in a lymph node or in the dermis without a previous cutaneous lesion or in distant sites such as the brain.

Melanoma more often involves the extremities in females and the head, neck and trunk in males. In dark-skinned people, malignant melanoma, when it does occur, tends to involve the palms and soles.

Suspicious pigmented areas are best examined in a good light with or without magnification and should be assessed using the seven-point checklist or ABCDE systems (see Table 37.4). The presence of any major feature in the seven-point checklist, or any of the features in the ABCDE system, is an indication for referral. The presence of minor features should increase suspicion.

Differential diagnosis of melanoma

The following can appear similar to MM.
- Basal cell papilloma (seborrhoeic keratosis).
- Pigmented basal cell carcinoma.
- Thrombosed angioma.
- Pyogenic granuloma.
- Dermatofibroma.

Investigation and staging

Dermatoscopy or epiluminescence microscopy (non-invasive 'microscopic' review of a suspicious lesion *in vivo*) can increase the diagnostic accuracy of melanoma in the hands of experienced clinicians.

The principal diagnostic investigation is excision of the lesion, which is critical to further management and determines prognosis. For smaller tumours, an excisional biopsy with a margin of 1–2 mm of normal skin is optimal. If the primary tumour is large and/

or the primary surgical therapy would be mutilating, an incisional biopsy is sometimes required. Although this specimen may not be representative of the whole for obtaining information on prognosis and there is a theoretical risk of disseminating MM cells, there is no evidence that this approach adversely affects the overall outcome (Roberts and Crosby, 2003). In either case, the biopsy should be taken with a view to a subsequent wider therapeutic excision if required; specimen orientation is required for correct histological interpretation.

The lymph nodes should be examined clinically in all cases. The role of sentinel lymph node biopsy (SLNB) as a staging investigation and treatment is discussed later in the chapter.

Routine staging investigations are not generally indicated and blood tests are unhelpful. However, in view of the significant improvements in treatment for advanced disease, it is possible, but unproven, that earlier detection of relapse could improve outcomes by earlier institution of effective therapies. In patients who are considered to have low-risk disease, those with stages I and IIA IIB and IIIA MM, staging CT scans should not routinely be done because of the low true-positive and high false-positive rates. In high-risk cases (stages IIC and IIIB or C) CT head, neck, thorax, abdomen and pelvis may be useful and radiological follow-up is considered, with CT scans 6-monthly for 3 years and annually thereafter to 5 years. Definitions of stages IIIA, B and C can be found in Balch *et al.*, 2009.

Stage classification

Reporting of certain histological features such as Clark's level and the presence of regression show high variability between pathologists, whereas other features such as Breslow thickness and ulceration show high concordance. In addition, tumour thickness, mitotic rate and the presence of ulceration are the most important histological prognostic indicators. This is reflected in the updated AJCC TNM staging classification and stage groupings (see Tables 37.5 and 37.6).

Treatment overview

The main aims of treatment are to detect MM as early as possible and to excise it with adequate margins but without unnecessarily mutilating the patient. Excisional surgery is very successful in the treatment of early or thin lesions. The extent of surgery and the role of routine lymph node dissection/biopsy have

Table 37.5 TNM staging classification for melanoma

Stage	Description
pTis	Melanoma *in situ*
pT1	Tumour ≤ 1.0 mm Breslow thickness
pT1a	With no ulceration and mitoses < 1/mm²
pT1b	With ulceration or mitoses ≥ 1/mm²
pT2	Tumour > 1.01–2.0 mm Breslow thickness
pT2a	Without ulceration
pT2b	With ulceration
pT3	Tumour 2.01–4.0 mm Breslow thickness
pT3a	Without ulceration
pT3b	With ulceration
pT4	Tumour > 4.0 mm Breslow thickness
pT4a	Without ulceration
pT4b	With ulceration
N1	Metastasis to one lymph node
N1a	Clinically occult (microscopic) metastasis
N1b	Clinically apparent (macroscopic) metastasis
N2	Metastasis to 2 or 3 regional nodes
N2a	Clinically occult (microscopic) metastasis
N2b	Clinically apparent (macroscopic) metastasis
N2c	Satellite or in-transit metastasis without nodal metastasis
N3	Metastasis in ≥ 4 regional nodes, or matted metastatic regional lymph nodes, or satellite or in-transit metastasis with metastasis in regional node(s)
M1	Distant metastasis
M1a	Metastasis to skin, subcutaneous tissues or distant lymph nodes
M1b	Metastasis to lung
M1c	Metastasis to all other visceral sites or distant metastasis at any site associated with an elevated serum lactic dehydrogenase

Adapted from Balch *et al.*, 2009.

been areas of active research and are discussed later. It is important to risk-stratify patients to identify those with high-risk disease who will benefit from both radiological and clinical follow-up. These patients should have access to oncology, surgery and dermatology if required.

Table 37.6 Stage groupings for melanoma

Stage group	Definition
0	Tis N0 M0
IA	T1a N0 M0
IB	T1b or T2a N0 M0
IIA	T2b or T3a N0 M0
IIB	T3b or T4a N0 M0
IIC	T4b N0 M0
III	Any T N1–3 M0
IV	Any T Any N M1

Adapted from Balch *et al.*, 2009.

Table 37.7 Excision margins recommended for cutaneous melanoma

Thickness of primary lesion (mm)	Margin of excision (cm)
≤ 1	1
1.01–2.0	1–2
2.01–4.0	2–3
> 4	3

From British Association of Dermatologists, UK guidelines for the management of cutaneous melanoma, http://www.sasds.co.za/images/Melanoma_Management_2010.pdf (accessed October 2014).

Metastatic melanoma is resistant to available standard cytotoxic therapy and radiotherapy. However, identifying the roles of BRAF and the immune system have led to significant advances in the treatment of advanced disease resulting in better survival. There is hope that these advances may lead to eradicating the disease in some patients with advanced disease.

Three agents have been approved by NICE in the last three years: ipilimumab, vemurafenib and dabrafenib (NICE, 2012a, 2012b, 2014a, 2014b).

New clinical guidelines incorporating these recommendations are due to be published by NICE during 2015.

Surgery

Surgery for the primary

Once a diagnosis of MM has been made, and in the absence of any evidence of metastatic disease, definitive surgery should be planned. Surgery involves a wide excision of the primary lesion. The epidermal margins taken depends on the Breslow thickness of the primary tumour. Current recommendations for surgical excision margins are based on five randomized controlled trials and a National Institutes of Health Consensus Panel and are shown in Table 37.7 (Marsden *et al.*, 2010).

Elective lymph node dissection (ELND)

Four RCTs including 1718 patients with no clinical evidence of lymph node metastases have investigated the role of ELND and concluded that there is no overall survival benefit for this procedure when it is used in addition to wide excision (Veronesi *et al.*, 1982; Sim *et al.*, 1986; Balch *et al.*, 1996, 2000). It is associated with greater short and long-term morbidity.

Elective completion node dissection is generally undertaken in the presence of a positive SLNB (below), and a therapeutic complete node dissection is the treatment of choice in patients with clinically palpable nodal disease (stages IIIB and IIIC).

Sentinel lymph node biopsy (SLNB)

SLNB involves the identification and biopsy of the first station lymph node that drains an affected area by the use of blue dye and/or radiolabelled colloid injected into the skin surrounding the primary lesion. The technique can successfully identify the sentinel node in up to 97% of cases. The current practice is that patients with a positive node should be offered radical node dissection.

The rationale for SLNB, followed by radical LN dissection if positive, is that early detection and removal of occult disease in regional nodes might improve regional disease control and possibly overall survival (Morton *et al.*, 2005; Ross, 2010). In many countries its value as a prognostic factor has made it part of the standard care of MM ≥ 1 mm Breslow thickness, but it is not universally accepted because there is no evidence that it does improve survival (Thomas, 2008; Boland and Gershenwald, 2012). In 2006, a large trial (MSTL-1) reported on 1269 patients who were randomised to either wide excision of the primary plus observation of the regional lymph nodes with lymphadenectomy if nodal relapse occurred, or wide excision and sentinel-node biopsy with immediate lymphadenectomy if nodal micrometastases were detected (Morton *et al.*, 2006). In the SLNB group, the presence of metastases in the sentinel node was the most important prognostic factor (5-year survival for the node-positive and node-negative groups was 72.3% versus 90.2%, HR for death = 2.48, $p < 0.001$).

The 5-year melanoma-specific survival rates were similar in the two groups (87.1% in the biopsy group, 86.6% in the observation group). However, a subgroup comparison showed that the rate of melanoma-specific deaths in the biopsy group was 26.2% among patients who underwent immediate lymphadenectomy compared with 48.7% in the observation group who underwent delayed lymphadenectomy. Ten-year follow-up of this trial with more than 2001 patients confirmed this result with improvement in disease-free survival in the biopsy group for both intermediate (HR = 0.76; $p = 0.01$) and thick tumours (HR = 0.70; $p = 0.03$). In the intermediate thickness group, melanoma-specific survival for patients with nodal metastasis was better for those in the biopsy group (HR 0.56; $p = 0.006$; Morton *et al.*, 2014).

The MSLT-1 also showed that, on completion lymphadenectomy, 88% of patients with a positive single sentinel node had no other affected lymph nodes. In the ongoing MSLT-2 trial, all patients undergo a biopsy and are then randomised to immediate node dissection or ultrasound monitoring.

Currently in the UK, SLNB may be considered in MM ≥ 1 mm Breslow thickness for prognostic information, or used in conjunction with adjuvant therapy trials, but it is not universally available. It clearly has an important role as a staging tool, but as yet there is no clear evidence for an overall survival benefit. Any patient being offered SNLB and ELND should be fully informed of the possible risks and benefits.

Adjuvant therapy

Interferon

Interferon is not generally offered as a standard adjuvant therapy for high-risk melanoma in the UK because of lack of evidence of a clinically significant survival benefit and its toxicity. It is sometimes offered to patients on the basis of improved relapse-free survival. However, a meta-analysis of 18 trials including over 10,000 patients found a statistically significant improvement in both disease-free (HR = 0.83; $p < 0.00001$) and overall survival (HR = 0.91; $p = 0.003$) (Mocellin *et al.*, 2013). Pegylated interferon is better tolerated than interferon A and has a licence in stage III disease, where it reduces relapse rates, and, for ulcerated primaries and microscopic node involvement, it improves overall survival (Eggermont *et al.*, 2012). An ongoing EORTC trial is evaluating pegylated interferon in this group of patients.

Adjuvant radiotherapy

Adjuvant radiotherapy (RT) has been used for several years after regional node dissection. Its proponents offer it to patients where the operative specimen shows multiple node involvement (3 or more), large size (3 cm or more) or with evidence of extracapsular involvement. Trial evidence suggests that it reduces local recurrence and improves disease-free survival but it does not improve overall survival (Burmeister *et al.*, 2012).

However, adjuvant RT causes significant morbidity with skin toxicity, lymphoedema and limb discomfort. Routine use of RT is not generally recommended, but an individualised approach based on the benefits and risks of treatment in selected patients may be appropriate.

Vitamin D

Based on the finding of low vitamin D levels in many melanoma patients and evidence that vitamin D may delay recurrence, draft recommendations of NICE guidelines suggest that newly diagnosed patients with low vitamin D levels should receive advice on supplementation.

Treatment for advanced disease

The management of advanced melanoma has changed significantly in recent years with the development and introduction of a number of new, effective agents. Current treatments and possible developments are based on inhibition of the BRAF oncogene in patients with a mutation (present in approximately 40–50% of cutaneous melanoma) and immunotherapy primarily with molecules acting on the immune regulatory mechanisms. As a result, all patients with metastatic melanoma and those falling into the high-risk groups should have their tumours evaluated for the BRAF mutation. The V600E mutation is by far the commonest of these mutations, although there are several others.

The success of these treatments has made the management of metastatic disease more complex and it is important that there is a multidisciplinary approach to treatment involving surgeons, dermatologists, physicians in other specialities, specialist and research nurses and oncologists. For example, managing the common skin toxicities of the BRAF inhibitors may require specialist advice by the dermatologist and managing high-grade colitis that can occur in about

15% of patients receiving ipilimumab therapy requires advice from a gastroenterologist.

Although the use of cytotoxic chemotherapy has reduced because of these more effective new treatments, it will continue to have a place in combination regimens, especially in patients with wild-type BRAF.

Surgery may be an option for managing patients with symptomatic solitary metastases, especially in the brain, but its use has not been shown to improve survival. The indications for surgery may increase to include resection of residual masses following immunotherapy treatment and/or resecting isolated progressive tumours when biological treatments have controlled disease elsewhere.

Decisions about the choice of initial systemic therapy for advanced disease depend on the BRAF mutation status, patient choice, quality of life and tumour kinetics. Sequential and cross-over trial designs aim to refine the clinical use of currently available drugs.

Choosing treatment

Melanoma is considered a heterogeneous disease and even in metastatic tumour specimens there is significant intra- and inter-tumour heterogeneity. Treatment decisions are based on genotyping because there are effective therapies that inhibit some of the commonest driver mutations. The BRAF activation mutation is found in between 40% and 60% of cutaneous melanomas, NRAS mutations occur in about 15% of cases (both being mutually exclusive). BRAF mutations occur in about 10% of mucosal melanomas but not in ocular melanoma, where GNAQ and GNA11 mutations have been found to occur in a high proportion of cases. In mucosal melanoma and in melanomas occurring in chronically sun-damaged skin, KIT mutations are found in about 20% of cases.

BRAF testing is done in several accredited genetic laboratories across the country and it is reasonable to test all high-risk primary melanomas and essential to do so in metastatic disease to aid management decisions.

BRAF and/or MEK inhibition

Two drugs are currently NICE-approved for stage IV metastatic melanoma patients harbouring the BRAF mutation: vemurafenib and dabrafenib. The BRIM 3 clinical trial established the role of vemurafenib and showed a 4-month improvement in overall survival compared to dacarbazine (McArthur et al., 2014). Dabrafenib has shown a similar survival improvement

(Hauschild et al., 2012). These small molecules have the advantage of crossing the blood–brain barrier and can treat brain metastases. Phase 3 trials have shown responses in the range of 50%, progression-free survival of 6–7 months and overall survival about 11 months. The BRAF inhibitors typically have a rapid onset of action, within a week, but the disease eventually becomes resistant. Common toxicities include cutaneous SCC and keratoacanthoma, skin rash, liver function abnormalities, arthralgia, asthenia, anorexia and a small chance of QT prolongation. They can be radiosensitising, and caution has to be exercised when giving concurrent radiotherapy.

To delay the onset of resistance, investigators have been evaluating the role of combining BRAF inhibitors with inhibitors of downstream molecules such as MEK. A large phase 3 trial comparing single-agent vemurafenib with combination of dabrafenib and tremetinib (a MEK inhibitor) has shown a survival improvement with the combination therapy and with fewer cutaneous SCC (the addition of a MEK inhibitor stops paradoxical activation of MAP kinase by BRAF inhibitors; Robert et al., 2015). Two other phase 3 trials have further confirmed the efficacy and safety of combination BRAF–MEK inhibitor therapy (Larkin et al., 2014; Long et al., 2014) with better progression-free survival rates compared to BRAF inhibitor monotherapy. Combination therapies improve the response rates to about 65–70%, PFS to 9 months and OS to 13–14 months.

It is likely that combination therapy will become an option for patients harbouring the BRAF mutation. The combination of dabrafenib and trametinib has been licensed but has yet to be evaluated by NICE.

Immunotherapy

The immune system is important in metastatic MM, as shown by lymphoid infiltration into tumour and surrounding tissues, and well-reported spontaneous remissions.

Immunotherapy as an option to treat MM has been investigated for decades with little success until recently.

In 2011, NICE approved the use of a CTLA4 monoclonal antibody, ipilimumab (a T-cell activator) on the basis of a phase 3 clinical trial that evaluated this agent in a pretreated cohort of metastatic melanoma patients. Ipilimumab showed low response rates of about 10% and was shown to improve overall survival by 3.6 months to 10 months (Hodi et al., 2010), but importantly longer-term follow-up data have shown approximately 20% of patients survive for 3 years or more. A pooled analysis of more than 1800 patients has shown that the flattening of the Kaplan–Meier survival curves at the 3-year time point has been durable with a significant proportion of these patients continuing to be alive for as long as 10 years (Schadendorf *et al.*, 2013).

Ipilimumab is also approved for use in the first-line setting. The commonest side effects are fatigue, rash and diarrhoea. The major complication of this therapy is the onset of immune-mediated toxicity, severe in 10–15% of treated patients. There are established guidelines for managing all such toxicities based on the reversal of the immune activation with the use of high-dose corticosteroids. All patients need to be advised to be proactive and maintain close contact with the treating team in managing potentially dangerous side effects such as diarrhoea (colitis), lethargy and visual disturbances (which may signify hypopituitarism and requires a high index of suspicion). Use of the drug is generally avoided in patients with pre-existing autoimmune conditions, and patients thought to be at risk generally have a hepatitis and HIV screen.

Two more new 'second-generation' immunotherapeutic molecules are the 'programmed death 1 protein' (PD-1) inhibitors, pembrolizumab and nivolumab. These are PD-1 and PD-L1 monoclonal antibodies which potentiate the T-cell anti-tumour response by impairing an inhibitory interaction between programmed death receptors on T cells and their ligands on cancer cells. This selectivity results in a better toxicity profile with fewer immunological adverse events. Responses are in excess of 50% with most being durable to 2 years and beyond, but early phase trials have shown these treatments to be very toxic. Evidence for the use of pembrolizumab in second line treatment following failure of ipilimumab and BRAF/MEK inhibition comes from a randomised phase 2 trial, where pembrolizumab showed improved progression free survival compared with investigator choice chemotherapy. It also showed a low incidence of toxicity such as fatigue, oedema, myalgia, colitis and diarrhoea, all of which occurred in 1% or fewer of patients (Ribas *et al.*, 2015). Pembrolizumab also had a superior response (33%), 6 month progression free survival (46%), 12 month overall survival and toxicity profile when compared to ipilimumab in the first line setting (Robert *et al.*, 2015).

Nivolumab, alone or in combination with ipilimumab, has been shown to be superior to ipilimumab alone in patients with advanced melanoma. The combination is however associated with a significant toxicity rate in excess of 50%. Tumour PD-L1 levels were not sufficiently effective at predicting response to nivolumab because responses were seen in patients with tumours that did not over express this protein (Larkin *et al.*, 2015). Nivolumab has been shown to be superior to ipilimumab and chemotherapy in other phase 3 trials in both untreated and treated patients (Robert *et al.*, 2015; Weber *et al.*, 2015).

Summary of PD-L1 inhibitors: Pembrolizumab and nivolumab Pembrolizumab and nivolumab have shown to be superior to ipilimumab with a shorter onset of action, better and more durable responses, improved progression free and overall survival and significantly better toxicity profiles. Response rates in excess of 70% (in tumours expressing PD-L1) have been demonstrated for the combination approach but with immune toxicities occurring in more than 50% of patients (Larkin *et al.*, 2015). It is likely that both these drugs will replace ipilimumab as the immunotherapy of first choice for most patients with advanced melanoma.

It is important to note that criteria to assess response to therapy such as RECIST v1.1 may be inadequate to assess responses seen with immunotherapeutic agents because there may be initial disease progression followed by a delayed response. It is recommended that immune response criteria be used by those evaluating responses to this drug (Wolchok *et al.*, 2009).

Chemotherapy

Despite the advances in biological treatments, chemotherapy is likely to continue to have a role in some patients such as those with BRAF wild-type tumours and those who have progressed or are not eligible for current standard treatments. Dacarbazine and more recently temozolomide have been standard treatments, but these have been replaced by the newer treatments. Several other cytotoxics such as the taxanes, platinum compounds and vinca alkaloids have some activity in MM. Current clinical interest is centred on the taxanes in combination with small molecules, which have shown responses in preclinical trials and are the subjects of ongoing study.

Isolated limb perfusion and limb infusion

Isolated limb perfusion, using melphalan with or without tumour necrosis factor, can be useful for peripheral, usually lower-limb, melanomas where the primary tumour is unresectable, are multiple, or has extensive in-transit metastases.

Electrochemotherapy

This may be useful for selected patients with troublesome cutaneous melanomatous deposits which are deemed inoperable. Patients are infused with a chemotherapeutic agent (usually bleomycin). Electrodes are then inserted into the tumour that requires treatment. The electrical charge disrupts cell membranes and aids delivery of the cytotoxic drug to the tumour cytoplasm. In melanoma, clinical trials have shown complete responses in the region of 56% and objective responses of 80.6% (Mali et al., 2013). The treatment is only available in specialist centres.

Radiotherapy

Radiotherapy can prevent or treat ulceration, bleeding and pain from unresectable lymph node disease, and subcutaneous or bone metastases. In this situation, relatively high-dose and hypofractionated regimens should be used to overcome the 'shoulder effect' seen in radioresistant cell survival curves (Steel, 2002); for example, 6 Gy per fraction given weekly for 5–6 weeks.

Stereotactic radiotherapy can be effective for treating isolated or a limited number of intracranial metastases, when surgery is not deemed possible or appropriate (Hanson et al., 2012). The best results are obtained in patients with small-volume intracranial disease, controlled extracranial disease and a good performance status. Whole-brain radiotherapy for multiple brain metastases is now reserved for symptomatic patients who have a good performance status and have controlled extracranial disease. BRAF inhibitors are now considered the most appropriate first-line treatment for those with multiple brain metastases which have the BRAF mutation.

Prognosis

With the introduction of newer treatments into routine clinical practice, a small but significant proportion of patients with metastatic disease can have a long remission. The survival of MM by stage is shown in Table 37.8. Historically, for stage IV, survival figures ranged from about 2–4 months for brain metastasis patients to about 12–18 months in those with skin and lymph node only disease. Only about 5% survived 5 years or more. However, with current treatments, around a fifth of patients treated can expect to survive 3 years or more.

Prognostic factors

Prognostic factors at time of presentation are as follows (Balch et al., 2004).

Table 37.8 Approximate 5-year survival for cutaneous melanoma by stage

Stage	Prognosis (approximate 5-year survival, %)
I	91
II	64
III	40

Adapted from Ben-Porat et al. (2006).

- Tumour thickness – the principal prognostic factors for patients with early MM (stages I–III) relate to the depth of invasion of the primary lesion. The level of invasion, or Clark level, is strongly correlated with outcome, but is not as reproducible among pathologists.
- Ulceration – the absence of an intact epidermis diagnosed histologically is associated with a doubling of the risk associated with the depth of penetration.
- Lymph nodes – the prognosis worsens with the number of nodes involved. A thin lesion (Breslow depth < 0.76 mm) without lymph node involvement has a 3% risk of metastasising in 5 years, whereas if regional lymph nodes are macroscopically involved there is a less than 20–50% chance of surviving 5 years.
- Gender – most studies have shown a better prognosis for females than males.
- Anatomical location – tumours on the extremities appear to have a better prognosis than those on the trunk.
- Age – older patients tend to have thicker lesions, are male with tumours on the head and neck and have ulcerated tumours at the time of diagnosis.

There is evidence that Vitamin D deficiency might lead to lower melanoma-specific survival and higher levels may be protective for disease relapse and survival (Newton-Bishop et al., 2009).

In metastatic disease, prognosis depends on age, number and extent of metastasis, with brain and large-volume visceral metastasis having worse outcomes.

Areas of current interest

Adjuvant therapy

The success of systemic therapy in stage IV disease has led to enthusiasm for clinical trials such as BRIM 8 examining the role of adjuvant vemurafenib and combination dabrafenib/trametinib. Adjuvant ipilimumab improves recurrence-free survival, but overall survival data are not yet available (Eggermont *et al.*, 2014).

Systemic therapy in stage IV metastatic disease

Despite recent advances in advanced stages of disease, the majority of patients die of their disease and there is a need to improve current treatments. Unanswered questions remain about the optimal sequence of treatments in the different BRAF-mutated cancers, and there are efforts to evaluate different combination treatments including BRAF/MEK inhibitors, checkpoint molecules (CTLA4 and PD-1/PD-L1) and radiotherapy.

Current and future clinical trials in cutaneous melanoma

In the adjuvant setting, the roles of biological therapies such as dabrafenib in combination with trametinib (COMBI-AD study) or vemurafenib (BRIM 8 study) are currently being studied in BRAF mutation-positive patients. Peginterferon alfa-2b is the subject of the adjuvant study EORTC 18081 in ulcerated melanoma greater than 1 mm Breslow thickness.

In the metastatic setting, the CHEKMATE study of ipilimumab versus nivolumab versus combination recruitment has completed and results are awaited. A trial of 3 mg versus 10 mg of ipilimumab has also completed recruitment.

The COLUMBUS study is looking a combination of LGX818 or LGX818 plus MEK162 compared with vemurafenib for patients with unresectable stage IIIC or stage IV melanoma with BRAF V600 mutations.

For advanced disease in the BRAF wild-type population, the NEMO study is evaluating MEK162 versus dacarbazine in patients with unresectable melanoma with NRAS mutation-positive melanoma and the PACMEL study is a randomised phase 2 study of paclitaxel with or without GSK1120212 or pazopanib in advanced BRAF melanoma.

Mucosal melanoma

Mucosal melanoma makes up around 1–2% of all melanomas. It is an aggressive form of melanoma that typically affects the head and neck aerodigestive tracts and the urogenital–rectal regions. It differs from cutaneous melanoma in its pathophysiology because 20% of patients have the KIT mutation and about 10% the BRAF mutation, and the modes of spread and prognosis

are different. Blood-borne metastases occur frequently by the time of presentation or shortly afterwards.

Surgery is the main treatment, with the aim of wide excision of the tumour with clear resection margins. In the head and neck region, consideration is often given to postoperative radiotherapy (when resection margins are involved or regional spread to lymph nodes in the neck have resulted in large nodes with extracapsular spread). The aim of radiotherapy is to reduce local recurrence, although this probably does not affect overall survival. Distant metastases typically lead to a poor prognosis, although recently KIT inhibitors such as imatinib have been used with some success. Immunotherapy has also been used, based on its activity in cutaneous melanoma, but cytotoxic therapy is largely ineffective.

Ocular melanoma

Incidence and epidemiology

After the skin, the eye is the second commonest site of melanoma, but it is still rare. The incidence is approximately 0.7 in 100,000 patients: fewer than 500 new cases are diagnosed each year in the UK, usually in patients in the fifth and sixth decades. Unlike cutaneous melanoma, the incidence has remained relatively stable over time. For ocular melanomas, 85% of tumours arise from melanocytes in the highly vascular, subretinal choroid (tumours in the iris, ciliary body and conjunctiva are much less common). It is associated with the dysplastic naevus syndrome, neurofibromatosis, basal cell carcinoma (Gorlin) syndrome and BRCA2 +ve breast/ovarian cancer. The tumours are usually a mixture of spindle and epithelioid cells, a predominance of the latter being associated with a poorer prognosis. As with cutaneous tumours, their colour may vary from deeply pigmented to amelanotic. They are usually dome-shaped tumours, but they may infiltrate in a mushroom-like growth pattern through the Bruch membrane.

Clinical features and spread

Patients may present with flashing lights, visual distortion or with a visual field defect; in general, the further away the tumour is from the optic nerve, the larger the defect before the patient notices a problem. Associated retinal detachment can cause more sudden vision loss. Other patients may present with a red eye due to anterior extension or a vitreous haemorrhage.

Metastatic disease is mainly blood-borne and the liver is the most common site, followed by the lungs, bone and brain. Distant spread often occurs by the time of diagnosis. Secondary disease may appear 10 years or longer after diagnosis of the primary, but is most common in the first 12 months.

Investigation

A diagnosis can usually be made by opthalmoscopy, but fluorescein angiography and ultrasound/MRI can help confirm the diagnosis. In experienced institutions, a correct diagnosis can be made without histological confirmation in 98% of cases. Biopsies are occasionally taken, particularly for more accessible anterior tumours.

Treatment

Patients are typically referred to one of four specialist centres in the UK for evaluation (Liverpool, Glasgow, Sheffield and London). For small tumours the preferred treatment is with brachytherapy (scleral plaque therapy). Proton beam radiotherapy is used for tumours that are too large to be treated with plaques or for those in locations where it is not possible to place a plaque, such as near the optic nerve. The optimal treatment for large choroidal tumours is enucleation. Observation may be preferable for slow-growing tumours which typically occur near the iris or for patients who are unfit for radiotherapy or surgery.

Scleral plaque therapy

Scleral plaques are sutured during a surgical procedure in which the tumour is located with transillumination. The dose is 80–100 Gy delivered to the apex of the lesion with low-energy gamma emitting isotopes, most commonly ^{125}I or ruthenium (^{106}Ru), shielded externally by gold. Treatment takes 2–10 days. The Collaborative Ocular Melanoma Study (COMS), which involved more than 1300 patients who were randomised to receive either enucleation or ^{125}I plaque brachytherapy, found no difference in survival between treatments (Diener-West et al., 2001). For patients receiving brachytherapy, there was a 10% risk of local treatment failure, 85% retained their eye and 37% had normal visual acuity 5 years after treatment. Patients eligible for brachytherapy in the COMS trial had tumours larger than 2.5 mm and smaller than 10 mm in diameter and less than 16 mm thick.

Charged particle therapy

Charged particle therapy (helium ions and proton beam) takes advantage of precisely focused pencil-beam radiation that has well-defined penetrating depths due to sudden decelerating energy dispersion (the Bragg peak) to deliver high doses to the target volume while sparing normal tissues. The target volume is defined by placing inert clips during surgery and accurately measuring tumour dimensions relative to these clips by studying retinal photographs and by performing ultrasound biometry of the globe prior to 3D planning. Patients require shell immobilisation. This procedure achieves local control that is comparable to that of brachytherapy, but the treatment is limited by the availability of equipment, which includes a cyclotron, to units such as Clatterbridge, Liverpool and is often reserved for patients with tumours thicker than 8–10 mm. Damato et al. (2005) reported a series of 349 patients treated in Liverpool with proton beam therapy to a dose of 53.1 Gy in 4 fractions. The 5-year local recurrence rate was 3.5% and 9.4% for subsequent enucleation. For conservation of vision, 79.1% retained counting of fingers or better and 44.8% retained vision of 20/40 or better.

Detection of metastatic disease

Patients with adverse histopathological and genetic features such as the presence of monosomy 3 have a worse 10-year survival than other patients. Prognostic information is routinely made available by the reference centres in the UK to help identify patients that may benefit from regular hepatic ultrasound or, more recently, MRI scans of the liver. Although it is not clear if early detection of liver metastasis this way will improve survival, earlier detection increases the chance of doing a surgical resection or other ablative treatment. There are many experimental therapies directed at the liver, but this is limited by general availability and it is useful to seek an opinion from large centres that have experience with these modalities.

Recently, the MEK inhibitor selumetinib has shown some activity in metastatic uveal melanoma, on the basis of which the SUMIT trial has opened. This is a randomised study to assess selumetinib in combination with dacarbazine compared with placebo plus dacarbazine as first systemic therapy in patients with metastatic uveal melanoma.

References

Balch, C. M., Soong, S. J., Bartolucci, A. A., *et al.* (1996). Efficacy of an elective regional lymph node dissection of 1 to 4 mm thick melanomas for patients 60 years of age and younger. *Ann. Surg.*, **224**, 255–266.

Balch, C. M., Soong, S., Ross, M. I., *et al.* (2000). Long-term results of a multi-institutional randomized trial comparing prognostic factors and surgical results for intermediate thickness melanomas (1.0 to 4.0 mm). *Ann. Surg. Oncol.*, **7**, 87–97.

Balch, C. M., Atkins, M. B. and Sober, A. J. (2004). Cutaneous melanoma. In *Cancer: Principles and Practice of Oncology*, Ed. V. T. Devita, Jr., S. Hellman and S. A. Rosenberg, 7th edn. Philadelphia, PA: JB Lippincott, pp. 1754–1808.

Balch, C. M., Gershenwald, J. E., Soong, S., *et al.* (2009). Final version of 2009 AJCC melanoma staging and classification. *J. Clin. Oncol.*, **27**, 6199–6206.

Ben-Porat, L., Panageas, K. S., Hanlon, C., *et al.* (2006). Estimates of stage-specific survival are altered by changes in the 2002 American Joint Committee on Cancer staging system for melanoma. *Cancer*, **106**, 163–171.

Boland, G. M. and Gershenwald, J. E. (2012). Sentinel lymph node biospy in melanoma. *Cancer J.*, **18**, 185–191.

Boniol, M., Autier, P., Boyle P, *et al.* (2012). Cutaneous melanoma attributable to sunbed use: systematic review and meta-analysis. *Br. Med. J.*, **345**, e4757.

Breslow, A. (1970). Thickness, cross-sectional areas and depth of invasion in the prognosis of cutaneous melanoma. *Ann. Surg.*, **172**, 902–908.

Burmeister, B. H., Henderson, M. A., Ainslie, J., *et al.* (2012). Adjuvant radiotherapy versus observation alone for patients at risk of lymph-node field relapse after therapeutic lymphadenectomy for melanoma: a randomised trial. *Lancet Oncol.*, **13**, 589–597.

Chapman, P. B., Einhorn, L. H., Meyers, M. L., *et al.* (1999). Phase III multicenter randomised trial of the Dartmouth regimen versus dacarbazine in patients with metastatic melanoma. *J. Clin. Oncol.*, **17**, 2745–2751.

Clark, W. H. Jr., From, L., Bernardino, E. A., *et al.* (1969). The histogenesis and biologic behaviour of primary human malignant melanomas of the skin. *Cancer Res.*, **29**, 705–726.

Coory, M., Baade,.P, Aitken, J., *et al.* (2006). Trends for in-situ and invasive melanoma in Queensland, Australia, 1982–2002. *Cancer Causes Control*, **17**, 21–27.

Damato, B., Kacperek, A., Chopra, M., *et al.* (2005). Proton beam radiotherapy of choroidal melanoma: the Liverpool-Clatterbridge experience. *Int. J. Radiat. Oncol. Biol. Phys.*, **62**, 1405–1411.

Diener-West, M., Earle, J. D., Fine, S. L., *et al.* (2001). The COMS randomized trial of iodine 125 brachytherapy for choroidal melanoma, III: initial mortality findings. COMS Report No. 18. *Arch. Ophthalmol.*, **119**, 969–982.

Eggermont, A. M., Suciu, S., Testori, A., *et al.* (2012). Long-term results of the randomized phase III trial EORTC 18991 of adjuvant therapy with pegylated interferon alfa-2b versus observation in resected stage III melanoma. *J. Clin. Oncol.*, **30**, 3810–3818.

Eggermont, A. M., Chiarion-Sileni, V., Grob, J. J., *et al.* (2014). Ipilimumab versus placebo after complete resection of stage III melanoma: Initial efficacy and safety results from the EORTC 18071 phase III trial. *J. Clin. Oncol.*, **32**(5), Suppl.; abstr. LBA9008.

Fitzpatrick, T. B., Rhodes, A. R., Sober, A. J., *et al.* (1988). Primary malignant melanoma of the skin: the call for action to identify persons at risk; to discover precursor lesions; to detect early melanomas. *Pigment Cell*, **9**, 110–117.

Fuss, M., Loredo, L. N., Blacharski, P. A., *et al.* (2001). Proton radiation therapy for medium and large choroidal melanoma: preservation of the eye and its functionality. *Int. J. Radiat. Oncol. Biol. Phys.*, **49**, 1053–1059.

Hanson, P. W., Elaimy, A. L., Lamoreaux, W. T., *et al.* (2012). A concise review of the efficacy of stereotactic radiosurgery in the management of melanoma and renal cell carcinoma brain metastases. *World J. Surg. Oncol.*, **10**, 176.

Hauschild, A., Grob, J. J., Demidov, L. V., *et al.* (2012). Dabrafenib in *BRAF*-mutated metastatic melanoma: a multicentre, open-label,phase 3 randomised controlled trial. *Lancet*, **380**, 358–365.

Hodi, F. S., O'Day, S. J., McDermott, D. F., *et al.* (2010). Improved survival with ipilimumab in patients with metastatic melanoma. *N. Engl. J. Med.*, **363**, 711–723.

Larkin, J., Ascierto, P. A., Dréno, B., *et al.* (2014). Combined vemurafenib and cobimetinib in BRAF-mutated melanoma. *N. Engl. J. Med.*, **371**, 1867–1876.

Larkin, J., Chiarion-Sileni, V., Gonzalez, R., *et al.* (2015). Combined nivolumab and ipilimumab or monotherapy in untreated melanoma. *N. Engl. J. Med.*, **373**, 23–34.

Lens, M. B. and Dawes, M. (2004). Global perspectives of contemporary epidemiogical trends of cutaneous malignant melanoma. *Br. J. Dermatol.*, **150**, 179–185.

Long, G. V., Stroyakovskiy, D., Gogas, H., *et al.* (2014). Combined *BRAF* and MEK inhibition versus *BRAF* inhibition alone in melanoma. *N. Engl. J. Med.*, **371**, 1877–1888.

MacKie, R. M. (1989). *Malignant Melanoma: A Guide to Early Diagnosis*. Glasgow: University of Glasgow.

Mali, B., Jarm, T., Snog, M., *et al.* (2013). Antitumor effectiveness of electrochemotherapy: a systematic review and meta-analysis. *Eur. J. Surg. Oncol.*, **39**, 4–16.

Marsden, J. R., Newton-Bishop, J. A., Burrows, L., *et al.* (2010). Revised U.K. Guidelines for the management of cutaneous melanoma 2010. *Br. J. Dermatol.*, **163**, 238–256.

McArthur, G. A., Chapman, P. B., Robert, C., *et al.* (2014). Safety and efficacy of vemurafenib in *BRAF*(V600E) and *BRAF*(V600K) mutation-positive melanoma (BRIM-3): extended follow-up of a phase 3, randomised, open-label study. *Lancet Oncol.*, **3**, 323–332.

Mocellin, S., Lens, M. B., Pasquali, S., *et al.* (2013). Interferon alpha for the adjuvant treatment of cutaneous melanoma. *Cochrane Database Syst Rev.*, **6**, CD008955.

Morton, D. L., Cochran, A. J., Thompson, J. F., *et al.* (2005). Sentinel node biopsy for early stage melanoma – accuracy and morbidity in MSLT-1, an international multi-centre trial. *Ann. Surg.*, **242**, 302–313.

Morton, D. L., Thompson, J. F., Cochran, A. J., *et al.* (2006). Sentinel-node biopsy or nodal observation in melanoma. *N. Engl. J. Med.*, **355**, 1307–1317.

Morton, D. L., Thompson, J. F., Cochran, A. J., *et al.* (2014). Final trial report of sentinel-node biopsy versus nodal observation in melanoma. *N. Engl. J. Med.*, **370**, 599–609.

Newton-Bishop, J. A., Beswick, S., Randerson-Moor, J., *et al.* (2009). Serum 25-hydroxyvitamin D3 levels are associated with Breslow thickness at presentation and survival from melanoma. *J. Clin. Oncol.*, **27**, 5439–5444.

NICE. (2012a). *Ipilumumab for Previously Treated Advanced (Unresectable or Metastatic) Melanoma. Technology Appraisal Guidance [TA268].* London: National Institute for Health and Care Excellence.

NICE. (2012b). *Vemurafenib for Treating Locally Advanced or Metastatic BRAF V600 Mutation-Positive Malignant Melanoma. Technology Appraisal Guidance [TA269].* London: National Institute for Health and Care Excellence.

NICE. (2014a). *Ipilumumab for Previously Treated Advanced (Unresectable or Metastatic) Melanoma. Technology Appraisal Guidance [TA319].* London: National Institute for Health and Care Excellence.

NICE. (2014b). *Dabrafenib for Treating Unresectable or Metastatic BRAF V600 Mutation-Positive Melanoma. Technology Appraisal Guidance [TA321].* London: National Institute for Health and Care Excellence.

Ribas, A., Puzanov, I., Dummer, R., *et al.* (2015). Pembrolizumab versus investigator-choice chemotherapy for ipilimumab-refractory melanoma.

(KEYNOTE-002): a randomised, controlled, phase 2 trial. *Lancet Oncol.*, **16**, 908–918.

Robert, C., Karaszewska, B., Schachter, J., *et al.* (2015). Improved overall survival in melanoma with combined dabrafenib and trametinib. *N. Engl. J. Med.*, **372**, 30–39.

Robert, C., Long, G. V., Brady, B., *et al.* (2015). Nivolumab in previously untreated melanoma without BRAF mutation. *N. Engl. J. Med.* **372**, 320–330.

Roberts, D. L., Anstey, A. V., Barlow, R. J., *et al.* (2002). U.K. guidelines for the management of cutaneous melanoma. *Br. J. Dermatol.*, **146**, 7–17.

Roberts, D. and Crosby, T. (2003). Cutaneous melanoma. In *BMJ Books. Evidenced Based Dermatology*, ed. H. Williams, M. Bigby, T. Diegpen *et al.* Oxford: Blackwell Publishing, Chapter 24.

Ross, M. I (2010). Sentinel node biopsy for melanoma: an update after two decades of experience. *Semin. Cut. Med. Surg.*, **29**, 238–248.

Schadendorf, D., Hodi, F. S., Robert, C., *et al.* (2013). Pooled analysis of long-term survival data from phase II and phase III trials of ipilimumab in metastatic or locally advanced, unresectable melanoma. *Eur. J. Cancer*, **49**, Suppl. 3, abstr. LBA 24.

Sim, F. H., Taylor, W. F., Pritchard, D. J., *et al.* (1986). Lymphadenectomy in the management of stage I malignant melanoma: a prospective randomized study. *Mayo Clin. Proc.*, **61**, 697–705.

Steel, G. G. (2002). *Basic Clinical Radiobiology*, 3rd edn. London: Arnold.

Thomas, J. M. (2008). Sentinel lymph node biopsy in malignant melanoma. *Br. Med. J.*, **336**, 902–903.

Veronesi, U., Adamus, J., Bandiera, D. C., *et al.* (1982). Delayed regional lymph node dissection in stage I melanoma of the skin of the lower extremities. *Cancer*, **49**, 2420–2430.

Weber, J. S., D'Angelo, S. P., Minor, D., *et al.* (2015). Nivolumab versus chemotherapy in patients with advanced melanoma who progressed after anti-CTLA-4 treatment (CheckMate 037): a randomised, controlled, open-label, phase 3 trial. *Lancet Oncol.*, **16**, 375–384.

Wolchok, J. D., Hoos, A., O'Day, S., *et al.* (2009). Guidelines for the evaluation of immune therapy activity in solid tumors: immune-related response criteria. *Clin. Cancer Res.*, **15**, 7412–7420.

Chapter 38

Management of cancer of the thyroid

Laura Moss

Introduction

Thyroid cancer is a diverse group of tumours with different clinical features and prognoses. It can occur at any age, but is uncommon in patients under the age of 25. Radiation exposure is the best-documented risk factor. Most thyroid cancers are carcinomas: papillary, follicular, medullary and anaplastic, in order of frequency. Thyroid lymphomas and sarcomas are rarer. The overall prognosis is related to the histological type. Well-differentiated thyroid cancer (papillary and follicular) has the best prognosis while anaplastic carcinoma progresses rapidly and has a very poor prognosis. There is limited evidence from prospective randomised controlled studies to guide management in differentiated thyroid cancer because it is an uncommon disease with a long natural history. Many areas of thyroid cancer management are controversial, including the extent of surgery and the indications for radioiodine ablation and radiotherapy. Evidence-based guidelines published in 2014 relied on large retrospective and cohort studies (Perros *et al.*, 2014).

This chapter focuses mainly on differentiated thyroid cancer, with shorter sections on medullary thyroid carcinoma (MTC), anaplastic thyroid cancer and thyroid lymphoma. There is also a short section on treatment of thyrotoxicosis at the end of the chapter.

Types of thyroid tumour

Thyroid tumours can be divided into benign, malignant primary and malignant secondary. Types of thyroid tumour are shown in Table 38.1.

The relative proportions of patients with differentiated thyroid cancer in a geographic area depend on dietary iodine intake, with the proportion of follicular cancers increasing where there is dietary iodine deficiency.

Table 38.1 The range of thyroid tumours

Type of tumour	Examples (approximate incidence %)
Benign	Follicular adenoma – single or multiple; variant = Hürthle cell adenoma
Malignant primary	*Differentiated thyroid cancer*
	Papillary (PTC: 80%)
	Follicular (FTC: 5–20%)
	Other carcinomas
	Medullary (8–12%, of which 75–80% are sporadic)
	Anaplastic (1–3%)
	Other malignant tumours
	Lymphoma (5%) (DLBCL and MALT types)
	Sarcoma
Malignant secondary	Melanoma
	Renal
	Breast
	Lung

DLBCL, diffuse large B-cell lymphoma; MALT, mucosa-associated lymphoid tissue.

Anatomy

The thyroid develops from an endodermal outgrowth from the midline of the pharyngeal floor, which then becomes the thyroglossal duct and elongates before developing into two lobes. The solid cord joining the gland to the tongue then disappears.

The thyroid consists of two lobes connected by the isthmus, and it weighs 15–20 g. It is very vascular and is surrounded by a sheath derived from the pretracheal

Practical Clinical Oncology, Second Edition, ed. Louise Hanna, Tom Crosby and Fergus Macbeth. Published by Cambridge University Press. © Cambridge University Press 2015.

fascia. The apex of each lobe can reach up to the oblique line on the thyroid cartilage and the base lies at the level of the fourth or fifth tracheal ring. The isthmus overlies the second, third and fourth tracheal rings. The pyramidal lobe is often present and extends up from the isthmus. The posterior aspect of each lobe is related to the four parathyroid glands, inside the fascial capsule of the thyroid gland behind the middle and inferior parts of the gland. The recurrent laryngeal nerve passes deep to the thyroid gland and is closely related to it, lying in the groove between the trachea and the oesophagus.

The first-station nodes are paralaryngeal, paratracheal and prelaryngeal within the central compartment or level VI. The central neck compartment is bounded superiorly by the hyoid, laterally by carotid arteries, anteriorly by the superficial layer of deep cervical fascia and posteriorly by the deep layer of deep cervical fascia. The inferior border is at the level of the innominate artery.

Pathology

Microscopically, the majority of the thyroid gland is made up of follicles filled with colloid. The parafollicular or C cells originate from the neural crest, produce calcitonin, and are located outside the follicles. They account for 0.1% of thyroid cells and they lie at the junction of the upper and lower two-thirds of the lobes.

Tumours can arise from the follicular epithelium (papillary, follicular and anaplastic), parafollicular or C cells (medullary), or non-epithelial stromal elements.

Papillary cancer

Papillary microcarcinoma is defined as a papillary cancer ≤ 10 mm. Incidental carcinomas refer to a tumour focus found solely on histological examination of the thyroid gland and not to any abnormality detected preoperatively.

Papillary cancers are often multifocal (the frequency of multifocality depends on method of pathological assessment). Orphan Annie nuclei and psammoma bodies are typical. The tall cell, columnar and diffuse sclerosing variants are more aggressive.

Follicular cancer

Cytology cannot distinguish adenomas from malignant tumours and so follicular cancers cannot be definitively diagnosed with FNAC. Histological confirmation requires invasion of the capsule and/or blood vessels.

Hürthle cell/oxyphil tumours

The majority of Hürthle cell/oxyphil tumours are benign; if malignant, they are usually well-differentiated. They produce thyroglobulin but may fail to take up radioiodine.

Anaplastic carcinoma

Anaplastic carcinoma arises from follicular cells. It can arise *de novo* or from differentiated thyroid cancer.

Medullary thyroid cancer (MTC)

MTC arises from parafollicular cells or C cells (neural crest/neuroendocrine origin), which can secrete calcitonin and carcinoembryonic antigen (CEA). Amyloid may be present.

Hereditary types

Tumours arising with MEN 2 and MEN 3 are often bilateral and multicentric. They are inherited in an autosomal dominant fashion and are associated with a germline mutation in the RET proto-oncogene on chromosome 10q, which codes for a receptor-like tyrosine kinase. C cell hyperplasia may be present.

Non-Hodgkin lymphoma

Many tumours are derived from mucosa-associated lymphoid tissue (MALT) and are therefore of low grade with a tendency for distant relapse. High-grade lymphomas can also occur.

Screening

There is currently no screening programme for the general population. For individuals with a strong family history of thyroid cancer or association with other cancers, genetic advice should be sought.

For MTC, all newly diagnosed patients, regardless of their family history, should be referred for germline RET mutation testing, which tests for exons 10, 11 and 13–15. Adult gene carriers are at high risk and are therefore recommended to have total thyroidectomy with central lymph node dissection (after excluding phaeochromocytoma). As a general guide, child gene carriers of MEN 3 should undergo surgery at an early age; in practice, thyroidectomy is often performed soon after the first year. Children carrying MEN 2 mutations typically have surgery by the age of 3 so that they are well established on thyroxine therapy by school age. The precise timing and extent of surgery is now dictated by the specific type of codon mutation.

Stage classification

TNM classification
The TNM classification is shown in Table 38.2.

Stage groupings
Papillary and follicular tumour subtypes are assigned to stage groupings depending on whether the patient is under age 45 or 45 years and older. All cases involving patients younger than 45 years, regardless of TNM categories, are stage I or II. All cases of anaplastic or undifferentiated thyroid cancer are stage IV. The stage groupings for thyroid cancer are shown in Table 38.3.

Differentiated thyroid cancer

Incidence and epidemiology
Differentiated thyroid cancer makes up < 1% of all malignancies but is the most common endocrine malignancy. In 2011, there were 2727 new cases of thyroid cancer in the UK, 28% in men and 72% in women and in 2012 there were 373 deaths in the UK. The UK crude incidence rate is 6 per 100,000 females and 2 per 100,000 males (CRUK: http://www.cancerresearchuk.org/cancer-info/cancerstats/types/thyroid/, accessed November 2014).

Thyroid cancer incidence rates in the UK, as in many Western countries, have been increasing since the mid-1970s. The rise has been more marked in women. The reason for the increase is unclear, with some studies concluding that increasing incidence reflects the increasing use of ultrasound to investigate thyroid nodules and the detection of subclinical disease rather than a true increase in incidence, and others suggesting that better and more frequent diagnostic activity cannot completely explain the increase.

Risk factors and aetiology
Risk factors for disease include the following.
- Increasing age and female gender.
- History of neck irradiation in childhood (particularly for papillary carcinomas).
- Nuclear fallout (age at exposure is important).
- Endemic goitre.

Table 38.2 The TNM classification of thyroid cancer

Stage	Papillary, follicular and medullary	Anaplastic and undifferentiated
T1	T1a: limited to thyroid < 1 cm T1b: limited to thyroid > 1 but ≤ 2 cm,	n/a
T2	> 2–4 cm, intrathyroidal	n/a
T3	> 4 cm or minimal extension	n/a
T4a	Subcutaneous, larynx, trachea, oesophagus, recurrent laryngeal nerve	Limited to thyroid
T4b	Prevertebral fascia, mediastinal vessels, carotid artery	Beyond thyroid capsule
N1a	Level VI	Level VI
N1b	Other regional (cervical, and upper/superior mediastinal)	Other regional

Adapted from UICC (2009).

Table 38.3 Stage groups for thyroid cancer

Stage	Papillary and follicular: age < 45 years	Papillary or follicular: age ≥ 45 years and medullary	Anaplastic/undifferentiated (all cases are stage IV)
Stage I	Any T any N M0	T1 N0 M0	–
Stage II	Any T any N M1	T2 N0 M0	–
Stage III	–	T3 N0 M0 or T1–3 N1a M0	–
Stage IVA	–	T1–3 N1b M0 or T4a any N M0	T4a any N M0
Stage IVB	–	T4b, any N, M0	T4b any N M0
Stage IVC	–	Any T any N M1	Any T any N M1

Adapted from UICC (2009).

- Gardner's syndrome.
- Cowden's syndrome.
- Familial adenomatous polyposis (FAP).
- Familial differentiated thyroid cancer.
- Turcot's syndrome.
- Carney complex.

Clinical presentation

Thyroid cancers may present as:

- asymptomatic thyroid nodule or cervical node;
- sense of fullness/pressure in neck;
- stridor, dysphonia, dysphagia, odynophagia, cough (more likely with lymphoma and anaplastic tumours);
- unexpected finding after thyroidectomy for presumed benign disease;
- unexpected finding on PET-CT scan performed for another indication;
- distant metastases – dyspnoea, haemoptysis, bone pain, etc.

Investigation and staging

General investigation

The majority of patients are diagnosed after undergoing neck USS and thyroid nodule FNAC.

FNAC is categorised by the Royal College of pathologists as Thy 1–5.

Thy1 – non-diagnostic. This includes poor operator or preparation technique as well as cyst fluid samples with insufficient colloid and epithelial cells (Thy1c).

Thy2 – non-neoplastic. For example, normal thyroid tissue, colloid nodule, thyroiditis. Cyst samples with abundant colloid are Thy2c.

Thy3 – neoplasm possible.

- **Thy3a –atypical** features but insufficient to place into any other category. May include inability to exclude a follicular neoplasm or papillary carcinoma or suboptimal specimens.
- **Thy3f – follicular neoplasm is suspected.** Histological possibilities include hyperplastic nodule, follicular adenoma or follicular carcinoma. These cannot be distinguished on cytology alone and a histology sample (e.g. diagnostic hemithyroidectomy) is need for diagnosis.

Thy4 – suspicious of malignancy but definite diagnosis of malignancy is not possible.

Thy5 – diagnostic of malignancy.

The likelihood of a malignancy increases with increasing Thy category and should be 100% for Thy5.

Although palpable thyroid nodules may be present in 3–7% of normal people, ultrasound-detectable nodules may be found in between 30% and 70%, the incidence rising with age.

The BTA 2014 guidelines have recently introduced an ultrasound scoring system for thyroid nodules whereby nodules are described as U1–U5 depending on their characteristics. Characteristic ultrasound signs for malignancy include the following.

- Papillary and medullary:
  - a solid hypo-echoic nodule;
  - hyper-echoic foci (i.e. microcalcification) within the nodule;
  - irregular margin;
  - intranodular vascularity;
  - absence of an associated halo;
  - an irregular margin and a 'taller than wide' shape has also been shown to be a good predictor of malignancy.
- Follicular lesions (including follicular adenoma and follicular carcinoma) are often:
  - hyperechoic;
  - homogenous;
  - with a well-defined halo.

Despite size of a nodule being used in some guidelines, evidence does not support this as a reliable indicator of malignancy.

Patients with locally advanced disease should undergo CT or MRI of neck and chest to assess local disease extent and to plan surgical treatment. Avoid iodinated contrast media for approximately 2 months before radioiodine (because of potential interference with radioiodine uptake).

Serum calcitonin and CEA should be checked if MTC is suspected.

Vocal cord mobility should be assessed pre- and postoperatively.

Radionuclide imaging with ^{123}I or ^{131}I is of limited use in the diagnosis of thyroid cancer. Malignant nodules are traditionally said to be 'cold', but they may also appear as 'warm' and 'hot' areas.

Serum thyroglobulin measurement is of no diagnostic value unless the thyroid has been removed.

Serum thyroglobulin (Tg)

Serum thyroglobulin is a glycosylated protein, which is a key substrate for biosynthesis and storage of thyroid hormones. It is secreted by normal and cancerous thyroid cells and its release is TSH-dependent. Detection sensitivity is increased when the TSH level is elevated. The serum Tg level is more sensitive than an ^{131}I whole-body scan in detecting recurrent or metastatic disease.

Serum Tg may be undetectable in 20% of patients with isolated lymph node metastases when they are on thyroxine. Thyroglobulin autoantibodies interfere with the ability to accurately measure and follow Tg. Autoantibodies are present in 4–27% of the general population and in 15–30% of thyroid cancer patients. In order to interpret the serum Tg level, it is necessary to know the TSH level and Tg antibody level. Serum Tg is not useful preoperatively as a diagnostic test.

Treatment overview

Although early cases of differentiated thyroid cancer may be cured with surgery alone, most patients are managed with a combination of surgery, radioiodine and TSH-suppressive doses of thyroxine. External beam radiotherapy may play a role in locally advanced and metastatic disease.

Surgery

Surgery is the mainstay of treatment but the extent of thyroid and nodal surgery needed for low-risk cases is controversial. Patients with follicular thyroid cancer < 4 cm with capsule invasion and no vascular invasion, in the absence of other adverse risk factors appear to have an excellent prognosis (O'Neill *et al.*, 2011; Sugino *et al.*, 2012). Therefore, clear recommendations cannot be made and the extent of surgery should be guided by MDT discussion.

Indications for hemithyroidectomy (removal of one lobe and isthmus)

Differentiated thyroid cancers (DTCs) ≤ 1 cm.

These patients have an extremely low risk of death from thyroid cancer (0.1–0.5%), and can be adequately treated by hemithyroidectomy provided that:

- the tumour does not extend beyond the thyroid capsule; and
- there is no evidence of multifocal/bilateral disease, overt lymph node metastases, distant metastases, vascular invasion.

The disadvantage of this approach is the difficulty of follow-up, because Tg measurements can be difficult to interpret and imaging shows residual thyroid tissue.

Indications for total thyroidectomy

The potential advantages of a total thyroidectomy include:

- the ability to follow up using serum Tg;
- eliminating the risk of a second thyroid cancer focus developing in the remaining lobe in multifocal papillary thyroid cancer;
- reducing the risk of local recurrence.

Total thyroidectomy is indicated if the tumour is larger than 1 cm, multifocal, with extrathyroidal spread or if there is familial disease, positive lymph nodes, previous neck irradiation or Hürthle cell subtype.

The rate of recurrent laryngeal nerve injury is 1–6% (higher following re-operation); 30% of patients require postoperative calcium supplementation. After 3 months, the rate of hypocalcaemia is only 2%.

Indications for completion thyroidectomy

If the diagnosis of thyroid cancer has been made after thyroid lobectomy completion, (contralateral) thyroid lobectomy should be carried out within 8 weeks of histological diagnosis of cancer.

Central compartment lymph node dissection

Whether *prophylactic* central compartment node surgery improves disease-specific survival or recurrence-free survival is not proven. It is uncertain when to do this in addition to a total thyroidectomy for patients with node-negative papillary thyroid cancer. The potential benefit of additional staging information and reduced local recurrence must be weighed against the increased risk of injury to the recurrent laryngeal nerves and parathyroid glands. Patients who are node-negative preoperatively and have high-risk features such as age > 45 years, tumours greater than 4 cm in diameter and extrathyroidal disease should be considered for prophylactic central neck node dissection

Patients with pre- or intraoperative evidence of central lymph node involvement should undergo a *therapeutic* central compartment dissection.

When lateral neck nodes are involved, a therapeutic selective neck dissection (levels IIa–Vb) is recommended, preserving the accessory nerve, sternocleidomastoid muscle and internal jugular vein. Dissection of levels I and IIb is not routinely recommended.

Role of levothyroxine

Supraphysiological doses of levothyroxine are used to reduce the risk of thyroid cancer recurrence.

A meta-analysis supports the effectivness of TSH suppression in preventing major adverse clinical events (McGriff *et al.*, 2002).

Levothyroxine (T4) should be used rather than liothyronine (T3) for long-term TSH suppression. Following initial treatment and before evaluating the response to treatment after 9–12 months, TSH should always be suppressed to below 0.1 mU/L. The average dose of thyroxine required to achieve TSH suppression is in the range 150–200 μg. Free T4 (FT4) is often above the normal range when significant TSH suppression is achieved.

After assessing treatment response 9–12 months after radioiodine remnant ablation, the risk of thyroid cancer recurrence should be reclassified according to the criteria for dynamic risk stratification and the degree of TSH suppression adjusted as below:

- incomplete response: the serum TSH should be suppressed below 0.1 mU/L indefinitely in the absence of specific contraindications;
- indeterminate response: maintain serum TSH concentrations between 0.1 and 0.5 mU/L for 5–10 years;
- excellent response: the serum TSH should be maintained in the low–normal range, e.g. between 0.3 and 2 mU/L.

Radioisotope therapy

Rationale

Radioisotope therapy allows the detection and earlier treatment of persistent/metastatic disease by destroying normal thyroid tissue and microscopic foci of cancer in the thyroid remnant, and by making the interpretation of Tg results during follow-up easier. It may be used to ablate the thyroid remnant or to treat residual or recurrent disease.

Indications for radioiodine remnant ablation (RRA)

Definite indication:

- tumour > 4 cm,
- any tumour size with gross extrathyroidal extension,
- distant metastases present.

No indication:

- tumour < 1 cm unifocal or multifocal,
- classic papillary or follicular variant papillary or follicular thyroid cancer without vascular invasion *and* no extrathyroid extension.

Uncertain indication: factors to be considered include:

- large tumour size,
- extrathyroid extension,
- unfavourable histological cell type, e.g. tall cell, columnar, insular, diffuse sclerosing papillary cancer, poorly differentiated elements,
- widely invasive follicular thyroid cancer,
- multiple metastatic lymph nodes,
- large lymph nodes, multiple involved lymph node levels, high ratio of positive to negative nodes, extracapsular nodal involvement.

Preparation for [131]I

Patients should be advised to eat a low-iodine diet for 1–2 weeks before receiving [131]I.

- [131]I should be avoided for 2 months after iodinated intravenous contrast.
- [131]I should be avoided if the patient is currently taking amiodarone or has taken amiodarone within the previous 12 months.

In order for ^{131}I to enter thyroid cells (normal or malignant), TSH levels must be high (> 30m U/L) and so patients must either receive recombinant human TSH or undergo thyroid hormone withdrawal. Elevated TSH level stimulates the sodium iodide symporter (membrane protein involved in active transport) and, hence, radioiodine uptake into thyrocytes.

Use of recombinant human TSH (rhTSH)

Randomised trials have shown that ^{131}I remnant ablation is equally successful after recombinant human thyroid-stimulating hormone (rhTSH), as after thyroid hormone withdrawal (THW) for selected patients with DTC (Mallick *et al.*, 2012; Schlumberger *et al.*, 2012).

The use of rhTSH is also associated with better quality of life and reduces radiation exposure to normal tissues compared to THW. rhTSH has not been evaluated in randomised controlled trials for remnant ablation in patients at high risk of recurrence, or for the treatment of recurrent or metastatic differentiated thyroid cancer (DTC) and is not currently licensed for this purpose. However, rhTSH is the recommended method of preparation for ^{131}I ablation in patients who have the following characteristics: T1 to T3, N0 or NX or N1, and M0 and R0 (no microscopic residual disease; Perros *et al.*, 2014).

Other indications for the use of rhTSH include hypopituitary function, functional metastases causing TSH suppression, severe IHD, a previous history of psychiatric disturbance precipitated by hypothyroidism, advanced disease or frailty where THW will either not be possible or will be poorly tolerated with potential exacerbation of comorbidities.

Injections of rhTSH are given as 0.9 mg deep i.m. injections into the buttock on days 1 and 2, with radioiodine administered on day 3, and thyroglobulin measured on day 5.

Side effects of rhTSH are infrequent and mild and include flu-like myalgia, mild nausea and headache. There is possible stimulation of metastases resulting in local symptoms, and so the use of prophylactic corticosteroids before rhTSH should be considered.

If rhTSH is unavailable, alternative methods for preparation are as follows.

- Liothyronine can be started immediately after surgery and withdrawn 14 days before [131]I. If thyroxine has been started postoperatively it should be substituted with liothyronine 28 days before ^{131}I and then liothyronine should be withdrawn 14 days before RRA or therapy.

Technique

[131]I remnant ablation activity

Two large multicentre randomised trials and a meta-analysis (Mallick *et al.*, 2012; Schlumberger *et al.*, 2012; Cheng *et al.*, 2013) have shown that 1.1GBq of ^{131}I is as effective as 3.7 GBq in ablating the thyroid remnant. The lower activity is associated with fewer adverse events.

Patients with T1–2, N0 with R0 resection should receive 1.1 GBq while the decision on optimal ^{131}I activity for patients with T3 and/or N1 disease should be decided by the MDT on an individual basis taking all prognostic factors into consideration.

[131]I therapy

The optimal ^{131}I therapeutic activity for persistent neck disease or metastatic disease is uncertain. [131]I activities of 3.7–5.5 GBq are recommended for patients with known residual local disease following RRA or distant metastases.

Whole-body radioiodine scans are performed after giving radioiodine for ablation or therapy to determine the sites of radioiodine uptake. The timing of the scan depends on the administered activity, the method of patient preparation (rhTSH versus thyroid hormone withdrawal), and the clinician's choice of the residual activity at which to image the patient. SPECT-CT imaging in addition to planar imaging is helpful to localise the anatomical site of ^{131}I uptake accurately (Barwick *et al.*, 2012).

If the patient has been withdrawn from hormones, thyroxine can be started 2–5 days after radioiodine has been administered. If the patient has been given rhTSH, he or she should stay on thyroxine throughout.

Radioiodine side effects

Side effects include neck discomfort and swelling (which are rare unless there is a large thyroid remnant), altered sense of taste, nausea (vomiting is uncommon), sialoadenitis, dry mouth, radiation cystitis, gastritis and bleeding/oedema in metastases. Male fertility may be affected and so sperm storage should be considered for high-risk cases who are expected to receive multiple radioiodine treatments. No significant adverse effect on female fertility, birth weights or prematurity rates have been found. There is a slight increase in miscarriage rate in the first year after treatment.

If there are miliary pulmonary metastases, there is a small risk of the patient developing pulmonary fibrosis and so serial lung function tests are recommended to look for signs of restrictive defects. The risk of leukaemia and second cancer (salivary gland, breast, bladder, colon) is 0.5% (risk is highest with high cumulative dose, i.e. greater than 18.5 GBq), and after external beam radiotherapy.

Consider the use of high-dose corticosteroids before radioiodine if there is bulky neck disease or metastatic disease.

Radiation protection issues

Radiation protection issues are as follows.

- Exclude pregnancy before administration.
- Discontinue breast feeding at least 8 weeks beforehand.
- The patient should avoid pregnancy/conception for 6 months.
- Visiting is restricted to non-pregnant adults, who must stay in a designated area.
- Clothing must be washed separately after the patient returns home, unless it is heavily soiled, in which case onsite storage or disposal may be needed.
- The patient should double flush the toilet; use separate cutlery and crockery.
- The patient must sleep alone.

Table 38.4 Dynamic risk stratification after total thyroidectomy and ^{131}I ablation

Response	Criteria	Risk
Excellent	All the following • Suppressed and stimulated Tg < 1 µg/L • Neck US without evidence of disease • Cross-sectional and/or nuclear medicine imaging negative (if performed)	Low risk
Intermediate	Any of the following • Suppressed Tg < 1 µg/L and stimulated Tg ≥ 1 and < 10 µg/L • Neck US with non-specific changes or stable subcentimetre lymph nodes • Cross-sectional and/or nuclear medicine imaging with changes of uncertain significance	Intermediate risk
Incomplete	Any of the following • Suppressed Tg ≥ 1 µg/L or stimulated Tg ≥ 10 µg/L • Rising Tg values • Persistent or newly identified disease on cross-sectional and/or nuclear medicine imaging	High risk

Adapted from Tuttle *et al.*, 2010.

- Restrict time and extend distance with personal contacts.
- The duration of restrictions to be followed around non-pregnant adults is shorter than that for children and pregnant or potentially pregnant women. Restrictions are individualised for each patient. The timing of return to work depends on the type of work and work personnel involved.

Assessment of remnant ablation success and dynamic risk stratification

Remnant ablation success is assessed by stimulated Tg (using a reliable assay, and in the absence of assay interference) and specialised neck ultrasound without needing a diagnostic ^{131}I whole-body scan.

Patients treated with total thyroidectomy and ^{131}I ablation should undergo dynamic risk stratification 9–12 months after ablation.

Patients should be stratified into three categories: (a) excellent response, (b) indeterminate response, (c) incomplete response, as shown in Table 38.4.

Patients with an incomplete response based on evidence of residual thyroid tissue should be considered for further ^{131}I therapy once any surgically resectable disease has been excluded.

Patients with an incomplete response based on a stimulated Tg ≥ 10 µg/L or rising Tg value and normal neck US should be assessed with cross-sectional imaging. If imaging is negative, ^{131}I therapy should be considered.

Patients with an indeterminate response need to be kept under observation with serial Tg assessments and intermittent imaging to ensure there is no evidence of a rising Tg level or progressive radiological changes indicative of persistent or progressive disease.

Patients with an excellent response should be considered for relaxation of TSH suppression and increase in the interval of follow-up.

External beam radiotherapy

External beam radiotherapy is rarely used. The main indications for use are unresectable disease, non-iodine-avid disease, gross local invasion with macro- or microscopic residual, recurrent neck disease not amenable to surgery, and palliation of inoperable metastatic disease.

The concave geometry and close proximity of the thyroid bed to critical normal structures such as the oesophagus, trachea, larynx, lungs, spinal cord, and in cases with level 2 cervical lymph node disease, parotid glands make delivery of high doses difficult.

The treatment volume usually includes the thyroid bed, cervical and supraclavicular nodes, and the superior mediastinum. Intensity-modulated radiation therapy (IMRT) offers a better dose distribution than conventional radiotherapy techniques and is recommended.

It is possible that radiotherapy may reduce the uptake of radioiodine into residual thyroid tissue, and so consider giving radioiodine therapy before external beam radiotherapy.

Radiotherapy technique for thyroid bed and locoregional nodes including superior mediastinal nodes

IMRT

- Compared to conventional RT techniques, IMRT reduces the dose to radiosensitive organs close to the PTV, in particular the spinal cord, and thereby improves the PTV coverage. An improved therapeutic index is seen with IMRT relative to other techniques and is associated with less-frequent severe late radiation morbidity.
- The patient is positioned using an immobilisation shell, supine, usually with chin extended.
- Suggested CTV and dose/fractionation (may vary among institutions):
  - CTV1 (high-dose volume): 63–66 Gy in 30 daily fractions to regions of grossly positive margins or gross residual disease.
  - CTV2 (intermediate dose volume): 60 Gy in 30 daily fractions to regions of the operative bed directly involved with disease, adjacent soft tissues and draining nodal basins.
  - CTV3 (adjuvant dose volume): 56 Gy in 30 daily fractions to all the surgical resection bed with a 1–2 cm (minimum 0.5 cm) margin.
  - CTV4 (prophylactic dose volume): 54 Gy in 30 daily fractions to at-risk cervical and mediastinal nodal stations.

Conventional RT technique

- The patient is positioned using an immobilisation shell, supine, usually with chin extended.
- The aim is to deliver 60 Gy in 30 fractions over 6 weeks. As the spinal cord dose should not exceed 46 Gy, a two-phase technique is required. The first phase is delivered via anterior and posterior parallel-opposed fields to the thyroid bed, bilateral cervical nodes and superior mediastinum, generally encompassing the area from the tip of the mastoid processes to the carina with mandibular and apical lung shielding. If level II nodes do not need to be irradiated, the superior border may lie at the level of the hyoid, reducing the dose to the parotids and the risk of xerostomia. When both the neck and superior mediastinum are treated, the patient contour can change significantly in the cranio-caudal axis and compensation may be required.

- The dose delivered in the first phase is 40–44 Gy in 2 Gy fractions to allow for the contribution to the spinal cord dose from the phase 2 CT planned volume. Phase 2 therefore needs to be planned before completing the first phase in order to calculate the spinal cord dose prospectively.
- This technique is suboptimal because:
  - the postoperative dose to lymph node regions at risk is often only 40–44 Gy, which may be inadequate for treatment of microscopic residual disease;
  - the thyroid bed lies close to the spinal cord and so the dose may be limited to 55–60 Gy, lower than that needed for macroscopic residual disease.

Chemotherapy

Chemotherapy is not routinely used in the treatment of thyroid carcinoma. Its use has largely been superseded by the introduction of targeted therapies.

Doxorubicin was the most frequently used drug, with a reported partial response rate of approximately 20–30%. There is no clear evidence that its use increases survival.

Targeted therapies

Targeted therapies are indicated when a patient has symptomatic progressive metastatic thyroid cancer. The agents demonstrating the most activity and clinical benefit are sorafenib and lenvatinib. Sorafenib, for example, has been shown to increase progression-free survival by 5 months compared to placebo.

Molecular profiling is increasingly being used in the research setting to assess tumour response to various targeted therapies, for example good response rates have been reported in BRAF V600E mutated papillary carcinoma with vemurafanib, a potent inhibitor of the oncogenic BRAF protein kinase. Currently, molecular profiling is not robust enough to reliably predict clinical response and benefit, so is not in routine clinical practice.

This is a rapidly changing area and recommendations for specific agents cannot be made because of pending licence applications and funding assessments.

Special clinical situations

Pregnancy

It is essential to consider the risk to both mother and foetus when thyroid cancer is diagnosed during pregnancy. Most cases of DTC are not aggressive and therefore it is feasible to allow the pregnancy to continue. Discussion of the case by the MDT, as well as counselling of the couple, is required.

Surgery is the treatment of choice and may be indicated if there is rapid tumour growth or significant lymph node metastases (Stagnaro-Green *et al.*, 2011; De Groot *et al.*, 2012). Thyroidectomy in the first trimester is associated with a very high risk of miscarriage. Thyroidectomy may be performed safely in the second trimester when complication rates for the mother and foetus are low. There is no evidence to allow recommendations for or against TSH suppression when surgery has to be postponed until after delivery.

Patients should avoid pregnancy for 6 months after receiving radioactive iodine (ARSAC, 2006). There may be an increased risk of miscarriage in the first year following radioactive iodine treatment.

Children

Papillary carcinoma is the most common form of thyroid cancer in children, with 30–40% of tumours multifocal; 40–90% are found to have involved cervical nodes at initial surgery. At presentation, 10–20% have lung metastases; bone metastases are rare (< 1%). The recurrence rate of thyroid cancer is higher in children than it is in adults, especially young children. Fewer than 10% die of their disease.

Metastatic disease

Treatment depends on the site of the tumour: if the lung and other soft tissue sites that are not amenable to surgery are involved, give ^{131}I 3.7–7.4 GBq at 6- to 12-month intervals. There is no maximum cumulative dose, but FBC and renal function should be monitored. The risk of a second malignancy increases with cumulative dose. Individual doses should not exceed 200 rem total-body exposure.

If solitary metastases that do not concentrate radioiodine can be resected, the 5-year post-metastasectomy survival is 40–50%.

Management of an elevated serum thyroglobulin

Occasionally the serum thyroglobulin (Tg) may be falsely elevated by Tg antibodies, which may not always be measurable.

It is a serial rise in Tg or thyroglobulin antibody titre that is of more significance than one elevated result.

Tumour is rarely located on imaging when the stimulated Tg is less than 2 µg/L.

^{131}I whole body scans are used less frequently now to investigate elevated serum Tg, because it is less sensitive in detecting locoregional disease than Tg and neck US. If the patients is US-negative and Tg-positive, the choice of which imaging modalities to use and in which order is uncertain. Scans to consider when the neck ultrasound is negative include:

- chest CT (without iodinated iv contrast if further ^{131}I planned),
- neck MRI,
- bone scan,
- spine MRI,
- ^{18}fluoro-deoxy-glucose (FDG)-positron emission tomography (PET). Thyroxine withdrawal or rhTSH administration have been shown to increase the sensitivity of ^{18}FDG-PET-CT scan. Patients with positive ^{18}FDG-PET scan has been shown to have a markedly reduced 3-year survival compared with ^{18}FDG-PET scan-negative patients. If PET imaging is positive, ^{131}I imaging is typically negative and the patient is radioiodine-refractory, the so-called 'flip-flop' phenomenon.

If an isolated lesion amenable to surgery or EBRT is found then this and ^{131}I therapy can be considered.

If diagnostic imaging fails to identify the source of raised Tg, empirical ^{131}I treatment may be given. Factors that should be considered in making this decision include the risk category of the patient and the rate of rise of the serum Tg.

There is no evidence from RCTs for or against using empirical ^{131}I. Non-randomised clinical trials have reported abnormal uptake on the post-treatment whole body scan in 61% of patients. The activity of empiric ^{131}I therapy used is usually 3.7–7.4 GBq, usually 5.5 GBq.

Follow-up

The frequency and type of follow-up depend on an individual's risk of recurrence. The aims of follow-up are to detect recurrence early, to monitor TSH suppression and to detect and manage hypocalcaemia. The duration of follow-up should be life-long (long natural history, late recurrences, late side effects of radioactive iodine, consequences of supraphysiological thyroxine replacement).

Prognosis

Of patients with well-differentiated thyroid cancer, 5–20% develop distant metastases (lung > bone

> liver and brain). Older age is associated with worse outcomes.

The most important predictors are the patient's age, the tumour's size, grade and extrathyroid spread, and distant metastases. For children, the outcome is worse if they are younger than 10 years because the disease behaves more aggressively and the risk of recurrence is higher. Recurrence is also more likely if the tumour is a tall cell/columnar/diffuse sclerosing subtype, is poorly differentiated, is large, or there is lymph node involvement.

There are many prognostic scoring systems in use for well-differentiated thyroid cancer, for example, AGES (PTC), AMES (PTC and FTC), MACIS (PTC), Ohio State University (differentiated), and the University of Chicago (PTC).

Dynamic risk stratification is the preferred tool for assessing an individual's risk of relapse and for deciding on appropriate investigation, treatments and degree and duration of TSH suppression as well as intensity of follow-up.

Areas of current interest/controversy

There is currently no prospective randomised trial investigating the extent of initial surgery. Other areas of current interest include the following.

- Extent of initial surgery for low-risk cases (lobectomy vs. total thyroidectomy)
- The role of adjuvant EBRT.
- Empirical versus dosimetry-derived ^{131}I use.
- Indications for prophylactic central lymph node dissection.
- Degree and duration of TSH suppression.

Current clinical trials

IoN: this study will determine whether RAI is necessary for low-risk differentiated thyroid cancer patients who have already undergone total thyroidectomy and optimal TSH suppression. Patients will be randomised into two groups. One group will receive ^{131}I ablation at an activity of 1.1 GBq, the other will not receive ablation.

Medullary thyroid cancer

Incidence and epidemiology

The sporadic form of medullary thyroid cancer (MTC) is most common in the fifth and sixth decades of life. The female-to-male incidence ratio is 1.5:1.

There are different familial forms. In the MEN type 2, the disease presents in the first and second decades and is associated with parathyroid hyperplasia and phaeochromocytoma. In the MEN type 3, the disease presents in the first decade and is aggressive and associated with phaeochromocytoma, mucosal neuromas (especially of the lip and tongue), Marfanoid habitus, and a high-arched palate. Familial non-MEN MTC patients present in the sixth decade and beyond. Familial forms of MTC have equal gender frequency.

Risk factors and aetiology

MEN types 2 and 3 are associated with MTC. They are inherited in an autosomal dominant fashion and associated with mutations in the RET proto-oncogene.

Germline testing of RET can be used to distinguish cases of sporadic from hereditary MTC, and the precise RET mutations may suggest a particular phenotype and clinical course. This is important because the patient may also require surveillance and management of phaeochromocytoma and hyperparathyroidism and additional family members may be at risk for developing MTC.

Knowledge of the particular RET mutation can guide decisions about prophylactic thyroidectomy and intraoperative management of the parathyroid glands. Approximately 95% of patients with MEN 2 and MEN 3, and 88%of those with familial MTC, will have an identifiable RET mutation and about 1–7% of apparently sporadic cases have identifiable RET mutations.

RET mutations are more likely to be identified in patients with multifocal disease and/or MTC at a young age.

Spread

MTC may spread to lymph nodes and via the blood stream.

Clinical presentation

Possible clinical presentations include the following.

- Detection during screening.
- Typically with thyroid mass and lymphadenopathy.
- Wheezing, secretory diarrhoea and flushing are involved with large-volume local or metastatic MTC. It is important to document the patient's family history to ascertain whether there are any

features to suggest MTC or MEN, including any history of sudden unexpected deaths.

Specific investigations for MTC include the following.

- Serum calcitonin should be measured preoperatively and during follow-up (it may be raised with chronic renal failure, pregnancy, pernicious anaemia, and in the neonatal period).
- CEA may be a useful marker.
- All new patients should be screened biochemically for phaeochromocytoma and hyperparathyroidism. A lack of family history does not exclude heritable disease because the disease can skip generations.

Treatment overview

Surgery is the mainstay of treatment and the role of external beam radiotherapy in locally advanced disease is unclear. There is no role for radioiodine therapy. Thyroxine is required as a replacement dose only.

Surgery

Surgery entails total thyroidectomy and central lymph node dissection (level VI). The lateral jugular nodes should be assessed; if they are positive, a modified radical or selective neck dissection is indicated.

Role of thyroxine

Thyroxine is required as a replacement dose only.

External beam radiotherapy

The role of postoperative RT is unclear because some studies report improved local control while others report no difference or a detrimental effect, probably because of selection bias. Consider postoperative RT if there is locally advanced disease, multiple involved lymph nodes, an elevated postoperative calcitonin level, or bulky inoperable tumour.

Treatment of recurrent disease

Recurrent cervical nodal disease

Recurrent nodal disease may be amenable to surgical excision.

Metastatic disease

Patients may experience frequent loose bowel actions, wheezing and flushing. The symptoms may respond to somatostatin analogue (e.g. octreotide) therapy.

Chemotherapy is rarely helpful unless there is rapidly progressive symptomatic disease and has largely been superseded by targeted therapies. Vandetanib has been licensed for use in symptomatic progressive metastatic or locally advanced MTC. Cabozantinib has also demonstrated activity in this clinical setting.

Raised calcitonin level

If the patient has a raised calcitonin level, imaging techniques may not be able to detect the site of recurrent disease until the serum calcitonin level is grossly elevated. Further guidance is provided below.

Follow-up

When the postoperative basal serum calcitonin is undetectable the risk of persistent or recurrent residual disease is low, and other tests including imaging techniques are not immediately required and the patient may enter into long-term follow-up.

Postoperative MTC patients with serum calcitonin levels $\geq$ 150 pg/mL should undergo neck US and additional imaging to look for distant metastases.

Postoperative MTC patients with serum calcitonin $\geq$ 150 pg/mL with symptomatic and/or progressive locoregional disease > 1 cm should be considered for locoregional therapy (e.g. surgery), while those with symptomatic distant metastases should be considered for clinical trials and palliative therapies such as surgery, EBRT, percutaneous interventions and hepatic embolisation.

Patients with detectable basal serum calcitonin levels postoperatively with negative imaging should have the basal calcitonin and CEA levels obtained approximately every 6 months initially to determine the doubling times (DTs). Ongoing follow-up of these tumour markers and physical examination should occur at one-quarter the shortest doubling time or annually, whichever is more frequent (i.e. follow the patient every 6 months if the shortest doubling time is 24 months).

Asymptomatic patients with small volume metastatic disease that is stable or slowly progressive on imaging, or with a calcitonin or CEA doubling time longer than 2 years, typically do not require systemic therapy, and the decision to start should be made only after a thorough discussion with the patient.

Patients with rapidly progressive disease on imaging or with a biochemical doubling time of less than 2 years should be considered for treatment with targeted therapy, ideally in the context of a clinical trial.

Prognosis

Young age, male gender, positive nodes and incomplete initial surgery are adverse factors. The 10-year survival in patients presenting with clinical disease rather than screened disease is 65% overall (stage I = 100%, stage II = 93%, stage III = 71% and stage IV = 20%).

Barbet *et al.* (2005) studied MTC patients with abnormal Ct levels after total thyroidectomy and bilateral lymph node dissection. When the Ct DT was less than 6 months, the 5- and 10-year survivals were 25% and 8%, respectively; when 6–24 months, the 5- and 10-year survivals were 92% and 37%, whereas all patients with Ct DT greater than 2 years were alive at the end of the study. TNM stage, European Organization for Research and Treatment of Cancer score, and Ct DT were significant predictors of survival by univariate analysis, but only the Ct DT remained an independent predictor of survival on multivariate analysis.

Areas of current interest/controversy

Areas of current interest include:

- the optimal management of calcitonin-positive cases;
- indications for postoperative radiotherapy;
- targeted therapy: optimal agent, when to start, duration of use.

Anaplastic thyroid cancer

Incidence and epidemiology

The incidence of anaplastic thyroid cancer has decreased. Disease occurrence peaks in the seventh decade of life. The female-to-male incidence ratio is 1.5:1.

Spread

For anaplastic carcinoma, spread is predominantly local, to form a large bulky mass.

Treatment overview

Many patients present with advanced disease and are of poor performance status making the treatment for the majority palliative. For those with localised disease and of good performance status, multimodality treatment may result in long-term control (Smallridge *et al.*, 2012).

Surgery

Surgery is rarely possible. If resection is being considered, it is important that the surgical intent is gross tumour resection and not just debulking.

External beam radiotherapy

Anaplastic thyroid cancer is the least radioresponsive thyroid cancer type.

Following an R0 or R1 thyroid resection in patients of good performance status and with no evidence of distant metastases, adjuvant radical radiotherapy ± concurrent chemotherapy should be considered.

If thyroidectomy is not appropriate but disease is localised, radical external beam radiotherapy, with or without concurrent chemotherapy, should be considered with the aim of local control. Concurrent chemoradiotherapy using a taxane (paclitaxel or docetaxel), and/or anthracyclines (doxorubicin) and/or platin (cisplatin or carboplatin) has been shown to improve patient survival in some studies.

Prognosis

The median survival is 6 months from development of symptoms; 75% of patients still die from local progression. In practice, some patients spend much of their remaining life receiving treatment and recovering from its acute toxicity.

Thyroid lymphoma

Lymphoma accounts for 1–5% of thyroid cancers and 1–2% of extranodal lymphomas. The most common types are diffuse large B-cell lymphoma (approx. 70%) and MALT lymphoma (approx. 25%). Other rarer subtypes include follicular lymphoma and classic Hodgkin lymphoma. Hashimoto's thyroiditis is associated with thyroid lymphoma in approximately 80% of cases, especially MALT type.

Incidence and epidemiology

The mean age of thyroid lymphoma occurrence is 60–65 years. The disease predominates in women; the female-to-male incidence ratio is 3:1 (ratio increases above 60 years). Annual incidence 1–2 cases per million population.

Clinical presentation

The patient typically presents with stage IE or stage IIE disease with a rapidly enlarging painless thyroid mass ± cervical lymphadenopathy. B symptoms occur in approximately 20%.

See Chapter 34 for the staging system. Most patients present with localised disease.

Investigation

US and FNAC using flow cytometry and immunohistochemistry are the main methods used to confirm a diagnosis. Core biopsy will yield more tissue and maintains the architecture. It can be difficult to diagnose thyroid lymphoma and occasionally open surgical biopsy is needed if less-invasive methods have failed to establish the lymphoma subtype.

Treatment

Overview

DLBCL tends to follow an aggressive clinical course and patients should be considered for multimodality treatment, whereas MALT lymphoma is usually indolent and single modality treatment is usually indicated. No randomised controlled trials have compared single with multimodality treatment for primary thyroid lymphoma and so guidance is based on small retrospective thyroid lymphoma series and extrapolation from extranodal lymphoma treatment.

Surgery

Thyroidectomy is not usually indicated.

Chemotherapy

DLBCL is usually treated with 3 cycles of R-CHOP (rituximab, cyclophosphamide, doxorubicin, vincristine, prednisolone) plus involved field radiotherapy. For bulky disease, up to 6 cycles of R-CHOP may be needed. Radiotherapy alone may, however, be indicated for localised MALT lymphoma.

External beam radiotherapy

For stage IE MALT type, the target volume should include the whole organ only. The dose is 24–30 Gy, in 12–15 fractions over 2.5–3 weeks.

For stage IE DLBCL, 3 cycles of systemic chemotherapy (R-CHOP) are given before involved site radiotherapy.

IMRT improves thyroid PTV coverage and reduces irradiation of normal tissue compared to conventional radiotherapy techniques. However, with the low doses indicated for the treatment of thyroid lymphoma,

there is no clear evidence that IMRT results in superior results.

Prognosis

The prognosis depends on the stage of disease. The majority of patients present with localised disease and have a favourable prognosis.

Thyrotoxicosis

Radioiodine may be given for hyperthyroidism due to Graves' disease or toxic multinodular goitre.

The recommended administered activity is 400–550 MBq of ^{131}I 3 days after stopping anti-thyroid medication, which can be restarted 3 days later. The patient should be advised to avoid close contact with young children or pregnant women for 21–24 days depending upon dose prescribed. Normal thyroid function returns in 50–70% of patients within 6 weeks; 15–20% develop hypothyroidism after 2 years, so these patients need long-term follow-up of thyroid function.

Severe thyrotoxicosis should be controlled first. Radioiodine is indicated after relapse on carbimazole or propylthiouracil. Prolonged use of anti-thyroid medication can be associated with irreversible agranulocytosis and hepatic dysfunction. Radioiodine should be used with great caution in patients with thyroid eye disease because of the risk of exacerbation (Bartalena et al., 1998).

The patient should be provided with written information. Precautions include restricting time spent in contact with people, especially children and pregnant women, avoiding sharing a bed, reducing time spent on public or shared private transport, avoiding sharing crockery or cutlery and taking time off work. The length that time restrictions apply is individualised depending on the dose of radioiodine and the nature of work, etc.

The management of thyroid eye disease is described on page 167.

References

ARSAC. (2006). *ARSAC Notes for Guidance*. Health Protection Agency for the Administration of Radioactive Substances Committee.

Barbet, J., Campion, L. and Kraeber-Bodéré, F. (2005). Prognostic impact of serum calcitonin and carcinoembryonic antigen doubling-times in patients with medullary thyroid carcinoma. *J. Clin. Endocrinol. Metab.*, **90**, 6077–6084.

Bartalena, L., Marcocci, C., Bogazzi, F., *et al.* (1998). Relation between therapy for hyperthyroidism and the course of Graves' ophthalmopathy. *N. Engl. J. Med.*, **338**, 73–78.

Barwick, T. D., Dhawan, R. T. and Lewington, V. (2012). Role of SPECT CT in differentiated thyroid cancer. *Nucl. Med. Commun.*, **33**, 787–798.

Cheng, W., Ma, C. and Fu, H. (2013). Low- or high-dose radioiodine remnant ablation for differentiated thyroid carcinoma: a meta-analysis. *J. Clin. Endocrinol. Metab.*, **98**, 1353–1360.

De Groot, L., Abalovich, M., Alexander, E.K., *et al.* (2012). Management of thyroid dysfunction during pregnancy and postpartum: an Endocrine Society clinical practice guideline. *J. Clin. Endocrinol. Metab.*, **97**, 2543–2565.

Mallick, U., Harmer, C., Yap, B., *et al.* (2012). Ablation with low-dose radioiodine and thyrotropin alfa in thyroid cancer. *N. Engl. J. Med.*, **366**, 1674–1685.

McGriff, N. J., Csado, G., Gourgiotis, L., *et al.* (2002). Effects of thyroid hormone suppression therapy on adverse clinical outcomes in thyroid cancer. *Ann. Med.*, **34**, 554–564.

O'Neill, C. J., Vaughan, L., Learoyd, D. L., *et al.* (2011). Management of follicular thyroid carcinoma should be individualized based on degree of capsular and vascular invasion. *Eur. J. Surg. Oncol.*, **37**, 181–185.

Perros, P., Colley, S., Boelaert, K., *et al.* (2014). British Thyroid Association guidelines for the management of thyroid cancer. *Clin. Endocrinol.*, **81**, Suppl. 1.

Schlumberger, M., Bastholt, L., Dralle, H., *et al.* (2012). 2012 European Thyroid Association guidelines for metastatic medullary thyroid cancer. *Eur. Thyroid J.*, **1**, 5–14.

Smallridge, R. C., Ain, K. B., Asa, S. L., *et al.* (2012). American Thyroid Association guidelines for management of patients with anaplastic thyroid cancer. *Thyroid*, **22**, 1104–1139.

Stagnaro-Green, A., Abalovich, M., Alexander, E., *et al.* (2011). Guidelines of the American Thyroid Association for the diagnosis and management of thyroid disease during pregnancy and postpartum. *Thyroid*, **21**, 1081–1125.

Sugino, K., Kameyama, K., Ito, K., *et al.* (2012). Outcomes and prognostic factors of 251 patients with minimally invasive follicular thyroid carcinoma. *Thyroid*, **22**, 798–804.

Tuttle, R. M., Tala, H. and Shah, J. (2010) Estimating risk of recurrence in differentiated thyroid cancer after total thyroidectomy and radioactive iodine remnant ablation: using response to therapy variables to modify the initial risk estimates predicted by the new American Thyroid Association staging system. *Thyroid*, **20**, 1341–1349.

UICC (2009). In *TNM Classification of Malignant Tumours (7th edition)*. Ed. L. H. Sobin, M. K. Gospodarowitc and Ch. Wittekind. Oxford: Wiley-Blackwell, pp. 58–62.

Further reading

ATA Guidelines Taskforce. (2009). Medullary thyroid cancer: management guidelines of the American Thyroid Association. *Thyroid*, **19**, 565–612.

ATA Guidelines Taskforce on Thyroid Nodules and Differentiated Thyroid Cancer. (2009). Revised American Thyroid Association management guidelines for patients with thyroid nodules and differentiated thyroid cancer. *Thyroid*, **19**, 1167–1214.

Castagna, M. G., Mainom, F., Cipri, C., *et al.* (2011). Delayed risk stratification, to include the response to initial treatment (surgery and radioiodine ablation), has better outcome predictivity in differentiated thyroid cancer patients. *Eur. J. Endocrinol.*, **165**, 441–446.

Iyer, N. G., Morris, L. G., Tuttle, R. M., *et al.* (2011). Rising incidence of second cancers in patients with low-risk (T1N0) thyroid cancer who receive radioactive iodine therapy. *Cancer*, **117**, 4439–4446.

Kim, K. B., Cabanillas, M. E., Lazar, A. J., *et al.* (2013). Clinical responses to vemurafenib in patients with metastatic papillary thyroid cancer harboring *BRAF*(V600E) mutation. *Thyroid*, **23**, 1277–1283.

Mazzaferri, E., Robbins, R., Spencer, C., *et al.* (2003). A consensus report of the role of serum thyroglobulin as a monitoring method for low-risk patients with papillary thyroid carcinoma. *J. Clin. Endocrinol. Metab.*, **88**, 1433–1441.

Nixon, I. J., Ganly, I., Patel, S. G., *et al.* (2013). The results of selective use of radioactive iodine on survival and on recurrence in the management of papillary thyroid cancer, based on Memorial Sloan-Kettering Cancer Center risk group stratification. *Thyroid*, **23**, 683–694.

Rubino, C., de Vathaire, F., Dottorini, M. E., *et al.* (2003). Second primary malignancies in thyroid cancer patients. *Br. J. Cancer*, **89**, 1638–1644.

Walsh, S., Lowery, A. J., Evoy, D., *et al.* (2013). Thyroid lymphoma: recent advances in diagnosis and optimal management strategies. *The Oncologist*, **18**, 994–1003.

Management of neuroendocrine tumours

Andrew Lansdown and Aled Rees

Introduction

Neuroendocrine tumours (NETs) constitute a heterogeneous group of neoplasms with significant variation in their mode of presentation and biological behaviour. They arise from neuroendocrine cells, which are widely distributed in the body; the spectrum of tumours that fall under this classification is accordingly diverse. Although tumours can arise within endocrine glands such as the pituitary and the parathyroids, tumours at these sites are typically benign, with limited growth potential, and are traditionally managed by endocrinologists. This chapter therefore focuses largely on NETs arising within the bronchial or gastroenteropancreatic systems, historically termed carcinoid tumours.

Management of these rare tumours is improving due to advances in imaging and to the increased use of multidisciplinary teams in specialist centres (Kaltsas et al., 2004; Ramage et al., 2012). Treatment options are diverse and should be tailored individually, but they may include one or more of surgery, medical therapy (somatostatin analogues, interferon alpha, sunitinib and everolimus), chemotherapy, radionuclide therapy, ablative therapy and embolisation. Current clinical trials are focused on defining the optimal use of existing therapies and exploring novel agents such as angiogenesis and MTOR inhibitors.

Tumour types

NETs are classified according to (1) histological differentiation and grading, and (2) staging, based on primary tumour site.

The WHO 2010 classification (Bosman et al., 2010) is based upon the concept that all NETs have malignant potential and is organised according to grade and stage.

Grading is based upon morphological criteria and the proliferative activity of the tumour, including the mitotic activity and/or Ki-67 labelling index. Well-differentiated tumours are divided into low-grade (G1) and intermediate-grade (G2) categories. All poorly differentiated NETs are classified as high-grade (G3) neuroendocrine carcinomas.

Staging systems in place include the Union for International Cancer Control (UICC) (7th edition) and the European Neuroendocrine Tumor Society (ENETS) staging systems (Rindi et al., 2007).

Incidence and epidemiology

The UK annual disease incidence is estimated at 2–5 cases/100,000 patients, with a slight female predominance. Disease incidence is thought to be increasing overall, possibly due to increased diagnostic awareness (Modlin et al., 2008). Autopsy studies indicate that small, clinically unrecognised NETs are relatively common (up to 10% for pancreatic NETs). There is no definite geographical variation in tumour incidence, although there are reported ethnic differences, with African-Americans having the highest incidence of 6.5 per 100,000 per year (Modlin et al., 2003). The average age at diagnosis is 61 years.

Risk factors and aetiology

The risk factors for NETs are poorly understood. Most are sporadic, but there is a small familial risk (4-fold increased risk with one affected first-degree relative, 12-fold with two affected first-degree relatives). A small proportion of NETs arise on a background of an inherited cancer syndrome, for example:

- multiple endocrine neoplasia type 1 (MEN1) – parathyroid and pituitary adenomas, pancreatic NETs, bronchial/gastric NETs;
- multiple endocrine neoplasia type 2 (MEN2) – hyperparathyroidism, medullary thyroid

Practical Clinical Oncology, Second Edition, ed. Louise Hanna, Tom Crosby and Fergus Macbeth. Published by Cambridge University Press. © Cambridge University Press 2015.

carcinoma (MTC), phaeochromocytoma. MTC is discussed in Chapter 38;

- type 1 neurofibromatosis (NF1) – neurofibromas, café-au-lait macules, optic glioma, phaeochromocytoma, and rarely duodenal somatostatinoma;
- Von Hippel Lindau syndrome (VHL) – renal cell carcinoma/cysts, phaeochromocytoma, cerebellar haemangioblastoma, retinal angioma, and pancreatic NETs;
- Carney complex – spotty skin pigmentation, cardiac myxomas, thyroid adenoma, nodular adrenocortical disease causing Cushing's syndrome, sertoli cell tumours and ovarian cysts.

A family history should be obtained and a clinical examination undertaken to look for an inherited cancer syndrome in all cases of NET.

Pathology and spread

Pathology

Macroscopically, NETs are typically solid and yellow in appearance, reflecting a high lipid content.

Microscopically, NETs are often trabecular, glandular, or form rosettes. The tumour cells typically have a granular cytoplasm and round nuclei, and the majority display low proliferative potential with infrequent mitoses. However, a proportion of NETs are poorly differentiated.

The neuroendocrine origin of tumours is confirmed by immunohistochemistry directed against a panel of general neuroendocrine markers, such as chromogranin A, synaptophysin and PGP9.5. A specific immunohistochemical analysis of hormone production (e.g. glucagon for glucagonomas, ACTH where ectopic ACTH production is suspected) may be valuable, depending on the tumour site and clinical presentation. All histological analyses should give an estimate of proliferative potential not only by mitotic rate but also by using an antibody to Ki-67 (MIB-1) to generate a Ki-67 index. This has prognostic relevance and may influence choice of therapy (e.g. chemotherapy in tumours with a high Ki-67 index).

Spread

NETs may be localised to the primary organ of origin, may invade regional lymph nodes, or may spread distantly to the liver, lungs or to bone. The tumour stage at presentation is dependent on the primary site

Table 39.1 Incidence of metastases at presentation according to primary site of NET

Site/type	Incidence of metastases at presentation (%)
Typical bronchial carcinoid	< 15
Atypical bronchial carcinoid	30–50
Thymus	80
Stomach	80 (for type III)
Duodenal	45
Small intestine	60–80
Appendix	< 2 cm: rare > 2 cm: 30
Ileocaecal	70
Rectal	< 1 cm: rare > 2 cm: majority
Insulinoma	< 10
Gastrinoma	70–80
VIPoma	50–60
Glucagonoma	80
Somatostatinoma	60–70
Non-functioning pancreatic	60–80

(Table 39.1). When present, bony metastases are generally a feature of advanced disease.

Clinical presentation

In keeping with the widespread distribution of these tumours, their modes of presentation vary considerably. Many are asymptomatic and are discovered incidentally as a part of investigations performed for other reasons.

Some patients present with symptoms suggestive of bowel obstruction even if abdominal radiology is normal.

Carcinoid syndrome

Classic carcinoid syndrome is a presenting feature in around 20% of cases of intestinal NETs and it occurs when vasogenic amines and peptides including serotonin and tachykinins gain access to the systemic circulation. This is usually seen in the context of intestinal NETs with liver metastases, although similar syndromes can occasionally occur in the absence of measurable peptide hormones or their products. The features of carcinoid syndrome include dry flushing

(90%), diarrhoea (70%), abdominal pain (40%), wheezing (25%), valvular heart disease (30%) and pellagra (5%). Some patients also describe increased lacrimation and rhinorrhoea.

The carcinoid flush is usually pink, lasts for a few minutes, and involves the face and upper trunk. Some patients are able to identify triggers such as alcohol, bananas, walnuts or chocolate.

Carcinoid crisis is an extreme presentation characterised by fluctuating blood pressure, tachycardia, arrhythmias, profound flushing and bronchospasm. It may be precipitated by tumour lysis (from embolisation, chemotherapy or radionuclide therapy), tumour handling or anaesthesia.

Carcinoid heart disease is present in up to 20% of patients at presentation and classically affects the right side of the heart in patients with carcinoid syndrome: tricuspid regurgitation is the most common valvular abnormality, but left-sided problems can also occur if a patent foramen ovale is present. In severe cases, valve replacement surgery is necessary.

Other presentations

Pulmonary NETs present with symptoms suggestive of bronchial obstruction (pneumonia, dyspnoea, pleuritic pain), cough or haemoptysis. Many of these are discovered incidentally on chest X-ray (Srirajaskanthan et al., 2009).

Bronchial, thymic and pancreatic NETs may also cause ectopic hormone production (e.g. Cushing's syndrome from ectopic ACTH secretion, acromegaly from ectopic growth hormone-releasing hormone production or syndrome of inappropriate anti-diuretic hormone secretion).

Pancreatic NETs present with either a hypersecretory syndrome or with symptoms directly related to the tumour mass (abdominal pain, weight loss) or to metastases. Their clinical features are shown in Table 39.2.

Investigation and staging

The diagnosis and staging of NETs is based on a combination of the following:

- clinical symptoms where present;
- biochemistry (general and specific neuroendocrine/hormone markers);
- radiological and nuclear imaging;
- histological confirmation (the gold standard and mandatory whenever possible).

Table 39.2 Incidence and clinical features of functioning pancreatic NETs

Tumour type	Incidence	Symptoms
Insulinoma	1–2 per million	Confusion
		Sweating
		Dizziness
		Relief with eating
		Weight gain
Gastrinoma	1 per million	Peptic ulceration
		Diarrhoea
Glucagonoma	1 per 5 million	Diabetes
		Weight loss
		Necrolytic migratory erythema
		Diarrhoea
		Stomatitis
VIPoma	1 per 5 million	Watery diarrhoea
		Marked hypokalaemia
Somatostatinoma	1 per 10 million	Steatorrhoea
		Cholelithiasis
		Weight loss
		Diabetes

Biochemistry

Biochemical tests comprise both general neuroendocrine markers and specific hormones for the underlying tumour type. They may be useful not only in establishing the diagnosis, but also in monitoring response to therapy.

Plasma chromogranin A (CgA) is a useful general tumour marker (Tomassetti et al., 2001). It retains high sensitivity in all types of NET with the highest levels often seen in metastatic intestinal NETs. Renal impairment, hypergastrinaemia and treatment with proton pump inhibitors are important causes of false-positive CgA elevation.

24-hour urinary 5-hydroxyindoleacetic acid (5-HIAA): many intestinal NETs secrete serotonin, and measurement of its metabolite 5-HIAA is useful, with up to 70% sensitivity in metastatic disease. Various drugs and foodstuffs affecting its measurement should be excluded for 3 days before and during urine collection.

Pancreatic polypeptide (PP) is secreted from a high proportion of pancreatic NETs and can be a useful additional marker in some cases, especially when CgA is in the normal range (Eriksson *et al.*, 2000).

Specific biochemical markers may also be useful in diagnosis depending on clinical presentation and index of suspicion for inherited disease (e.g. prolactin, calcium and PTH where MEN1 is suspected).

A fasting gut hormone profile should complement plasma CgA measurement in suspected pancreatic NETs. Blood should be collected in a lithium heparin bottle containing trasylol, spun and frozen prior to subsequent analysis. To avoid false-positive gastrin elevation, patients should discontinue proton-pump inhibitors (for at least 2 weeks) and H2 blockers (for at least 3 days) prior to testing.

Patients with suspected insulinoma require a supervised inpatient fast in a specialist endocrine unit.

Radiological and nuclear imaging

A number of imaging modalities are employed in the evaluation of NETs. Determining an appropriate imaging strategy in an individual patient requires close liaison with radiologists and nuclear medicine physicians but is partly dependent on whether the imaging is undertaken for screening at-risk populations, the initial detection of the disease, for determining tumour extent where neuroendocrine disease is already confirmed or for follow-up and assessing response to treatment.

CT scans are useful for identifying bronchial NETs, in assessing liver metastases (where triple-phase scanning enhances sensitivity), and identifying primary abdominal NETs, especially when somatostatin receptor scintigraphy (SSRS) is negative.

MRI and CT are both useful in imaging pancreatic NETs, although EUS is particularly sensitive, especially for identifying tumours within the pancreatic head where it can also enable fine needle aspiration for histological diagnosis (Anderson *et al.*, 2000). The procedure has low complication rates and shows good correlation with postoperative histology (Baker *et al.*, 2008).

Somatostatin receptor scintigraphy (SSRS; 'Octreo-Scan®'; ^{111}In-octreotide) has high sensitivity in locating primary NETs and in assessing the extent of metastatic disease (Chiti *et al.*, 2000; Kaltsas *et al.*, 2001; Schillaci *et al.*, 2003). The exception is for insulinomas, where sensitivity falls to less than 50%. Modern nuclear imaging centres now use SSRS in combination with single positron emission computed tomography

(SPECT) and fusion imaging with CT (Schillaci *et al.*, 1999). Demonstration of clear uptake on SSRS also predicts a response to somatostatin analogue therapy and determines suitability for peptide-receptor radionuclide therapy.

^{123}I-MIBG has significantly lower sensitivity than ^{111}In-octreotide (Kaltsas *et al.*, 2001), but may be useful when radiolabelled MIBG therapy is being considered.

PET scanning is increasingly used to image NETs, although its use is currently limited by scanner availability in the UK. A number of ^{68}Ga-labelled somatostatin analogues have been produced for diagnostic imaging, including DOTA octreotide (DOTATOC), DOTA octreotate (DOTATATE) and DOTA-NaI-octreotide (DOTANOC). ^{68}Ga-DOTATOC has high sensitivity and specificity in detecting unknown primary tumours, and in staging and follow-up after therapy compared with CT or SSRS (Gabriel *et al.*, 2007; Versari *et al.*, 2010; Treglia *et al.*, 2012). [18]FDG (fluorodeoxyglucose)-PET has a useful role in the staging of primary bronchial and poorly differentiated NETs.[18]F-DOPA and ^{11}C-5-HTP (hydroxytryptophan) PET/CT are emerging imaging techniques which appear to show high sensitivity for gastrointestinal and pancreatic NETs, but these are not yet routinely available.

Selective angiography with secretagogue (calcium) injection may be particularly useful in localising small gastrinomas or insulinomas, but palpation at laparotomy may occasionally be necessary in small functioning pancreatic NETs where imaging has been unhelpful. This is typically combined with intraoperative ultrasound.

Treatment

Treatment overview

NETs are rare; consequently, randomised trial data to form a robust evidence base to guide management are comparatively limited. All cases should thus be managed in the context of a multidisciplinary team (MDT) whose members may vary according to local expertise and interests but should include representation from endocrinology, gastroenterology, surgery, oncology, radiology/nuclear medicine and histopathology. This facilitates accurate diagnosis and staging, develops consensus on management, ensures individualised treatment planning, and improves interdisciplinary education. Increasingly, such groups should form part of a larger network of clinicians with interests in these tumours at national (UKINETS) and international (European Neuroendocrine Tumor Society, ENETS) levels, thereby facilitating multicentre studies and the development of consensus guidelines.

Treatment should aim to cure the patient if possible, but is often palliative because most patients have evidence of metastases at presentation. In patients with incurable disease, treatment should aim to maintain a good quality of life (QOL) for as long as possible, recognising that this can be achieved for a number of years in many NETs, even in the presence of metastatic disease. A specific QOL questionnaire, QLQ-GINET21, has recently been validated for patients with gastrointestinal NETs (Yadegarfar *et al.*, 2013).

Surgery

Surgery is currently the only treatment that can achieve a cure. Although metastatic disease at presentation frequently precludes a cure, surgery may still have a role in debulking the primary tumour, or in minimising the risk of bowel obstruction. For intestinal NETs it should be recognised, however, that marked fibrosis around the tumour (a desmoplastic reaction) may make surgical resection technically challenging and can run the risk of vascular compromise.

Preoperatively, patients with known functioning midgut NETs should be carefully assessed for the presence of carcinoid heart disease and should be treated in the pre-, peri- and postoperative periods with an intravenous infusion of octreotide (50 μg/hour) to minimise the risk of carcinoid crisis.

Patients with pulmonary NETs should undergo lung or wedge resection with lymph node dissection (Lim *et al.*, 2008).

The surgical management of gastroenteropancreatic NETs is dependent on the primary site, mode of presentation (elective versus emergency) and extent of disease (Sutton *et al.*, 2003).

Emergency presentations usually demand a resection sufficient to correct the immediate problem, but may need to be followed by a further, more definitive procedure; for example, in patients presenting with appendicitis where prognosis can be improved by performing a subsequent right hemicolectomy in appendiceal tumours greater than 2 cm in size or those that are 1–2 cm where the macro- or microscopic appearances are unfavourable (Plockinger *et al.*, 2008).

Small intestinal and colorectal NETs (> 2 cm) should be resected together with locoregional lymph node dissection. Resection should be considered even in patients with metastatic disease because it may improve prognosis in addition to minimising the risk of future intestinal obstruction (Ramage *et al.*, 2012).

Gastric NETs should be managed according to their type: type 1 (associated with chronic atrophic gastritis) and type 2 (associated with Zollinger–Ellison syndrome/MEN1) NETs occur in patients with hypergastrinaemia and require medical therapy (e.g. with proton-pump inhibitors for Zollinger–Ellison syndrome); endoscopic resection and surveillance may also be required but the risk of metastases is very low. Type 3 gastric NETs occur sporadically, are more aggressive, and frequently show evidence of metastasis at presentation. They are not associated with hypergastrinaemia. Most require gastrectomy and regional lymph node clearance.

Surgery for pancreatic NETs should be performed only by specialists and the extent of disease can vary from enucleation only for superficial or easily localised insulinomas (which have low malignant potential) to distal or total pancreatectomy or even pancreatoduodenectomy in more extensive disease.

Surgical resection of liver metastases may prolong survival and can offer symptomatic relief in carefully selected cases. Liver surgery with 'curative intent' may be considered for resectable well-differentiated liver disease, in the absence of right heart failure, extra-abdominal or diffuse peritoneal disease (Pavel *et al.*, 2012).

Whenever abdominal surgery is contemplated for NETs, consideration should always be given to cholecystectomy in order to prevent gallstone formation in patients who subsequently commence somatostatin analogues.

Drug therapy: somatostatin analogue therapy

Somatostatin analogue therapy forms the mainstay of symptomatic control in gastroenteropancreatic NETs.

Endogenous somatostatin has a very short circulatory half-life, making it unsuitable for use. Octreotide has a half-life of several hours and may be administered subcutaneously in doses of 50–100 μg, 2–3 times daily. Sustained-release preparations, administered every 4 weeks and usually given in preference, are also available, allowing dosing every 2–4 weeks. These include

Lanreotide Autogel® and Sandostatin LAR®, both of which have been shown to improve QOL (including reduced frequency of flushing and diarrhoea) with equivalent or improved efficacy compared with short-acting octreotide (Rubin *et al.*, 1999; Tomassetti *et al.*, 2000; Toumpanakis *et al.*, 2009).

Long-acting somatostatin analogues are thus used as standard practice in symptomatic treatment of NETs, although shorter-acting analogues may still have a role in symptomatic breakthrough and in the management of carcinoid crisis. In addition to good symptomat control, which occurs in the majority of patients, biochemical response (inhibition of hormone production) occurs in 30–70% and tumour stabilisation (or rarely even shrinkage) may occur. Indeed, the PROMID study confirmed that octreotide LAR® slowed the time to tumour progression in well-differentiated metastatic intestinal NETs to a median of 14 months compared to 6 months with placebo (Rinke *et al.*, 2009). More recently, the CLARINET study (Controlled study of Lanreotide Antiproliferative Response In NET) randomised patients with advanced, well/moderately differentiated, asymptomatic NETs to Lanreotide Autogel® 120 mg monthly or placebo (Caplin *et al.*, 2014). Lanreotide was associated with significantly prolonged progression-free survival (hazard ratio for progression or death 0.47), an effect which was observed in patients with grade 1 and grade 2 tumours, and irrespective of hepatic tumour load. Thus, somatostatin analogues should now also be considered as anti-proliferative treatments in non-functioning as well as functioning NETs.

Patients should be warned of side effects (diarrhoea, steatorrhoea, abdominal discomfort, flatulence, anorexia and nausea) at the start of therapy. These are usually mild and diminish with continued use. In addition, patients with diabetes may need to adjust their insulin dosage.

Long-term use can result in gallstones (10–50%), although these are rarely symptomatic; hence, ultrasonographic surveillance is no longer considered necessary.

Somatostatin analogues are also effective in controlling clinical syndromes associated with unresectable pancreatic NETs, including VIPomas, glucagonomas and occasionally insulinomas, although 50% of the latter demonstrate a paradoxical fall in blood glucose levels due to a suppression of counter-regulatory hormones such as glucagon.

Newer somatostatin analogues are emerging. Pasireotide is a novel somatostatin analogue that binds more broadly to somatostatin receptors compared with octreotide and lanreotide. In a phase I study, long-acting pasireotide was well tolerated in patients with advanced gastrointestinal NETs refractory to other somatostatin analogues (Wolin *et al.*, 2013).

Proton-pump inhibitors form the mainstay of medical therapy in gastrinomas with no evidence for added benefit from somatostatin analogue therapy.

Diazoxide may be used short-term for patients with insulinomas awaiting surgery or longer-term for unresectable or metastatic disease.

Drug therapy: interferon

Interferon alfa in a dose of 3–5 MU, 3–5 times weekly, is employed in the treatment of NETs. However, its use is not widespread, in part related to conflicting data as to its efficacy in addition to difficulties with tolerability and high cost. Nevertheless, biochemical and symptomatic response may be seen in 40–70% of patients. It may be used alone or in combination with somatostatin analogue therapy.

Drug therapy: chemotherapy

The precise role of chemotherapy, and the most effective chemotherapeutic regimen in NETs remains uncertain. It is clear, however, that chemotherapy has little therapeutic value in well-differentiated, slowly proliferating intestinal NETs. A detailed histological profile of the proliferative potential of a tumour is therefore mandatory in selecting patients who are appropriate for treatment.

Poorly differentiated or anaplastic NETs may demonstrate up to a 70% response rate with cisplatin and etoposide-based combinations, although the duration of response may not extend beyond 8–9 months (Mitry *et al.*, 1999).

Pulmonary NETs, which often share pathological and behavioural characteristics with small-cell lung cancers, are also often treated with combinations of a platinum and etoposide, although again, treatment decisions should be based individually on tumour characteristics and radiological progression.

Pancreatic NETs are often chemosensitive, with reported response rates of 40–70%, although the optimal regimen has not yet been determined and various combinations of streptozocin, 5-fluorouracil, doxorubicin, cisplatin, dacarbazine and adriamycin are in use. Temozolomide, which is orally available, has been used in combination with capecitabine, with up to 70% response rate reported (Strosberg *et al.*, 2011). Where possible, such patients should be incorporated into clinical trials of new or existing agents.

Drug therapy: new agents

Two new treatment options have emerged for patients with advanced, progressive, well-differentiated pancreatic NETs.

The oral tyrosine kinase inhibitor sunitinib and the MTOR inhibitor everolimus have both been approved as licensed therapies for patients with advanced, unresectable pancreatic NETs. In a multicentre, randomised, double-blind, placebo-controlled phase III trial of patients with advanced, well-differentiated pancreatic NETs, daily sunitinib improved progression-free and overall survival. Treatment was well tolerated, but toxicities included neutropenia and hypertension (Raymond *et al.*, 2011). Everolimus was also shown to improve progression-free survival in a prospective, randomised phase III study in patients with advanced low-grade or intermediate-grade pancreatic NETs. Treatment was well tolerated, but adverse events included glucose intolerance, stomatitis, diarrhoea and infections (Yao *et al.*, 2011). The optimal position for sunitinib or everolimus in the treatment of metastatic pancreatic NETs is unclear at present, but they are typically considered in patients with well-/moderately differentiated tumours who progress post-somatostatin analogue therapy or after cytotoxic chemotherapy.

Radionuclide therapy

Indolent NETs are relatively radioresistant and so there is a limited role for conventional external beam radiotherapy in treating NETs other than for its analgesic benefits in bony metastases. However, by targeting radioisotopes directly at the tumour sites, higher doses of radiation can be administered than with beam irradiation, multiple sites can be treated simultaneously and non-target damage can be minimised.

Peptide-receptor radionuclide therapy (PRRT) can be used for symptomatic patients with unresectable or metastatic progressive disease when abnormally increased uptake of the corresponding imaging compound is evident. ^{131}I-MIBG, ^{90}Y-DOTATOC, ^{90}Y-DOTATATE and ^{177}Lu-DOTATATE have all been used, with beneficial effects on symptom palliation,

improved QOL and disease stabilisation (Krenning *et al.*, 2005; Cwikla *et al.*, 2010). Treatment is well tolerated: although mild haematological toxicity is common, renal toxicity is rare. In a recent retrospective analysis of patients with progressive metastatic NETs receiving ^{90}Y-DOTATOC or ^{90}Y-DOTATATE PRRT, radiological responses were observed in 71% patients (24% partial response, 47% stable disease; Vinjamuri *et al.*, 2013).

Embolisation and ablation techniques

Embolisation of the hepatic artery may be indicated for patients with multiple and hormonally active liver metastases that are not amenable to surgical resection (Eriksson *et al.*, 1998). The aim of therapy is to control symptoms and reduce tumour size. The methods used vary considerably, but the technique can use different combinations of embolising particles, chemotherapeutic agents and radionuclides, and in-house guidelines should be developed at each centre. Symptomatic response may occur in 40–80% of patients, but the potential therapeutic benefit should be balanced against a mortality of up to 4–7% and possible side effects including postembolisation syndrome (fever, abdominal pain and nausea), carcinoid crisis (the risk of which should be minimised by octreotide infusion, judicious use of fluids, antibiotics and allopurinol) and hepatic abscess formation (5%).

Radiofrequency ablation, which may be performed laparoscopically or percutaneously, improves symptoms when at least 90% of the visible tumour is ablated, and reduces hormone secretion and tumour size. The main limitation is the size, accessibility and number of tumours.

Selective Internal Radiation Microsphere Therapy (SIRT) is an emerging treatment for patients with NET liver metastases. Radioactive ^{90}Y resin microspheres are administered through a percutaneous hepatic artery catheter. Symptomatic and radiological responses may be seen in 50% of patients (King *et al.*, 2008).

Prognosis

Prognosis in NETs is dependent on histological features (worse with poorly differentiated tumours and those with high Ki-67 index), tumour size, location, and stage. The overall 5-year survival varies from 20% to 80% depending on these factors and the treatment employed. For any given site, the 5-year survival worsens with increasing stage of disease (4–35% with distant metastases, 20–70% with regional spread, and 40–95% for localised disease). Rectal NETs carry the best prognosis of tumours arising from the gut (74–88% 5-year survival rate). Bronchial NETs also carry a favourable prognosis if the histology is typical (80–90% 5-year survival), although atypical carcinoids have 5-year-survival rates of 40–70% (Fink *et al.*, 2001). The prognosis for pancreatic NETs is variable and depends on tumour type (Table 39.1), although overall 5-year survival is in the order of 30–45%.

Areas of current interest and clinical trials

Areas of current interest

The molecular biology of NETs is poorly understood at present. Conventional searches for mutations, rearrangements or amplifications in known candidate oncogenes, or loss of tumour suppression gene activity (with the exception of MEN1) have largely been disappointing (Zikusoka *et al.*, 2005). Large-scale genomic approaches using exome sequencing, genome-wide DNA methylation, RNA expression and copy number analyses may identify new pathways as the basis for novel diagnostic and treatment strategies. Research studies are also exploring biomarkers, such as circulating tumour cells, as prognosticators and early markers of response to therapy.

Clinical trials

There are a number of clinical trials in NETs which are open or in development on the National Cancer Research Network Upper GI portfolio. These include the NET01 study, a randomised phase II study comparing capecitabine plus streptozocin with or without cisplatin in the treatment of unresectable or metastatic gastroenteropancreatic neuroendocrine tumours, which is due to report shortly.

RADIANT-4 is a multi-centre, randomised, double-blind, phase III study of everolmius plus best supportive care versus placebo plus best supportive care in the treatment of patients with advanced NETs of gastrointestinal or lung origin.

Acknowledgements

The authors would like to acknowledge the contribution of Atul Kalhan to this chapter.

References

Anderson, M. A., Carpenter, S., Thompson, N. W., *et al.* (2000). Endoscopic ultrasound is highly accurate and directs management in patients with neuroendocrine tumors of the pancreas. *Am. J. Gastroenterol.*, **95**, 2271–2277.

Baker, M. S., Knuth, J. L., DeWitt, J., *et al.* (2008). Pancreatic cystic neuroendocrine tumors: preoperative diagnosis with endoscopic ultrasound and fine-needle immunocytology. *J. Gastrointest. Surg.*, **12**, 450–456.

Bosman, F. T., Carneiro, F., Hruban, R. H., *et al.* (2010). *WHO Classification of Tumours of the Digestive System.* Lyon: IARC.

Caplin, M. E., Pavel, M., Cwikla, J. B., *et al.* (2014). Lanreotide in metastatic enteropancreatic neuroendocrine tumors. *N. Engl. J. Med.*, **371**, 224–233.

Chiti, A., Briganti, V., Fanti, S., *et al.* (2000). Results and potential of somatostatin receptor imaging in gastroenteropancreatic tract tumours. *Q. J. Nucl. Med.*, **44**, 42–49.

Cwikla, J. B., Sankowski, A., Sekecka, N., *et al.* (2010). Efficacy of radionuclide treatment DOTATATE Y-90 in patients with progressive metastatic gastroenteropancreatic neuroendocrine carcinomas (GEP-NETs): a phase II study. *Ann. Oncol.*, **21**, 787–794.

Eriksson, B. K., Larsson, E. G., Skogseid, B. M., *et al.* (1998). Liver embolizations of patients with malignant neuroendocrine gastrointestinal tumors. *Cancer*, **83**, 2293–2301.

Eriksson, B., Oberg, K. and Stridsberg, M. (2000). Tumor markers in neuroendocrine tumors. *Digestion*, **62** (Suppl. 1), 33–38.

Fink, G., Krelbaum, T., Yellin, A., *et al.* (2001). Pulmonary carcinoid: presentation, diagnosis, and outcome in 142 cases in Israel and review of 640 cases from the literature. *Chest*, **119**, 1647–1651.

Gabriel, M., Decristoforo, C., Kendler, D., *et al* (2007). 68Ga-DOTA-Tyr3-octreotide PET in neuroendocrine tumors: comparison with somatostatin receptor scintography and CT. *J. Nucl. Med.*, **48**, 508–518.

Kaltsas, G., Korbonits, M., Heintz, E., *et al.* (2001). Comparison of somatostatin analog and meta-iodobenzylguanidine radionuclides in the diagnosis and localization of neuroendocrine tumors. *J. Clin. Endocrinol. Metab.*, **86**, 895–902.

Kaltsas, G. A., Besser, G. M. and Grossman, A. B. (2004). The diagnosis and medical management of advanced neuroendocrine tumors. *Endocr. Rev.*, **25**, 458–511.

King, J., Quinn, R., Glenn, D. M., *et al.* (2008). Radioembolization with selective internal radiation microspheres for neuroendocrine liver metastases. *Cancer*, **113**, 921–929.

Krenning, E. P., Teunissen, J. J., Valkema, R., *et al.* (2005). Molecular radiotherapy with somatostatin analogs for (neuro-)endocrine tumors. *J. Endocrinol. Invest.*, **28** (Suppl. 11), 146–150.

Lim, E., Goldstraw, P., Nicholson, A. G., *et al.* (2008). Proceedings of the IASLC International Workshop on Advances in Pulomnary Neuroendocrine Tumors 2007. *J. Thorac. Oncol.*, **3**, 1194–1201.

Mitry, E., Baudin, E., Ducreux, M., *et al.* (1999). Treatment of poorly differentiated neuroendocrine tumours with etoposide and cisplatin. *Br. J. Cancer*, **81**, 1351–1355.

Modlin, I. M., Lye, K. D. and Kidd, M. (2003). A 5-decade analysis of 13,715 carcinoid tumors. *Cancer*, **97**, 934–959.

Modlin, I. M., Oberg, K., Chung, D. C., *et al.* (2008). Gastroenteropanreatic neuroendocrine tumours. *Lancet Oncol.*, **9**, 61–72.

Pavel, M., Baudin, E., Couvelard, A., *et al.* (2012). ENETS consensus guidelines for the management of patients with liver and other distant metastases from neuroendocrine neoplasms of foregut, midgut, hindgut and unknown primary. *Neuroendocrinology*, **95**, 157–176.

Plockinger, U., Couvelard, A., Falconi, M., *et al.* (2008) Consensus guidelines for the management of patients with digestive neuroendocrine tumours: well-differentiated tumour/carcinoma of the appendix and goblet cell carcinoma. *Neuroendocrinology*, **87**, 20–30.

Ramage, J. K., Ahmed, A., Ardill, J., *et al.* (2012). Guidelines for the management of gastroenteropancreatic neuroendocrine (including carcinoid) tumours (NETs). *Gut*, 61, 6–32.

Raymond, E., Dahan, L., Raoul, J. L., *et al.* (2011). Sunitinib malate for the treatment of pancreatic neuroendocrine tumors. *N. Engl. J. Med.*, **364**, 501–513.

Rindi, G., Klöppel, G., Couvelard, A., *et al.* (2007). TNM staging of midgut and hindgut (neuro) endocrine tumors: a consensus proposal including a grading system. *Virchows Archiv.*, **451**(4), 757–762.

Rinke, A., Müller, H. H., Schade-Brittinger, C., *et al.* (2009). PROMID Study Group. Placebo-controlled, double-blind, prospective, randomized study on the effect of octreotide LAR in the control of tumor growth in patients with metastatic neuroendocrine midgut tumors: a report from the PROMID Study Group. *J. Clin. Oncol.*, **27**, 4656–4663.

Rubin, J., Ajani, J., Schirmer, W., *et al.* (1999). Octreotide acetate long-acting formulation versus open-label subcutaneous octreotide acetate in malignant carcinoid syndrome. *J. Clin. Oncol.*, **17**, 600–606.

Schillaci, O., Corleto, V. D., Annibale, B., *et al.* (1999). Single photon emission computed tomography procedure improves accuracy of somatostatin receptor scintigraphy in gastroenteropancreatic tumours. *Ital. J. Gastroenterol. Hepatol.*, **31** (Suppl. 2), S186–189.

Schillaci, O., Spanu, A., Scopinaro, F., *et al.* (2003). Somatostatin receptor scintigraphy in liver metastasis detection from gastroenteropancreatic neuroendocrine tumors. *J. Nucl. Med.*, **44**, 359–368.

Srirajaskanthan, R., Toumpanakis, C., Karpathakis, A., *et al.* (2009). Surgical management and palliative treatment in bronchial neuroendocrine tumours: a clinical study of 45 patients. *Lung Cancer*, **65**, 68–73.

Strosberg, J. R., Fine, R. L., Choi, J., *et al.* (2011). First-line chemotherapy with capecitabine and temozolamide in patients with metastatic pancreatic endocrine carcinomas. *Cancer*, **117**, 268–275.

Sutton, R., Doran, H. E., Williams, E. M., *et al.* (2003). Surgery for midgut carcinoid. *Endocr. Relat. Cancer*, **10**, 469–481.

Tomassetti, P., Migliori, M., Corinaldesi, R., *et al.* (2000). Treatment of gastroenteropancreatic neuroendocrine tumours with octreotide LAR. *Aliment. Pharmacol. Ther.*, **14**, 557–560.

Tomassetti, P., Migliori, M., Simoni, P., *et al.* (2001). Diagnostic value of plasma chromogranin A in neuroendocrine tumours. *Eur. J. Gastroenterol. Hepatol.*, **13**, 55–58.

Toumpanakis, C., Garland, J., Marelli, L., *et al.* (2009). Long-term results of patients with malignant carcionoid syndrome receiving octreotide LAR. *Aliment. Pharmacol. Ther.*, **30**, 733–740.

Treglia, G., Castaldi, P., Rindi, G., *et al.* (2012). Diagnostic performance of Gallium-68 somatostatin receptor PET and PET/CT in patients with thoracic and gastroenteropancreatic neuroendocrine tumours: a meta-analysis. *Endocrine*, **42**, 80–87.

Versari, A., Camellini, L., Carlinfante, G., *et al.* (2010). Ga-68 DOTATOC PET, endoscopic ultrasonography, and multidetector CT in the diagnosis of duodenopancreatic neuroendocrine tumors: a single-centre retrospective study. *Clin. Nucl. Med.*, **35**, 321–328.

Vinjamuri, S., Gilbert, T. M., Banks, M., *et al.* (2013). Peptide receptor radionuclide therapy with (90) Y-DOTATATE/(90)Y-DOTATOC in patients with progressive metastatic neuroendocrine tumours: assessment of response, survival and toxicity. *Br. J. Cancer*, **108**, 1440–1448.

Wolin, E. M., Hu, K., Hughes, G., *et al.* (2013). Safety, tolerability, pharmacokinetics, and pharmacodynamics of a long-acting release (LAR) formulation of pasireotide (SOM230) in patients with gastoenteropancreatic neuroendocrine tumours: results from a randomized, multicenter, open-label, phase I study. *Cancer Chemother. Pharmacol.*, **72**, 387–395.

Yadegarfar, G., Friend, L., Jones, L., *et al.* (2013). Validation of the EORTC QLQ-GINET21 questionnaire for assessing quality of life of patients with gastrointestinal neuroendocrine tumours. *Br. J. Cancer*, **108**(2), 301–310.

Yao, J. C., Shah, M. H., Ito, T., *et al.* (2011). Everolimus for advanced pancreatic neuroendocrine tumours. *N. Engl. J. Med.*, **364**, 514–523.

Zikusoka, M. N., Kidd, M., Eick, G., *et al.* (2005). The molecular genetics of gastroenteropancreatic neuroendocrine tumors. *Cancer*, **104**, 2292–2309.

Chapter

40

Management of cancer in children

Owen Tilsley

Introduction

This chapter aims to provide the reader with an introduction to the management of children with cancer. Contemporary reviews and resources will be referred to as appropriate. Radiotherapy is an important component of the treatment for many childhood tumours and this may involve advanced techniques including brachytherapy or protons, sometimes requiring referral to another centre or even abroad. Many different healthcare professionals are involved in the delivery of care, coordinated in the UK by specialised multidisciplinary teams (MDTs) at one of 19 principal treatment centres, often in collaboration with shared care units closer to home.

Paediatric cancer is uncommon. Of the 280,000 patients diagnosed with cancer in England in 2012, only 1303 were children (0.5%). The incidence of some childhood cancers has increased marginally over the last 40 years, but death rates have declined dramatically for all non-CNS childhood cancers. With cure rates now over 70%, the prevalence of paediatric cancer survivors in the population is increasing rapidly, posing challenges for the management of cancer survivorship and the late effects of treatment. The incidence of cancer between the ages of 10 and 65 is well modelled by a 10% increase per annum, which equates to a 10-fold increase every 25 years. Given the relative rarity of paediatric cancer, it is still unusual to encounter an adult survivor of paediatric malignancy, but will become more common.

An important challenge in treatment is to minimise toxicity while maximising the chance of cure, leading to a risk-based stratification of treatment intensity, including for radiotherapy. As a result, most paediatric cancer is delivered using nationally or internationally agreed protocols. Radiotherapy has significant late toxicity as it reduces the natural growth seen in childhood, and, because of the long life expectancy of survivors, it may cause radiotherapy-induced second malignancies.

The radiotherapy pathway

Giving radiotherapy to children is complex and requires a team of clinical oncologists, therapeutic radiographers, mould room staff and play specialists, together with nurses, anaesthetic staff, physicists, dosimetrists, and psychologists or psychotherapists.

Play therapy

Play therapy is important in preparing children for radiotherapy. If the trust and cooperation of a younger child can be gained, treatment may not require a general anaesthetic. Play therapy should occur early, often before the child visits the radiotherapy department. It may reduce anxiety and misconceptions, and it can introduce strategies such as distraction to help the child cope with being still and alone during radiotherapy. It may also help children to express their wishes and feelings, and can provide emotional support, advocacy and sibling support.

Initial consultation

The initial consultation will usually introduce a new team to the family. It should be pre-arranged so that the child and family can decide who they want to bring with them. It should explain the reason for the radiotherapy and be long enough for the family's questions to be answered. The child's ability to cope without anaesthetic should be assessed and any specific health or support needs identified. Discussion of late effects is often the hardest part of the consultation, and so it is better to discuss these and obtain consent at a further appointment. The extent of the late effects may not be

Practical Clinical Oncology, Second Edition, ed. Louise Hanna, Tom Crosby and Fergus Macbeth. Published by Cambridge University Press. © Cambridge University Press 2015.

fully known until the radiotherapy has been planned and so a number of separate consultations may be needed. Verbal information should be supplemented with written information. The paediatric therapeutic radiographer may also wish to meet the family, and a visit to view the department may be arranged. Ways of mitigating the effects of radiation on fertility before treatment should be discussed, if appropriate.

Anaesthesia

Children older than three to four will usually lie still with good play therapy input, but anaesthesia is required for younger children and some older ones with learning difficulties or behavioural problems. It is more often needed when shells or prone positioning are used. The child is usually anaesthetised in the radiotherapy department because once they are asleep they should be moved as little as possible. This may be away from immediately available medical support in the event of a problem and it therefore requires an experienced anaesthetic team which needs to be available daily for the duration of the radiotherapy course. As the child has to fast before the anaesthetic, it is usual to treat the child at the start of the morning to reduce the disruption to the child's routine and eating.

Immobilisation and scanning

A pre-planning discussion should be held before this visit to reduce delays and minimise the discussion of planning uncertainties in front of the child and family. They should be fully informed about the procedure before it begins and an action plan should be discussed and agreed. This will include the removal of clothes, marking with pens and sticking radio-opaque markers on the skin and the possible use of permanent skin markers. If an immobilisation device is to be made, the child should understand the procedure and be happy to cooperate. The scanning procedure should be explained, as it is possible that previous scans were performed under anaesthetic. The number of staff present should be kept to a minimum, but as well as the planning staff and the family, the play therapist and paediatric therapeutic radiographer may need to be present for support. The child and family should understand the role of each staff member. The clinical room where the immobilisation device is fitted and the scan performed should be child-friendly and safe and should have distraction tools such as music or light projectors.

Planning

Craniospinal radiotherapy and total body irradiation are techniques requiring special competence, and planning paediatric radiotherapy requires an understanding of its effects on growth and development. Specialisation in the planning department is useful but the low demand for paediatric radiotherapy means that full-time specialisation is unlikely to be necessary.

Consent

This should involve a discussion of the acute and late effects of treatment and, depending on the age and wishes of the child, it may not always be appropriate for the child to be present. Sometimes the discussion should include the late effects on sexual and reproductive function, neurocognitive deficits, hormonal deficiencies and the need for hormone replacement therapy, effects on bone and soft tissue growth, vision and hearing and the risk of second malignancies.

The legal age of capacity is 18 in England, Wales and Northern Ireland, and 16 in Scotland. At this age, only the individual can give consent unless they are deemed to lack capacity under the provision of the Mental Capacity Act 2005 (England and Wales) or the Adults with Incapacity (Scotland) Act 2000. There is no formal statutory instrument in Northern Ireland. Children under this age can consent to medical treatment if the doctor believes they understand the procedure and its consequences (Gillick or Fraser competent). If a child is under 16 and is not yet competent, any person or body with parental responsibility may consent, even if the child is refusing treatment. If the doctors believe that parental refusal of consent is detrimental to the child, legal advice is required as it may be possible to obtain a court order for treatment. It is necessary to obtain consent only from one individual with parental responsibility, but it would be wise to seek the advice of colleagues if the parents disagree. A competent child is legally entitled to withhold consent to treatment. However, if the parents and treating doctor believe that refusing treatment is not in the child's best interest, legal advice should be obtained and the correct way forward may need to be established by judicial process.

Radiotherapy treatment

Children may benefit from seeing the treatment machine in advance. They should understand what is involved and have their anxieties allayed. They should understand that for short periods of time they need to be alone in the room. The use of a long ribbon through the maze held by both the child and family member may help. The room should be child-friendly with distraction devices, music and an intercom. The use of a bedspread over the bed and the concealment of unnecessary devices such as other patients' shells may help. Ideally, the same staff should treat the child each day on the same machine and the number of staff should be kept to a minimum.

In the case of machine failure or service, these staff should, if possible, treat the child on a different machine. The child should understand each staff member's role. Suitable time should be allowed in radiotherapy appointments because gaining the trust and cooperation of children may take longer than for adults. The waiting area should also be a child-friendly and safe environment, with suitable play and recreational equipment. Some radiotherapy departments operate a no-wait policy for children.

Radiotherapy techniques

Conformal radiotherapy

Scoliosis, epiphyseal slippage, avascular necrosis and abnormalities of craniofacial growth may be seen after radiation exceeding around 20 Gy to bones, and the child's age at the time of treatment and the site may affect any adverse effects. Traditionally, paediatric radiotherapy was given 'symmetrically' to bones to avoid asymmetric growth and these principles remain for the low-dose radiotherapy given in Wilms' tumour following tumour spillage at surgery and in high-risk neuroblastoma. However, the increased conformality and ability to spare appreciable amounts of normal tissue obtained with high-quality conformal, 3D CT-planned radiotherapy with multiple beams and multi-leaf collimation may outweigh the benefit of a symmetrical reduction in bone growth, especially for the older child.

Intensity-modulated radiation therapy (IMRT)

In rhabdomyosarcoma and Ewing sarcoma, radiotherapy to a high dose, typically 54 Gy, is given when surgery is impracticable or too morbid. These are often large tumours in the trunk and head and neck. Delivering this dose of radiotherapy can be challenging when also trying to keep the dose to important organs at risk within tolerance, and so IMRT techniques may be required. It is generally believed that the benefits of increased conformality outweigh the potential increase in second malignancy arising from the 'low-dose bath' and the possible higher integral dose given.

Protons

Protons and X-rays have equivalent radiobiological effects in both normal and malignant tissue, so protons are not believed to be inherently superior. However, the Bragg peak of a proton beam and a near-zero dose beyond it have clear dosimetric advantages over a megavoltage beam, and it is often possible to reduce the dose of radiation given to tissues surrounding a planning target volume significantly. Two high-energy proton facilities are planned in the UK in London and Manchester, but, while these are being planned and built, children for whom proton therapy is deemed suitable are sent abroad, usually to the USA.

The proton treatment centre needs to be able to administer chemotherapy as well because this is often given during radiotherapy. If the local clinical oncologist believes proton therapy may be beneficial and practicable, an application is made to the UK Paediatric Proton Clinical Reference Panel which reviews the case and associated imaging, and, if appropriate, approves NHS funding of the treatment together with travel and accommodation for the child and up to two carers. Treatment abroad is inconvenient and expensive, and normally recommended only for children at particular risk of late effects which could be reduced by proton beam treatment. Generally, inclusion criteria include treatment with curative intent, absence of metastases, performance status of either 0 or 1, and with no other additional diagnosis likely to limit 5-year survival. Re-treatment cases are rejected. The current UK list of indications is dominated by paediatric indications. Currently these are non-metastatic pelvic sarcoma, spinal and paraspinal 'adult-type' sarcoma, rhabdomyosarcoma of the pelvic, head and neck, para-meningeal and orbital locations, Ewing sarcoma, ependymoma, optic pathway and other selected low-grade gliomas, craniopharyngioma, pineal parenchymal tumours (not pineoblastoma), retinoblastoma, and base of skull chordomas and chondrosarcomas. It is proposed that the list be expanded, and is likely to increase further when high-energy proton facilities become available in the UK. It is anticipated that medulloblastoma will be added, because proton therapy completely removes the significant exit dose of the spinal megavoltage fields and long-term survival appreciably exceeds the 40% which many consider appropriate grounds for referral. However, the delivery of proton radiotherapy abroad within an optimal 4 weeks of surgery may be impracticable, especially given the transient postoperative neurological deficits associated with posterior fossa surgery.

Brachytherapy

Brachytherapy has a limited role in paediatric radiotherapy, but is well suited for the treatment of small accessible tumours, usually soft tissue sarcomas of the pelvis and head and neck. It may also be used to treat a local recurrence in a previously treated radiation volume. The steep fall in radiation dose away from the target volume may result in fewer late effects in surrounding tissue than with external beam therapy and the overall treatment time is shorter. There may also be radiobiological advantages to a short treatment time. Brachytherapy is usually delivered by remote after-loading and so is often not appropriate for the larger volumes that most paediatric cancers require. Given its limited application and the skills required, brachytherapy service in the UK is highly centralised.

Molecular radiotherapy

Molecular radiotherapy, also called unsealed source radiotherapy or radionuclide therapy, involves the administration of a radiolabelled drug. Oral iodine-131 is given for thyroid cancer and iodine-131 radiolabelled meta-iodobenzylguanidine [MIBG, a catecholamine] may be given for neuroblastoma and neuroendocrine tumours. In the UK, only a few centres have appropriate facilities and support for the administration of unsealed sources to children. Twenty-four-hour paediatric medical and nursing support is required, with general childcare provided by relatives or family friends who need to be accommodated in a separate but adjoining room. They are recognised under radiation protection legislation as 'comforters and carers', they must not be pregnant and they need to give informed consent before undertaking their role.

Cancers commonest among infants

These tumours share similar age distributions with the peak age at less than 1, Wilms' tumour and neuroblastoma become rare beyond the age of 8. Hepatoblastoma, retinoblastoma and infant germ cell tumours exhibit an even more rapid decline in incidence with age, becoming rare beyond the age of 3.

Neuroblastoma

In 2012, 85 childhood neuroblastomas were diagnosed in England. Neuroblastomas may arise from anywhere in the sympathetic nervous system; 40% are adrenal, 25% abdominal, 15% thoracic, 5% cervical and 5% from pelvic sympathetic ganglia. Neuroblastoma metastasises to lymph nodes, bone marrow, bone, dura, orbits, liver, and skin, and less commonly to the lung and CNS. Patients present with symptoms caused by the volume of the primary or secondaries, with systemic upset or paraneoplastic hypertension or vasoactive intestinal peptide induced secretory diarrhoea. Auto-immune opsoclonus myoclonus ataxia syndrome occurs in 2%. Neuroblastoma may occur prenatally and be diagnosed with obstetric ultrasound. Investigation includes cross-sectional imaging, bone scan, bone marrow, an iodine-123 MIBG scan, 24-hour urinary catecholamines and tumour biopsy. Treatment is with risk-stratified chemotherapy and radiotherapy given to the tumour bed in high-risk cases. Risk stage is allocated according to the International Neuroblastoma Pathology Classification (INPC) (Shimada et al., 1999) by a combination of: age; the number of n-myc copies; the presence of certain chromosomal deletions; the presence of intraspinal neuroblastoma occupying more than 1/3 of the spinal canal; pain requiring opiates; diarrhoea requiring nasogastric or IV fluid support; respiratory distress; cardiovascular, renal or liver impairment; hypertension; tumour encasing major arteries, veins, nerves or the trachea on imaging. Treatment varies from observation only to cyclophosphamide and vincristine, with further additions of etoposide/carboplatin and doxorubicin as risk increases. For those deemed to be at even higher risk, cisretinoic acid, a differentiating agent, anti GD2 (ganglioside-2) monoclonal antibodies and high-dose chemotherapy are given. For intermediate- and high-INPC risk-stratified patients, local radiotherapy is given to the primary site. The CTV is the prechemotherapy tumour volume and any residual enlarged areas after induction chemotherapy plus 1–2 cm, and the dose is 21 Gy in 14 fractions. The radioisotopes iodine-131 MIBG and lutetium-177 dotatate, a somatostatin analogue, may be used at relapse.

Wilms' tumour

In 2012, 79 childhood Wilms' tumours were diagnosed in England. There is a difference in practice between the American Children's Oncology Group

(COG) treatment of immediate nephrectomy with histology guiding the stratification of subsequent chemotherapy, and the European SIOP approach, which is biopsy and 4 weeks of preoperative vincristine and dactinomycin for localised tumours and an additional 2 weeks of chemotherapy including doxorubicin for metastatic disease, aimed at reducing the tumour size and the possibility of intraoperative tumour rupture. The previous UKW3 trial evaluated both approaches and found equivalent outcomes, thereby providing neither group with an imperative for change (Mitchell *et al.*, 2006). In Europe, treatment is stratified according to the stage of the tumour after initial chemotherapy and post-chemotherapy histology. Stage I tumours are localised to the kidney; stage II tumours extend beyond the kidney but are completely removed; stage III tumours are those where there is incomplete removal, where nodal or peritoneal spread has occurred, or where the tumour has ruptured. Stage IV disease represents haematogenous spread. The histological risk group is determined by the presence of higher-grade elements, especially blastemal elements and the degree of necrosis in the nephrectomy specimen. Low-risk stage I tumours receive no further therapy. Chemotherapy with vincristine and dactinomycin is given in stages II and III low-risk and stages I, II and III intermediate-risk histology. Flank radiotherapy is given for intermediate-risk stage III tumours. The dose is 14.4 Gy in 8 fractions with a boost of 10.8 Gy in 6 fractions to macroscopic residual disease. High-risk tumours receive vincristine, dactinomycin and doxorubicin and, for stage II and III tumours, additional drugs and flank radiotherapy to a dose of 25.2 Gy in 14 fractions are given. Sites of metastatic disease are also irradiated.

Retinoblastoma

In 2012, 42 childhood retinoblastomas were diagnosed in England. In 40% of cases, retinoblastoma occurs in association with germline loss of one of the RB1 gene alleles. Germline mutations may give rise to multiple, often bilateral retinoblastomas, and siblings of affected patients should be screened. It usually presents as leukocoria, a white pupil rather than red-eye on flash photography, but squint, nystagmus and an inflamed eye are also possible. At 50 years follow-up of heritable retinoblastoma, there was a 51% incidence of subsequent malignancy, mostly sarcoma. Treatment is centralised

in two UK centres, Birmingham and London. In the past, external beam radiotherapy was used for medium and large tumours or where vision was threatened. However, late cosmetic deformity, pituitary dysfunction and second malignancy mean that it is now reserved for salvage where other modalities have failed. Treatment is with chemotherapy, at times given into the vitreous or opthalmic artery. Surgery, including enucleation, laser photocoagulation, cryotherapy and iodine-125 or ruthenium-106 plaques may be used at relapse. Five-year survival is 95%.

Hepatoblastoma

In patients younger than 5 years, hepatoblastoma is the commonest liver tumour: hepatocellular carcinoma is very rare. Hepatoblastoma is associated with a number of genetic syndromes. Alpha feto-protein levels are markedly elevated and are useful as a tumour marker. The child usually presents with a rapidly enlarging mass. Treatment is with initial biopsy, preoperative risk-stratified chemotherapy, and complete surgical excision which, if necessary, may involve hepatectomy and liver transplant. Cisplatin monotherapy is given for those at standard risk, cisplatin and doxorubicin (PlaDo) for high-risk, and dose-dense weekly cisplatin and doxorubicin for very high-risk. There is no role for radiotherapy.

Infant germ cell tumours (GCTs)

Most childhood extragonadal GCTs arise in mid-line sites, usually sacrococcygeal, mediastinal or retroperitoneal. The large majority are benign. Most malignant GCTs contain yolk sac elements and have elevated αFP levels. Treatment is with surgery and observation, and with carboplatin, etoposide and bleomycin at relapse.

Cancers commonest among children

Acute lymphoblastic leukaemia

Leukaemia was diagnosed in 429 children in England in 2012 and the majority were acute lymphoblastic leukaemias (ALL). The use of multi-agent chemotherapy results in cure rates of 98% in low-risk ALL, and 86% in high-risk ALL. Patient therapy is stratified by risk. Low-risk patients are 1 to < 10 years old at diagnosis and with a maximum white cell count before starting treatment of < 50 × 10^9/L; all other patients are stratified as high-risk. Bone marrow assessment at either days 8 or 15, day 29 and at week 14 is used to stratify further treatment according to response. Current chemotherapy regimens consist of an early induction phase with dexamethasone, a consolidating phase with dexamethasone, vincristine, mercaptopurine, systemic and intrathecal methotrexate and, at times, asparaginase, a maintenance phase of vincristine, dexamethasone, mercaptopurine and methotrexate which may also be given intrathecally, and a late intensification phase in poor responders. Infants younger than one year do less well and are treated with more intensive chemotherapy.

The central nervous system (CNS) and testes have been considered sanctuary sites for lymphoblasts and, historically, craniospinal and testicular radiotherapy have been used in first-line treatment. However, there is now no role for radiotherapy in the first -line treatment of ALL as intrathecal methotrexate is as effective and without the late sequelae of radiation, and craniospinal radiation or testicular radiation can still be used at relapse at these sites with a dose of 24 Gy in 12 fractions. The current UKALL2011 trial will look at the scheduling of dexamethasone given in the first 4 weeks of treatment and the addition of high-dose methotrexate. It will also examine whether vincristine and pulsed dexamethasone can be omitted during the maintenance phase and whether intrathecal methotrexate to prevent CNS relapse can be omitted in those who received high-dose methotrexate. Total body irradiation with allogenic (matched donor) stem-cell transplant continues to be used in relapsed patients responding poorly to chemotherapy. Doses in the range 10–14.4 Gy, typically 12 Gy, is given in 6 fractions over 3 days.

Acute myeloid and other leukaemias

Acute myeloid leukaemia (AML) accounts for 15% of childhood leukaemia and comprises a group of relatively well-defined haemopoietic malignancies. Treatment is shorter and more intensive than for ALL, and consists of remission induction with 1 or 2 cycles of mitoxantrone, cytarabine and etoposide with intrathecal methotrexate or cytarabine, followed by post-remission or consolidation therapy with 2–3 further blocks of the same chemotherapy (Rubnitz, 2012). In the UK, the MyeChild trial will examine induction and consolidating chemotherapy. AML occurs with increased frequency in Down's syndrome, where the outlook is less favourable, and specific multi-agent

treatment protocols exist. Chronic myeloid leukaemia is treated with imatinib. Radiotherapy is not used.

Cancers in adolescents

Hodgkin lymphoma

In 2012, 164 lymphomas were diagnosed in children in England. Hodgkin lymphoma presents with an enlarging mass, pressure effects if the tumour is in the thorax or abdominal cavity, or with constitutional symptoms of fever, night sweats and weight loss. Diagnosis is made by lymph node biopsy. Adequate amounts of tissue and an assessment of lymph node architecture are required and so a FNA is inadequate. A staging CT scan of the neck, thorax, abdomen and pelvis, PET scan and bone marrow aspiration should be undertaken in those with stage IIB and above. Treatment is with chemotherapy that is adapted to response as assessed by FDG-PET, with the addition of involved field radiotherapy for the 50% or so who are deemed to be poor responders. All patients receive two cycles of vincristine, etoposide, prednisolone and doxorubicin (OEPA) and then undergo repeat PET assessment. Favourable stage I and IIA patients receive no further chemotherapy, but local field radiotherapy to any sites remaining FDG-PET-positive. Patients with stage IIB and above, or those with bulky disease, extranodal spread or a high erythrocyte sedimentation rate (ESR) receive a further 2 or 4 blocks of chemotherapy, dependent on stage, with cyclophosphamide, vincristine, prednisolone and dacarbazine (COPDAC) and involved field radiotherapy to all sites at presentation only if the FDG-PET scan was positive after the first 2 cycles. Radiotherapy is given to all involved nodes with a 1–2-cm margin, treating to 19.8 Gy in 1.8 Gy fractions, with an additional 10 Gy in 5 fractions to those with bulky disease or a very poor PET response. This strategy was evaluated in the EuroNet-Paediatric Hodgkin Lymphoma Group EuroNet-PHL-C1 study. Oopexy should be considered if pelvic nodal irradiation is planned.

Non-Hodgkin lymphoma

Non-Hodgkin lymphoma (NHL) is rare in children. The presenting symptoms are similar to Hodgkin lymphoma, but usually with rapid onset. The commonest subtypes are Burkitt lymphoma, diffuse large B-cell lymphoma, lymphoblastic T- or B-cell lymphoma, and anaplastic large cell lymphoma. Almost all are high-grade. B-cell NHL usually involves abdominal and head and neck lymph nodes while T-cell NHL usually affects mediastinal nodes. Investigation is with nodal biopsy, CT scanning of the neck, thorax, abdomen and pelvis, bone marrow biopsy and lumbar puncture (CNS involvement occurs in 6% of cases). Treatment is with multi-agent chemotherapy. Radiotherapy is not used. Outcomes are generally good.

Bone sarcoma

Bone sarcomas are discussed in Chapter 33.

Adolescent germ cell tumours

Before the introduction of platinum-based chemotherapy, survival of children with adolescent malignant germ cell tumours was poor. Two standard regimens are used internationally: cisplatin, etoposide, bleomycin (BEP) and cisplatin, etoposide and ifosfamide (PEI). To minimise oto- and nephrotoxicity associated with cisplatin, the UK has used carboplatin, etoposide and bleomycin (JEB) instead. The GC8901 (GC2) trial recruited from 1989 to 1997 and reported similar survival but reduced toxicity with carboplatin (Mann *et al.*, 2000). The GC 2005 04 (GC3) continued with JEB, with the number of courses determined by risk determined by tumour site, stage and αFP level. The results are awaited. Current practice is to give 4 cycles of JEB, but this may be inadequate for higher-risk tumours in post-pubertal children, and adult protocols may be followed instead.

'Adult-type' sarcoma

Non-rhabdomyosarcomatous sarcoma accounts for only 5% of paediatric sarcomas, and it tends to occur in older children. Clear cell, synovial and fibrosarcoma are the commonest types. Treatment is with surgery, with postoperative radiotherapy added for incomplete or marginal excision. Although not supported by high-quality evidence, adjuvant chemotherapy with doxorubicin and ifosfamide is offered in paediatric soft tissue sarcomas as higher response rates have been observed and chemotherapy may be better tolerated than in adults.

Carcinoma and melanoma

These tumours occur only in older children, but are still rare. They are treated in line with their adult counterparts.

Cancers with no clear peak age

Rhabdomyosarcoma

In England in 2012, 93 soft tissue sarcomas were diagnosed in children and the majority were rhabdomyosarcomas. Rhabdomyosarcoma is characterised by the presence of rhabdomyoblasts which are malignant cells containing striated muscle. They may arise anywhere in the body, and not just where skeletal muscle is present. It is associated with Li–Fraumeni syndrome, pleuropulmonary blastoma, neurofibromatosis type 1, Beckwith–Wiedemann, Costello and Noonan syndromes. Patients present with an enlarging lump, pressure effects associated with the tumour, or with distant disease. Lymph node metastases are common, and haematogenous spread can occur to lung, liver, bone and bone marrow. Investigation is with cross-sectional imaging of the trunk, a bone scan, a bone marrow and a biopsy. Patients with parameningeal disease require imaging of the craniospinal axis and a lumbar puncture. Patients who will receive doxorubicin require an echo assessment of cardiac function.

If possible, an initial complete excision is undertaken, but this should not be too mutilating because second-look surgery is encouraged after chemotherapy for incomplete excisions. Patients are grouped by the extent of initial surgery into Intergroup Rhabdomyosarcoma Studies stages (IRS) 1, 2 or 3. IRS1 is a complete microscopic excision (R0), IRS2 is excision with microscopic residual (R1) or with a primary complete resection with involved nodes, and IRS3 is a macroscopically incomplete excision (R2) or a biopsy only. IRS4 represents metastatic disease.

Prognosis and therapy are dictated by age, tumour size, site, morphology, the completeness of the initial surgery and the presence of metastatic disease. Poor prognostic factors are alveolar morphology, age 10 or above and tumour size 5 cm or greater. Favourable sites are the orbit, genitourinary non-bladder/prostate (i.e. paratesticular and vagina/uterus) and non-parameningeal head and neck, with all other sites being unfavourable.

The European Paediatric Soft Tissue Study Group EpSSGrms 2005 study has recently closed to accrual and stratified therapy into low-, standard-, high- and very high-risk strategies depending on prognostic factors. Low-risk patients received only vincristine and dactinomycin and surgery if a complete response was not achieved. Radiotherapy was not given.

Standard-risk patients received ifosfamide, vincristine and dactinomycin (IVA), and, unless the initial surgery resulted in a complete excision (IRS1), radiotherapy was given to the primary site at doses ranging between 36 and 50.4 Gy in 1.8 Gy fractions depending on resection margins and chemotherapy response. High-risk patients were randomised to IVA ± doxorubicin (IVA versus IVADo) and maintenance or no maintenance chemotherapy, and patients received radiotherapy as above. Very high-risk patients (alveolar disease and nodal spread and any patient with metastatic disease) received IVADo and radiotherapy to doses ranging between 41.4 and 50.4 Gy, again depending on resection margins and response. A boost of 5.4 Gy in 3 fractions may be given in large tumours with poor response to chemotherapy. The radiotherapy CTV is the initial tumour extent and any clinically involved nodes generally plus 1–2 cm. Metastatic sites may also be irradiated. Radiotherapy was given after the first 4 blocks of IVA or IVADo chemotherapy, but during the first of 5 blocks of IVA. Dactinomycin should be omitted during radiotherapy to the trunk, abdomen or head and neck. The next EpSSG trial will explore further the use of maintenance chemotherapy and compare 41.4 and 50.4 Gy radiation doses.

CNS malignancies

A wide range of benign and malignant tumours may arise in the CNS, and unlike most other paediatric tumours, it has not been possible to exclude radiotherapy from effective treatment. The late effects of radiation on cognitive and endocrine function are significant and they increase with reducing age of the child. Because of this, it is unusual to offer radiotherapy to children less than 3 years old. CNS tumours were diagnosed in 260 children in England in 2012.

Medulloblastoma and other PNETs

Medulloblastoma is a primitive neuroectodermal tumour (PNET) arising in the posterior fossa, almost always around the fourth ventricle. It may present with ataxia which is sometimes dismissed as clumsiness, headache, or often an acute emergency with profound deterioration due to the development of obstructive hydrocephalus. An MRI scan will reveal a mass in the posterior fossa. The differential diagnosis includes ependymoma.

Treatment is with surgery. A postoperative residual tumour of more than 1.5 cm^2 has been shown to be a poor prognostic factor, and, although untested in a randomised fashion, further surgery is encouraged if more tumour can be removed. MRI imaging of the craniospinal axis and a lumbar puncture for CSF cytology at least 14 days after surgery are required to exclude metastatic disease. CSF may be falsely positive if it is taken from a port or too soon after surgery. Other adverse prognostic indicators are n-myc gene amplification, large cell anaplastic morphology and a delay of more than 6 weeks from surgery to the start of radiotherapy.

The traditional radiation dose for craniospinal radiotherapy was around 35 Gy in 21 fractions, but a COG study in the USA showed high survival rates with a lower craniospinal dose plus chemotherapy with vincristine and cisplatin and either cyclophosphamide or lomustine. The latter approach is used widely in the UK. The UK-led PNET3 study compared immediate radiotherapy with 4 cycles of pre-radiation chemotherapy, alternating vincristine and etoposide with cyclophosphamide and carboplatin, which improved 5-year survival from 65% to 77% (Taylor et al., 2003). The next multicentre randomised study to be run in the UK compared conventional and hyperfractionated radiotherapy. Craniospinal radiotherapy to 23.4 Gy in 13 fractions with a posterior fossa boost to a total of 55.8 Gy in 31 fractions was compared to 36 Gy in 36 fractions, with a posterior fossa boost of 24 Gy in 24 fractions and a further 8 Gy in 8 fraction boost to the tumour bed to a total of 72 Gy treating twice daily. This revealed equivalent toxicity and overall 5-year survival at 86% and event-free survival at 79%. It is possible that long-term toxicity differences may become apparent with continued follow-up (Lannering et al., 2012).

Metastatic medulloblastoma and PNETs arising outside the posterior fossa have a worse prognosis, and in addition to 35 Gy of craniospinal radiotherapy with a boost to around 55 Gy, high-dose chemotherapy is given. The current UK approach follows the St Jude's MB03 protocol with risk-adapted standard craniospinal RT post-surgery and 4 courses of high-dose cyclophosphamide/cisplatin (Gajjar et al., 2006). The PNET5 study will run in the UK and will explore daily carboplatin concurrently with radiotherapy. In low-risk patients the craniospinal dose will be reduced to 18 Gy. Pineoblastomas, PNETs of the pineal, have an outlook similar to localised medulloblastoma and receive craniospinal radiotherapy to 35 Gy, with a tumour boost to 55.8 Gy and standard-risk medulloblastoma chemotherapy. Given the profound effects of craniospinal radiotherapy in those less than

2–3, high-dose chemotherapy with focal radiotherapy is used in preference to craniospinal radiotherapy.

Craniospinal techniques vary, and they now include proton beam and tomotherapy. Conventionally, it was simulator planned and administered prone with a cranial shell using a direct spinal field and a pair of lateral head fields to cover the entire neuro-axis. The lateral fields were centred on the outer canthus to avoid the anterior divergence of a more posteriorly based cranial field into the contralateral eye. A collimator rotation was chosen to match the superior (rostral) divergence of the posterior spinal field, and a couch angle applied to each lateral to remove the inferior (caudal) divergence of the lateral fields. The field edge was shaped with blocks to be 5 mm below the anterior cranial fossa and 1 cm below the middle and posterior fossae to treat the meningeal extensions along cranial nerves. The posterior neck was not shielded in order to ensure treatment of any postoperative meningocele. The match to the posterior field was as low as the shoulders permitted to spare as much anterior neck, thyroid and pharynx as possible. The posterior field extended from the bottom of the head field to the bottom of S2, and extended 1 cm lateral to the pedicles to allow for meningeal extension along the spinal nerves. The use of wedged fields, a spinal compensator or field-within-field technique were used to ensure dose homogeneity. The spinal field dose was prescribed to the anterior edge of the spinal canal. Given the uncertainties of matching, it was usual to have three otherwise identical plans but with the junction between head and spine fields moved at least 1 cm. Planning is now usually by CT planning and virtual simulation, and may be performed supine. Verification is required by portal imaging, cone beam CT or equivalent. Lens doses should be confirmed by thermoluminescence dosimetry (TLD), placed on at the outer canthus, which will overestimate the lens dose, and on the closed eyelid, which will underestimate the dose. If the lens dose cannot be reduced, except by compromising the planning volume, no changes should be made, but the increased risk of cataract should be discussed with the family.

Ependymoma

Of paediatric ependymomas, 90% arise in the brain and 60% in the posterior fossa. The median age of presentation is 5 years old. A space-occupying lesion in the brain may present with a focal deficiency, seizure or pressure effects, either headache or a fall in conscious level. Many ependymomas occur around the fourth ventricle, and so the presentation may be similar to that of a medulloblastoma. Investigation is with an MRI scan. Dissemination by CSF is reported in 10–20% cases, and so imaging of the entire craniospinal axis is necessary. Management is with surgical excision and postoperative radiotherapy. Long-term survival is 80% in those for whom a complete excision (as assessed on a postoperative scan) can be achieved, and 0–22% in those where a complete excision cannot be achieved. The prognosis at relapse is very poor. Radiotherapy is given postoperatively, traditionally to 54 Gy, although better survival rates have been reported with a dose of 59.4 Gy. The role of chemotherapy in ependymoma is still uncertain. The first ependymoma study, SIOP99, which ran until 2008 in the UK, showed that vincristine, etoposide, cyclophosphamide followed by second-look surgery was able to achieve a complete resection in just over half of patients. The SIOP Ependymoma 2 study is randomising those who have undergone a complete macroscopic excision to postoperative radiotherapy to 59.4 Gy and then either observation or chemotherapy with vincristine, etoposide, cyclophosphamide and cisplatin (VEC-CDDP). Those for whom complete excision is not possible will be randomised to chemotherapy with VEC with or without high-dose methotrexate, with assessment of response determined radiologically. If possible, second look surgery will be undertaken, and, if not possible, radiation to 59.4 Gy with an 8 Gy stereotactic boost will be given with further VEC-CDDP chemotherapy postoperatively. Children less than 12 months will be offered dose-dense chemotherapy. Historically, craniospinal or whole brain radiotherapy has been given, but this is no longer felt to be necessary. A typical CTV will be the postoperative tumour bed with a 1-cm margin. Appropriate cases may be referred for proton therapy abroad.

Diffuse intrinsic pontine glioma

Approximately 80% of paediatric brainstem gliomas arise within the pons, and the majority of these are diffuse intrinsic pontine gliomas, with characteristic appearances on imaging so that biopsy is not usually necessary. Patients present with cranial nerve palsies or hydrocephalus. Radiotherapy is the only treatment that appears to alter the course of this illness and may transiently significantly improve symptoms, but the median survival is only 10 months and the 2-year overall survival rate is less than 10%. Adjuvant temozolomide as given in high grade glioma failed to improve survival

(Cohen *et al.*, 2011). Discrete and exophytic tumours of the brainstem are usually low-grade tumours and have a much more favourable outlook.

Low-grade glioma (LGG)

Glial tumours account for 75% of primary childhood CNS tumours. Low-grade astrocytomas are the largest group of CNS tumours in children and pilocytic astrocytoma is the commonest. Other low-grade astrocytomas include diffuse astrocytomas, oligodendroglial tumours and gangliogliomas. Despite long-term survival in many patients, 50–75% of patients with LGG eventually die of either progression of a low-grade tumour or transformation to a malignant glioma. The time to progression can vary from a few months to several years, with the median survival among patients with LGG ranging from 5 to 10 years. As in adults, the treatment is surgical, with radiotherapy reserved for recurrent inoperable tumour. However, given the toxicity of CNS radiotherapy in younger children, chemotherapy is tried first, and for certain indolent but inoperable tumours such as optic pathway gliomas in the context of neurofibromatosis type 1, radiation is not recommended. Appropriate cases may be referred for proton therapy abroad. The SIOP LGG2 study closed to recruitment in 2012, and evaluated a strategy of observation after first surgery and, at recurrence, children over the age of 7 proceeded to radiotherapy while those less than 7 received carboplatin and vincristine and were randomised to receive etoposide or not. The results are awaited.

High-grade glioma (HGG)

Paediatric HGGs are significantly less common than LGGs and comprise only 20% of all hemispheric gliomas and approximately 6–10% of all newly diagnosed primary intracranial neoplasms (MacDonald *et al.*, 2011). Although the biology of paediatric and adult HGG differ, their treatment and outlook are similar. Children with glioblastoma fare far worse than those with anaplastic astrocytoma, with a median survival of 9–12 months (Mueller and Chang, 2009), and a 5-year survival of 5–15%. For anaplastic astrocytoma the 5-year survival is 20–40%. The most important determinant of outcome is the extent of the resection. Postoperative radiotherapy is given to a dose of 54 Gy in those over the age of 3 with a CTV encompassing the tumour bed with 25-mm margins. Escalating the dose to 72 Gy did not improve outcome (Fulton *et al.*, 1992). A randomised phase III trial showed a survival advantage with the addition of adjuvant chemotherapy with lomustine, vincristine and prednisolone (Spostol *et al.*, 1989), but subsequent studies have failed to confirm this, and no other chemotherapy regimen has shown effectiveness in a randomised trial. Following the favourable results of a randomised trial of temozolomide in adults (Stupp *et al.*, 2009) and the observation that temozolomide appears active in children, this has become standard therapy in children as well, but a COG study in the USA failed to show an improvement compared to historical controls (Cohen *et al.*, 2011). A UK and European randomised trial of bevacizumab in high-grade glioma has recently been completed and the results are awaited.

Craniopharyngioma

UK recommendations for the treatment of craniopharyngioma and other endocrine malignancies have been published (Spoudeas, 2005). Craniopharyngiomas are rare, slow-growing, congenital, mid-line epithelial tumours arising embryologically from maldevelopment in the pituitary stalk. Patients may present with visual, endocrine or hypothalamic symptoms or obstructive hydrocephalus. Treatment is with surgery, but complete excision can be difficult. Aggressive surgery may cause significant endocrine, visual and cognitive damage, and minimally invasive surgery is preferred for larger tumours with observation of any residual tumour. They tend to recur and invade locally causing pituitary, visual and hypothalamic problems. Further minimally invasive surgery should then be followed by local radiotherapy in the older child, and referral for proton therapy should be considered.

Intracranial germ cell tumours

These account for 4% of paediatric tumours, and constitute dysgerminomas, also called germinomas or non-secretory germ cell tumours (60%) and non-germinomatous germ cell tumours including embryonal carcinoma, endodermal sinus tumour (yolk sac tumour), choriocarcinoma, teratomas and mixed tumours (40%). The majority of CNS germ cell tumours arise in the pineal gland, suprasellar region, basal ganglia and hypothalamus. Patients present with local pressure effects including pituitary failure and hydrocephalus. Diagnosis is usually made on imaging and biopsy, but the presence of elevated blood or CSF αFP or βHCG is diagnostic and may prevent the need for biopsy. They are highly radiosensitive, with a tendency to spread via the cerebrospinal fluid and so systemic craniospinal radiation has been the standard treatment for many decades and outcomes are excellent. Malignant teratoma outcomes, although good, are inferior. Teratomas are less radiosensitive, and are treated with chemotherapy and focal radiotherapy. In the UK and Europe, the SIOP CNS GCT 96 study evaluated craniospinal radiotherapy to 24 Gy in 15 fractions, with a 16 Gy in 10-fractions boost to the tumour or 2 courses of carboplatin and etoposide alternating with etoposide and ifosfamide, followed by local radiotherapy, determined by patient and physician choice. This showed poorer event-free survival (97% versus 88%) with chemotherapy and local irradiation, but, with salvage, no difference in an overall survival of 98% (Calaminus et al., 2013). The current European trial, SIOP CNS GCT, is recruiting in the UK. Patients with dysgerminoma will receive the same chemotherapy, and 24 Gy whole ventricular radiotherapy, and, if a complete response is not achieved, 16 Gy consolidating radiotherapy. Patients with malignant teratoma receive 4 cycles of cisplatin, etopside and ifosfamide followed by local radiotherapy to 54 Gy while those with metastatic teratoma receive 30 Gy craniospinal radiotherapy and a 24 Gy tumour boost.

Meningioma

Meningioma is rare in children, accounting for only 2.6% of paediatric brain tumours, and is treated with surgery. Radiotherapy may be considered after multiple recurrences. There is no role for chemotherapy.

Late effects of treatment

Late effects related to treatment for cancer may occur soon after treatment is complete or may take many decades to develop. Life-long follow-up of survivors is recommended to ensure early diagnosis, counselling and treatment. A comprehensive guide to long-term follow-up and the management late effects has recently been published in Scotland (SIGN, 2013).

Fertility

The testis and ovary are sensitive to the effects of both chemotherapy and radiotherapy. Before puberty the ovary may be less affected by chemotherapy. A transient drop in spermatogenesis occurs at 0.5 Gy. Azoospermia occurs at 2–3 Gy, but recovers within 3 years. At 4–6 Gy recovery is not certain and may take 5 years. Beyond 6 Gy there is a high risk of permanent sterility. Total body irradiation will sterilise men. Testosterone production

declines beyond 15 Gy and falls to zero at doses above 24 Gy. The likelihood of ovarian failure increases with age and concurrent chemotherapy. At aged 20, immediate ovarian failure occurs at 16.5 Gy with menopause brought forward at lower doses. Menstruation continues with uterine doses up to 40 Gy, but the ability of uterine tissues to hypertrophy and vascularise during pregnancy is reduced beyond 20–30 Gy, leading to an increased risk of miscarriage. Management guidance on fertility has been written jointly by the Royal College of Obstetricians and Gynaecologists, Physicians and Radiologists (Mead, 2007).

Second malignancy

The American Childhood Cancer Survivor Study reported a 30-year cumulative incidence of second malignancy of 20.5%, 6 times higher than that seen in the general population (Friedman et al., 2010) and at 25 years it exceeds all other causes of death. The risk is increased in those who received extensive chemotherapy, especially with alkylating agents, and in those with a genetic predisposition to cancer. The British Childhood Cancer Survivor Study, a population-based cohort of 17,981 5-year survivors of childhood cancer diagnosed with cancer before age 15 years between 1940 and 1991, found that beyond 45 years from diagnosis, recurrence accounted for 7% of the excess number of deaths observed while second primary cancers and circulatory deaths together accounted for 77% (Reulen et al., 2010).

Endocrine function and the breast

Hypothalamic and anterior pituitary function may be more sensitive to the effects of radiation in children and late failure may occur after doses of 24–35 Gy with an effect on growth and puberty. Precocious puberty may be seen following hypothalamic irradiation which may need to be delayed with depot LHRH superagonists such as leuprolide or goserelin to allow skeletal growth to continue. Long-term specialist endocrine follow-up is required for children receiving sizeable pituitary radiation. Direct irradiation of the thyroid gland can lead to hypothyroidism, a condition more likely to occur in younger females. There is also an increased risk of developing thyroid nodules. Irradiation of the breast bud leads to impaired development of the breast, ranging from agenesis to modest loss of volume depending on the dose and stage of development at the time of irradiation. Second malignancy may occur, and

NICE recommends annual mammographic screening of women who received more than 30 Gy of supradiaphragmatic irradiation as a child.

Cognitive function

There are appreciable late cognitive effects following the treatment of many of these tumours, and although the tumour itself, surgery and missed schooling are contributory factors, radiotherapy is the major cause. Chemotherapy- or radiotherapy-induced hearing loss may further compromise a child's schooling if it is unrecognised and not corrected. The effects are less pronounced in older children, but are severe in children less than 3, and amount to a decline of approximately 4 IQ points per year as the child fails to progress as quickly as would have been expected (Ris *et al.*, 2001). It is not yet known what effect childhood radiotherapy may have on the incidence of neurodegenerative diseases when old, but long-term survivors do score highly on frailty assessments.

Eyes, ears and teeth

The eyes of children and adults are equally sensitive to radiation damage, but a combination of high-dose steroids and chemotherapy increases the chance of cataract formation. Cataracts are almost inevitable after TBI. The developing ear is at risk of radiation damage to the sensorineural pathways at doses above 30–40 Gy. The risk is increased by the use of high-dose platinum compounds, aminoglycosides and the presence of a shunt. The size, shape and quality of teeth can be affected by doses as low as 20 Gy in children under age 5, and xerostomia has lasting effects on dental health. Irradiation of the facial bones in younger children leads to craniofacial abnormalities that may require surgery at a later stage for cosmetic reasons but also to correct malocclusion. Chronic sinusitis can also be a problem following doses over 30 Gy.

References

Calaminus, G., Kortmann, R., Worch, J., *et al.* (2013). SIOP CNS GCT 96: final report of outcome of a prospective, multinational nonrandomized trial for children and adults with intracranial germinoma, comparing craniospinal irradiation alone with chemotherapy followed by focal primary site irradiation for patients with localized disease. *Neuro. Oncol.* **15**, 788–796.

Cohen, K. J., Pollack, I. F., Zhou, T., *et al.* (2011). Temozolomide in the treatment of high-grade gliomas in children: a report from the Children's Oncology Group. *Neuro. Oncol.*, **13**, 317–323.

Friedman, D. L., Whitton, J., Leisenring, W., *et al.* (2010). Subsequent neoplasms in 5-year survivors of childhood cancer: the Childhood Cancer Survivor Study. *J. Natl Cancer Inst.*, **102**, 1083–1095.

Fulton, D. S., Urtasun, R. C., Scott-Brown, I., *et al.* (1992). Increasing radiation dose intensity using hyperfractionation in patients with malignant glioma. *J. Neurooncol.*, **14**, 63–72.

Gajjar, A., Chintagumpala, M., Ashley, D., *et al.* (2006). Risk-adapted craniospinal radiotherapy followed by high-dose chemotherapy and stem-cell rescue in children with newly diagnosed medulloblastoma (St Jude Medulloblastoma-96): long-term results from a prospective, multicentre trial. *Lancet Oncol.*, **7**, 813–820.

Lannering, B., Rutkowski, S., Doz, F., *et al.* (2012). Hyperfractionated versus conventional radiotherapy followed by chemotherapy in standard-risk medulloblastoma: results from the randomized multicenter HIT-SIOP PNET 4 trial. *J. Clin. Oncol.*, **30**, 3187–3193.

MacDonald, T. J., Aguilera, D. and Kramm C. M. (2011). Treatment of high-grade glioma in children and adolescents. *Neuro. Oncol.*, **13**, 1049–1058.

Mann, J. R., Raafat, F., Robinson, K., *et al.* (2000). The United Kingdom Childrens Cancer Study Groups second germ cell tumor study: carboplatin, etoposide, and bleomycin are effective treatment for children with malignant extracranial germ cell tumors, with acceptable toxicity. *J. Clin. Oncol.*, **18**, 3809–3818.

Mead, G. (2007). The effects of cancer treatment on reproductive functions. *Clin. Med.*, **7**, 544–545.

Mitchell, C., Pritchard-Jones, K. and Shannon, R. (2006). Immediate nephrectomy versus preoperative chemotherapy in the management of non-metastatic Wilms' tumour: results of a randomised trial (UKW3) by the UK Children's Cancer Study Group. *Eur. J. Cancer*, **42**, 2554–2562.

Mueller, S. and Chang, S. (2009). Pediatric brain tumors: current treatment strategies and future therapeutic approaches. *Neurotherapeutics*, **6**, 570–586.

Reulen, R. C, Winter, D. L., Frobisher, C., *et al.* (2010). Long-term cause-specific mortality among survivors of childhood cancer. *J. Am. Med. Ass.*, **304**, 172–179.

Ris, M. D., Packer, R. and Goldwein, J. (2001). Intellectual outcome after reduced-dose radiation therapy plus adjuvant chemotherapy for medulloblastoma: a Childrens Cancer Group study. *J. Clin. Oncol.*, **19**, 3470–3476.

Rubnitz, J. E. (2012). How I treat pediatric acute myeloid leukemia. *Blood*, **119**, 5980–5988.

SIGN. (2013). *SIGN 132. Long Term Follow up of Survivors of Childhood Cancer.* Edinburgh: Scottish Intercollegiate Guidelines Network.

Shimada, H., Ambros, I. M., Dehner, L. P., *et al.* (1999). The International Neuroblastoma Pathology Classification (the Shimida system). *Cancer*, **86**, 364–372.

Spostol, R., Ertel, I. E., Jenkin, R. D., *et al.* (1989). The effectiveness of chemotherapy for treatment of high grade astrocytoma in children: results of a randomized trial. *J. Neurooncol.*, **7**, 165–177.

Spoudeas, H. A. (2005). *Paediatric Endocrine Tumours.* Crawley, West Sussex: Novo Nordisk Ltd. Available at: http://www.bsped.org.uk/clinical/docs/rareendocrinetumour_final.pdf, accessed January 2015.

Stupp, R., Hegi, M. E., Mason, W. P., *et al.* (2009). Effects of radiotherapy with concomitant and adjuvant temozolomide versus radiotherapy alone on survival in glioblastoma in a randomised phase III study: 5-year analysis of the EORTC-NCIC trial. *Lancet Oncol.*, **10**, 459–466.

Taylor, R. E., Bailey, C. C., Robinson, K., *et al.* (2003). Results of a randomized study of preradiation chemotherapy versus radiotherapy alone for nonmetastatic medulloblastoma: The International Society of Paediatric Oncology/United Kingdom Childrens Cancer Study Group PNET-3 Study. *J. Clin. Oncol.*, **21**, 1581–1891.

Multiple choice questions

1. A 20-year-old man presents with a metastatic testicular tumour. Which of the following features would put him into the poor-risk category?
   (a) Pure seminoma with 20 lung metastases
   (b) Pure seminoma with hCG 50× upper limit of normal (ULN)
   (c) Choriocarcinoma with 20 lung metastases
   (d) Embryonal germ cell tumour (GCT) with αFP 50× ULN
   (e) Mixed GCT with 10 lung and 2 liver metastases

2. With regard to cancer-related emergencies, which of the following statements is correct?
   (a) Syndrome of inappropriate anti-diuretic hormone (SIADH) gives rise to hyponatraemia and reduced plasma osmolarity in the presence of inappropriately dilute urine
   (b) In patients with SIADH who do not respond to fluid restriction, cautious administration of intravenous sodium chloride should be considered
   (c) The addition of surgery to radiotherapy has been shown to improve functional outcome compared to surgery alone in the treatment of spinal cord compression
   (d) In good-performance-status patients with solitary intracerebral metastases, radiotherapy with 12 Gy in 2 fractions is equivalent to 30 Gy in 10 fractions
   (e) Patients at high risk from neutropenic sepsis should receive intravenous ciprofloxacin and co-amoxiclav on admission to hospital

3. A 45-year-old man presents with an enlarging mass on the penis. Biopsy reveals invasive squamous carcinoma. The tumour is invading the corpus cavernosum and there are two mobile, palpable inguinal node metastases. What is the stage?
   (a) T3 N1 MX
   (b) T1 N1 MX
   (c) T3 N2 MX
   (d) T2 N1 MX
   (e) T2 N2 MX

4. Xeroderma pigmentosa is associated with which of the following?
   (a) Autosomal dominant inheritance
   (b) Jaw cysts
   (c) Medulloblastoma
   (d) A defect of nucleotide excision repair
   (e) A decreased risk of skin cancer

5. A patient presents with multiple bilateral pulmonary opacities suggestive of malignancy but with no obvious underlying primary site of disease. A CT-guided biopsy reveals adenocarcinoma on which the following immunohistochemical tests are performed: cytokeratin-7 (CK7) positive, cytokeratin-20 (CK20) negative, thyroid transcription factor (TTF-1) positive, thyroglobulin negative. The most likely underlying primary site of disease is which of these?
   (a) Colon
   (b) Bladder
   (c) Lung
   (d) Thyroid
   (e) Pancreas

6. A 53-year-old woman presents with a painless right-sided thyroid nodule and normal TFTs. There is no family history of thyroid disease or endocrine malignancy. US confirms a solitary 3 × 2 cm hypoechoic nodule with no abnormal nodes. FNA is reported as showing a follicular neoplasm. The next most appropriate step is:
   (a) Serum thyroglobulin measurement
   (b) Repeat FNAC
   (c) To request CT scan of the neck, thorax and abdomen with intravenous contrast

(d) To advise a right-sided thyroid lobectomy

(e) Total thyroidectomy and central lymph node dissection

7. A 54-year-old man presents with a 6-month history of a hoarse voice and no other ENT symptoms. Clinic room examination reveals a proliferative lesion on the left false cord with normal true cord mobility and palpable lymphadenopathy in level II on the ipsilateral side. EUA and CT scan confirm involvement of the false cord with extension along the aryepiglottic fold towards the epiglottis and involvement of the pre-epiglottic space. There is a left level II lymph node measuring 3 cm. There is no evidence of distant metastases. Biopsy from the false cord shows moderately differentiated squamous carcinoma. According to the 7th edition TNM classification, what stage disease is this?

(a) T2 N1 M0

(b) T2 N2a M0

(c) T2 N2b M0

(d) T3 N1 M0

(e) T3 N2a M0

8. A 54-year-old patient has hepatocellular carcinoma associated with hepatitis C infection. Investigations reveal three tumours in the right lobe of the liver: 2 cm, 2 cm and 3 cm in size. There is no evidence of metastatic disease. Which of the following options is the treatment of choice?

(a) Radiofrequency ablation

(b) Liver transplantation

(c) Transarterial chemoembolisation

(d) External beam radiotherapy

(e) None of the above is superior to the others

9. In electron therapy, which of the following statements is correct?

(a) The therapeutic range (on the central axis) is approximately $E/2$ cm (where E is the energy of the incident electron beam in MeV)

(b) Unlike kV photons, electron treatments rarely require the use of bolus

(c) The 80% isodose is wider at depth than at the surface

(d) Hot and cold spots caused by inhomogeneities can be easily corrected for, provided their position is known

(e) The 10% isodose is wider at depth than at the surface

10. Which of the following conditions is most typically associated with an increase in colorectal adenocarcinomas?

(a) Neurofibromatosis

(b) Xeroderma pigmentosa

(c) A germline mutation in BRCA1

(d) Turcot's syndrome

(e) A genetic defect in the Hedgehog pathway

11. A 62-year-old woman presents with postmenopausal bleeding. A hysteroscopy shows a tumour in the uterus which on biopsy is found to be a well-differentiated adenocarcinoma. An MRI scan suggests that the tumour is invading 3 mm into the myometrium, with a myometrial thickness of 7 mm. What initial treatment would you recommend?

(a) TAH, BSO and pelvic lymphadenectomy

(b) TAH, BSO

(c) Radical radiotherapy

(d) Intrauterine progesterone

(e) TAH, BSO and infracolic omentectomy

12. A 54-year-old woman presents with an enlarging mass on the vulva that has been present for 12 months. A biopsy confirms this is squamous carcinoma. There is no other finding on examination. The tumour involves the right side of the vulva, measures 8 cm in maximum diameter and extends to within 3 mm of the anal margin. She does not wish to have an anovulvectomy. What is the most appropriate treatment?

(a) Local excision

(b) Radical vulvectomy and groin node dissection

(c) Radical radiotherapy to include the primary tumour with an electron field to the perineum

(d) Radical chemoradiotherapy to the vulva and groin nodes

(e) Symptomatic treatment

13. A 65-year-old man with pancreatic carcinoma undergoes a Whipple's operation. Final histology shows a T3 N1 (5 of 15 nodes positive) grade 3 adenocarcinoma with vascular invasion, distance to

closest resection margin is 1 mm. Based on current evidence (and outside the context of a clinical trial), what is the most appropriate management?

(a) No adjuvant therapy

(b) Adjuvant 5-FU chemotherapy

(c) Adjuvant gemcitabine chemotherapy

(d) Adjuvant chemoradiation

(e) Re-operation

14. A patient presenting with SVCO is given oxygen, commenced on high-dose steroids and his condition stabilises. CT scanning confirms the presence of a large superior mediastinal mass. What is the most appropriate management at this stage?

(a) Radiotherapy to the mediastinum using parallel opposed anterior and posterior fields; dose 20 Gy in 5 fractions over 5 days

(b) Chemotherapy with BEP

(c) Referral for biopsy

(d) Anticoagulation

(e) Insertion of a percutaneous stent into the IVC

15. For someone on MST 60 mg b.d., what should the breakthrough dose of oral morphine be?

(a) 20 mg

(b) 10 mg

(c) 30 mg

(d) 40 mg

(e) 60 mg

16. An otherwise fit and well 61-year-old man presents with dysphagia and is found to have an adenocarcinoma of the oesophagus. A CT scan shows no evidence of metastatic disease. An EUS confirms the tumour to be from 36 to 39 cm *ab oral*, extending into the right crus of the diaphragm together with two malignant lymph nodes in the peritumoural region. What stage is this and what is the standard treatment in the UK?

(a) Stage T3 N1 M0: 4 cycles epirubicin, cisplatin and capecitabine (ECX) chemotherapy prior to surgery

(b) Stage T3 N1 M1b: definitive chemoradiotherapy

(c) Stage T4 N1 M0: 2 cycles cisplatin and 5-FU followed by surgery

(d) Stage T4 N1 M1b: 2 cycles cisplatin and 5-FU followed by surgery

(e) Stage T3 N1 M0: 2 cycles cisplatin and capecitabine followed by surgery

17. The age-specific incidence in England and Wales is decreasing for which of these cancers?

(a) Pancreatic cancer

(b) Gastric cancer

(c) Colorectal cancer

(d) Oesophageal cancer

(e) Testicular germ cell tumours

18. Criteria for urgent referral with suspicion of colorectal cancer include:

(a) Rectal bleeding with anal symptoms in a 62-year-old

(b) Eight weeks change in bowel habit without rectal bleeding in a 45-year-old

(c) Persistent rectal bleeding without anal symptoms in a 35-year-old

(d) Unexplained iron deficiency anaemia in men Hb < 110 g/L

(e) Left iliac fossa mass

19. A previously fit 46-year-old woman is found to have a 4 cm basaloid carcinoma of the anal canal. On examination she has a palpable lymph node in her left groin. There is no evidence of distant metastatic disease. An FNA of the groin node is negative for malignancy. What is the correct initial treatment?

(a) Surgery alone because basaloid tumours are not radiosensitive

(b) Cisplatin/5-FU concurrent with radiotherapy to the GTV plus 3 cm

(c) 5-FU plus mitomycin concurrent with radiotherapy to the GTV plus 3 cm

(d) 5-FU and mitomycin concurrent with radiotherapy to the stage-defined CTV

(e) Cisplatin and 5-FU concurrent with radiotherapy to the stage-defined CTV

20. Regarding radical radiotherapy for prostate cancer, which of the following statements is correct?

(a) The GTV to PTV margin is usually 2 cm

(b) 3D conformal radiotherapy allows dose escalation to 64 Gy

(c) If included in the treatment, an appropriate seminal vesicle dose is 56 Gy

(d) The use of neoadjuvant hormone therapy causes greater rectal toxicity

(e) A three-field plan with an anterior field and two laterals causes greater rectal toxicity than a three-field plan with an anterior field and two posterior obliques

21. An otherwise fit 45-year-old woman presents with epigastric discomfort. An endoscopy reveals a smooth 3 cm submucosal lesion at the gastric cardia. A CT scan is consistent with a gastrointestinal stromal tumour. What would you recommend next?

(a) Wide local surgical resection

(b) Endoscopic ultrasound-guided FNA

(c) Imatinib

(d) A D2 total gastrectomy

(e) A PET scan

22. The MRC CR07 study has demonstrated:

(a) An improvement in overall survival with preoperative radiotherapy

(b) A reduction in CRM positivity with pre- over postoperative radiotherapy

(c) A significant reduction in local recurrence confined to lower-third tumours in patients receiving preoperative radiotherapy

(d) A significant reduction in local recurrence in patients receiving selective postoperative chemoradiotherapy

(e) A significant reduction in local recurrence in patients receiving preoperative radiotherapy

23. An 84-year-old woman presents to an ophthalmologist with diplopia and reduced visual acuity in her left eye. A CT scan shows a left retro-orbital mass. She had a mastectomy 10 years previously for a left breast cancer, followed by tamoxifen for 5 years. Other staging scans are negative. The CA15-3 is 310 u/mL. The original tumour was ER+ve. The most appropriate management now is:

(a) Anastrozole

(b) Urgent palliative radiotherapy to orbit

(c) Urgent palliative radiotherapy to orbit and anastrazole

(d) Palliative chemotherapy

(e) Surgical excision of the mass

24. Which of the following statements about opioids is correct?

(a) Morphine is glucuronated in the liver, so renal impairment does not lead to opioid toxicity

(b) Tachycardia is a characteristic feature of opioid toxicity

(c) Patients with opioid toxicity may think they have seen animals running under their bed

(d) Low-dose morphine is classed as a 'weak opioid' on the WHO analgesic ladder

(e) Opioid toxicity typically causes pupil dilatation

25. A fit 60-year-old woman undergoes surgery for a carcinoma of the tranverse colon. Histology shows a grade 2 adenocarcinoma, T3 N2 (4 out of 14 nodes involved) with vascular invasion and perineural invasion. There is no evidence of metastatic disease. What is the most appropriate management?

(a) Weekly 5-FU/folinic acid

(b) Modified de Gramont 5-FU

(c) Oxaliplatin–fluoropyrimidine-based regimen

(d) Oxaliplatin–capecitabine

(e) Irinotecan–modified de Gramont

26. A 45-year-old man presents with gradual onset of right-sided weakness. An MRI scan of the brain shows an enhancing tumour in the right frontal and parietal region. The tumour is excised surgically and histology shows a glioma with frequent mitoses and necrosis. It is decided to treat with radical postoperative radiotherapy. Which of the following statements is correct?

(a) Treating each field each day, Monday to Friday, 5 days a week, the dose to the ICRU reference point should be 54 Gy in 30 fractions

(b) Craniospinal axis radiotherapy improves survival by reducing the risk of recurrence elsewhere in the central nervous system

(c) CT and MRI image co-registration is not usually helpful in planning because of difficulties correcting for scale, rotation and lateral translation

(d) The GTV is the contrast-enhancing tumour as seen on imaging

(e) If megavoltage photons are used, alopecia is unlikely because of the skin sparing in the build-up region

27. Which of the following is associated with a poor prognosis in neuroendocrine tumours?
    (a) Well-differentiated tumour
    (b) High Ki-67 index
    (c) Origin in the appendix
    (d) Bronchial origin
    (e) Absence of atypical cells

28. Which of the following statements about radiotherapy for thyroid eye disease is correct?
    (a) It should be given prophylactically
    (b) Proptosis usually pushes the lenses so far forward that their radiation dose can be ignored
    (c) NICE recommends avoiding radiotherapy because of the risk of long-term side effects
    (d) The long-term risk of cataract is 10%
    (e) The usual dose is 40 Gy in 20 fractions over 4 weeks

29. Which of the following statements regarding retinoblastoma is correct?
    (a) 40% of cases are associated with a germline loss of one of the *RB1* alleles
    (b) External beam radiotherapy is the treatment of choice
    (c) Chemotherapy should be avoided because of the risk of significant toxicity
    (d) Enucleation is the treatment of choice
    (e) Small tumours do not require immediate treatment and can be observed

30. A 43-year-old man presents with a swelling in the right thigh. Investigations show a soft tissue mass within the quadriceps muscle. A biopsy is undertaken, followed by surgery to remove the tumour. Histology shows a leiomyosarcoma with 20 mitoses per high-power field and more than 50% necrosis. The tumour measured 3 cm diameter and had an excision margin of 25 mm. According to the TNM 7th edition classification, what stage is the tumour?
    (a) pT1 NX MX
    (b) pT2 N0 M0
    (c) pT1 N0 M0
    (d) R1 NX MX

(e) G3 T2 N0 M0

31. A 63-year-old male is being planned for potentially curative definitive platinum-based chemoradiation for a squamous cell carcinoma starting at 30 cm *ab oral* using a two-phase technique: phase 1 with anterior–posterior parallel-opposed fields; phase 2 with three fields, one anterior and two posterior obliques. You are asked to review the plans: $PTV_{max} = 106\%$; $PTV_{min} = 95\%$; the spinal cord V45 = 20%; combined lung V20 = 10%; and heart V30 = 70%. What action do you recommend?
    (a) Accept the current plan
    (b) Increase the dose contribution from phase 2
    (c) Increase the contribution of the anterior field during phase 1
    (d) Increase the dose contribution from phase 1
    (e) Increase the contribution of the posterior field during phase 1

32. A 45-year-old maths teacher has just completed adjuvant treatment for a right breast cancer. She had a 2.0 cm grade 3 tumour, with 1 of 17 nodes involved. The tumour was ER +ve but HER-2 –ve. She has had 6 cycles of FEC chemotherapy and radiotherapy to the conserved breast. She has started tamoxifen. She wants to know what her prognosis is. According to the Nottingham prognostic index, what is her 10-year survival likely to be?
    (a) 51%
    (b) 41%
    (c) 61%
    (d) 71%
    (e) 31%

33. A 57-year-old fit woman presents with abdominal distension, poor appetite and weight loss. CT scan shows bilateral ovarian masses and an omental 'cake'. Her CA125 is 763 U/mL. She undergoes laparotomy and debulking. Tumour deposits are found in the ovaries and on the omentum and surface of the liver measuring 2.5 cm. What stage is her ovarian cancer?
    (a) FIGO stage IIIC
    (b) FIGO stage IVA
    (c) FIGO stage IIC

(d) FIGO stage IIIB

(e) FIGO stage IIIA

34. Which of the following statements about radiotherapy for vulval cancer is correct?

(a) The dose of concurrent weekly cisplatin is 50 mg/m²

(b) Moist desquamation of the vulval skin can occur, but it is not usually painful

(c) The vulva does not tolerate radiotherapy well, so radiation doses in excess of 60 Gy cannot be given

(d) The clinical target volume in advanced vulval cancer includes the primary tumour, vulva, groin and pelvic nodes

(e) Postoperative radiotherapy does not reduce the local recurrence rate in patients with a resection margin of less than 8 mm

35. Which of the following statements about radiotherapy for mesothelioma is correct?

(a) Wide-field palliative radiotherapy can alleviate pain in around 60% of patients

(b) Palliative radiotherapy to the chest for mesothelioma usually alleviates shortness of breath

(c) The dose for prophylactic needle-track radiotherapy can be kept as low as 50 Gy in 25 fractions because only microscopic disease is being treated

(d) In postoperative radiotherapy following extrapleural pneumonectomy, the GTV is the entire hemithorax

(e) Symptomatic disease in the thorax should be treated with high-dose palliation

36. Which of these is the correct estimated 5-year overall survival following an Ivor–Lewis oesophagectomy on a fit patient with a T3 N1 adenocarcinoma?

(a) 60%

(b) 40%

(c) 5%

(d) 20%

(e) 0%

37. In megavoltage photon therapy, which of the following statements is correct?

(a) The width of the radiation beam increases linearly with distance from the treatment head because of the inverse-square law

(b) The beam penumbra is the distance between the 30% and 70% depth doses

(c) As the energy increases, the d_{max} decreases

(d) When the distance from the treatment machine to the patient increases, the inverse-square law causes percentage depth doses below the d_{max} to increase

(e) As the field size increases, the central axis receives less radiation per monitor unit because of reduced scatter from the machine head and within the patient

38. Which of the following aspects of reporting trials can actually lead to less reliable conclusions?

(a) Ensuring as complete a follow-up as possible

(b) Reporting trials whether or not they show a 'positive' or 'negative' result

(c) Stressing to readers those outcomes where there is a difference between subgroups

(d) Performing a meta-analysis

(e) Reporting treatment effects and confidence intervals

39. Which one of the following cytotoxic drugs is a vesicant when extravasated – that is, is associated with a high risk of causing inflammation and blistering of local skin and underlying tissue leading to tissue death and necrosis?

(a) Carboplatin

(b) Bleomycin

(c) Paclitaxel

(d) Etoposide

(e) Methotrexate

40. Which of the following statements relating to the cervical lymph nodes is correct?

(a) Level II contains the submandibular nodes

(b) Preauricular and intraparotid nodes are included in level I

(c) Lower jugular nodes lie in level III

(d) Level III extends from the hyoid bone superiorly to the lower border of the cricoid cartilage

(e) Level VI contains the anterior central compartment nodes and extends between the hyoid bone superiorly and the carina inferiorly

41. Whose law states that a palpable non-tender gallbladder is a typical feature of an obstructive tumour of the lower biliary tree?
    (a) Kruckenberg
    (b) Courvoisier
    (c) Trousseau
    (d) Bismuth
    (e) Virchow

42. Which of the following genetic defects is most commonly associated with the adenoma–carcinoma sequence for colorectal carcinoma?
    (a) A loss of heterozygosity in the RB gene
    (b) DNA mismatch repair
    (c) Chromosome 22 loss
    (d) HER 2 amplification
    (e) DNA hypomethylation

43. Regarding carcinoma of the anus, which of the following statements is correct?
    (a) Anal-margin tumours have a worse prognosis than tumours in the anal canal
    (b) Patients with HIV/AIDS are at reduced risk of toxicity from treatment
    (c) Anal fissure is a risk factor for anal cancer
    (d) A history of intraepithelial neoplasia of the cervix, vagina or vulva is a risk factor for anal cancer
    (e) Patients who are treated with radical chemoradiotherapy have a significantly better life expectancy than patients treated with radical surgery

44. Osteolytic bone metastases are a typical feature of:
    (a) Prostate cancer
    (b) Gastric cancer
    (c) Renal cell cancer
    (d) Carcinoid tumours
    (e) Bladder cancer

45. A man presents with a grade 3, pT1 bladder cancer. The most appropriate management is transurethral resection of bladder tumour (TURBT) followed by:

    (a) Radical radiotherapy with regular cystoscopic follow-up
    (b) Radical cystectomy
    (c) Neoadjuvant chemotherapy and radical cystectomy
    (d) Systemic chemotherapy with regular cystoscopic follow-up
    (e) Intravesical BCG with regular cystoscopic follow-up

46. Which one of the following statements about bone scans is true?
    (a) Bone scans are very useful for diagnosing myeloma deposits
    (b) Bone scans are not useful for showing metastases from bladder cancer
    (c) The isotope used is ^{123}I
    (d) Bone scans show osteoblast activity
    (e) Bone scans show high activity in the brain and heart

47. A 58-year-old man presents with an enlarging mass on the penis. A biopsy confirms this is squamous carcinoma. Clinical examination and staging investigations are otherwise normal. The tumour is staged as T2 invading the corpus carvernosus, grade 3. What is the most appropriate management?
    (a) Brachytherapy
    (b) External beam radiotherapy to the penis and groin nodes
    (c) Sentinel node biopsy, partial amputation of the penis and inguinal node dissection if sentinel node is positive
    (d) Partial amputation of the penis and prophylactic radiotherapy to the groin nodes
    (e) Topical chemotherapy with 5-FU

48. A 25-year-old man with stage II non-seminomatous germ cell cancer undergoes treatment with four cycles of BEP chemotherapy. After treatment, a CT scan shows a significant response, but the presence of a residual mass measuring 4 cm diameter. The treatment should be:
    (a) Give a further two cycles of BEP and rescan
    (b) Observe with serial CT scans
    (c) Surgery to remove the mass

(d) Observe with serial CT scans and tumour markers

(e) Radiofrequency ablation of the mass

49. A 57-year-old fit woman presents with abdominal distension, poor appetite and weight loss. A CT scan shows bilateral ovarian masses and an omental 'cake'. Her CA125 is 763 U/mL. She undergoes laparotomy and debulking. Tumour deposits are found in the ovaries and on the omentum and surface of the liver measuring 2.5 cm. There is 0 cm residual disease. Of available cytotoxic chemotherapy agents, which would you recommend now?

(a) Offer single-agent carboplatin chemotherapy

(b) Discuss options of platinum-based chemotherapy alone or platinum-based chemotherapy with paclitaxel

(c) Discuss options of platinum-based chemotherapy alone or paclitaxel alone

(d) Offer cisplatin, doxorubicin and cyclophosphamide chemotherapy

(e) Offer single-agent cisplatin

50. A 65-year-old woman presents with postmenopausal bleeding. A hysteroscopy shows polyps and biopsy confirms adenocarcinoma. She undergoes TAH and BSO and histology shows a FIGO stage IA grade I tumour and there is adenomyosis extending into the deep myometrium. What management would you recommend?

(a) Adjuvant progestin

(b) Radiotherapy with external beam and obturator

(c) External beam radiotherapy alone

(d) Clinical follow-up only

(e) Radiotherapy with obturator alone

51. A patient with cervical cancer is undergoing radical chemoradiotherapy and has received five cycles of cisplatin chemotherapy. She developed paraesthesiae, muscle cramps, tremor and hyperreflexia. Her calcium level was 1.89 mmol/L. She was given calcium supplements and her most recent serum calcium is within the normal range but her symptoms have not resolved. What is the most likely biochemical cause of her symptoms?

(a) Hypercalcaemia

(b) Hypokalaemia

(c) Hypomagnesaemia

(d) Hyponatraemia

(e) Hyperphosphataemia

52. Which statement regarding patients with small-cell lung cancer and a good performance status (PS 0–1) is correct?

(a) Platinum-based systemic chemotherapy in patients with limited disease does not prolong survival

(b) Single-agent chemotherapy is as effective as combination chemotherapy

(c) Prophylactic cranial irradiation in patients with limited disease and a complete response to chemotherapy does not prolong survival

(d) There is no survival benefit from thoracic radiotherapy in patients with extensive disease.

(e) Consolidation thoracic radiotherapy in patients with limited disease and a complete response to chemotherapy prolongs survival

53. A 43-year-old man presents with a swelling in the right thigh. Investigations show a soft-tissue mass within the quadriceps muscle. A biopsy is undertaken, followed by surgery to remove the tumour. Histology shows a leiomyosarcoma with 20 mitoses per high-power field and with more than 50% necrosis. The tumour measured 3 cm diameter and had an excision margin of 25 mm. What is the most appropriate management?

(a) Clinical follow-up with chest X-ray every 3 months

(b) Adjuvant chemotherapy with ifosphamide and doxorubicin

(c) Re-excision

(d) Postoperative radiotherapy

(e) Sentinel node lymph node biopsy followed by groin-node dissection if positive

54. A 30-year-old woman presents with an enlarging mass of lymph nodes in the right neck. It is mobile, measures 5 cm in diameter, and has a rubbery feel. She has no 'B' symptoms. A lymph node biopsy confirms classical Hodgkin lymphoma. There is no evidence of any other sites of disease and the ESR was 16. Out of the options listed, what is the most appropriate treatment?

(a) Six cycles of CHOP chemotherapy

(b) Mantle radiotherapy with a radiotherapy dose of 40 Gy in 20 fractions

(c) Six cycles of ABVD chemotherapy

(d) Two cycles of ABVD chemotherapy followed by involved field radiotherapy (20 Gy)

(e) Surgery to remove the rest of the mass followed by involved field radiotherapy

55. A 75-year-old woman develops small-volume lymphadenopathy in the left axilla and left neck. A CT scan shows no other sites of disease. Her haemoglobin is 12.5 g/dL and her LDH is in the normal range. Biopsy of one of the lymph nodes shows grade 1 follicular lymphoma. What is the best management?

(a) CHOP chemotherapy

(b) Single-agent chlorambucil

(c) Surveillance

(d) ABVD chemotherapy

(e) Single-agent fludarabine

56. A 70-year-old man, who is on warfarin for atrial fibrillation, presents with a slowly enlarging lesion at the inner canthus of his left eye. On examination, the lesion diameter is 0.75 cm and depth is 0.5 cm. Biopsy confirms a basal cell carcinoma. The most appropriate management is:

(a) Surgical excision

(b) Radiotherapy with 90 kV X-rays

(c) Radiotherapy with 6 MeV electrons

(d) Radiotherapy with 170 kV X-rays

(e) Radiotherapy with 9 MeV electrons

57. A patient has an excisional biopsy for an ulcerated pigmented cutaneous lesion. The histology is of a 4.2-mm thick nodular melanoma completely excised. Which of the following options would be considered as standard to offer the patient?

(a) A further 5-cm wide excision

(b) Sentinel lymph node biopsy followed by lymph node dissection

(c) Elective lymph node dissection

(d) Adjuvant low-dose interferon α

(e) A staging CT scan

58. A 39-year-old man with medullary thyroid cancer underwent surgery with total thyroidectomy and lymph node dissection. Postoperatively, serum calcitonin was 163 pg/mL, but imaging studies showed no evidence of disease. The patient is asymptomatic. What is the most appropriate course of action?

(a) Postoperative radiotherapy to the neck

(b) Treatment with vandetanib

(c) Treatment with octreotide

(d) Measure serum calcitonin and CEA and perform physical examination every 6 months initially

(e) Therapeutic radioiodine

59. A 51-year-man old undergoes an ileal resection and right hemicolectomy for a locally advanced, node-positive, well-differentiated carcinoid tumour. Five years later the patient presents with flushing and palpitations and a CT scan reveals three tumours in segments 2 and 3 of the liver. What is the most appropriate next investigation?

(a) Twenty-four-hour urine 5-HIAA

(b) Serum chromogranin A

(c) PET scan

(d) Somatostatin receptor scintigraphy (OctreoScan®)

(e) ^{123}I-MIBG scan

60. Which of the following is an 'unfavourable' subset of carcinoma of unknown primary site?

(a) Poorly differentiated carcinoma in the midline

(b) Female patient with papillary serous adenocarcinoma of the peritoneal cavity

(c) Female patient with axillary lymphadenopathy

(d) Adenocarcinoma of the pleura

(e) Squamous cell cervical lymphadenopathy

61. Regarding heterotopic bone formation, which of the following statements is correct?

(a) It causes clinical problems in 43% of patients after a hip replacement

(b) It typically develops 6 months after hip surgery

(c) Prophylactic radiotherapy is effective if given up to 4 days after re-operation of the hip

(d) Prophylactic radiotherapy is ineffective if given just before re-operation

(e) Fractionated radiotherapy is more effective than a single fraction

62. Which of the following statements is correct?

(a) The oesophageal pharyngeal syndrome of oxaliplatin is made worse by exposure to heat

(b) Palmar–plantar erythrodysaesthesia caused by liposomal doxorubicin is made worse by exposure to cold

(c) Scalp warming can reduce alopecia caused by some chemotherapy drugs

(d) An anthracycline extravasation is best treated with a cold compress

(e) A vinca alkaloid extravasation is best treated with a cold compress

63. A 74-year-old woman presents with a painless smooth swelling in the right neck (3 × 4 cm). There are no ENT symptoms and no abnormalities detectable in clinic. She has been a smoker of 20 cigarettes a day for 40 years. There is no comorbidity and her WHO PS = 0. US of the neck shows a solitary cystic mass at level II only. FNAC shows squamous carcinoma cells. What would you do next?

(a) Contrast-enhanced CT neck

(b) FDG-PET scan

(c) Panendoscopy of upper aerodigestive tract

(d) Right modified radical neck dissection

(e) Excision of cystic mass for definitive pathology

64. A 65-year-old man underwent abdominoperineal resection in January 2004 for a T3 N0 M0 rectal carcinoma. At routine follow-up in January 2005, his CEA was found to be elevated at 25 U/mL and a CT scan showed a solitary liver metastasis that was resectable on radiological grounds. Based on current evidence, the standard treatment outside of a clinical trial is:

(a) Liver resection only

(b) Preoperative modified de Gramont chemotherapy followed by liver resection

(c) Preoperative oxaliplatin-based chemotherapy followed by liver resection

(d) Preoperative irinotecan-based chemotherapy followed by liver resection

(e) Radiofrequency ablation

65. A fit 66-year-old man presents with a bilateral cT3a prostate cancer, PSA = 25 ng/mL and Gleason 4 + 4 = 8 in all eight cores, maximum core length = 12 mm. MRI/bone scan confirm T3a N0 M0 disease. The most appropriate management is:

(a) Radical prostatectomy, lymph node dissection and adjuvant radiotherapy

(b) Radical prostatectomy, lymph node dissection and 2 years of adjuvant hormonal therapy

(c) Radical external beam radiotherapy with a high-dose-rate brachytherapy boost

(d) Neoadjuvant androgen deprivation and radical external beam radiotherapy

(e) Neoadjuvant and adjuvant androgen deprivation and radical external beam radiotherapy

66. A patient is to receive a course of definitive chemoradiation for an inoperable carcinoma of the tail of the pancreas. Both kidneys are functioning. You are given a radiotherapy plan for approval that has an anterior and two lateral fields. The liver V30 = 40%, small bowel D_{max} = 45 Gy, left kidney V30 = 90%, the right kidney V20 = 25%. What do you do?

(a) Reduce the dose to the PTV

(b) Accept the plan

(c) Reduce the margin given to the GTV

(d) Add a posterior field

(e) Increase the weight to the anterior field

67. With regard to brachytherapy for carcinoma of the cervix, which of the following statements is correct?

(a) For practical purposes, Manchester point A is sometimes defined as 1 cm above and 1 cm lateral to the flange at the lower end of the uterine tube

(b) Manchester point B is 3 cm from the midline

(c) The ICRU 38 bladder point is the anterior surface of the bladder balloon

(d) The ICRU 38 rectal point is 5 mm behind the posterior vaginal wall at the level of the lower end of the intrauterine tube

(e) The rectal dose should be less than half of the dose to point A

68. You are shown a plan for a radical lung treatment for CHART radiotherapy (54 Gy in 36 fractions over 12 days). The V20 for the lung is 45%. The dose to the PTV lies between 95% and 107%. The maximum spinal cord dose is 15 Gy. What action should you take?

(a) Accept the plan

(b) Accept the plan but reduce the prescribed dose of radiotherapy

(c) Treat the patient with 60 Gy in 30 fractions over 6 weeks instead

(d) Move one or more beams so they pass through the spinal cord rather than the lung

(e) Move one or more beams so they pass through lung rather than spinal cord

69. Which of the following is important for minimising measurement bias in clinical studies?

(a) Meta-analysis

(b) Adjusted analyses

(c) Blinding

(d) Per protocol analysis

(e) A transparent randomisation process

70. The ICRU reference point should be:

(a) Always at the centre of the tumour

(b) Representative of the PTV dose

(c) At the isocentre if there is one

(d) At the point of maximum dose within the PTV

(e) At the point of minimum dose within the PTV

71. A patient has a 5 cm squamous cancer of the lower anal canal. An MRI demonstrates evidence of left-sided internal iliac lymphadenopathy. No other disease is found. The correct stage is:

(a) T2 N1 M0

(b) T2 N2 M0

(c) T3 N1 M0

(d) T3 N1 M1

(e) T2 N1 M1

72. Which of the following statements about gastrointestinal stromal tumours is correct?

(a) They arise from the intestinal cells of Jacal

(b) They are associated with dysregulation of the tumour suppressor gene, KIT

(c) An increase in size of the tumour can occur when responding to imatinib

(d) Standard treatment for patients whose tumours have been resected is adjuvant imatinib

(e) GIST tumours stain positively with CD119

73. A 56-year-old woman undergoes breast screening. A 1.5 cm abnormality is detected in the left breast, which is biopsied and shows lobular carcinoma *in situ*. She has a very strong family history of breast cancer and does not wish to accept observation alone. What surgical treatment would you recommend?

(a) Wide local excision followed by postoperative radiotherapy

(b) Wide local excision alone

(c) Unilateral mastectomy

(d) Bilateral mastectomy

(e) Bilateral mastectomy with unilateral axillary lymph node dissection

74. A 62-year-old man undergoes a radical nephrectomy for renal cell carcinoma. Histology confirms an 8 cm tumour confined to the kidney with three positive regional lymph nodes. What stage is this?

(a) T2 N1b

(b) T3 N2

(c) T3 N1b

(d) T2 N2

(e) T2 N3

75. A man is discussed at the multidisciplinary meeting following TURBT. A large papillary mass was fully resected. Pathology shows a grade 3 transitional cell carcinoma with invasion of the muscularis propria. What stage is he?

(a) T2a

(b) pT2a at least

(c) pT1b

(d) pT2b

(e) pT3a

76. A man with metastatic NSGCT is being treated with his first course of chemotherapy with standard 5-day BEP. When he attends for his third cycle of chemotherapy, he mentions some mild exertional dyspnoea. What is the most appropriate management?

(a) Delay chemotherapy for 1 week to allow the patient time to improve

(b) Stop chemotherapy after two cycles

(c) Stop BEP and change to TIP for the remaining cycles

(d) Treat with oxygen, antibiotics and high-dose intravenous steroids and continue with the third cycle of BEP without delay.

(e) Investigate with CXR, CT of the chest and pulmonary function tests, proceeding with EP for a total of four cycles if bleomycin toxicity is suspected

77. Which of the following is a risk factor for ovarian cancer?

 (a) Breast feeding
 (b) Tubal ligation
 (c) Use of the oral contraceptive pill
 (d) A germline mutation in the HNPCC gene
 (e) Early menopause

78. A 45-year-old woman presents with FIGO stage IB1 carcinoma of the cervix. Following radical hysterectomy and lymph node dissection, she is found to have a 6 cm tumour with extension into the parametrium with negative lymph nodes. There is no evidence of distant metastases. What stage is the tumour?

 (a) FIGO IIA
 (b) pT2b pN0
 (c) FIGO IIB
 (d) pT1b2 pN0
 (e) FIGO IIIB

79. In vaginal cancer, which of the following statements is correct?

 (a) Vaginal cancer is a rare disease, so treatment should always follow the standard protocol
 (b) Radiotherapy phase 1 includes the pelvic and paraaortic lymph nodes
 (c) The radiotherapy field for carcinoma of the upper third of the vagina should include the inguinal nodes
 (d) Vaginal cancers in the lower vagina usually have a worse prognosis than those in the upper vagina
 (e) There is a strong evidence base for the use of concurrent chemoradiotherapy for squamous carcinoma of the upper vagina

80. A 53-year-old man had a left upper lobectomy for a moderately differentiated pT2 pN1 M0 squamous cell carcinoma of the lung. Resection margins were reported as clear, with a medial resection margin of 6 mm. What further therapy is it appropriate to offer him (outside a clinical trial)?

(a) Adjuvant radiotherapy to the mediastinum
(b) Adjuvant chemotherapy
(c) Adjuvant radiotherapy to the mediastinum followed by adjuvant chemotherapy
(d) Further surgical resection
(e) Concomitant chemoradiotherapy

81. Which of the following statements about Ewing sarcoma is correct?

 (a) Relapsed disease can often be cured with second-line intensive chemotherapy
 (b) The incidence of distant metastases is low
 (c) It is a chemoresistant tumour
 (d) Radiotherapy should not be given in inoperable disease because of the risk of fracture when the tumour responds
 (e) Radiotherapy is indicated for sites of metastases, including the whole lung

82. A 59-year-old woman presents with vague abdominal symptoms of nausea, weight loss, leg oedema and urinary pressure. Her serum CA125 level is 2537 U/mL. A CT scan shows bilateral pelvic masses with para-aortic lymphadenopathy. A biopsy and immunohistochemistry are performed. The tumour is found to be cytokeratin negative, CD19 positive, and CD20 positive and Ki-67 of 95%. What is the most appropriate initial treatment?

 (a) Laparotomy, debulking, total abdominal hysterectomy, bilateral salpingo-oophorectomy, omentectomy
 (b) Chemotherapy with carboplatin and paclitaxel
 (c) Rasburicase then chemotherapy with R-CHOP
 (d) Radiotherapy to sites of bulky disease
 (e) Allopurinol then chemotherapy with ABVD

83. Which statement best describes the role of chemotherapy in primary tumours of the central nervous system?

 (a) Concurrent chemotherapy with radical radiotherapy has been shown to more than double the 2-year survival in patients with grade IV gliomas
 (b) The improvement seen with concurrent chemotherapy and radical radiotherapy

is greatest in patients with a poor performance status

(c) Radiological features of primary CNS lymphoma are typical, so that patients should receive chemotherapy without the need for histological confirmation

(d) Adjuvant chemotherapy has been shown to double median survival in grade gliomas

(e) The usual dose of temozolamide is 20 mg/m^2

84. An 85-year-old lady presents with a non-healing ulcer on the left lower leg. It measures 6 cm in maximum diameter, 1 cm in depth, and has a rolled edge. Clinical examination reveals no other tumours. A biopsy is undertaken that shows moderately differentiated squamous carcinoma. What is the optimal management?

(a) Observation

(b) Radiotherapy with 170 kV photons, 40 Gy in 8 fractions over 8 days

(c) Radiotherapy with 9 MeV electrons and 1 cm bolus, 60 Gy in 30 fractions over 6 weeks

(d) Surgical excision and healing with secondary intention

(e) Surgical excision and skin grafting

85. Concerning malignant melanoma, which of the following statements is true?

(a) Nodular melanoma is the most common subtype

(b) Sunscreens have been shown to reduce the risk of malignant melanoma

(c) A 10 mm choroidal melanoma can be treated with scleral plaque therapy instead of enucleation

(d) Adjuvant low-dose interferon α has been shown to improve survival

(e) The addition of carmustine, tamoxifen and cisplatin to dacarbazine improves survival over dacarbazine alone in advanced melanoma

86. A 51-year-old woman develops appendicitis. During surgery, it is noted that the appendix forms a mass that is locally invasive. The mass is excised and shows a carcinoid tumour with atypical cells. Four years later she develops some mild right upper quadrant discomfort and an ultrasound shows a 3 cm mass in segment 8 of the liver. Further investigations show no other sites of disease. What is the optimal management?

(a) Capecitabine and streptozocin

(b) Interferon α

(c) ^{90}Y octreotide isotope therapy

(d) ^{131}I MIBG isotope therapy

(e) Surgical resection

87. A 4-year-old boy presents with painless swelling of the abdomen. An abdominal ultrasound shows a large tumour in the right flank. A CT scan shows that this is arising from the right kidney and is invading the perinephric structures. A biopsy is not undertaken because of the risk of tumour rupture. What is the most likely diagnosis?

(a) Neuroblastoma

(b) Wilm's tumour

(c) Rhabdomyosarcoma

(d) Non-Hodgkin lymphoma

(e) Teratoma

88. Which of the following statements about keloids is correct?

(a) Keloids should not be excised before radiotherapy because this would increase the risk of recurrence

(b) Radiotherapy should be given within 1 month of excision

(c) Radiotherapy is effective in about half of all cases

(d) Keloids are unsuitable for treatment with brachytherapy

(e) A single fraction of 6 Gy with 100 kV photons is adequate for small keloids

89. A 59-year-old fit woman has a 10 mm mass in the upper outer quadrant of the right breast. Biopsy shows poorly differentiated cancer; CK7+, CK20−, TTF-1 focally+, ER−. CT scan shows multiple lung and liver metastases. Which of the following is the most appropriate chemotherapy regimen?

(a) FEC

(b) gemcitabine and carboplatin

(c) modified de Gramont

(d) R-CHOP

(e) Ifosfamide and doxorubicin

90. A 56-year-old man in previously excellent heath has been referred to you for a second opinion about management of his epithelioid malignant mesothelioma. Which statement is correct?

    (a) Pleuropneumonectomy followed by postoperative chemotherapy and radiotherapy has been shown to improve survival compared to no surgery for stage I disease

    (b) The median survival for all patients is 18 months

    (c) The epithelioid variant has the best prognosis

    (d) The response rate to chemotherapy is more than 50%

    (e) The presence of pleural plaques significantly increases the chance of developing mesothelioma in patients exposed to asbestos

91. A 36-year-old woman is undergoing surveillance after a molar pregnancy. Her hCG fails to fall into the normal range and her pretreatment level was 913 IU/L. What management would you recommend?

    (a) Chemotherapy with intramuscular methotrexate

    (b) Chemotherapy with actinomycin-D, methotrexate and etoposide

    (c) Chemotherapy with actinomycin-D, methotrexate, etoposide, vincristine and cyclophosphamide

    (d) Observation

    (e) Hysterectomy

92. A 45-year-old man has had a right hemicolectomy for a mucinous carcinoma of the caecum as an emergency. The stage was T2 N0, grade II, completely resected with no lymphovascular infiltration; what further management would you advise?

    (a) A complete total colectomy

    (b) An adjuvant course of oxaliplatin and 5-FU chemotherapy

    (c) An adjuvant course of capecitabine chemotherapy

    (d) Postoperative staging including colonoscopic review of the remaining bowel

    (e) Postoperative CEA

93. Which of the following statements is true about choosing wide or restrictive entry criteria to a trial?

    (a) With wide entry criteria it is impossible to work out what the trial population was

    (b) With restrictive entry criteria there is more chance of a significant result

    (c) Wide entry criteria make it more difficult to recruit patients to the trial

    (d) Restrictive entry criteria give more clinically meaningful results

    (e) Restrictive entry criteria mean that it is often impossible to determine if a treatment works for all people, or just some

94. What is the definition of high-dose-rate brachy-therapy?

    (a) Dose rate greater than 6 Gy/hr

    (b) Dose rate greater than 8 Gy/hr

    (c) Dose rate greater than 10 Gy/hr

    (d) Dose rate greater than 12 Gy/hr

    (e) Dose rate greater than 14 Gy/hr

95. Which of the following statements about hormonal treatments is correct?

    (a) Aromatase inhibitors should not be given to premenopausal women after ovarian function suppression

    (b) Tamoxifen is less likely than an aromatase inhibitor to cause thromboembolic events

    (c) Aromatase inhibitors are less likely than tamoxifen to cause osteoporosis

    (d) Tamoxifen is less likely than aromatase inhibitors to cause endometrial hyperplasia

    (e) Tamoxifen is less likely than aromatase inhibitors to cause arthralgia

96. Which of the following statements about postoperative adjuvant radiotherapy for stage IC, grade 3, carcinoma of the endometrium is correct?

    (a) It should be combined with concurrent chemotherapy with weekly cisplatin

    (b) A reasonable dose is 45 Gy in 25 fractions to the whole pelvis followed by 9–18 Gy as an external beam boost to the GTV

    (c) It should be followed by adjuvant hormonal therapy with a progestin

(d) An acceptable dose for the boost would be 20 Gy LDR to the whole vagina

(e) The lower border of the radiation field should cover the obturator foramina

97. Which of the following statements regarding carboplatin and paclitaxel is correct?

(a) Carboplatin and paclitaxel have different routes of excretion so the order in which they are given does not matter

(b) Paclitaxel is given before carboplatin; otherwise there is a 20% reduction in paclitaxel clearance

(c) Paclitaxel is given after carboplatin to reduce the risk of myelosuppression

(d) Paclitaxel and carboplatin are given simultaneously to reduce the treatment time for the patient

(e) Scalp cooling should be offered because it reduces the risk of alopecia due to carboplatin

98. Which of the following statements about trastuzumab is correct?

(a) It has been shown to improve overall 20-year survival when used in patients with HER2-positive breast cancers as adjuvant therapy in combination with chemotherapy

(b) It is a chimeric IgM antibody

(c) It causes symptoms of heart failure in approximately 10% of patients

(d) It should always be preceded by the administration of antihistamines and steroids

(e) It is recommended with docetaxel as first-line therapy in patients with HER2-positive mestastatic breast cancer who are unsuitable for an anthracycline

99. Regarding pineal tumours, which of the following statements is correct?

(a) Due to the site of these tumours, biopsy is rarely indicated before treatment

(b) Germ cell intracranial tumours rarely produce elevated serum βhCG and/or αFP

(c) Pineocytomas are less chemosensitive than oligodendrogliomas

(d) Pineoblastomas should be considered for stereotactic radiotherapy

(e) The dose recommended for craniospinal axis radiotherapy is lower for germ cell tumours than for parenchymal tumours

100. A 55-year-old woman with stage 3C ovarian cancer relapses 4 months after carboplatin and paclitaxel chemotherapy. What would be the recommended chemotherapy treatment now?

(a) Liposomal doxorubicin

(b) Topotecan

(c) Single-agent carboplatin

(d) Carboplatin and paclitaxel

(e) Carboplatin and gemcitabine

101. Which cancer is the most common in the UK?

(a) Uterus

(b) Oesophagus

(c) Larynx

(d) Bladder

(e) Carcinoma of unknown primary site

102. A patient has recently been diagnosed with carcinoma of the pancreas. Investigations reveal a 3 cm mass in the head of the pancreas invading the second part of the duodenum. There is evidence of coeliac lymphadenopathy but no other evidence of metastatic disease. The stage is:

(a) T2 N1 M0

(b) T3 N1 M0

(c) T4 N1 M0

(d) T3 N1 M1a

(e) T4 N1 M1a

103. A 45-year-old woman weighs 73 kg and her serum creatinine is 95 mM/L. Using the Cockcroft-Gault formula, what is the best estimation of her creatinine clearance in mL/min?

(a) 36

(b) 56

(c) 76

(d) 96

(e) 116

104. Radiotherapy doses as low as which level can affect sperm production?

(a) 3 Gy

(b) 16 Gy

(c) 10 Gy

(d) 5 Gy

(e) 1 Gy

105. A 66-year-old electrician presents with shortness of breath. His chest X-ray shows pleural thickening and an ultrasound shows this to be solid with an associated pleural effusion. A CT scan shows thickening of the mediastinal pleura and loss of lung volume. Out of the following, what investigation would be most likely to give the diagnosis?

(a) Bronchoscopy

(b) CT-guided fine-needle aspiration cytology

(c) Thoracoscopic biopsy

(d) Cytology of pleural fluid

(e) Sputum cytology

106. Which of the following statements about hormonal treatments is correct?

(a) Tumours that develop resistance to tamoxifen are very unlikely to respond to an aromatase inhibitor

(b) Aromatase inhibitors act primarily on steroid synthesis in the adrenal gland

(c) In patients with prostate cancer who are starting treatment with an LHRHa, an anti-androgen is also required to prevent tumour 'flare'

(d) Ovarian cancer is not a hormonally sensitive disease

(e) Tumours that are oestrogen-receptor negative and progesterone-receptor positive should not be treated with tamoxifen

107. A 54-year-old man undergoes a left nephrectomy for renal cell cancer. Eight months later he feels short of breath and has back pain. CXR and CT scan confirm the presence of a local recurrence and two peripheral lung metastases. His Karnofsky performance status is 50. His Hb is 10.5 g/dL and his serum-corrected calcium is 2.7 mM/L. What management would you recommend?

(a) Symptomatic treatment only

(b) Interferon α

(c) Interleukin-2

(d) Chemotherapy with the Atzpodien regimen

(e) Attempted surgical resection of the lung metastases in an attempt to control the local recurrence

108. The MRC ST02 (MAGIC) trial was recently published. This trial demonstrates that:

(a) Preoperative epirubicin, cisplatin and capecitabine (ECX) followed by surgery is superior to surgery alone

(b) Postoperative epirubicin, cisplatin and 5-fluorouracil (ECF) has no proven role in gastric cancer

(c) Preoperative chemotherapy is superior to postoperative chemotherapy in gastric cancer

(d) Pre- and postoperative ECF chemotherapy is superior to surgery alone

(e) Capecitabine is equivalent to 5-FU in the adjuvant therapy of gastric cancer

109. A 49-year-old woman had radical chemoradiotherapy for cervical carcinoma 2 years ago. She now presents with back pain radiating down the right leg with pain and numbness of the left knee. What is the most likely site of recurrence?

(a) L3 vertebra

(b) L4 vertebra

(c) Left psoas muscle

(d) Left para-aortic nodes

(e) Pelvic nodes

110. A 60-year-old male smoker presents with a 6-week history of cough and swelling of the face and upper limbs. Examination findings are consistent with SVCO and CXR shows right paratracheal lymphadenopathy. What is the most likely underlying diagnosis?

(a) Thymoma

(b) High-grade NHL

(c) Lung cancer

(d) Metastatic germ cell tumour

(e) Hodgkin lymphoma

111. A 55-year-old man complains of back pain. Examination is unremarkable, but spinal MRI reveal a 3 cm extradural soft tissue mass at the level of T12. Biopsy shows malignant plasma cells, but staging investigations for multiple myeloma are negative. He is referred for radiotherapy. What is the optimum PTV and dose schedule?

(a) GTV plus 10 cm margin, 50 Gy in daily 2 Gy fractions

(b) GTV plus 2 cm margin, 60 Gy in daily 2 Gy fractions

(c) GTV plus 2 cm margin, 40 Gy in daily 2 Gy fractions

(d) GTV plus 5 cm margin, 30 Gy in daily 3 Gy fractions

(e) GTV plus 2 cm margin, 20 Gy in daily 4 Gy fractions

112. A laboratory assessment of the α/β ratio for a malignant melanoma cell line demonstrated an average value of approximately 2. Taking this information into account, which of the following radiotherapy regimens is likely to be the most effective in cancer control of melanoma?

(a) 30 Gy in 10 fractions

(b) 21 Gy in 3 fractions

(c) 10 Gy in a single fraction

(d) 30 Gy in 5 fractions

(e) 35 Gy in 15 fractions

113. A 35-year-old man with a smoking history of 20 pack years presents with chest discomfort and shortness of breath. He has lost weight and has been having night sweats. He is found to have a poorly differentiated carcinoma in the mediastinum. What is the most appropriate chemotherapy regimen?

(a) BEP

(b) R-CHOP

(c) FOLFOX

(d) ABVD

(e) ICE

114. Which of the following statements about erlotinib is correct?

(a) It is a monoclonal antibody directed against EGFR

(b) It is given intravenously

(c) Patients who develop a rash typically have a worse response than those who do not

(d) The recommended dose is 200 mg daily

(e) The rash responds to topical clindamycin

115. Which of the following statements about oestrogen is correct?

(a) In premenopausal women, oestrogens are mainly synthesised in the theca cells of the ovary

(b) In women, oestrogens are produced in the adrenal gland by the action of the aromatase enzyme

(c) Oestrogen-receptor-positive breast cancers invariably respond to hormonal treatment

(d) Oestrogens reduce low-density lipoproteins

(e) Oestrogens are anticoagulants

116. In radiotherapy planning, which of the following statements is correct?

(a) The internal margin accounts for the uncertainties and lack of reproducibility in setting up the patient day by day

(b) The treated volume is the tissue volume that receives a dose considered significant in relation to normal tissue tolerance

(c) Reducing the planning CT-scan slice thickness reduces the distance required to be added to the gross tumour volume to make the clinical target volume

(d) CTV + IM + SM = PTV

(e) The function of 'parallel' organs may be seriously affected even if a small portion is irradiated above a tolerance dose, and the effect of radiation on the function of 'serial' organs is more dependent on the volume irradiated.

117. A 64-year-old man develops jaundice with pale stools and dark urine. He also has some vague right upper quadrant pain and weight loss. There are no masses palpable on examination. An ultrasound scan suggests the presence of a distal tumour in the biliary tract. Out of the following options, what is the most appropriate investigation to perform next?

(a) Percutaneous transhepatic cholangiograph

(b) MRI scan

(c) ERCP

(d) CT scan

(e) Doppler ultrasound

118. In vaginal cancer, which of the following statements is correct?

(a) The most common malignant tumour is squamous carcinoma of the vagina

(b) The lymphatic drainage from the lower two-thirds of the vagina is to the pelvic nodes and from the upper third to the inguinal nodes

(c) Carcinoma of the vagina is associated with procidentia

(d) Previous abnormal cervical cytology is not associated with an increased risk of vaginal cancer

(e) Vaginal cancer accounts for 10% of all gynaecological malignancy

119. Regarding malignant forms of gestational trophoblastic tumour, which statement is correct?

(a) Choriocarcinoma occurs with a frequency of about 1 per 500,000 live births

(b) The most widely used standard therapy for low-risk patients is intravenous actinomycin-D

(c) The overall survival in the low-risk group is good at around 75%

(d) Patients with high-risk disease should be offered EMA-CO chemotherapy (etoposide, methotrexate, actinomycin-D, cisplatin and vinorelbine)

(e) The rare placental site trophoblast tumour can usually be cured if patients present within 4 years of pregnancy

120. A 45-year-old homosexual man presents with a 2-week history of multiple, painless, purple macules on his hard palate. He is found to be HIV-positive on testing. What is the most appropriate management?

(a) Intralesional chemotherapy with vinblastine

(b) Optimise antiretroviral therapy for 3 months and review

(c) Radiotherapy to hard palate using parallel opposed 6 MV photons, 20 Gy in 10 fractions over 2 weeks

(d) Radiotherapy to hard palate using parallel opposed 6 MV photons, 16 Gy in 4 fractions over 4 days

(e) Systemic chemotherapy with liposomal doxorubicin 20 mg/m^2 every 3 weeks

Multiple choice answers

1.	e	41.	b	81.	e
2.	c	42.	e	82.	c
3.	e	43.	d	83.	a
4.	d	44.	c	84.	e
5.	c	45.	e	85.	c
6.	d	46.	d	86.	e
7.	d	47.	c	87.	b
8.	b	48.	c	88.	e
9.	e	49.	b	89.	b
10.	d	50.	d	90.	c
11.	b	51.	c	91.	a
12.	d	52.	e	92.	d
13.	c	53.	d	93.	e
14.	c	54.	d	94.	d
15.	a	55.	c	95.	e
16.	c	56.	b	96.	e
17.	b	57.	e	97.	b
18.	d	58.	d	98.	e
19.	d	59.	d	99.	c
20.	c	60.	d	100.	a
21.	a	61.	c	101.	d
22.	e	62.	d	102.	b
23.	c	63.	c	103.	c
24.	c	64.	a	104.	e
25.	c	65.	e	105.	c
26.	d	66.	b	106.	c
27.	b	67.	d	107.	a
28.	d	68.	d	108.	d
29.	a	69.	c	109.	a
30.	a	70.	b	110.	c
31.	b	71.	b	111.	c
32.	a	72.	c	112.	d
33.	a	73.	d	113.	a
34.	d	74.	d	114.	e
35.	a	75.	b	115.	d
36.	d	76.	e	116.	d
37.	d	77.	d	117.	c
38.	c	78.	b	118.	c
39.	c	79.	d	119.	e
40.	d	80.	b	120.	b

Index